THE Woman's BOOK OF
Healing Herbs

THE Woman's
BOOK OF
Healing Herbs

HEALING TEAS, TONICS, SUPPLEMENTS, AND FORMULAS

BY SARÍ HARRAR
AND SARA ALTSHUL O'DONNELL

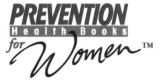

Rodale Press, Inc.
Emmaus, Pennsylvania

Copyright © 1999 by Rodale Press, Inc.

Illustrations copyright © 1998 by Virge Kask and Wendy Smith

Prevention Health Books for Women is a trademark of Rodale Press, Inc.

The face-cream recipe on page 108 and the yoni powder recipe on page 370 were adapted from *Herbal Healing for Women: Simple Home Remedies for Women of All Ages*. Copyright © 1993 by Rosemary Gladstar. Permission granted by Fireside, a division of Simon & Schuster, Inc.

Printed in the United States of America on acid-free ∞, recycled paper ♻

Library of Congress Cataloging-in-Publication Data
Harrar, Sarí.
      The woman's book of healing herbs : healing teas, tonics, supplements, and formulas / by Sarí Harrar and Sara Altshul O'Donnell.
          p.   cm.
      Includes index.
      ISBN 0–87596–510–5   hardcover
      1. Herbs—Therapeutic use.   2. Herbal cosmetics.   3. Women—Health and hygiene.
   I. O'Donnell, Sara Altshul.   II. Title.
   RM666.H33H37   1999
   615'.321'082—dc21   98–34254

      ISBN 1–57954–214–X   paperback

Distributed to the book trade by St. Martin's Press

      4   6   8   10   9   7   5   hardcover

   2   4   6   8   10   9   7   5   3   1   paperback

Visit us on the Web at www.rodalebooks.com, or call us toll-free at (800) 848-4735.

──── OUR PURPOSE ────

We inspire and enable people to improve their lives and the world around them.

The Woman's Book of Healing Herbs Staff

MANAGING EDITOR: Sharon Faelten
WRITERS: Sarí Harrar, Sara Altshul O'Donnell
CONTRIBUTING WRITERS: Alisa Bauman, Julia VanTine, Selene Yeager
ASSOCIATE RESEARCH MANAGER: Anita C. Small
LEAD RESEARCHERS: Carol J. Gilmore, Teresa A. Yeykal
EDITORIAL RESEARCHERS: Jennifer Abel, Christine Dreisbach, Jennifer Fiske, Laura Goldstein, Grete Haentjens, Lois Guarino Hazel, Jennifer L. Kaas, Sherry Weiss Kiser, Mary Kittel, Terry Sutton Kravitz, Sandra Salera Lloyd, Mary S. Mesaros, Paris Mihely-Muchanic, Staci Ann Sander
SENIOR COPY EDITOR: Jane Sherman
ART DIRECTOR: Darlene Schneck
COVER AND BOOK DESIGNER: Lynn N. Gano
COVER PHOTOGRAPHER: Mitch Mandel
PHOTO DIRECTORS: Lynn N. Gano, Sandy Freeman
PHOTO EDITORS: James A. Gallucci, Geoff Semenuk
PHOTO STYLIST: Melissa Hamilton
ILLUSTRATORS: Virge Kask, Wendy Smith
BOTANICAL ILLUSTRATION CONSULTANT: Nancy Ondra
LAYOUT DESIGNER: Donna G. Rossi
DIGITAL IMAGING CONSULTANT: Dale Mack
MANUFACTURING COORDINATOR: Patrick T. Smith
OFFICE MANAGER: Roberta Mulliner
OFFICE STAFF: Julie Kehs, Mary Lou Stephen

RODALE HEALTH AND FITNESS BOOKS

VICE-PRESIDENT AND EDITORIAL DIRECTOR: Debora T. Yost
EXECUTIVE EDITOR: Neil Wertheimer
DESIGN AND PRODUCTION DIRECTOR: Michael Ward
MARKETING MANAGER: Kristine Siessmayer
RESEARCH MANAGER: Ann Gossy Yermish
COPY MANAGER: Lisa D. Andruscavage
PRODUCTION MANAGER: Robert V. Anderson Jr.
STUDIO MANAGER: Leslie M. Keefe
ASSISTANT STUDIO MANAGER: Thomas P. Aczel
BOOK MANUFACTURING MANAGER: Mark Krahforst

Contents

PART ONE
Our Herbal Heritage

PART TWO
Top Healing Herbs for Women

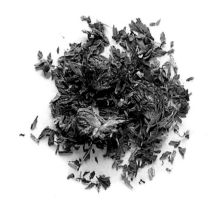

PART THREE

Teas, Tinctures, Techniques, and More

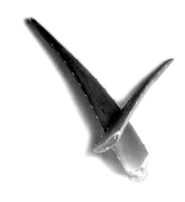

PART FIVE

Staying Healthy with Herbs

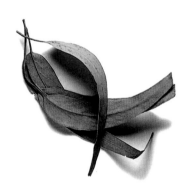

PART SIX

The Healing Power of Herbs

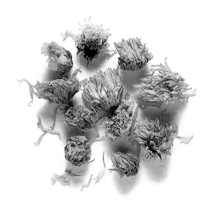

PART FOUR

Aromatherapy and Flower Essences

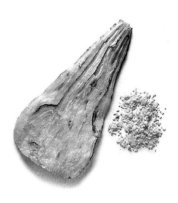

PART SEVEN

Herbs for Beautiful Skin, Hair, and Nails

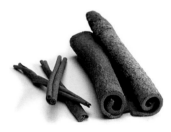

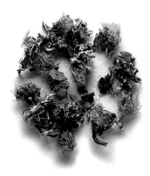

PART EIGHT

Herbs for Emotional Healing

PART NINE

Your Herbal Resource Guide

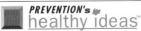

PREVENTION's *for*
healthy ideas™
For the best interactive guide to healthy active living,
visit our Web site at **http://www.healthyideas.com**

Acknowledgments

The authors are grateful to the many professionals who shared their expertise in the use of medicinal herbs as this book was being researched and written. In particular, we'd like to acknowledge the following individuals, who gave considerably of their time.

☙ Betzy Bancroft, a professional member of the American Herbalists Guild and manager of Herbalist and Alchemist, an herbal medicine company in Washington, New Jersey.

☙ Mary Bove, N.D., a naturopathic physician, midwife, and member of Britain's National Institute of Medical Herbalists who practices at the Brattleboro Naturopathic Clinic in Vermont.

☙ James A. Duke, Ph.D., a botanical consultant, former ethnobotanist with the U.S. Department of Agriculture, and author of *The Green Pharmacy*.

☙ David Edelberg, M.D., chairman and founder of the American WholeHealth Centers in Boston, Chicago, Denver, and Bethesda, Maryland, and section chief of holistic medicine at Illinois Masonic Medical Center and Grant Hospital, both in Chicago.

☙ Margi Flint, a professional member of the American Herbalists Guild who teaches herbal approaches to health at Tufts University School of Medicine in Boston and is a practicing herbalist at AtlantiCare Hospital in Lynn, Massachusetts.

☙ Cascade Anderson Geller, an herbal educator and consulting herbal practitioner in Portland, Oregon.

☙ Rosemary Gladstar, director of the Sage Mountain herbal education center in East Barre, Vermont, and author of *Herbal Healing for Women*.

☙ Amanda McQuade Crawford, a practicing herbalist in Ojai, California, professional member of the American Herbalists Guild, member of Britain's National Institute of Medical Herbalists, president of the American College of Integrative Medicine in Albuquerque, and author of *Herbal Remedies for Women*.

☙ Lisa Murray-Doran, N.D., a naturopathic physician and instructor at the Canadian College of Naturopathic Medicine in Toronto.

☙ Aviva Romm, a certified professional midwife and herbalist who practices in Bloomfield Hills, Michigan, professional member of the American Herbalists Guild, and author of *The Natural Pregnancy Book* and *Natural Healing for Babies and Children*.

☙ Douglas Schar, a practicing medical herbalist In London, editor of the *British Journal of Phytotherapy*, and author of *Backyard Medicine Chest*.

☙ Susun S. Weed, an herbalist and herbal educator from Woodstock, New York, and author of the *Wise Woman* series of herbal health books.

☙ David Winston, a professional member of the American Herbalists Guild, founder of Herbalist and Alchemist, an herbal medicine company in Washington, New Jersey, and head of the Herbal Therapeutic Research Library.

Introduction

ADVENTURES IN HERBAL HEALING

You'd think that after writing and editing articles and books on health for 20 years, I'd be in perfect health. Well, not quite. I'm not immune to the kinds of health complaints that sometimes hit out of the blue. A back strain. Migraines. And asthma, which I inherited. Plus the occasional cut, scrape, bruise, muscle ache, and other stuff that any woman is likely to encounter.

I hate getting sick. But I hate taking medicine, too. Every drug I've ever taken has disagreed with me. So when I started editing *The Woman's Book of Healing Herbs,* I got very excited. Herbal medicine opens up a whole new realm of healing possibilities for me. Feverfew for migraines. Grindelia for asthma. And, of course, like most women who don't have time to be sick, I'm very enthusiastic about echinacea, which has gotten a lot of press due to its ability to boost immunity and prevent colds.

If you're like me—and so many other women who are curious about the healing power of herbs—you've probably been looking for a reliable, practical, comprehensive source of information on herbs for women. When a national survey asked 1,008 men and women to identify their top source of herbal information, only 9 percent said that they consulted their doctors, and just 4 percent mentioned pharmacists. In contrast, 41 percent relied on friends and family for advice, and 72 percent said that they turned to magazines and books.

That's why I'm so pleased to introduce *The Woman's Book of Healing Herbs.*

This is the one book on which women like us can rely to help us explore nature's pharmacy and select remedies for our unique needs. To research this book, the authors traveled widely and studied with some of the most experienced herbalists in the country. Sarí Harrar attended a conference at the Southwest College of Naturopathic Medicine in Tempe, Arizona. Both Sarí and Sara O'Donnell participated in the annual Medicines from the Earth conference in Asheville, North Carolina, one of the largest botanical medicine conferences in the country. The authors attended workshops with Susun S. Weed and other herbalists who are well-respected for their innovative use of herbs for women's health concerns. And they consulted at length with David Winston, Douglas Schar, and dozens of other authorities in herbal medicine. These herbalists are among the experts whom doctors consult when fielding questions from patients who are eager to try herbal treatments.

I'm guessing that this isn't the first book on herbal healing you've had in hand. If you're like a lot of women, you have a personal library of books on natural healing. Some may be dog-eared from heavy use. Others may go unopened for months. Whether this is the first herb book that you've ever picked up or one of many you've seen, I think you'll be pleased with what we offer: the thoroughly researched explanations of why herbs work, written in everyday language. The depth of the information—detailed but not tedious. The rich language used to describe the history and philosophy of herbal healing. And best of all, the emphasis on the special role that herbs have always played in women's health.

Highly practical, the advice that this book offers takes the guesswork out of knowing what herbs have to offer, how much you should take, how to use them safely, and when to consult a medical doctor or other qualified health-care practitioner for health concerns that go beyond self-help. Both medical experts and alternative healers welcome this kind of information. With each passing year, more and more doctors and pharmacists are reading about herbal medicine in their professional journals and crowding into workshops and seminars on botanical remedies.

"Once again, consumers are leading the way," says Fredi Kronenberg, Ph.D., director of the Richard and Hilda Rosenthal Center for Complementary and Alternative Medicine at Columbia University College of Physicians and Surgeons in New York City. "As people use more herbs, and as companies produce more and more herbal products, doctors and pharmacists are realizing that they need to learn about this. In a sense, they're going back to their roots—back to herbal medicine."

We hope you agree that this book helps you find your own path of healing with herbs.

Sharon Faelten

Sharon Faelten
Editor

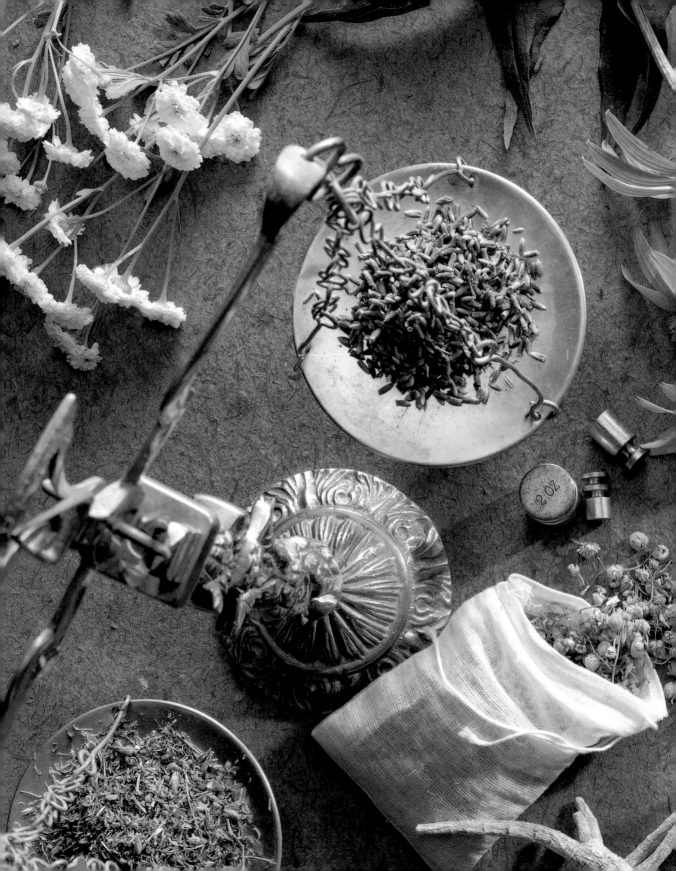

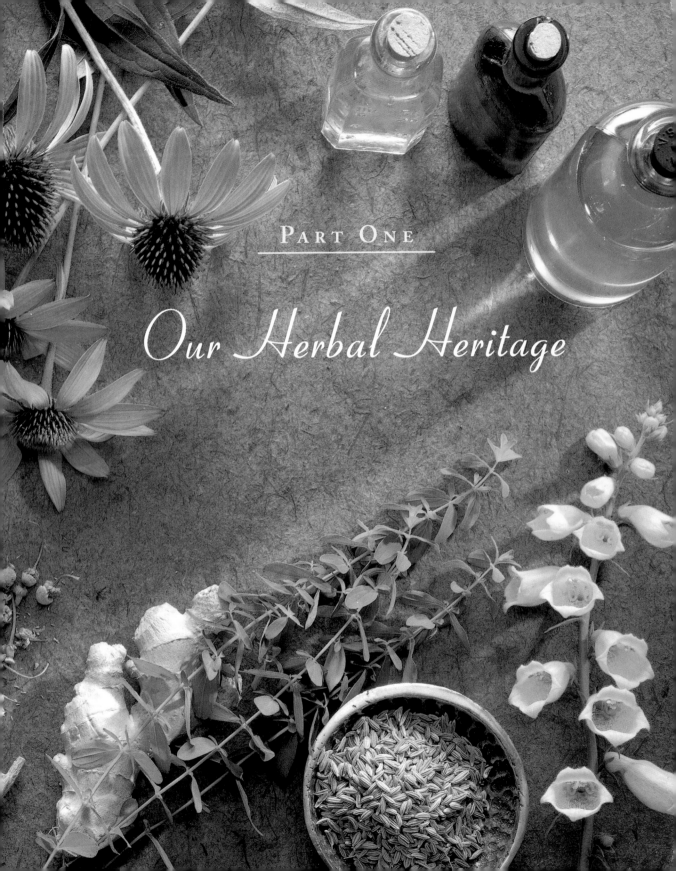

PART ONE

Our Herbal Heritage

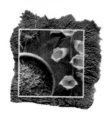

A Renaissance in Natural Healing

Thousands of years before chemists in high-tech laboratories invented potent pharmaceutical drugs, over-the-counter drugstore remedies, and commercial beauty products, women around the world visited Mother Nature's pharmacy for all of their health-care needs.

In China, women unearthed the pale, gnarled root called dang gui to soothe menstrual difficulties and mixed angelica into age-defying complexion creams. In North America, Native American women steeped black cohosh tea to ease menopausal discomforts and sipped a steaming echinacea brew for colds and flu. They created colorful cosmetics with flower pollen and petals and washed their hair with fragrant yarrow, white sage, and meadow rue. In Europe, women gathered sunshine yellow St.-John's-wort flowers for healing wounds and relied on lavender to relieve stress. The women of ancient Greece soothed irritated skin with calendula petals and regulated their menstrual cycles with chasteberry leaves soaked in wine.

Since the earliest days of the human race, plant remedies have been our medicines, our allies in maintaining emotional balance, and the key ingredients in our skin- and hair-care formulas. Today, millions of women are re-discovering this nourishing connection to the Earth, reviving a tradition that was very much alive as recently as the days of our great-grandmothers and grandmothers.

Paradise Lost?

"Until the early part of this century, herbalism was the primary system of healing in the United States," says herbalist Rose-mary Gladstar, director of the Sage Mountain herbal education center in East Barre, Vermont, and author of *Herbal Healing for Women*. "Many of our great-grandmothers knew something about plant home remedies. Pharmacies sold dried herbs and herbal prod-

Is There an Herbalist on Your Family Tree?

Call it the legacy of "Dr. Mom." For thousands of years, women have kept their households and communities healthy, relieving day-to-day health concerns with home remedies. Until the early part of the twentieth century, many of Dr. Mom's treatments were herbal remedies, according to medical historians.

"If you ask around in your family, you may learn that your own grandmother or great-grandmother knew a lot about herbs," says Sharol Tilgner, N.D., a naturopathic physician, herbalist, professional member of the American Herbalists Guild, and president of Wise Woman Herbals in Cresswell, Oregon.

"After I became an herbalist, I was surprised to learn that my own great-grandmother had been an herbalist and midwife," Dr. Tilgner says. "And *her* mom came to Oregon on a wagon train. My great-grandmother dried herbs in her home and under the trees in her yard, and she took a bag of remedies with her to deliver babies. But I never heard these stories from her; later in her life, she was embarrassed about that kind of healing. In the era of scientific medicine and an era where men practiced medicine and women did not, she didn't want to talk about herbs. I'm glad that attitude is changing today."

ucts. Women grew and gathered medicinal herbs for themselves and their families. And they passed the information on to their daughters and to their daughters' daughters. We lost this link when most people in this country stopped using herbs. But fortunately, we're rebuilding our connections to this wonderful tradition."

In small ways, traces of that old link remain. Think back. Did your mother, grandmother, or great-grandmother ever slather your chest with a mustard plaster to relieve congestion? Or suggest eating onions to reduce a fever? Or recommend cold, wet tea bags to revive tired eyes? If folk remedies like those sound familiar, you've experienced a connection with this ancient healing art, Gladstar notes.

Maybe you've used herbal remedies without realizing it. Perhaps you've relaxed with a calming mug of chamomile tea, for example. But even if you haven't, that doesn't mean that you haven't been benefiting from the healing powers of the plant kingdom. The fact is, a lot of modern-day health care is based on nature's enduring pharmacy.

"It's surprising to realize that 30 to 40 percent of all prescription medicines are derived from plants or were developed from clues about the way plant substances affect the human body," says Larry Walker, Ph.D., associate director of the National Center for the Development of Natural Products at the University of Mississippi in Oxford. Commonly prescribed plant-based medicines include digoxin, a treatment for congestive heart failure originally derived from foxglove, and atropine, a substance that comes from the nightshade plant and is used by ophthalmologists to dilate the pupils of the eyes before testing for glaucoma.

"For over-the-counter remedies, the percentage is the same, or perhaps even higher," says Dr. Walker. One of our most commonly used drugs, for example—aspirin—has roots in the green world. Aspirin was originally derived from willow, meadowsweet, and wintergreen, plants rich in pain-relieving compounds called salicylates.

Mouthwashes such as Listerine contain the active ingredient thymol, a powerful antiseptic that researchers have found in herbs such as thyme and wild bergamot. And some commercial creams used for muscle aches and arthritis contain tiny amounts of capsaicin, a powerful compound derived from red peppers that triggers the release of the body's natural painkillers.

"Plant-based remedies are used in every therapeutic area, from depression to heart disease and from cancer to gynecological problems," Dr. Walker notes. "And we're still looking to the natural world for important new treatments."

Paradise Found

Today, women are returning to the source of this healing power—Mother Nature's healing garden, the world's oldest health-care system.

Dismissed a couple of decades ago as the domain of hippies and the back-to-nature crowd, herbal remedies have become quite mainstream again. At least one-third of American adults—almost 60 million women and men—have used herbal remedies to treat common health concerns such as colds,

headaches, allergies, insomnia, PMS, and menopausal discomforts. Among the favored remedies are echinacea (which was also an herbal best-seller nearly 80 years ago), garlic, ginkgo, kava-kava, and St.-John's-wort.

Why the stampede back to the green pharmacy? Why try herbal remedies when we already have access to more than 9,500 prescription medications and 100,000 over-the-counter health products in various dosage forms and strengths, and when we can call on a health-care system staffed with more than 730,000 medical doctors? Professional herbalists who have been practicing for 10, 15, 20, or more years see many reasons.

Touching nature, again. "I think people have an inherent trust in nature," says Cascade Anderson Geller, an herbal educator and consulting herbal practitioner in Portland, Oregon. "Even people who are just coming to herbs, who may be a little nervous about taking something that doesn't come from a pharmacy, want to trust that inborn sense that nature is the right place to start the healing process."

Gentle, effective, and affordable healing. "Women are finding out that the quick fixes offered by chemical-laden drugs don't always work," says Sharol Tilgner, N.D., a naturopathic physician, herbalist, professional member of the American Herbalists Guild (AHG), and president of Wise Woman Herbals in Cresswell, Oregon. "They want something less expensive than prescription drugs, and with far fewer side effects—something that works for everyday health problems and helps chronic conditions, too."

Enhanced well-being. "Women want to hold on to good health. And herbs have the unique ability to support our life force—to work with our bodies to restore and enhance health," Gladstar says. "Women are finding that herbs can do some things that most conventional medicines cannot do—build and strengthen natural immunity and help us adapt to the incredible stresses of modern-day life."

The power of self-care. "Women and men have a strong desire these days to take better care of themselves," says ethnobotanist Rob McCaleb, president and founder of the Herb Research Foundation in Boulder, Colorado. "We're no longer willing to delegate responsibility for our health to other people. We don't want to be told what to do or what to take. We want to make informed choices about our own health and to know all the options, from conventional drugs to herbs to all forms of alternative medicine."

"When a woman picks herbs from her garden for a remedy or even makes a cup of herbal tea, she is helping herself become well," says Chanchal Cabrera, a member of Britain's National Institute of Medical Herbalists (NIMH) and a professional member of the AHG who practices in Vancouver.

In the Healing Garden

Healing herbs grow everywhere—in your backyard and deep in the Amazon rain forest, high on remote mountain ridges and in sun-baked deserts, in shady woodlands, and even in the sea. Some, like dandelion, are often scorned as weeds; others, such as red clover, alfalfa, and oats, are common farm crops. Still others, such as thyme, garlic, and cayenne pepper, may be sitting in your kitchen spice rack right now. And still others, such as some forms of ginseng, are exotic, costly, and rare—in some places, endangered to the point of extinction.

To a cook, herbs are flavor enhancers. But herbal healers define herbs more broadly. "To an herbalist, any plant used for medicinal purposes is an herb," Cabrera says. "Any leaf, flower, bark, root, seed, sap, berry, mushroom, or seaweed used for healing is considered a healing herb."

Whether an herb is in the form of a tasty leaf or a crunchy seed, its healing power originates with scores of natural substances contained within the plant—substances that herbalists and researchers say may work together like a ballet troupe or an orchestra. These compounds, which include minerals, vitamins, and a wide variety of natural chemicals, work in a woman's body to improve her health, Cabrera says. They may balance hormones to relieve hot flashes or PMS, improve fertility, reduce breast tenderness, stimulate the immune system to fight a cold or battle an infection, help knit torn skin back together, relieve anxiety, lift mild depression, or lull you into restful sleep, to cite just a few examples.

Each herb has a unique chemical fingerprint that may include hundreds or perhaps even thousands of different substances, says James A. Duke, Ph.D., a botanical consultant, former ethnobotanist with the U.S. Department of Agriculture, and author of *The Green Pharmacy*, who specializes in medicinal plants. "We know now that a well-researched herb like licorice contains more than 600 different compounds, and there are still more to discover," Dr. Duke says. "I think we will one day know that each herb actually contains thousands. And that's one of the keys to an herb's healing potential."

A Chemical Potpourri

Thanks to this chemical richness, an herb can have more than one action in the body,

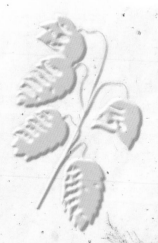

The Wise Woman Tradition
Hands-On Health Care

"Knowledge of plants is old knowledge and easily accessible. Some women simply 'remember' how to find it buried in the fertile soil of their own hearts."

—Rosemary Gladstar, herbalist, author, and teacher

From the first grandmother who brewed herb tea for a child's tummyache to a modern working woman who stays up all night tending to a feverish two-year-old, the Wise Woman tradition is the oldest tradition of healing known on our planet," says Susun S. Weed, an herbalist and herbal educator from Woodstock, New York, and author of the *Wise Woman* series of herbal health books. This durable yet invisible tradition specializes in nourishing the unique individual—and preventing disease—with the use of dooryard weeds, simple ceremony, and compassionate listening, Weed notes.

Historical records from as long ago as 500 B.C. often use "feminine" forms of the words *pharmacist* and *herbalist*. "That indicates that women were often the herbal healers of their day," notes medical historian John M. Riddle, Ph.D., chairman of the history department at North Carolina State University in Raleigh and author of *Eve's Herbs*. "Later, in the Middle Ages, women were expected to have medicinal herb gardens. There's a famous statement that the garden nourishes and heals. Women were the healers who used the garden when they practiced domestic, at-home medicine, and when they attended births as midwives."

The Wise Woman tradition has weathered two great "challenges" and survived, Dr. Riddle and Gladstar note. The first was the Inquisition, which included midwives among its targets during the sixteenth, seventeenth, and eighteenth centuries in Europe, Dr. Riddle says. The second came early in the twentieth century, when modern pharmaceutical medicines pushed herbal remedies off drugstore shelves and out of home medicine chests.

"Our great-grandmothers and great-great-grandmothers most likely knew about herbal remedies, but they put the knowledge aside as old-fashioned," Gladstar says. "Now, women are finding that herbs still have an important place in nurturing good health. We are rediscovering our links to this ancient tradition."

Dr. Duke says. Garlic fights infection, for example. But it can also lower high cholesterol and high blood pressure. Pungent fennel seeds can relieve digestive discomfort. But they're also a traditional milk booster for nursing mothers. Valerian can help you sleep, but taken with other herbs, it may also relieve menstrual cramps. Lavender has an antimicrobial effect: When used on the skin, it kills germs. But its scent can reduce feelings of stress as well. St.-John's-wort lifts mild to moderate depression when taken internally, but the blood red oil made from its flowers may help heal burns.

"Your body knows how to use the chemicals in the plants because human beings evolved using plants as food and medicine," Dr. Duke notes. "When you take an herbal remedy, your body makes good use of what it needs from this chemical potpourri and up to a point ignores what it doesn't need. Our bodies work well with plants as our food and as our medicine."

The chemical complexity of herbs can sometimes puzzle researchers. "Often, we know that an herb works, but research can't figure out exactly why. Scientists keep looking, but the explanation remains an elusive mystery," says Ed Smith, a professional member of the AHG and founder of Herb Pharm in Williams, Oregon. "Researchers offer three or four different explanations for why valerian relaxes people and helps them sleep, for example. As they continue to look further, they find still more active ingredients."

Various groups of researchers have tried to pinpoint the active ingredient in echinacea, the popular cold-and-flu herb, and they've identified at least three different classes of compounds that may be responsible, Dr. Walker says. "If you isolate individual pure compounds, you can see some interesting activity, but none of them alone seems to account for the effect. The complex mixture found in the plant seems to show a combination of actions that result in a boost for the immune system," he says.

Herbs' chemical versatility makes them valuable medicines, says Mary Bove, N.D., a naturopathic physician, midwife, and member of the NIMH who practices at the Brattleboro Naturopathic Clinic in Vermont.

Trusting Tradition

The first researchers to study herbs weren't university-trained scientists in white lab coats bending over bubbling beakers or computer printouts. Medical historians can only guess at how the first herbal medicines were discovered. But they do know that human beings were probably using botanicals 12,000 years ago, and possibly even earlier than that. Cave remains in the current Iran/Iraq region that contain residue of the medicinal ephedra species have been dated back 60,000 years.

Prehistoric women and men learned to use herbal remedies by experimenting with wild plants for thousands of years, swallowing this and tasting that, sometimes with good results and other times with tragic endings if a plant was toxic, Dr. Duke says. "By trial and error, our ancestors picked out the best medicines," he says. "It took them many, many generations. And the effort probably cost many lives as men and women sampled almost all of the leaves, flowers, roots, barks, and seeds of the plants growing around them."

The result was a completely human-tested system of herbal medicine—or rather, many systems—developed by people living in different cultures, with different local plants, all around the world. "Humans have existed for

Traditional Chinese Medicine
Health in Harmony

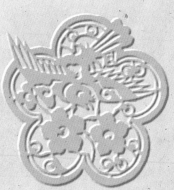

"The utmost in the art of healing can be achieved when there is unity."

—*The Yellow Emperor's Classic of Internal Medicine*

Its origins veiled in myth and mystery, China's 2,500-year-old healing system is alive and well today. Just ask the one-quarter of the world's population who rely on it for health care, or simply peek at the herbs for sale in your local pharmacy.

Practitioners trained in Traditional Chinese Medicine work with about 500 herbal remedies, which are prescribed in combinations that range from simple 3-herb formulas to complex 100-herb mixtures. Now, many of these botanicals have traveled to the West. From energizing ginseng to dang gui (a menstrual-cycle regulator) and from vitality-enhancing licorice to memory-boosting ginkgo, dozens of ancient Chinese healing herbs are widely used in the United States today.

Traditional Chinese Medicine uses herbs, acupuncture, and lifestyle changes to help restore health by re-establishing balance in the body and mind. Practitioners view disease as a sign of disharmony that thwarts the body's natural healing abilities. Using basic principles first outlined in the world's oldest medical text, the 2,500-year-old *The Yellow Emperor's Classic of Internal Medicine*, practitioners sleuth for signs of imbalance: They study your tongue, interpret nuances in the speed and strength of your pulse, and grill you about what you like to eat, your sleep habits, your bowel habits, and your sex life.

From the traditional Chinese view, health is profoundly influenced by the balance of yin and yang—the opposite but complementary qualities that exist in every aspect of life, such as cold and heat, water and fire, earth and heaven, rest and activity—and by the interaction of five natural elements: fire, earth, metal, water, and wood. Each is associated with specific organ systems, colors, and emotions. Herbs can help harmonize these elements and can also bolster all-important *qi* or *chi* (pronounced *chee*), the essential life force.

2.5 million years in Africa; a million years in China, India, and Indonesia; about 40,000 years in Australia; and about 25,000 years in the Americas," Dr. Duke says. "That makes herbal medicine the longest-running clinical study in the history of the world."

Herbal folklore, often dismissed as inaccurate and even silly, guides the recommendations of today's herbalists. Moreover, it has provided the clues for a great deal of modern medicine, Dr. Duke says. "Ninety percent of drugs that come from plants were discovered by looking into traditional uses," he says. "Even today, when botanists search for new medicinal plants in the rain forest, they are more successful when they get information from local people about the way they use plants."

Of particular interest to herbalists and ethnobotanists like Dr. Duke are the cases where more than one culture uses the same or very similar herbs for the same purpose. There are about 100 similar herbs used in parallel ways by Chinese and Native American healers, for example, including ginseng and several plant species containing the bitter yellow antiseptic compound called berberine that is found in goldenseal, says Dr. Duke. "When two groups of people independently come to the same conclusion about an herb, that's strong evidence that it may really work," he says.

Ancient Discoveries, Modern Remedies

Today's herbal remedies draw on "prescriptions" developed by many cultures and employ plants that historians know were used by some of the world's earliest civilizations.

In Egypt, where healers included everything from leeks to hippopotamus fat to pomegranates in medicines, hieroglyphic writings from 1500 B.C. describe the use of myrrh and castor oil, among many other herbs. Herbalists still recommend these herbs today.

In Greece in the third century B.C., the physician Hippocrates used the healing herbs elder, garlic, horehound, rosemary, sage, fennel, hawthorn, mint, cloves, and rose, among others. Later, in A.D. 100, the Greek healer Dioscorides wrote an herbal healing classic called *De Materia Medica*, a book that covers approximately 500 medicinal plants, including cinnamon, mustard, and a bramble that helped regulate women's menstrual periods.

China's oldest herbal handbook, *The Yellow Emperor's Classic of Internal Medicine*, dating to 300 B.C., includes ginseng, ginger, water lily, witch hazel, and mugwort.

Practitioners of India's 5,000-year-old healing system, called Ayurveda, have long used at least 700 plant medicines, including garlic, ginseng, and birch bark.

A Roman medical text from A.D. 100 lists catnip, garlic, mint, dill, dock, and thyme among its healing herbs.

Herbs used by the Aztecs in A.D. 1552 included dioscorea (now called wild yam) and nettle juice.

Native Americans used a wide variety of herbal medicines to treat hundreds of conditions, including fever, constipation, pain, and respiratory problems. Among the thousands of medicinal herbs still in use today among Native Americans are passionflower, black cohosh, echinacea, and partridgeberry.

In colorful herbal remedy books dating to the Middle Ages, European healers discussed the virtues of hundreds of herbs, in-

(continued on page 13)

Healing Herbs: As Near as Your Backyard

From weeds such as dandelion to easy-growing garden favorites such as mint, garlic, and calendula flowers, a potpourri of medicinal herbs is growing right in your own backyard.

"Women can do so much with the safe, common herbs already coming up in the yards and fields near their own homes," notes Betzy Bancroft, a professional member of the American Herbalists Guild and manager of Herbalist and Alchemist, an herbal medicine company in Washington, New Jersey. "Some of the best remedies I make and use come from local plants."

Here are some healing herbs that you might discover on a ramble close to home and the ways in which herbalists believe they may help. (One note of caution, however: Pick and use only those herbs that you have positively identified. Use a good field guide. When in doubt, leave a plant alone, Bancroft says. And use only herbs grown in a clean environment away from pesticide and herbicide sprays, lawn-care chemicals, and other sources of pollution such as heavy metals, which often occur along roadsides. If you can't ask whether an area is treated or untreated by chemicals, don't collect there, Bancroft says.)

1. Dandelion (common weed). Leaves and roots are good for water retention, digestive problems (stimulates digestion), constipation, and liver health.

2. Nettle (common weed). Leaves are good for a mineral-loaded "tonic" that may ease water retention and increase breast milk. Cooked or dried nettles lose their sting; handle fresh stinging nettles with care—and a pair of gloves.

3. Red clover (common lawn weed and agricultural crop). Flowering tops are good for balancing hormones during menopause, relieving menstrual problems, and fertility.

4. Mint (garden tea herb). Leaves are good for digestive spasms and nausea.

5. Yarrow (common field weed and ornamental plant). Leaves and flowers are good for cuts and scrapes.

6. Lavender (ornamental garden herb). Flowers and leaves are good for reducing nervous stress and tension.

7. Garlic (edible herb). Bulbs are good for reducing cholesterol and fighting infection.

8. Calendula (garden flower). Petals are good for treating wounds and burns.

9. Red raspberry (common garden shrub). Leaves are good for reproductive health. May relax and strengthen uterus, ease menstrual cramps, and normalize hormones.

10. Lemon balm (common herb garden ornamental). Leaves are good for spasms of the digestive tract, insomnia, and herpes simplex.

11. Thyme (easy-to-grow culinary herb). Leaves are good for congestion and respiratory infections.

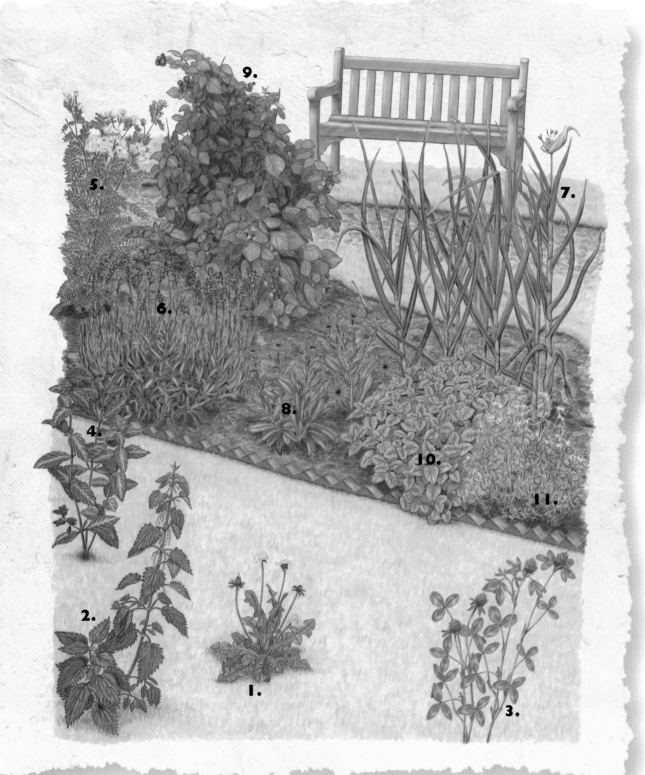

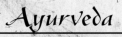

Ayurveda

India's Ancient Science of Life

"In Ayurveda, truth is being, pure existence, the source of all life."

—Vasant Lad, director of The Ayurvedic Institute
in Albuquerque

About 5,000 years ago, India's wise men first recorded the tenets of a health system still widely practiced today: Ayurveda—from the words *ayur* (life) and *veda* (knowledge).

Embracing more than medicine, this ancient healing philosophy aims to help people live healthfully and harmoniously, aided by diet, breathing exercises, and herbal formulas. Ayurveda has sent botanical emissaries to America in the form of herbs found in health food stores and on kitchen spice racks. These include the familiar nutmeg, cloves, saffron, and coriander—all used in Ayurveda to strengthen the body's energy centers—as well as lesser-known healing herbs such as gotu kola, ashwaganda, guggul, and shatavari.

At the heart of Ayurveda's healing philosophy is *prana*, the unseen primal energy that brings life to mind and body. Ayurvedic practitioners may suggest special breathing exercises that are said to draw more of this life energy into the body, where it can promote healing.

Ayurveda emphasizes individuality while stressing that all of existence reflects the ever-changing relationships between five elements: ether (or space), air, fire, water, and earth. Within every human being, these five elements combine to form specific personality types, called *doshas*, that profoundly influence physical and psychological makeup. The three basic doshas are *vata*, a restless, active, alert personality; *pitta*, a fiery, competitive, creative type; and *kapha*, a strong, slow-moving sort. A person's constitution may reflect varying levels of any or all of the three doshas.

Practitioners often prescribe special herbs and food plans to rebalance the doshas, prevent disease, and enhance healing. Classic Ayurvedic healing texts recommend herbal remedies, called *rasayanas*, that contain 10 to 20 different botanicals, sometimes mixed with fruits and minerals and taken as teas, pills, jellies, or pastes or powders mixed with food.

cluding valerian, lady's-mantle, and chaste-berry. European settlers who sailed to the New World brought the seeds of these and other medicinal plants with them. Some of the weeds that we find in our own backyards—non-native varieties such as mullein and English plantain—may be descendants of these early medicinal gardens, Dr. Duke notes.

Herbal Wisdom
More Than Health in a Bottle

"Anything that connects a woman with the food she eats or the herbal medicine she takes connects her to the Earth. That's very healing. We need to move away from looking at medicine as health in a bottle. Instead, cook with healthy plants. Make teas from safe back-yard weeds. That's joyful—and much deeper healing than just using a bottle of something."

—*Jill Stansbury, N.D., naturopathic physician and herbalist*

New Evidence for Old Truths

Tradition says that herbs work. And today, much to the delight of herbalists, scientific researchers are discovering *how* botanical medicines heal. "Finally, natural products research is coming close to discovering what traditional herbalists have been saying about herbs all along," says David Hoffman, a founding and professional member of the AHG, a fellow of the NIMH, assistant professor of integral health studies at the California Institute of Integral Studies in Santa Rosa, and author of *The New Holistic Herbal*. "This scientific information is giving people a new reason to trust plant medicines."

Laboratories in Europe, Russia, India, Japan, China, and the United States are uncovering clues about the natural chemistry of plants that often validate traditional medicine, says Dr. Duke. Here are just a few examples.

Aloe. The gooey gel from aloe's spiny leaves has been used to treat cuts, burns, and scrapes for at least 2,500 years. Studies now show that substances in the gel penetrate damaged tissue, promote healing activity, increase blood flow to injured areas, and relieve pain and inflammation.

Chamomile. Slovakian folklore advises people to bow before this daisylike herb, used for hundreds of years for upset stomachs and insomnia and to heal cuts and bruises. Research suggests that two compounds in chamomile—alpha-bisabolol and chamazulene—partially account for its antiseptic, anti-inflammatory, and sedative actions.

Feverfew. Seventeenth-century English herbalist Nicholas Culpeper wrote that this herb "is very effectual for all pains in the head." Three centuries later, several British studies have confirmed that feverfew can reduce the frequency and severity of migraine headaches.

Garlic. Extolled by the Greek naturalist Pliny in the first century A.D. for quieting coughs and expelling parasites, garlic has been the subject of more than 2,500 scientific studies that confirm its benefits for lowering blood pressure, reducing cholesterol, and fighting off yeast infections, colds, and flu.

(continued on page 17)

Plant Medicine: The Inside Story

Pluck a sprig of gorgeously scented lavender from a summer garden. Pull a long, bitter-tasting dandelion root from the earth. Both are healing herbs, but that's where the similarity ends. Inside each is a unique blend of active chemical ingredients, scientists say, with special medicinal benefits for humans.

But why do the plants produce these useful substances in the first place? Why does lavender grow scented leaves and dandelion develop a harsh-flavored root? "Phytochemists are still trying to understand all the reasons that plants create these compounds," notes Steven Dentali, Ph.D., a chemist and owner of a natural-products consulting service in Troutdale, Oregon. "Many play a beneficial role in the life of the plant. It's still something of a mystery, but we know these chemicals have been healing people for thousands of years."

Here's a look at the major active ingredients in healing herbs, where they're found, and how they may be of use to the plants—and to you.

Bitters. Often found in roots (1) and leaves (4). *Possible benefit for the plant:* The bitter taste may discourage hungry predators. *Potential benefit for you:* Bitters such as dandelion root and leaf, burdock, and yellow dock root improve digestion by stimulating bile flow and digestive juices (enzymes in the stomach and intestines).

Flavonoids. Often found in flowers (5), leaves (4), stems (3), fruit (7), and roots (1). *Possible benefit for the plant:* They're responsible for the rich yellows and oranges found in flower petals and fruits—colors that may help attract pollinating insects as well as animals that will eat the fruit and scatter the seeds. *Potential benefits for you:* Strengthening of blood vessel walls, protection from cell damage caused by oxidation, and easing of water retention, inflammation, and muscle spasms.

Volatile oils. Often found in leaves (4), flowers (5), bark (9), and fruit (7). *Possible benefits for the plant:* They give herbs such as rosemary, lavender, ginger, and mint their "signature" scents. They may help attract pollinators, repel predators, and—thanks to their antimicrobial action—protect against disease. *Potential benefits for you:* Antiseptic action and stress relief (when scents are inhaled as aromatherapy essential oils). Various herbs rich in volatile oils may also enhance appetite, stimulate circulation, and relieve water retention.

Alkaloids. Often found in roots (1), leaves (4), and seeds (2). *Possible benefits for the plant:* These potent compounds may repel predators and are thought by some to also help regulate plant growth. Coffee, black tea, tobacco, and opium all contain alkaloids, as do goldenseal, ephedra, and Oregon grape root, among others. *Potential benefits for you:* Some alkaloid-rich herbs fight bacterial and fungal infections. Many others are very strong substances that should not be used as home remedies.

Gums and resins. Often found in the trunks and branches (6) of trees and shrubs. *Possible benefit for the plant:* Gums and resins such as myrrh, pine resin, and guggul are forms of sap and act as the blood of the plant's circulatory system, transporting nutrients wherever needed. *Potential benefit for you:* Some gums, like guggul, which is extracted from a plant related to myrrh, may lower cholesterol.

Mucilage. Often found in seeds (2), roots (1), and inner bark (8). *Possible benefit for the plant:* Mucilage is a water-retaining agent that helps seeds germinate. *Potential benefit for you:* Mucilage-rich seeds such as psyllium and flax gently ease constipation. Marshmallow root and slippery elm bark, also high in mucilage, soothe irritated mucous membranes.

Saponins. Often found in roots (1) and leaves (4). *Possible benefit for the plant:* Botanists speculate that saponins, which can lather like soap when mixed with water, may discourage predators from feeding on plant parts. *Potential benefits for you:* Some can work as expectorants to reduce coughs, while others strengthen blood vessels, regulate hormones, or counteract stress. Saponin-rich herbs include mullein, partridgeberry, black cohosh, wild yam, and licorice.

Tannins. Often found in bark (9), roots (1), and leaves (4). *Possible benefits for the plant:* This is as yet unclear to scientists. *Potential benefit for you:* Tannin-rich herbs, such as witch hazel, oak bark, and black tea, have an astringent action that protects and heals skin and mucous membranes.

Anthraquinones. Often found in roots (1) and leaves (4). *Possible benefit for the plant:* Protection against fungal and bacterial infections. *Potential benefits for you:* These yellow compounds, found in yellow dock and other plants, stimulate bile production, aiding digestion and nudging a sluggish liver. They are recommended only for short-term use.

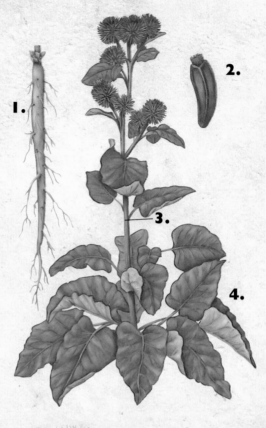

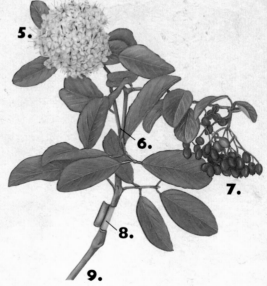

Old European Herbalism
Color and Controversy

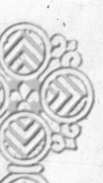

"You may see plainly without a pair of spectacles . . . the virtues of plants."

—Herbalist Nicholas Culpeper, 1616–54

For more than 1,000 years, European herbalism has been an amalgam—a patchwork of remedies from ancient Greece, the Roman Empire, and India as well as from churchyard "physic gardens" and village herbalists who gathered healing herbs in wild meadows, woods, and hedgerows in England, Germany, and other areas.

This colorful healing tradition has even produced a few herbalist-rebels who opposed the growing power of physicians and apothecaries and sought to put herbal healing back in the hands of the common people. Among them was the sixteenth-century German physician Paracelsus, who condemned the modern medicine of his day and advocated a return to a simpler system called the Doctrine of Signatures, which drew connections between a plant's appearance and its healing potential.

This fanciful-sounding doctrine was at times surprisingly accurate. St.-John's-wort, for example, was identified as a wound healer because its leaves contain tiny, woundlike oil sacs and its extracts are blood red. Today, wound healing is still one of its main uses. Yellow-flowered plants such as dandelion were linked with jaundice and used as liver remedies, as dandelion leaf and root are today.

Other renegade natural healers published illustrated herbal remedy books in English (instead of scholarly Latin) that were aimed at helping ordinary people gather and concoct their own remedies instead of relying on outrageously expensive medicines from apothecary shops.

One, the seventeenth-century author Nicholas Culpeper, enraged England's newly organized College of Physicians by translating their herbal remedy guide into layman's language. *Culpeper's Complete Herbal*, subtitled *A Comprehensive Description of Nearly All Herbs*, is still available today.

Among its poetic and opinionated entries is this one, for spearmint: "It is good to repress the milk in women's breasts. . . . Taken in wine, it helps women in their sore travail in child-bearing."

Ginger. A standby in Traditional Chinese Medicine, this spicy root was used traditionally in Europe against nausea. Four of six studies have found ginger useful against motion sickness, while others suggest that it may reduce morning sickness, perhaps by absorbing and neutralizing stomach acid.

Ginseng. Two thousand years ago, a Chinese herbalist noted that using ginseng can foster longevity, soothe the spirit, enlighten the mind, and bring "brightness" to the eyes. Today, some studies show that ginseng may sharpen your mental powers by shortening reaction time, boosting alertness, improving concentration, and tuning up hand-eye coordination.

Uva-ursi. A long-time remedy for bladder infections, uva-ursi has been shown to contain two substances, arbutin and methylarbutin, that undergo chemical changes during digestion and form substances that kill or inhibit bacteria in the urinary tract.

"As we apply science to these traditional herbal remedies, we see how trustworthy they are," Dr. Duke says. "The more I study medicinal herbs, the more convinced I am that our ancestors knew exactly what they were doing. The more I look, the more I see that the actions of chemicals discovered in the plants, in most cases, correspond to what our ancestors said the herbs do."

Europe Leads the Way

Herbal medicine is not a passing fad. Experts estimate that 80 percent of the world's people rely on herbal medicine for their health care. In France, for example, 30 to 40 percent of doctors prescribe chiefly botanical medicines. In Germany, 7 out of 10 doctors prescribe herb-based remedies, called phytomedicines, to their patients.

Also in Germany, nearly 300 herbal medicines have been reviewed for safety and effectiveness by a government-appointed panel called Commission E, which is made up of physicians, pharmacologists, and other herbal medicine experts. Herbal experts in the United States are increasingly turning to the Commission E reports and to newer research for trustworthy information about herbal side effects and effectiveness.

The Commission E reports, coupled with research under way in the United States and around the world, will give doctors, pharmacists, and consumers even more information for making sound choices about herbal remedies, says Mark Blumenthal, executive director of the American Botanical Council in Austin, Texas.

Natural healers such as Dr. Bove say that herbs offer many compelling benefits for women. Here are just a few.

Benefit #1: A Nondrug Approach That Works

Research shows that herbal remedies are effective alternatives to prescription and over-the-counter drugs for treating a variety of common complaints, from minor first-aid needs to insomnia, from PMS to depression, and from eczema to acne, according to Dr. Duke.

"Herbs aren't weak substitutes for drugs—they are extraordinarily effective in many kinds of situations," says David Winston, a professional member of the AHG and founder of Herbalist and Alchemist, an herbal medicine company in Washington, New Jersey, where he maintains one of the largest private herb libraries in the United States. Ginger, for example, rivals the most popular medication sold as a preventive for motion sickness. Here are some other examples.

Cranberry. A traditional bladder infection fighter, this tart red fruit has been shown to keep bacteria from sticking to the inner walls of the bladder. And when germs can't stick, they are washed out of the body, so infections don't worsen. The potential benefit is fewer rounds of antibiotics for repeat episodes.

Ginkgo. Studies suggest that an extract made from ginkgo's elegant, fan-shaped leaves may effectively treat symptoms associated with Alzheimer's disease in as little as three months.

Horse chestnut. A West German study has found that this herb may restore elasticity to varicose veins, possibly avoiding the need for expensive and risky surgery.

Milk thistle. The seeds of this spiny, purple-flowered plant may repair liver cells and protect them against further damage— something that few, if any, synthetic drugs can do. Researchers credit the active ingredient silymarin.

Valerian. The premier anti-insomnia herb, pungent valerian root was shown in one Swiss study to improve sleep for 89 percent of those with sleep problems. Forty-four percent reported "perfect sleep" after using valerian.

But herbal healing isn't simply an alternative to conventional medicine. "Plant medicines and conventional Western medicine fit together beautifully, like a hand in a glove," Winston says. "Where Western medicine is strong, such as in handling emergencies and life-or-death conditions, herbalism is weak. And where herbalism is strong, such as in

dealing with day-to-day health problems and building strong health, Western medicine is weaker."

It's always wise to check with your physician and with an experienced herbal practitioner before combining herbal treatments with prescription medications, Winston says. But for nagging health problems or while recovering from a major illness, herbs can be a welcome addition to a comprehensive healing strategy.

Benefit #2: Fewer Side Effects

Chosen wisely and taken in the right doses, herbal remedies have a trustworthy safety record, says Geller. "Most of the cases of toxicity come from long-term use (months) of the same herb or formula. Do not continue to take something past the time of need, and take breaks of days or weeks from products," she says. Generally, the side effects of herbs are much milder than the side effects caused by drugs.

The complex chemistry of plants may be a buffer against harmful side effects, say herbal experts like Geller, Winston, and Dr. Duke. For example, while diuretic drugs that treat water retention can also deplete the body's important stores of potassium, herbs such as dandelion leaf are effective diuretics and good sources of potassium as well. And while commercial anti-inflammatory drugs such as aspirin can also cause stomach bleeding, the herbal anti-inflammatory meadowsweet is thought to contain antacid-like substances that soothe the digestive tract.

Women who take herbs find that they can treat common health concerns without experiencing the unwanted side effects that often

Native American Herbal Healing
Listening to the Plant Teachers

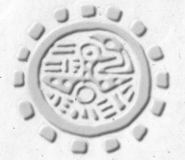

"We return thanks for all herbs, which furnish medicines for the cure of our diseases."

—Iroquois prayer

Over thousands of years, North America's original inhabitants developed more than 200 different herbal medicine traditions, giving us natural healing secrets that Americans use today to ease dozens of health concerns, including colds, coughs, cuts, indigestion, and menstrual problems.

From the Delaware to the Cherokee, from the Ojibwa to the Potawatomi, Native American peoples and their healing practices are varied and unique. Yet most share a core philosophy that health is regained when a person is reconnected with the Great Spirit—with the Earth, with family, and with the community. Plants, born of Mother Earth, are seen as teachers that help the body remember how to function in healthy ways.

From local plants arose many remedies. Relief from the common cold came with pine-bark tea for the Cree and with yarrow tea for the Abnaki and Cheyenne. For menstrual cramps, Paiute women relied on juniper berries, the Cherokee chose partridgeberry, and the Kiowa brewed dandelion-leaf tea. Headache? The Chippewa eased head pain by inhaling steam from yarrow-leaf tea, while the Omaha sipped a brew made with crushed wild columbine seeds.

Here are some herbs that come to us from Native American traditions.

✔ Echinacea, used by the Cheyenne, Dakota, Lakota, and others for sore throats, snakebites, wounds, burns, and tonsillitis.

✔ Witch hazel, used by the Potawatomi and Mohegan peoples for cuts, bruises, insect bites, and sore muscles.

✔ Black cohosh, used by the Cherokee for rheumatism, menstrual problems, and backaches.

✔ Blue cohosh, used by the Cherokee, Chippewa, and others for menstrual problems, childbirth, indigestion, and to calm overexcitement.

✔ Slippery elm, used by the Mohegan and Ojibwa to ease coughs and dry, sore throats.

A Medieval–And Thoroughly Modern– Herbal Healer

*H*ildegard von Bingen, the twelfth-century German nun who wrote two well-respected herbal remedy books and composed poetry and ethereal music, may well have been one of the world's most astonishing, and busy, women. Abbess of a religious community overlooking the Rhine Valley, she was highly regarded as a theologian, philosopher, and prophet by popes and emperors alike.

"Hildegard was a Renaissance woman long before the Renaissance," notes historian Joyce Suellentrop, associate professor of history at Kansas Newman College in Wichita. "Her accomplishments were vast, despite the fact that she was a woman living in the Middle Ages."

Little is known about her first 30 years as a Benedictine nun and later as an abbess. But when Hildegard reached her forties, something changed. In words and in colorful "illuminations" drawn by an unknown artist under her direction, Hildegard made public the visions that she said God had been sending her since childhood.

Today, Hildegard is best remembered for her soaring vocal music and her visionary writings. But in her day, this medieval woman of the cloth was revered as a healer, too. Her botanical medicine books, titled *Physica* and *Causae et Curae* in Latin, describe more than 500 herbs and detail the causes and symptoms of and remedies for 47 diseases.

"Hildegard's favorite herb was fennel," Suellentrop says. "She recommended it for eye problems, water retention, and disorders of the stomach, liver, and lungs.

For arthritis, Hildegard recommended chewing pulverized mint leaves steeped in wine. For liver problems, she suggested hyssop. And for low sexual desire, she suggested inhaling the scents of a potpourri of dried geranium, mallow, and plantain. "Hildegard was unique in the attention she paid to the emotional and sexual dimensions of women's lives," Suellentrop notes. "She writes about sexual pleasure, conception, and birth in a positive way. And she saw the connection between emotional health and physical health. In so many ways, she was a very modern healer."

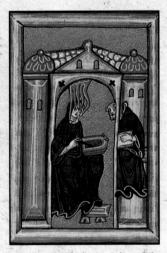

A self-portrait of Hildegard von Bingen—abbess, composer, philosopher, and healer.

come with pharmaceutical drugs, herbal experts say. Here are some examples.

Colds and flu. Over-the-counter decongestants and antihistamines may simply suppress symptoms like sneezing, coughing, and congestion. Plus, they can make you too drowsy to drive or get your work done. But if you take echinacea or fresh garlic for colds and flu, you can ease the symptoms—and battle the bugs that made you sick in the first place—without feeling sleepy, says Dr. Duke. Using herbs strengthens you, while using antibiotics may, in the long run, strengthen the enemy, he notes.

Depression. Studies show that St.-John's-wort is as effective as prescription antidepressants for relieving mild to moderate depression, with none of the side effects of medication, such as loss of interest in sex and digestive disturbances.

Infections. While taking antibiotics for long periods of time can lead to the development of dangerous, drug-resistant bacteria, herbal "antibacterial agents" such as garlic don't seem to create resistant strains, Winston says.

Sleeplessness. Sip a mug of insomnia-melting herbal tea (a combination of valerian, chamomile, and lemon balm works well), says Gladstar, and you won't wake up in the morning with that groggy, hung-over feeling that can come with over-the-counter and prescription sleeping pills.

For more about safety and side effects when using herbs, see "Using Herbs Wisely and Safely" on page 112.

Benefit #3: Preventive Medicine

Are you feeling tired all the time? Stressed beyond your limits? Do you catch a cold whenever someone in your office sneezes? Are you coping with a chronic problem such as acne or digestive trouble? Herbs may help these problems, too. In fact, herbalists say that botanical remedies shine when it comes to restoring vitality, raising low resistance, rebuilding your body's cushion against stress, and addressing the root causes of nagging health conditions.

"This is the true power of healing herbs," Gladstar explains. "More than providing quick fixes for symptoms, herbs can improve underlying health so that you can overcome fatigue or low immunity or improve an ongoing problem so that it isn't such an ordeal."

"Everybody knows that we're better off preventing health problems than dealing with illness," says McCaleb.

For health protection, herbalists recommend using tonic herbs—gentle botanicals that can be taken for weeks or months at a time.

"These herbs feed the body and may contain essential vitamins and minerals," says Kathleen Maier, a physician's assistant, professional member of the AHG, director of the Dreamtime Center for Herbal Studies in Flint Hill, Virginia, and former advisor on botanical medicine to the National Institutes of Health. "Often, the best way to take tonic herbs is as gentle herbal teas or even cooked into foods such as soups and stir-fries."

Combined with a healthy eating plan and regular physical activity—as little as a 30-minute walk two or three times a week—"it's amazing what you can accomplish with herbs," notes Geller.

For more about protecting your health with herb tonics, see "Herbal Tonics" on page 152.

The Herbal Medicine Chest: Handy Fixes for Everyday Ills

At home or on the road, herbs may offer effective treatment when an emergency arises, notes Sharleen Andrews-Miller, faculty member at the National College of Naturopathic Medicine in Portland, Oregon, and associate medicinary director at the college's public clinic. If assembled in advance, an herbal first-aid kit will save the day when the need arises, whether the problem is a cut, scrape, or bruise, indigestion or insomnia.

For your basic herbal first-aid kit, follow these suggestions from Andrews-Miller and Jenny McFeely, a member of Britain's National Institute of Medical Herbalists and a professional member of the American Herbalists Guild, who teaches courses on herbalism at her Herbal Healing and Research Center in Scottsdale, Arizona.

Aloe. For minor burns, sunburn, and rashes. At home, keep a plant on a sunny windowsill. For travel, carry a tube of aloe gel.

Antiseptic herbal mix. In advance, combine ½ ounce (about 1 tablespoon) each of tinctures of echinacea, St.-John's-wort, Oregon grape root, and calendula. For preventing infection in wounds, apply topically. The mixture can also be taken in water or juice for colds, flu, sore throats, and other infections. This remedy should not be taken internally over a long period of time.

Bentonite clay or baking soda/ ground oatmeal mix. To make a healing pack, mix the clay or baking soda and oatmeal with water and an anti-infection herb (such as garlic, thyme, or calendula) or an herbal tincture. Apply to pimples, boils, and wounds.

Dried calendula flowers. Make a strong tea with 1 tablespoon of petals per cup of boiling water, steep for 20 minutes, strain, and cool. Use to wash cuts and scrapes.

Dried chamomile flowers. Chamomile tea eases digestive problems, calms anxiety, and relieves mild insomnia. Strained through a coffee filter and cooled, it can be used as a wash for eye infections such as pinkeye.

Eucalyptus essential oil. For congestion, add a few drops to a bowl of steaming water and breathe the vapors gently.

Gingerroot or capsules. For nausea, motion sickness, or morning sickness, take as tea or capsules or chew crystallized ginger.

Goldenseal powder in capsules. For infections. The powder can also be used in salves or mixed with water and bentonite clay or a baking soda/oatmeal mix to soothe external infections.

Echinacea tincture. For colds, flu, and infections.

Rescue Remedy. A combination of Bach flower essences that some herbalists say can quickly soothe anxiety, stress, and fear. "This is great to have on hand during an emergency, when the last thing you need is people getting upset," Andrews-Miller says.

Tea tree essential oil. Dilute with vegetable oil to fight fungal and bacterial infections in cuts, abrasions, and athlete's foot.

Witch hazel tincture. For rashes and minor burns. It cleans and helps heal wounds.

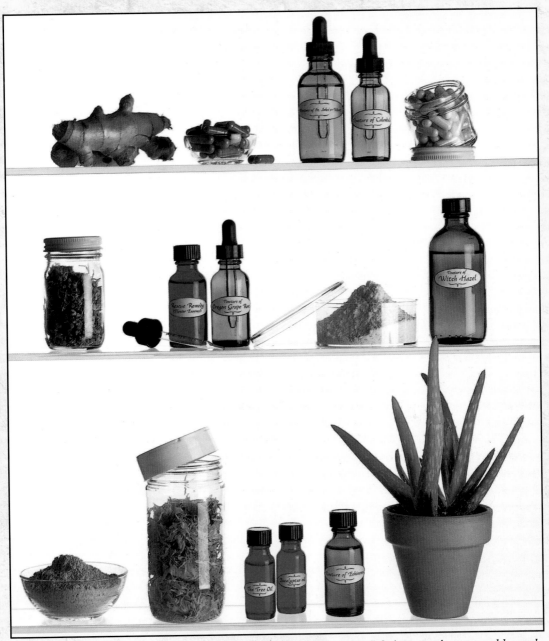

From top left: Gingerroot, ginger capsules, calendula tincture, St.-John's-wort tincture, goldenseal capsules, chamomile flowers, Rescue Remedy, Oregon grape root tincture, bentonite clay, witch hazel, oatmeal and baking soda, calendula flowers, tea tree oil, eucalyptus oil, echinacea tincture, and aloe vera.

Herbal Wisdom
Medicines That Prevent Disease

"Preventive medicine is where herbal medicine makes its greatest contribution. There are no orthodox drugs available that prevent heart disease the way garlic or hawthorn can. There are no synthesized pharmaceuticals that can prevent the common cold the way echinacea or maitake can. These fascinating substances represent herbal medicine's unique contributions to the world of medicine and, indeed, the future of medicine in general. If you have appendicitis, take yourself to the emergency room. If you want to avoid getting appendicitis, investigate herbal medicine."

—*Douglas Schar, herbalist and author*

Benefit #4: Perfectly Suited to Women

Women are at the forefront of the herbal renaissance. They outnumber men in their use of plant remedies, visits to professional herbalists, and attendance at herb conferences and workshops. There are more women among the ranks of professional herbalists as well.

And it's no wonder: Herbalists say that plants seem to have an affinity for the female body, effectively correcting problems with a woman's reproductive system, supporting her emotions, and delighting her senses with skin- and hair-friendly botanicals like lavender and rose petals.

"The real connection for women and herbs is the cycles of life," Maier says. "Women go through many cycles as they mature, creating different needs for their bodies. Energy levels change, along with dreams, visions, and aspirations. Herbs are perfect for women's changing needs."

That means that herbs have the ability to meet a woman's physical needs by balancing hormones, relieving menstrual discomforts, maintaining the health of the breasts and reproductive system, and providing safe remedies for everyday discomforts during pregnancy, herbalists say. There's chasteberry to ease PMS. Cramp bark tea to relieve—what else?—menstrual cramps. False unicorn root to enhance fertility. Dang gui to diminish menopausal hot flashes. Cleavers and milk thistle to ease breast tenderness.

Herbs also may support women's emotional needs, an important benefit for those who find themselves stressed out or emotionally drained. Chamomile lessens anxiety. St.-John's-wort relieves mild depression. A cup of tea made with nettle, clover, blue violet, oatstraw, and raspberry gives a pleasant energy lift. Botanical remedies can also help support a woman during an emotional crisis and leave her stronger and healthier when the crisis passes, says Maier.

Herbs are not the right choice for all emotional problems, of course. But when they are, they may work with fewer side effects. Using them can be an elegant, nurturing experience: Taking the time to brew a cup of delicious herbal tea or snip a sprig of lavender can be calming in and of itself, she says.

Flowers, essential oils, and herbal scents can delight us and enhance our natural beauty, too. How about a yarrow and peppermint steam for oily skin? A lavender and jojoba-oil deep-conditioning treatment for oily hair? Or a horsetail and dill soak for dull, brittle nails? Homemade skin- and hair-care "potions" may soothe and beautify skin, hair, and nails—without stripping away your body's natural, protective moisture barrier or exposing skin to colorings, additives, or synthetic chemicals. Creating your own beauty products with luxurious oils and scented herbs is lots of fun, too.

"Women are the nurturers in our society. Often we give a lot, and we could use more nurturing ourselves," Maier says. "Herbs give us the nourishment we need. When women are working with herbs, there's this overall sense of peacefulness, relaxation, and reconnection."

Benefit #5: A Renewed Connection to Nature

For many women, life is a blur of technology, whirring at the speed of light. We rush from home to office, with stops at school, day care, and soccer practice. Day and night, life's basic needs depend on machines—cars and coffee makers, computers and microwave ovens, answering machines and electric toothbrushes. Our fast-paced, high-tech lives often leave little time or opportunity for walking barefoot on the grass, contemplating a growing garden or a patio flowerpot, or enjoying the sensual pleasures of the changing seasons—spring blossoms, summer thunderstorms, autumn leaves, a winter snowfall. Getting in touch with na-

ture happens in fleeting moments or on summer vacations.

"As we move more into the technological age, there's a tremendous longing in human beings to connect with nature," Gladstar notes. "It reminds us of what' is human about us."

Brewing a soothing cup of simple herbal tea and taking a moment to enjoy the variety of natural colors, textures, shapes, and tastes in the herbs and the finished product can be the first step on a journey closer to the natural world, Cabrera says. "It's not just the chemistry of the herbs that's healing," she says. "It's also having a relationship with nature again."

Many women herbalists say that they notice a change when the women they counsel begin using this earth medicine. "A woman can feel more rooted," says herbalist Amanda McQuade Crawford, a practicing herbalist in Ojai, California, professional member of the AHG, member of the NIMH, president of the American College of Integrative Medicine in Albuquerque, and author of *Herbal Remedies for Women*. "Drinking herb tea, or even taking an herbal extract, puts her in touch with the Earth where she belongs, an Earth that cares for her."

The result is physical *and* emotional healing. "Something shifts," Maier notes. "There's excitement. Joy. The first thing a lot of women say after adopting herbal medicine is, 'I can't wait to tell my daughter,' or 'I can't wait to tell my grandmother.'"

It only takes a moment to make this connection, Gladstar suggests. "If you hold your herbal remedy in your hands for just an instant and give thanks to the plants that are helping you and to the people who collected and prepared them, you will be involved with a deeper kind of healing," she says.

Herbs for Mind, Body, and Beauty

Think of herbs as the world's first holistic healing aids. There's a botanical remedy for nearly every health concern a woman could possibly face, from day-to-day health problems to minor first-aid emergencies, from skin- and hair-care needs to stress relief and emotional support.

This list is a brief overview of just some of the healing herbs from Mother Nature's vast pharmacy that are recommended by top herbalists and that you will find throughout this book.

Hair. Henna, lavender, lemongrass, rosemary, and sage.

Ear pain and headaches. Feverfew, mullein, and willow bark.

Complexion and lips. Burdock, calendula, elderflower, usnea, and yellow dock.

Mouth, teeth, and gums. Black tea, cardamom, cayenne, cloves, echinacea, fennel, goldenseal, mint, myrrh, and stevia.

Heart. Garlic, ginger, guggul, hawthorn, and onions.

Respiratory health. Echinacea, elderberry, elecampane, eucalyptus, eyebright, garlic, ginger, goldenseal, grindelia, horehound, horsetail, mullein, pleurisy root, and thyme.

Breasts. Blessed thistle, burdock, castor oil, dandelion, evening primrose oil, fennel, goat's-rue, and yellow dock.

Digestion. Chamomile, gentian, ginger, fennel, and peppermint.

Kidneys and urinary tract. Corn silk, cranberry, and dandelion leaf.

Reproductive and sexual health. Black cohosh, chasteberry, damiana, dang gui, false unicorn root, lady's-mantle, partridgeberry, red raspberry leaf, rose essential oil, and wild yam.

Joints. Agrimony, black cohosh, burdock, dandelion, ginger, St.-John's-wort, and sandalwood.

Muscles. Arnica, cramp bark, white willow bark, and witch hazel.

Varicose veins. Butcher's broom, hawthorn, and witch hazel.

Skin. Aloe, burdock, calendula, chamomile, *Coleus forskohlii*, comfrey, echinacea, St.-John's-wort, and sarsaparilla.

Whole-Body Health

Energy. Basil essential oil, birch essential oil, ginseng, lemon balm, mint, nettle, and oatstraw.

Immunity. Astragalus, reishi mushrooms, and Siberian ginseng.

Stress, memory, and emotions. Chamomile, ginkgo, kava-kava, lemon balm, passionflower, St.-John's-wort, skullcap, and valerian.

Weight control. Cayenne, green tea, schisandra, and seaweed.

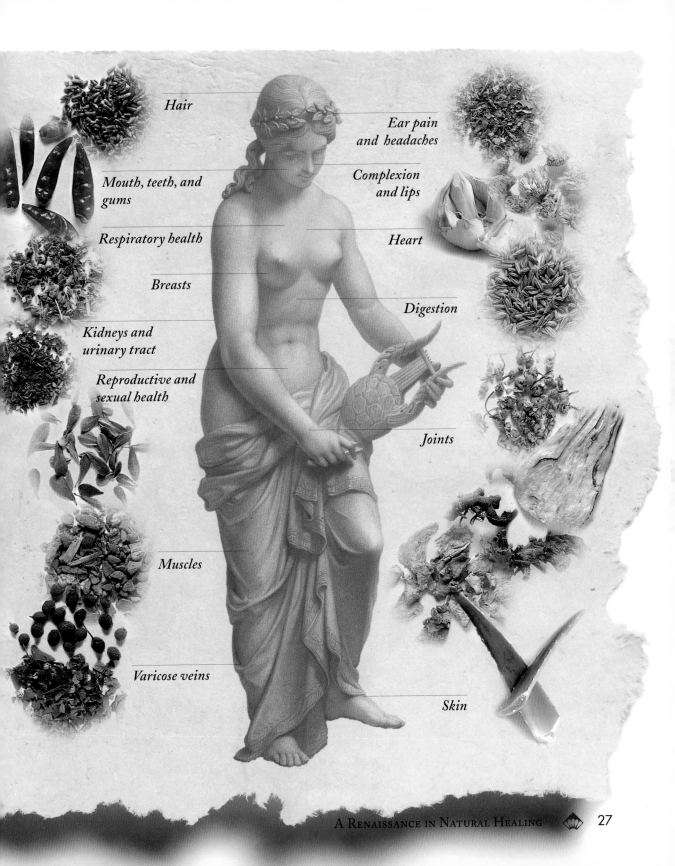

Hair

Ear pain
and headaches

Mouth, teeth, and
gums

Complexion
and lips

Respiratory health

Heart

Breasts

Digestion

Kidneys and
urinary tract

Reproductive and
sexual health

Joints

Muscles

Varicose veins

Skin

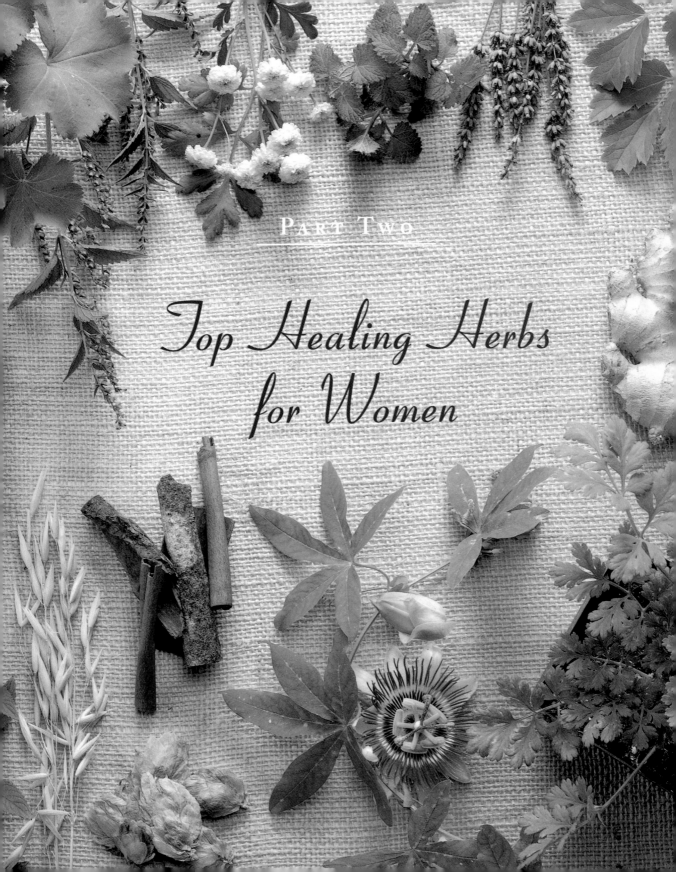

PART TWO

Top Healing Herbs
for Women

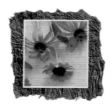

The Beauty, Tradition, and Science of 50 Nurturing Botanicals

knowledgeable herbalist may draw on 1,000 to 2,000 healing plants in nature's pharmacy. A health food store or pharmacy may stock dozens upon dozens of herbal products. But how many herbs does a woman need for physical and emotional well-being? These 50 safe, easy-to-find herbs are considered by top American and British practitioners to be among the best choices for problems that concern women the most, from PMS to menopause, indigestion to colds and flu, and first-aid to beauty. So they're a great place to begin your journey into the ancient and nurturing world of botanical home remedies.

A Field Guide to the Herbs

We wish that we could take you on a guided tour of the forests, fields, riverbanks, and gardens around the world where these important healing herbs thrive. As living plants, these healing botanicals have a natural beauty and unique personalities that are captured in colorful botanical portraits throughout this section. As you read each herb's profile, note the shape of its leaves, the graceful curve of its stem, or the color of its flowers. Herbal healers say that experiencing the beauty and living presence of plants can be an important part of the healing process, reconnecting us with the natural world and rekindling feelings of awe and serenity that feed the soul. We hope that the illustrations will inspire you to go out and get acquainted with healing herbs growing in your own lawn or garden or a nearby field.

In this section, you'll also learn what makes each herb valuable and unique. Each profile highlights useful information about the herb.

Botanical name and other common names. Herbs have many names. Black cohosh, for example—a menstrual pain reliever—gets its best-known common name from a Native American word for its knobby, rough roots. But it is also known as black snakeroot and even bugbane. Botanists, meanwhile, refer to black cohosh by its Latin name, *Cimicifuga racemosa.*

Knowing a plant's Latin name is important to help ensure that you gather or purchase the right herbal remedy, because it's the name by which it will be known no matter where you are. An herb's common name can vary from region to region or from country to country, making it hard to be sure what you're using.

These scientific-sounding, two-part Latin names reveal fascinating clues to the herbs' role in history and medicine. The species name *officinalis* or *officinale,* for example, indicates herbs that have long been recognized and used by healers.

History and traditional uses. In this section, you'll discover how people throughout history—from the ancient Greeks to Native Americans, from Europeans of the Renaissance to early twentieth-century practitioners—used each herb, tracing the link between ancient healing arts and the ways women use herbal remedies today.

Healing potential. Natural healers have known how to use beneficial herbs for thousands of years, but science is just beginning to explain *why* these ancient healing herbs work. You'll be intrigued to read about the collage of chemical compounds that may be responsible for an herb's healing potential—compounds such as chamazulene, a substance found in chamomile blossoms that may relieve stomach pain, and gingerols and shogaols found in ginger that may be responsible for this spicy root's anti-nausea actions.

Use information. Herbs come in a number of forms, and herbalists often recommend particular forms for specific conditions. You'll learn what's available and how different types of herbs and herbal products are commonly used.

Safety. Herbs are real medicine, so they need to be used wisely. How much is safe to take? Can they interact with medications? (Details on the use of herbs during pregnancy and other safety issues also appear elsewhere in the book.)

Purchasing and growing information. Like vitamins, some herbs are more widely available than others. And like vegetables, they grow better in certain circumstances than in others. So you'll find tips on where to buy herbs and herbal products as well as seeds or seedlings.

Parts used. Often, a plant's medicinal powers are concentrated in a particular part or in several different parts. Close-up photographs help you identify which part or parts of a particular herb are used, such as flowers, leaves, stalks, seeds, roots, or even bark.

Savvy herb users know which part of the plant is used medicinally. If you're trying to combat menstrual irregularities, for example, you'll use chasteberry berries, not leaves. Chasteberry leaves are fit for the compost pile, whereas the berries work on the hormonal system.

Use these handy profiles to get acquainted with herbs before you explore their use. And refer to them often to refamiliarize yourself with the herb's potential benefits.

Aloe

Aloe barbadensis
ALSO KNOWN AS ALOES; ALOE VERA

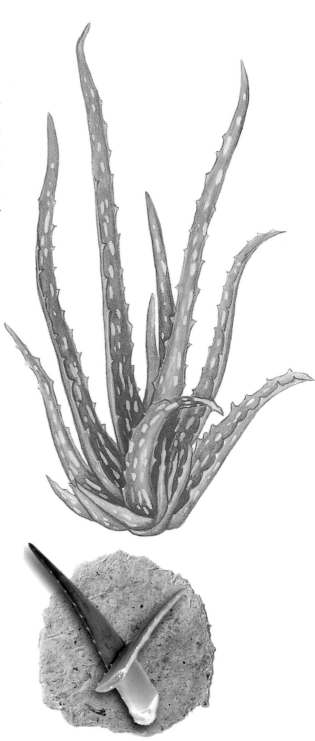

HISTORY AND TRADITIONAL USES   The spiky, spiny aloe plant was hailed as a skin soother by ancient Egyptian medics, and in its native Africa, aloe was the treatment of choice for wounds from poisoned arrows. Today, aloe is one of the most widely used herbs for skin problems, and it is found in a dizzying array of cosmetics and hair-care and first-aid products.

HEALING POTENTIAL   The transparent gel that oozes out of a broken aloe leaf is effective first-aid treatment for skin irritations, cuts, and minor burns: Studies show that it enhances wound healing and promotes cell growth and attachment. Other studies point to aloe's potential as a treatment for psoriasis and frostbite.

USING ALOE   For minor skin rashes, scrapes, cuts, or burns, herbalists suggest cutting off a lower leaf near the center stalk and removing any spines, then splitting the leaf in half and scraping the gel that oozes out directly onto your wound. Experts say that because aloe's healing power may be lost when the plant is processed, aloe gel fresh from the plant is a better bet than first-aid products containing aloe.

SAFETY   Aloe leaves also produce a bitter latex that, when dried and taken internally, is a potent, potentially toxic laxative. Because ingesting aloe leaf can cause intense cramping, experts advise against internal use. Also, don't apply aloe vera gel to abdominal incisions after a cesarean delivery or laparotomy, as it could delay healing.

PURCHASING AND GROWING ALOE   You can buy aloe anywhere houseplants are sold, including supermarkets. Aloe likes lots of sun and a minimum temperature of 41°F. A hardy houseplant, it isn't too picky about soil, doesn't need much water, and requires little care. To propagate, separate and repot the rooted suckers at the plant's base.

PART USED   Fresh gel from leaves.

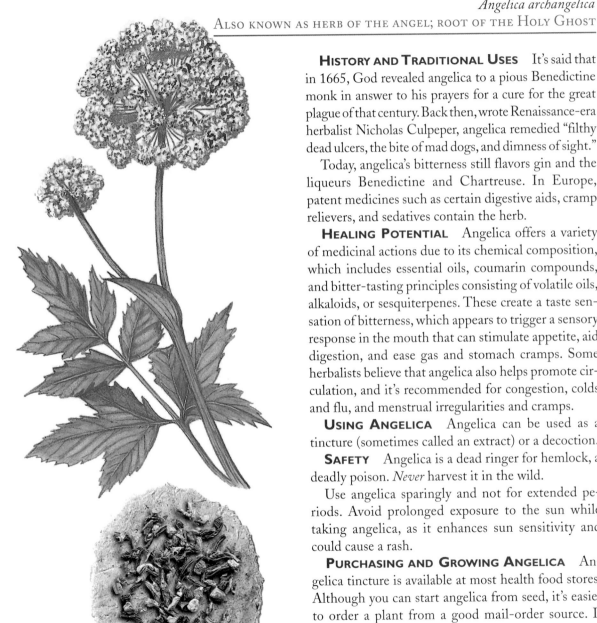

Angelica

Angelica archangelica

HISTORY AND TRADITIONAL USES   It's said that in 1665, God revealed angelica to a pious Benedictine monk in answer to his prayers for a cure for the great plague of that century. Back then, wrote Renaissance-era herbalist Nicholas Culpeper, angelica remedied "filthy dead ulcers, the bite of mad dogs, and dimness of sight."

Today, angelica's bitterness still flavors gin and the liqueurs Benedictine and Chartreuse. In Europe, patent medicines such as certain digestive aids, cramp relievers, and sedatives contain the herb.

HEALING POTENTIAL   Angelica offers a variety of medicinal actions due to its chemical composition, which includes essential oils, coumarin compounds, and bitter-tasting principles consisting of volatile oils, alkaloids, or sesquiterpenes. These create a taste sensation of bitterness, which appears to trigger a sensory response in the mouth that can stimulate appetite, aid digestion, and ease gas and stomach cramps. Some herbalists believe that angelica also helps promote circulation, and it's recommended for congestion, colds and flu, and menstrual irregularities and cramps.

USING ANGELICA   Angelica can be used as a tincture (sometimes called an extract) or a decoction.

SAFETY   Angelica is a dead ringer for hemlock, a deadly poison. *Never* harvest it in the wild.

Use angelica sparingly and not for extended periods. Avoid prolonged exposure to the sun while taking angelica, as it enhances sun sensitivity and could cause a rash.

PURCHASING AND GROWING ANGELICA   Angelica tincture is available at most health food stores. Although you can start angelica from seed, it's easier to order a plant from a good mail-order source. It thrives in deep, moist loam, likes partial shade, and grows to eight feet tall.

PARTS USED   Leaves and root.

Astragalus

Astragalus membranaceous
ALSO KNOWN AS HUANG QI

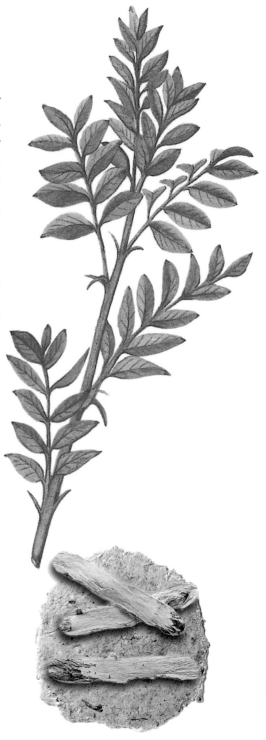

HISTORY AND TRADITIONAL USES Two thousand years ago, astragalus was listed in *Shen Nung's Herbal* as a tonic. Healers believed then, as they do today, that astragalus increases the body's resistance to disease.

Practitioners of Traditional Chinese Medicine often combine astragalus with other herbs because astragalus is believed to help promote their healing power. One of the most popular traditional Chinese tonics, which is still used today, was created in the thirteenth century during the Yuan Dynasty. Simply called Ginseng and Astragalus Combination (Chinese name: *Buzhong Yiqi Tang*), this tonic also contains licorice, ginger, black cohosh, and other Chinese herbs. It reportedly increases strength and endurance.

HEALING POTENTIAL Evidence indicates that astragalus works in the bone marrow to produce white blood cells and helps the body produce antibodies and interferon, which means that it enhances immune function. For people who are debilitated, stressed out, and seem to catch every cold or virus that comes along, top herbal healers frequently recommend astragalus.

Astragalus is high in polysaccharides, large molecules composed of chains of sugar subunits. Although scientists aren't quite sure why, they believe that polysaccharides have significant anti-cancer action.

USING ASTRAGALUS Because astragalus takes several weeks to establish activity in the body, herbal healers recommend using it for periods of from three months to two years.

SAFETY Astragalus is generally regarded as safe.

PURCHASING AND GROWING ASTRAGALUS
You'll find astragalus tinctures, tonics, and capsules in health food stores. This herb is tricky to grow without expert advice.

PART USED Root.

Black Cohosh

Cimicifuga racemosa

ALSO KNOWN AS BLACK SNAKEROOT; BUGBANE; RATTLEROOT

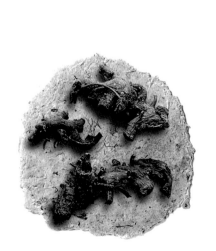

HISTORY AND TRADITIONAL USES   The name of this herb, which was introduced to early settlers by Native Americans, comes from the Algonquin word *cohosh*, meaning "knobby, rough roots." Native American women traditionally relied on black cohosh for "women's diseases."

By the 1800s, herbal healers became convinced that black cohosh was a panacea and used it to treat everything from snakebite to smallpox to hypochondria. By 1912, black cohosh was one of the medicinal herbs most frequently prescribed by American physicians.

HEALING POTENTIAL   Black cohosh supplies estrogenic sterols and glycosides (chemicals that help the body produce and use a variety of hormones) and a host of micronutrients. According to Commission E, the expert panel that judges the safety and effectiveness of herbal medicines for the German government, black cohosh is effective for treating PMS, painful menstruation, and problems associated with menopause. In fact, studies indicate that it can be as effective as hormone replacement therapy for relieving hot flashes and other menopausal difficulties.

USING BLACK COHOSH   Black cohosh can be taken in the form of a decoction or a tincture (sometimes called an extract) or in capsules.

SAFETY   Commission E recommends that black cohosh not be used for more than six months. Do not use this herb if you suspect that you are pregnant, because it stimulates the uterus and can cause premature contractions. Do not use while nursing.

PURCHASING AND GROWING BLACK COHOSH The dried herb as well as the handsome plant can be purchased through mail-order sources. Black cohosh is easy to grow in rich, moist soil in light shade.

PART USED   Rhizome.

Black Haw

Viburnum prunifolium
ALSO KNOWN AS STAG BUSH; SWEET VIBURNUM

HISTORY AND TRADITIONAL USES   Black haw's reputation as an herbal aid for preventing miscarriage goes back to the time of early Native Americans and pioneers.

Black haw comes from the bark of a decorative shrub that is native to North America. It is a kissing cousin to cramp bark (*V. opulus*), which has similar healing properties.

HEALING POTENTIAL   Black haw bark contains salicin, the compound that is responsible for aspirin's pain-relieving and anti-inflammatory abilities. Other chemical components of this herb include scopoletin, which is known as a powerful uterine relaxant, and valerianic acid, which is a sedating substance.

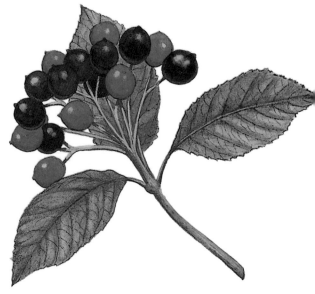

Herbalists believe that because of these active ingredients, black haw relieves menstrual cramps, helps normalize irregular uterine contractions during labor, and eases bleeding after childbirth. Finally, black haw is rich in steroidal saponins, steroidlike compounds that supposedly serve as raw material for the production of hormones by the liver. Herbalists say that these components make black haw very useful for easing menopausal symptoms.

USING BLACK HAW   Black haw bark can be boiled down, or decocted, into a hot drink or taken in the form of a tincture (sometimes called an extract).

SAFETY   Because black haw contains oxalates, which can cause kidney stones, individuals with a history of kidney stones should consult a physician before using this herb.

PURCHASING BLACK HAW   Dried black haw bark can be purchased from mail-order sources. Tinctures are available at health food stores.

PART USED   Bark.

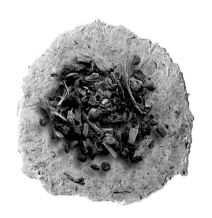

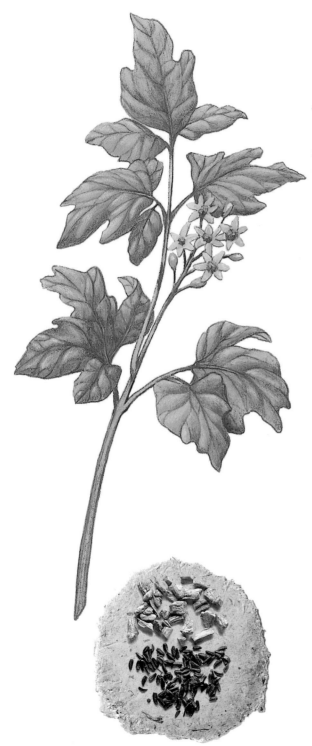

Blue Cohosh

Caulophyllum thalictroides
ALSO KNOWN AS PAPOOSE ROOT

HISTORY AND TRADITIONAL USES Sometimes referred to as woman's best friend, blue cohosh is one of the oldest known American herbal remedies. First introduced as medicine in 1828, it was renowned primarily for its powerful ability to promote menstruation and labor.

Native Americans used blue cohosh for everything from hiccups to hysterics. Its nickname, papoose root, speaks to its reputation as a Native American labor-inducing herb. In 1852, blue cohosh was included as an official drug in the *American Dispensatory*, an early remedy reference for physicians. Soon afterward, demand for its healing powers began to build. The Eclectics—American physicians in the mid-1800s to early 1900s who combined herbal remedies with mainstream medicine—used blue cohosh as a tonic during the last several weeks of pregnancy, especially for "delicate" women and those who had long, painful labors. Their experience showed that the herb would—in their words— "facilitate labor and relieve much suffering."

HEALING POTENTIAL Blue cohosh contains the chemical caulosaponin, which actively stimulates uterine contractions and promotes blood flow to the pelvic region. Leading herbalists consider blue cohosh among the best uterine and menstrual stimulants available and agree on its use for helping to ease and speed labor or relieve menstrual cramps.

USING BLUE COHOSH Blue cohosh can be taken as a decoction or a tincture (sometimes called an extract) or in capsules.

SAFETY Because it can cause uterine contractions, do not use this herb during pregnancy. The berries are poisonous.

PURCHASING BLUE COHOSH Tinctures, teas, and capsules are sold in health food stores.

PARTS USED Root and rhizome.

Burdock

Arctium lappa

ALSO KNOWN AS BEGGAR'S-BUTTONS; CLOTBUR; FOX'S CLOTE

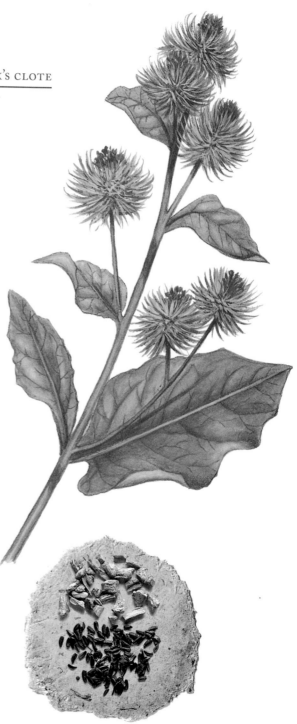

HISTORY AND TRADITIONAL USES   Despite its utterly weedy appearance and fierce, tenacious burrs, burdock is a nutritious, deliciously edible plant—and it boasts a convincing, 3,000-year-old reputation for purifying the blood and boosting immunity.

Traditionally, herbalists used burdock for burns, kidney problems, rheumatism, and lung infections. And should someone be unlucky enough to be bitten by "serpents or mad dogs," burdock root worked wonderfully, wrote seventeenth-century herbalist Nicholas Culpeper.

HEALING POTENTIAL   Among its active ingredients, burdock root contains inulin, an immune-system booster with anti-diabetic properties.

In Traditional Chinese Medicine, burdock is called *niu bang*. Chinese researchers report it to be effective against inflammation, tumors, and bacterial and fungal infections.

Burdock's diuretic and mild laxative properties may help to remove toxins from the system. Reputable herbal experts say that skin problems such as psoriasis, eczema, acne, and others all can be treated effectively with burdock.

USING BURDOCK   Burdock is used in the form of a tea or tincture (sometimes called an extract), both made from dried burdock root, or taken in capsules. The Japanese call the root *gobo* and cook with it frequently; its flavor fuses those of celery and potato. Burdock's tender leaves can be served raw, steamed, or sautéed. Peel the tender stalks and eat them raw or cook them like asparagus.

SAFETY   Burdock is generally regarded as safe.

PURCHASING BURDOCK   Dried burdock root, seeds, tincture, tea, and capsules are available at health food stores or through mail order.

PARTS USED   Leaves, root, and seeds.

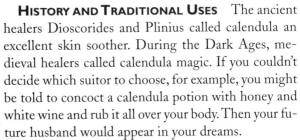

Calendula

Calendula officinalis

ALSO KNOWN AS POT MARIGOLD; MARYBUD; GOLD-BLOOM

HISTORY AND TRADITIONAL USES The ancient healers Dioscorides and Plinius called calendula an excellent skin soother. During the Dark Ages, medieval healers called calendula magic. If you couldn't decide which suitor to choose, for example, you might be told to concoct a calendula potion with honey and white wine and rub it all over your body. Then your future husband would appear in your dreams.

HEALING POTENTIAL Calendula is related to burdock and chamomile, herbs that are also used by herbalists for their skin-soothing properties. Among calendula's chemical ingredients are factors that reduce inflammation and combat infection from bacterial, fungal, and viral sources. In addition, factors in calendula actually help the skin knit itself back together after a wound. In Germany, calendula is specifically recommended for treating hard-to-heal wounds, leg ulcers, and mouth and throat irritations.

Russian research indicates that tincture of calendula may have promise as a treatment for herpes simplex outbreaks and certain flu viruses. It may even have promise as a cancer fighter—specifically, skin cancer. Research suggests that the plant stimulates the immune system and shows anti-cancer properties.

USING CALENDULA Calendula is made into teas, creams, ointments, infusions, and tinctures (sometimes called extracts). It's most effective to make a cream that combines both infused calendula and tinctured calendula.

SAFETY Calendula is generally regarded as safe.

PURCHASING AND GROWING CALENDULA Calendula teas, tinctures, and skin-care products are sold in health food stores. Seeds and dried calendula blossoms are available by mail order. Calendula likes well-drained soil and full sun.

PARTS USED Flowers.

Cayenne

Capsicum annuum; C. frutescens

ALSO KNOWN AS TABASCO PEPPER; CHILI PEPPER; HOT PEPPER

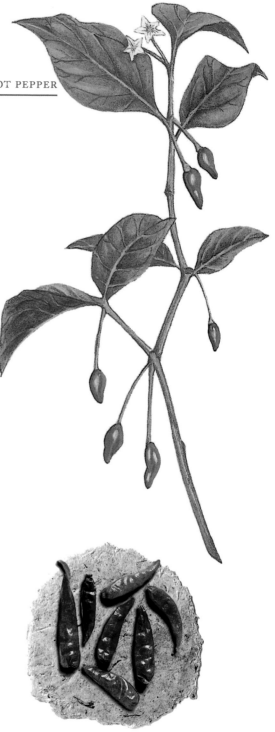

HISTORY AND TRADITIONAL USES   Cayenne, or capsicum, comes from the Greek *kopto*, meaning "I bite." Bite into a hot pepper, and you'll know in a flash how powerfully stimulating this herb can be.

In sixteenth-century England, cayenne was noted as a remedy for what was then known as king's evil, an infection of the lymph nodes in the neck. And later, among American herbalists, cayenne was an herb of choice for treating everything from cold feet to dropsy (fluid accumulation) to rheumatism.

HEALING POTENTIAL   Cayenne contains vitamins A and C along with the alkaloid capsaicin. Considered a powerful stimulant and irritant, capsaicin produces an intense burning sensation when it touches the mouth, eyes, or tender skin. The sensation signals the brain to secrete endorphins, feel-good substances that block pain, induce well-being, and sometimes create euphoria.

Evidence shows that creams containing capsaicin effectively relieve a variety of painful conditions, including shingles, post-mastectomy pain, nerve pain caused by diabetes, and even cluster headaches.

Added to food, cayenne perks up appetite, improves digestion, and relieves gas, nausea, and indigestion. The herb thins phlegm and eases its passage from the lungs, thus helping to prevent and treat coughs, colds, and bronchitis.

USING CAYENNE   Medicinally, cayenne is used as a tincture (or extract), an infusion, or capsules.

SAFETY   Wear plastic or latex gloves when you chop hot peppers, and avoid touching your eyes or nose.

PURCHASING CAYENNE   Capsaicin creams are sold in drugstores without a prescription, and cayenne capsules and tincture are available at health food stores.

PARTS USED   Pods (seeds removed)

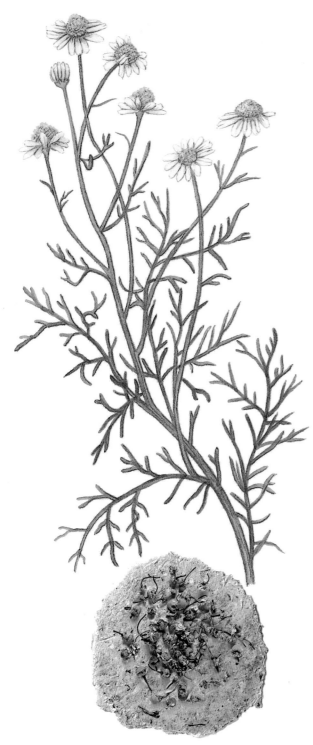

Chamomile

Matricaria recutita

ALSO KNOWN AS GERMAN CHAMOMILE

HISTORY AND TRADITIONAL USES　It counter-acts irritation. It soothes troubled tummies. It protects against ulcers. It eases muscle spasms. Time and time again, its action against bacterial and fungal infections has been shown in the laboratory. It's German chamomile, and it's been healing humans for more than 2,000 years.

In nineteenth-century America, German chamo-mile was recommended for painful and sluggish men-struation, especially when accompanied by "nervous or hysterical" symptoms.

HEALING POTENTIAL　A member of the daisy family, German chamomile is related to calendula, echinacea, and blessed thistle. The herb contains a complex collage of chemicals that work individually and collectively on the body. To soothe an irritated stomach, for example, one chemical, A-bisabolol, speeds the mending of torn tissue to heal any ulcera-tion. Another, chamazulene, shrinks the swollen stomach tissue that creates pressure on nerve endings to cause pain. Yet another, azulene, kills staphylo-coccus and streptococcus infections, preventing or curtailing bouts of food poisoning or intestinal flu.

USING CHAMOMILE　German chamomile is usu-ally taken as a tea. (Don't confuse German chamomile with Roman chamomile, which is used in shampoos and cosmetics.)

SAFETY　People with allergies to closely related plants like ragweed, asters, and chrysanthemums could be allergic to chamomile, too.

PURCHASING AND GROWING CHAMOMILE Look for whole dried flowers, not powdered or pul-verized chamomile. You can grow this fragrant, daisy-like annual from seeds or seedlings in full sun to partial shade and in sandy, dry, well-drained soil.

PARTS USED　Flowers.

Chasteberry

Vitex agnus-castus
ALSO KNOWN AS VITEX; MONK'S PEPPER

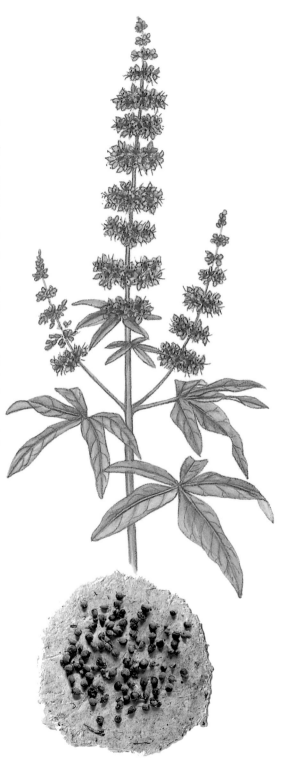

HISTORY AND TRADITIONAL USES Ancient Athenian women used chasteberry to quell sexual passion and sacrificed it to the goddess Ceres as a symbol of chastity. The medieval herbalist Gerard called chasteberry the perfect herb for celibates. In nineteenth-century France, chasteberry syrup was given to "suppress the desires of Venus." Its Latin name means pure, innocent, or chaste.

Modern herbalists don't buy the notion that chasteberry dampens a woman's desire; some say, in fact, that it might have precisely the opposite effect.

HEALING POTENTIAL Chasteberry has been studied extensively, and it appears to work by evening out hormone imbalances that occur during the menstrual cycle. Specifically, it influences the pituitary gland to stem secretion of the hormone prolactin. When prolactin is reduced, an irregular menstrual cycle usually normalizes. This makes chasteberry useful for women who, month after month, experience premenstrual syndrome, menstrual cramps, and menstrual irregularities.

During menopause, chasteberry is recommended for flooding, spotting, severe hot flashes, and dizziness. Acne caused by menopausal changes might also be relieved with chasteberry.

USING CHASTEBERRY Chasteberry is taken as a tea or tincture (sometimes called an extract). This is a slow-acting herb, so take it regularly for months or more to reap its benefits.

SAFETY Chasteberry may counteract the effectiveness of birth control pills.

PURCHASING AND GROWING CHASTEBERRY Health food stores sell dried whole chasteberries, tea, and tinctures. You can buy this handsome perennial bush by mail order. Plant it in a sunny spot.

PARTS USED Berries.

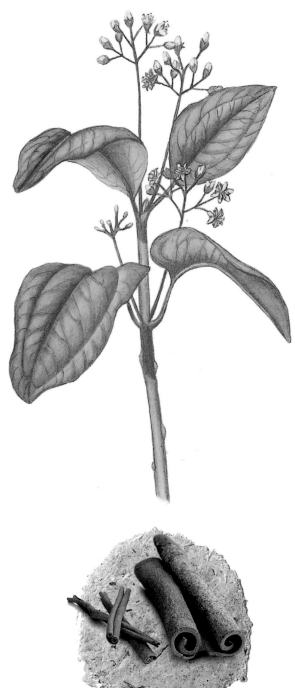

Cinnamon

Cinnamomum zeylanicum
<small>No other common names</small>

HISTORY AND TRADITIONAL USES Cinnamon was once deemed as rare as frankincense and as costly as gold, and the desire for it made it a hot commodity among ancient spice traders.

For the Chinese, cinnamon is a native herb, cultivated from the bark of a small evergreen tree, that has been used medicinally for 4,700 years. Today, it is still one of the most commonly used herbs in Chinese herbal remedies. Chinese healers believe that the daily use of cinnamon makes one look and feel younger. They also use cinnamon to reduce fevers, and in folk medicine, it was used to combat infection.

HEALING POTENTIAL Cinnamon bark contains an oily chemical called cinnamaldehyde that kills a variety of illness-causing bacteria, including the dreaded *Escherichia coli*, *Salmonella*, and *Staphylococcus aureus*. Research shows that cinnamon is able to stop the growth of these and several other types of bacteria, as well as the Asian flu virus.

Herbalists report that cinnamon bark also helps regulate the menstrual cycle and checks flooding during menopause. And cinnamaldehyde has a tranquilizing effect that helps reduce anxiety and stress. Finally, in China, researchers have discovered that cinnamon tea stops attacks of bronchial asthma.

USING CINNAMON Cinnamon is used as a tea or tincture (sometimes called an extract) or can be sprinkled directly on food. Cinnamon sticks can be chewed.

SAFETY Do not use cinnamon in medicinal amounts during pregnancy.

PURCHASING CINNAMON Ground cinnamon and cinnamon sticks are sold at supermarkets everywhere, and cinnamon tincture is available at health food stores.

PART USED Bark.

<small>The Beauty, Tradition, and Science of 50 Nurturing Botanicals</small> <small>43</small>

Coltsfoot

Tussilago farfara

ALSO KNOWN AS COUGHWORT; HORSE-HOOF; FOAL-FOOT

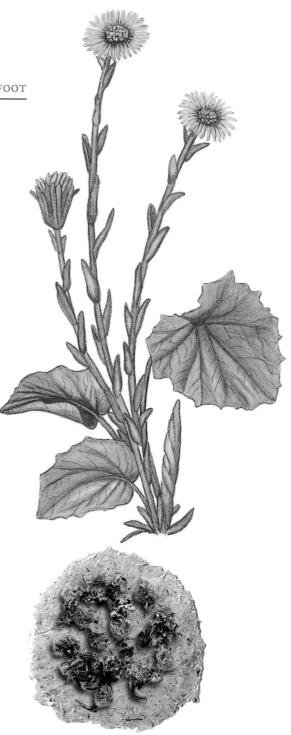

HISTORY AND TRADITIONAL USES   Its botanical name, *Tussilago*, means "to chase coughing fits" in Latin. "The smoke of this plant is said to cure an inveterate cough," wrote the Roman naturalist Pliny in the first century A.D. Centuries later, British herbalists were still insisting that smoking coltsfoot would relieve coughs, and the herb was even nicknamed British tobacco.

HEALING POTENTIAL   Although the notion of therapeutic smoking strains modern-day credulity, traditional healers were right about one thing. As a tea or tincture, coltsfoot is a recommended cough remedy, particularly for chronic problems like emphysema. The herb contains the soothing substance mucilage; flavonoids, plant pigments that provide healthy benefits; and zinc, a trace mineral that is essential to fast healing.

Another component, tussilagone, has been tested on dogs and found to ease breathing difficulty. Working in concert, it appears that coltsfoot's constituents reduce inflammation and respiratory distress.

USING COLTSFOOT   Coltsfoot is used in tea or as a tincture (sometimes called an extract).

SAFETY   Women should avoid coltsfoot during pregnancy and while nursing unless guided by a qualified health-care practitioner, and coltsfoot should not be used long-term except under supervised care.

PURCHASING AND GROWING COLTSFOOT
Coltsfoot tincture and tea can be found in health food stores, and the dried herb is available through mail-order sources. You can also buy coltsfoot plants by mail, but beware: This hardy herb with a daisylike flower can overrun your garden. Confine it to naturalistic settings.

PARTS USED   Flowers and leaves.

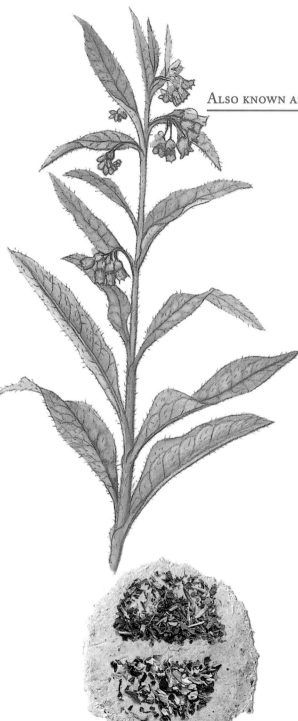

Comfrey
Symphytum officinale

HISTORY AND TRADITIONAL USES Comfrey means "to grow together" in Latin and Greek, and for good reason—this herb has been healing wounds since at least the first century B.C. The Greek physician Dioscorides praised comfrey's wound-healing powers in the first superstition-free medicinal herbal. Seventeenth-century healers called on comfrey to mend broken bones and to remedy back pain for men who overindulged in the pleasures of the flesh. Later, comfrey was used for a variety of problems, from coughs and congestion to diarrhea and dysentery.

HEALING POTENTIAL Comfrey contains allantoin, a medicinal ingredient that reduces inflammation and, according to herbalists, stimulates the immune system and eases asthma, ulcers, and lung ailments. Other ingredients include rosmarinic acid, an inflammation reducer; mucilage, which protects and soothes irritated tissue; and tannins, which kill bacteria.

However, comfrey also contains pyrrolizidine alkaloids, compounds that may cause liver damage and cancer, according to long-term studies in rats. German scientific literature concludes that taking comfrey for respiratory problems, gastrointestinal disorders, arthritis, or gout isn't worth the potential risk. So in Germany, the herb is recommended for external use only for bruises, sprains, and dislocations.

USING COMFREY Comfrey is primarily used externally in ointments, poultices, or compresses.

SAFETY Use dried comfrey only; avoid fresh, young leaves. Do not use during pregnancy. If you take comfrey internally, do not use it for extended periods.

PURCHASING COMFREY Dried comfrey, seeds, and plants are available through mail-order sources, and comfrey tincture and other preparations are sold in health food stores.

PARTS USED Leaves and root.

Cramp Bark

Viburnum opulus

ALSO KNOWN AS GUELDER ROSE; HIGH CRANBERRY; RED, ROSE, OR WATER ELDER

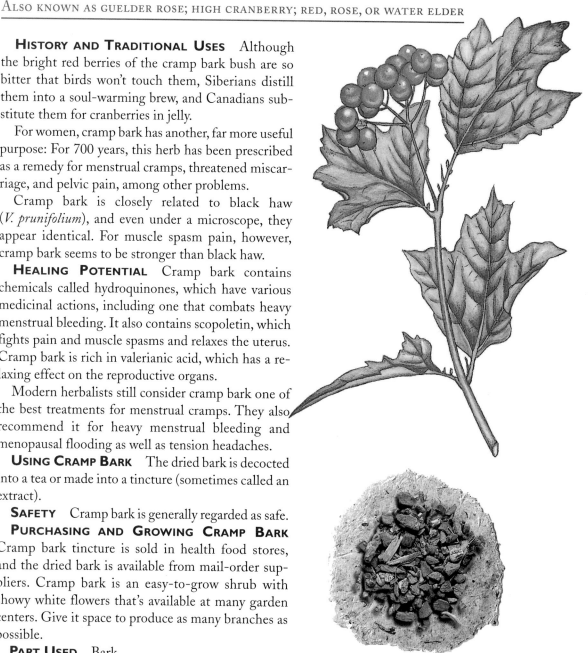

HISTORY AND TRADITIONAL USES Although the bright red berries of the cramp bark bush are so bitter that birds won't touch them, Siberians distill them into a soul-warming brew, and Canadians substitute them for cranberries in jelly.

For women, cramp bark has another, far more useful purpose: For 700 years, this herb has been prescribed as a remedy for menstrual cramps, threatened miscarriage, and pelvic pain, among other problems.

Cramp bark is closely related to black haw (*V. prunifolium*), and even under a microscope, they appear identical. For muscle spasm pain, however, cramp bark seems to be stronger than black haw.

HEALING POTENTIAL Cramp bark contains chemicals called hydroquinones, which have various medicinal actions, including one that combats heavy menstrual bleeding. It also contains scopoletin, which fights pain and muscle spasms and relaxes the uterus. Cramp bark is rich in valerianic acid, which has a relaxing effect on the reproductive organs.

Modern herbalists still consider cramp bark one of the best treatments for menstrual cramps. They also recommend it for heavy menstrual bleeding and menopausal flooding as well as tension headaches.

USING CRAMP BARK The dried bark is decocted into a tea or made into a tincture (sometimes called an extract).

SAFETY Cramp bark is generally regarded as safe.

PURCHASING AND GROWING CRAMP BARK Cramp bark tincture is sold in health food stores, and the dried bark is available from mail-order suppliers. Cramp bark is an easy-to-grow shrub with showy white flowers that's available at many garden centers. Give it space to produce as many branches as possible.

PART USED Bark.

Dandelion

Taraxacum officinale

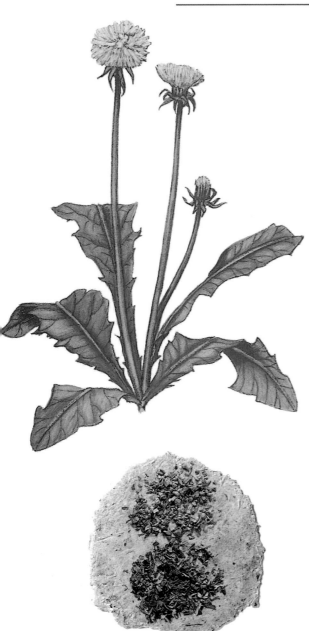

HISTORY AND TRADITIONAL USES Dandelion probably originated in ancient Greece, and its botanical name comes from the Greek words for "disorder" and "remedy." Its tiny, parachute-tufted seeds have helped dandelion blow itself to the four corners of the globe, and wherever it lands, people usually eat it or make it into medicine (or both).

In China, dandelion has been used to treat breast cancer for more than a thousand years. Today, doctors add dandelion to a Chinese herb formula for people with AIDS. In Costa Rica, the herb is sold as a diabetes remedy.

HEALING POTENTIAL Dandelion contains chemicals called eudesmanolides, which are found in no other herb. Other components include sterols, flavonoids, and mucilage. As a result, dandelion stimulates the flow of bile, a fluid that aids fat digestion, which is why it's used for liver and gallbladder disorders. Dandelion is also recommended for digestive complaints, specifically for the incomplete digestion of fat.

USING DANDELION Add tender young dandelion leaves to your salads. To remove the bitter taste from older leaves, steam them. Dried dandelion root and leaves are used for tea, but you can also take a dandelion tincture (sometimes called an extract) or capsules.

SAFETY Do not take dandelion root if you have gallbladder disease.

PURCHASING AND GROWING DANDELION Dried leaves, tinctures, and capsules of dandelion are available in health food stores. Dried dandelion root is available by mail order. Before harvesting dandelion from your lawn, make sure that the ground is insecticide- and herbicide-free.

PARTS USED Leaves and root.

Dang Gui

Angelica sinensis

ALSO KNOWN AS DONG QUAI

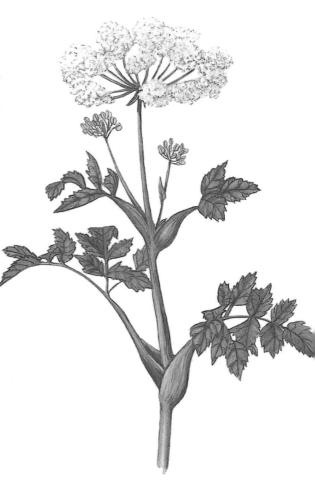

HISTORY AND TRADITIONAL USES One of the first Chinese drugs mentioned in ancient medical books, dang gui dates back to 400 B.C. and is the most popular of all Chinese herbs, especially for women.

In Traditional Chinese Medicine, doctors treat allergies, arthritis, nervousness, and high blood pressure with dang gui, and they believe the herb has the power to prevent cancer. Because it's also believed that dang gui helps a woman retain her youthful glow long past her youth, dang gui is an ingredient in Chinese beauty creams.

Angelica (*A. archangelica*) is dang gui's Euro-American cousin (see page 33).

HEALING POTENTIAL Dang gui contains vitamins B_{12} and E and other active components, including ferulic acid, which eases menstrual cramps, muscle spasms, and other types of pain. Its B_{12} content, along with folate and biotin, stimulates the formation and development of red blood cells in the bone marrow, effectively remedying a type of anemia that commonly accompanies menstrual problems.

Herbalists report that dang gui regulates menstruation, eases cramps, relaxes the uterus, clears up psoriasis and eczema, reduces hot flashes, and eases vaginal dryness.

USING DANG GUI Dang gui root can be taken in the form of tea or a tincture (sometimes called an extract) or in capsules. Herbalists recommend that you stop taking this herb one week before your menstrual period and resume at the end of your period.

SAFETY Do not use this herb if you are pregnant.

PURCHASING DANG GUI Dang gui is best purchased, not grown. The root is available from mail-order sources; capsules and tinctures are available at health food stores.

PART USED Root.

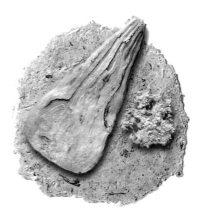

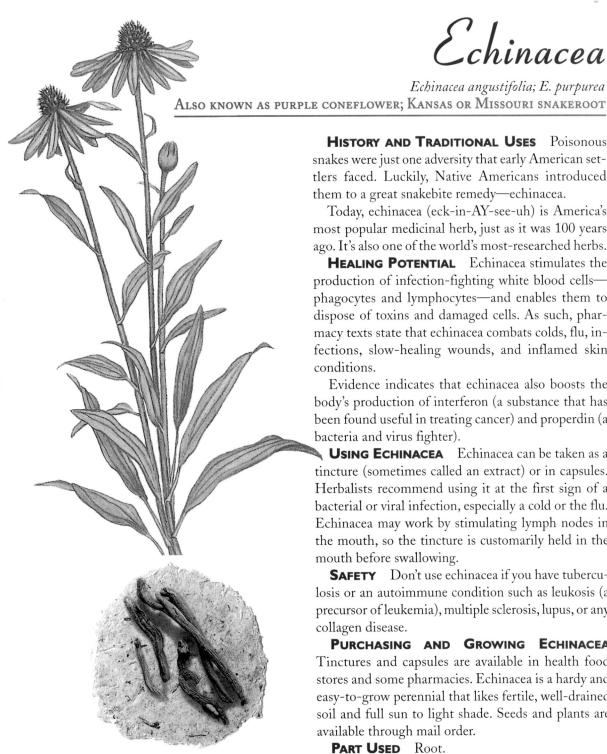

Echinacea

Echinacea angustifolia; E. purpurea

ALSO KNOWN AS PURPLE CONEFLOWER; KANSAS OR MISSOURI SNAKEROOT

HISTORY AND TRADITIONAL USES Poisonous snakes were just one adversity that early American settlers faced. Luckily, Native Americans introduced them to a great snakebite remedy—echinacea.

Today, echinacea (eck-in-AY-see-uh) is America's most popular medicinal herb, just as it was 100 years ago. It's also one of the world's most-researched herbs.

HEALING POTENTIAL Echinacea stimulates the production of infection-fighting white blood cells—phagocytes and lymphocytes—and enables them to dispose of toxins and damaged cells. As such, pharmacy texts state that echinacea combats colds, flu, infections, slow-healing wounds, and inflamed skin conditions.

Evidence indicates that echinacea also boosts the body's production of interferon (a substance that has been found useful in treating cancer) and properdin (a bacteria and virus fighter).

USING ECHINACEA Echinacea can be taken as a tincture (sometimes called an extract) or in capsules. Herbalists recommend using it at the first sign of a bacterial or viral infection, especially a cold or the flu. Echinacea may work by stimulating lymph nodes in the mouth, so the tincture is customarily held in the mouth before swallowing.

SAFETY Don't use echinacea if you have tuberculosis or an autoimmune condition such as leukosis (a precursor of leukemia), multiple sclerosis, lupus, or any collagen disease.

PURCHASING AND GROWING ECHINACEA Tinctures and capsules are available in health food stores and some pharmacies. Echinacea is a hardy and easy-to-grow perennial that likes fertile, well-drained soil and full sun to light shade. Seeds and plants are available through mail order.

PART USED Root.

Eucalyptus

Eucalyptus globulus
ALSO KNOWN AS BLUE GUM; FEVER TREE

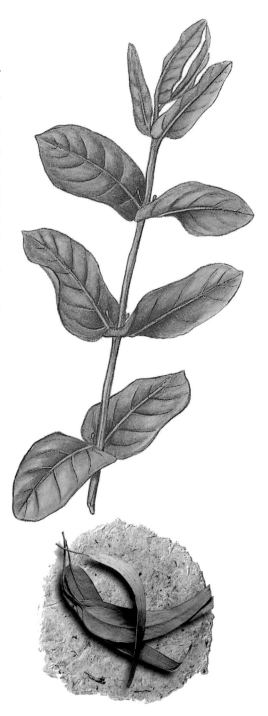

HISTORY AND TRADITIONAL USES   Without eucalyptus trees, Australia would be a pretty barren continent with little greenery, since eucalyptus covers more than three-quarters of the place. Its roots store water, a boon to thirsty aborigines and early Australian settlers. In America, the Eclectic physicians, who practiced a combination of conventional and herbal medicine from the mid-1800s to the mid-1900s, used eucalyptus to ease respiratory infections—a treatment that is still used today.

HEALING POTENTIAL   The key to eucalyptus's healing power is a chemical called cineole, or eucalyptol. Evidence shows that it may relieve nasal and bronchial congestion, ease sore throats and coughs, and fight infection. Eucalyptus tea is especially good for bronchitis and throat inflammations. As the tea is sipped, its aromatic oils are excreted through the lungs, where they act as an expectorant to help loosen and eject mucus. The oils also act as an antiseptic to fight infection. In addition, eucalyptus leaf tea contains tannins, which help relieve throat inflammation.

USING EUCALYPTUS   Eucalyptus leaves can be brewed into a tea. Essential oil of eucalyptus is a common ingredient in cough drops, nasal inhalers and sprays, sore-muscle rubs, and other preparations.

SAFETY   Too much eucalyptus may cause nausea, vomiting, and diarrhea. Don't use this herb if you have inflammatory disease of the bile ducts (such as gallbladder disease) or severe liver disease. Do not use eucalyptus preparations on areas of the face—especially the nose—in infants and young children.

PURCHASING EUCALYPTUS   Eucalyptus leaves are available by mail order and at some health food stores. To be effective, the leaves must contain 70 to 85 percent cineole (eucalyptol).

PARTS USED   Leaves.

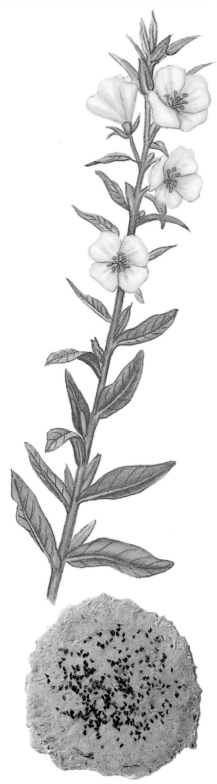

Evening Primrose

Oenothera biennis

ALSO KNOWN AS TREE PRIMROSE; SCABBISH; CURE-ALL

HISTORY AND TRADITIONAL USES Evening primrose has a long history as a wild edible plant and has served as food and medicine for Native Americans and Europeans. The Cherokee drank evening primrose tea as a slimming tonic and used the hot root externally as a hemorrhoid remedy. For the Iroquois, evening primrose also served as a hemorrhoid remedy. At the turn of the century, it was occasionally used for digestive problems and frequent urination.

HEALING POTENTIAL Today, the oil extracted from evening primrose seeds is recommended by mainstream physicians and herbalists alike for easing a variety of problems, some specific to women.

Evening primrose oil is rich in essential fatty acids (EFAs), including gamma-linolenic acid. EFAs are substances that help the body produce prostaglandins, which in turn can lower blood pressure, regulate stomach acids and body temperature, and control inflammation. They also stimulate uterine contractions and regulate the effects of sex hormones. Women who don't have enough EFAs can suffer menstrual cramps, breast tenderness, and symptoms of premenstrual syndrome.

Evening primrose oil helps mitigate menopausal problems and may be recommended for chronic inflammatory conditions, including eczema, hay fever, asthma, and arthritis. In Britain, herbal practitioners use evening primrose oil for multiple sclerosis and other autoimmune diseases.

USING EVENING PRIMROSE The oil is usually taken in capsule form.

SAFETY Evening primrose is generally regarded as safe.

PURCHASING EVENING PRIMROSE Evening primrose oil capsules are sold in health food stores.

PART USED Oil from seeds.

Fennel

Foeniculum vulgare
ALSO KNOWN AS SWEET FENNEL

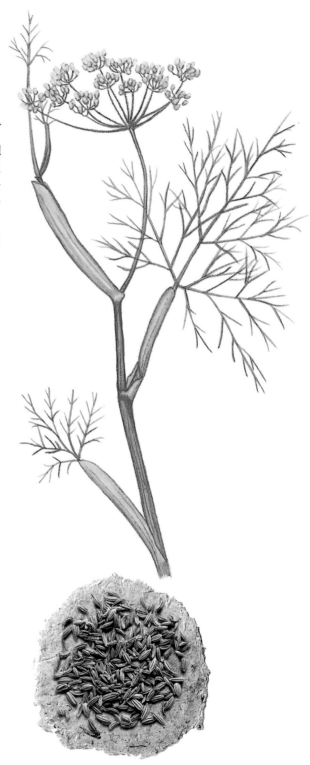

HISTORY AND TRADITIONAL USES   Long loved for their culinary as well as their medicinal uses, fennel seeds taste faintly of licorice and are used to flavor pickles, liqueurs, breads, and candies. Fennel stems or bulbs are often used in salads or cooked as a vegetable.

Roman physicians reportedly relieved everything from lethargy to frenzy with fennel, and in modern China, a poultice of powdered fennel seeds is said to speedily heal snakebites. In African countries, fennel tincture serves as a remedy for cramps, diarrhea, and stomachaches, and Jamaicans use it to relieve colds.

Sixteenth-century herbalists used fennel to increase a nursing mother's milk—a use still favored today.

HEALING POTENTIAL   Rich in volatile oils, fennel is what's known as a carminative herb, meaning that it has soothing activity in the large and small intestines that eases gas and gas pains. According to experts, one of fennel's volatile oils, anethole, has specific properties that increase breast milk production, stimulate appetite and digestion, and combat infection.

USING FENNEL   Fennel seeds can be brewed into a tea or added to foods. Fennel tincture (or extract) and capsules are also used.

SAFETY   Fennel stimulates the uterus, so avoid it during pregnancy unless directed otherwise by a qualified health-care practitioner. Commission E, the expert panel that judges the safety and effectiveness of herbal medicines for the German government, advises that fennel not be used for a prolonged time without direction from a qualified herbalist.

PURCHASING AND GROWING FENNEL   Fennel tincture, tea, and capsules are available in health food stores. You can grow fennel from seeds or buy plants from a nursery. Plant in humus-rich soil in full sun.

PARTS USED   Seeds and fresh stems and bulbs.

Feverfew

Chrysanthemum parthenium; Tanacetum parthenium
ALSO KNOWN AS FEATHERFEW; FLIRTWORT; VETTER-VOO

HISTORY AND TRADITIONAL USES Use of feverfew reaches back to the ancient Greeks, but it was seventeenth-century herbalist Nicholas Culpeper who wrote that "it is very effectual for pains in the head." Although he published his book, *Culpeper's Complete Herbal*, 400 years ago, he knew then what science knows now: Feverfew is a good herb for bad headaches.

HEALING POTENTIAL The active constituent of feverfew is parthenolide, which may inhibit the release of serotonin from blood platelets. Serotonin is a hormone that helps to constrict blood vessels, and that action could potentially stop a throbbing vascular headache—like a migraine—in its tracks.

British medical journals have spotlighted feverfew as a treatment for migraine headaches and possibly arthritis, and studies support its benefits. Scientists theorize that its active constituents may inhibit inflammation-inducing prostaglandins and histamines.

USING FEVERFEW In feverfew, parthenolide levels can vary from product to product. In order to be effective, a commercial product must contain at least 0.2 percent parthenolide. (British feverfew has the highest parthenolide content.) Fresh feverfew leaves can be chewed, added to salads, or infused into vinegar or oil and used daily to prevent migraines. Feverfew can also be brewed into tea or taken freeze-dried in capsules.

SAFETY Feverfew can cause mouth sores in sensitive people. Also, it stimulates the uterus, so don't use it during pregnancy unless it's specifically recommended by a qualified health-care practitioner.

PURCHASING FEVERFEW Teas and capsules are available at health food stores. Feverfew seeds and plants are available by mail order.

PARTS USED Leaves.

Garlic

Allium sativum

ALSO KNOWN AS STINKING ROSE

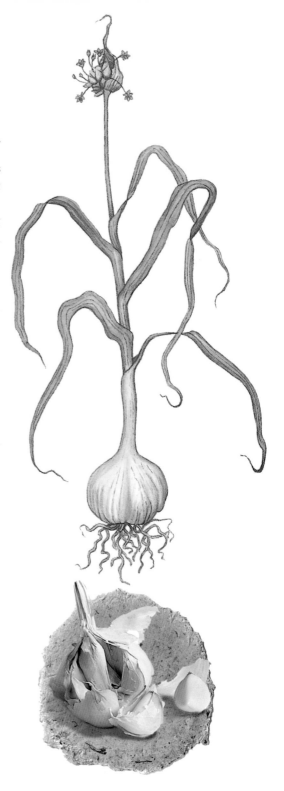

HISTORY AND TRADITIONAL USES Garlic has had more folklore and scientific research devoted to it than any other herb. This humble little gray bulb was, and still is, used globally by all three classic healing systems—Traditional Chinese Medicine, traditional European medicine, and Ayurveda. As far back as the first century B.C., the Greek physician Dioscorides stated that garlic "clears the arteries and opens the mouths of the veins"—a fact that science affirmed nearly a thousand years later.

HEALING POTENTIAL Intact garlic cloves contain an odorless, sulfur-containing amino acid called alliin. When the garlic is crushed, alliin becomes allicin, a potent but unstable antibiotic that produces garlic's famous pungent taste and smell. Allicin, research shows, helps lower cholesterol and blood pressure and helps prevent blood clots. Eating fresh, raw garlic or taking certain dried garlic preparations can reduce the risk of developing atherosclerosis (hardening of the arteries) and other risk factors for coronary disease.

Research indicates that garlic is effective against bacterial and fungal infections, digestive ailments, and high blood pressure. What's more, studies suggest that this familiar food may even help prevent cancer.

USING GARLIC When garlic is cooked, the odor diminishes because allicin is unstable, so cooked garlic may not contain much. When garlic is eaten raw, however, allicin is quickly released in the mouth during chewing and is converted in the stomach to other active compounds. So to get garlic's full healing power, experts urge that you eat it raw.

SAFETY Avoid using fresh garlic while nursing, as it may give the baby gas or indigestion.

PARTS USED Cloves.

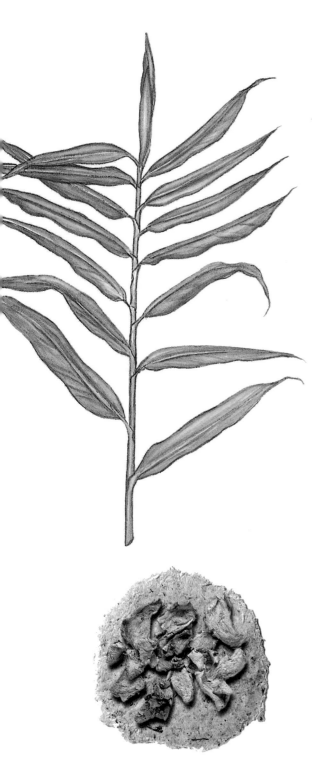

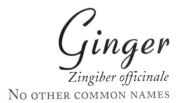

Ginger

Zingiber officinale

NO OTHER COMMON NAMES

HISTORY AND TRADITIONAL USES According to an ancient Indian proverb, "Every good quality is contained in ginger." Immortalized in the *Pen Tsao Ching* (*The Classic Book of Herbs*), which was penned in 3,000 B.C. by Emperor Shen Nung, ginger is one of the most widely used medicinal herbs in China today. And Chinese cooks use fresh ginger in most of their meals to prevent indigestion.

HEALING POTENTIAL When it comes to quelling the queasiness of motion sickness, ginger has no equal, say herbalists. In fact, researchers have demonstrated that ginger beats dimenhydrinate, the main ingredient in motion sickness drugs like Dramamine, for controlling symptoms of seasickness and motion sickness.

Ginger contains various essential oils—the exact composition depends on where the plant was grown. Two types of substances—gingerols and shogaols—are considered responsible for ginger's effectiveness as an anti-nausea remedy. Ginger stimulates saliva flow and digestive activity, settles the stomach, relieves vomiting, and eases pain from gas and diarrhea.

Herbalists also use ginger to remedy painful ovulation and relieve menstrual cramps.

USING GINGER Ginger can be used fresh or dried, but the fresh root tastes best. Keep it refrigerated. Grate some into tea or add it to other recipes. Sucking on candied ginger can relieve motion or morning sickness, experts say. You can also take it in capsule form.

SAFETY Do not use dried gingerroot during pregnancy, although fresh ginger and the powdered spice are fine. Because ginger may increase bile secretion, anyone with gallstones should consult a qualified health-care practitioner before using the dried root.

PART USED Root.

Ginkgo

Ginkgo biloba

ALSO KNOWN AS MAIDENHAIR TREE

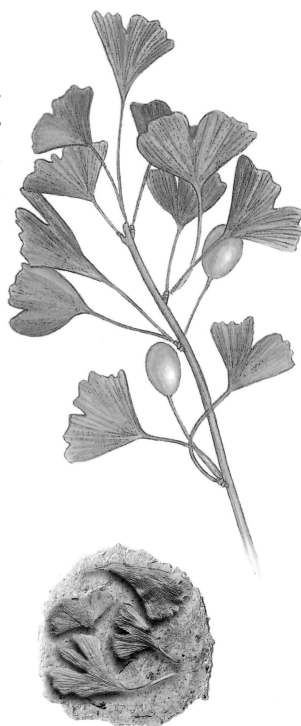

HISTORY AND TRADITIONAL USES Ginkgo trees were often planted in Japanese temple gardens. And in Asian healing traditions, ginkgo nuts have an ancient reputation for strengthening the kidneys, lungs, and digestive system and for restoring vitality to people recovering from long illnesses.

HEALING POTENTIAL Today, standardized extracts of ginkgo leaves have been shown to sharpen memory, boost concentration, reduce anxiety, lessen the distressing symptoms of Alzheimer's disease, and improve a host of circulation problems, making this herb a best-seller in Europe. Herbalists call ginkgo the perfect remedy for aging because it profoundly benefits organs that are usually diminished by time: the eyes, brain, blood vessels, and cardiovascular system.

Herbalists believe that ginkgo gently dilates blood vessels, improving circulation in the arteries, veins, and tiny capillaries. Laboratory research indicates that ginkgo lowers blood pressure and sends more blood to the brain and to the body's extremities. As a result, say proponents, forgetfulness fades, mood improves, and walking is easier for people with circulation problems in their legs.

USING GINKGO Researchers studying the benefits of ginkgo use concentrated leaf extracts containing standardized amounts of a substance called ginkgolide. Quantities in commercial products may vary, so effectiveness can vary from brand to brand. Some herbalists say tinctures (liquid extracts) made from whole ginkgo leaves can also be beneficial but work more slowly than concentrated extracts.

SAFETY Taking too much concentrated ginkgo extract (more than 240 milligrams) can cause dermatitis, diarrhea, and vomiting. The usual dose is 120 milligrams a day.

PARTS USED Leaves.

Ginseng

Panax ginseng (Korean ginseng); P. quinquefolium (American ginseng)
ALSO KNOWN AS SANG; ROOT OF LIFE; A DOSE OF IMMORTALITY

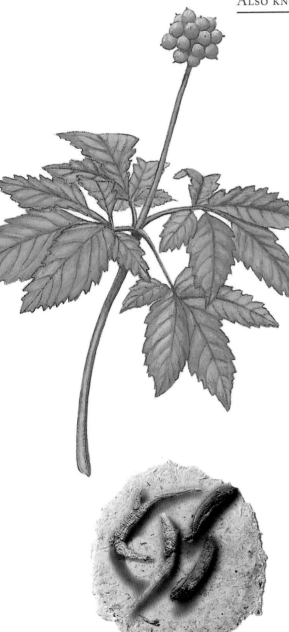

HISTORY AND TRADITIONAL USES   Ginseng has enjoyed a near-mythical reputation for thousands of years. This sweet and faintly aromatic root occupied a place of honor in China's 2,000-year-old medical manual, *The Herbal Classic of the Divine Plowman*. Today, ginseng is still widely used by Asians to rejuvenate, increase sexual desire, and ease difficult childbirth, among other uses.

Native Americans relied on American ginseng for menstrual problems, headaches, exhaustion, fever, colic, vomiting, and earaches. Growing in popularity in both the United States and China is Siberian ginseng, which is not a true form of ginseng but the root of a plant called *Eleutherococcus senticosus* that shares certain properties with true ginseng.

HEALING POTENTIAL   Ginseng root contains a banquet of active ingredients, including at least 18 different hormonelike saponins called ginsenosides that botanists say fight stress and fatigue, protect the liver, and guard against memory loss. Proponents say this herb can be of special help to women by easing exhaustion during childbirth and relieving stress-related hot flashes at menopause.

USING GINSENG   The root can be chewed or made into a tea. Ginseng is also taken in the form of capsules, tablets, and liquid extracts.

SAFETY   To avoid irritability, avoid consuming caffeine and other stimulants while using ginseng.

PURCHASING GINSENG   Figuring out exactly what quantity of ginsenosides an American or Korean product contains can be tricky, since the amount is given in percentages, not total weight, and the product may contain other ingredients in addition to ginseng. Read the label carefully and do the math, or call the manufacturer.

PART USED   Root.

Goldenseal

Hydrastis canadensis

ALSO KNOWN AS YELLOW ROOT; ORANGE ROOT; JAUNDICE ROOT; EYE BALM

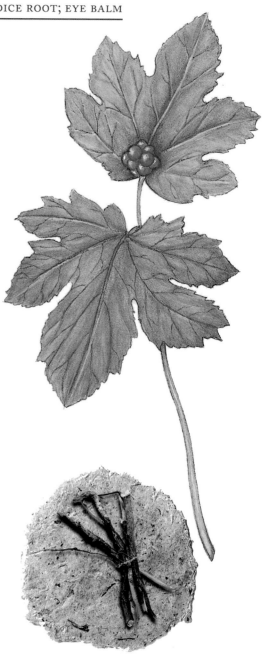

HISTORY AND TRADITIONAL USES Once abundant in North America's shady woodlands, goldenseal's wrinkled, chrome yellow root was a well-known Native American remedy. The Cherokee used it to soothe inflammation and stimulate appetite. The Iroquois washed sore eyes with goldenseal, and the Micmac applied the herb to chapped lips. Eagerly adopted by white settlers in the 1700s, goldenseal quickly became popular in Europe, too. In the nineteenth and twentieth centuries, America's Eclectics prescribed it for digestive and respiratory problems.

HEALING POTENTIAL Goldenseal root contains two alkaloids, hydrastine and berberine, both of which are potent natural antibiotics, inflammation fighters, uterine tonics, and digestive aids. Today, herbalists call on goldenseal to alleviate sinus infections, colds and flu, laryngitis, sore throats, earaches, gastritis, and colitis. Used in the form of a douche, goldenseal is considered by herbalists to be a remedy for vaginal infections.

USING GOLDENSEAL This herb may be used in various ways—as a tea or tincture (sometimes called an extract), in capsules, as an eyewash or gargle, in eardrops, as a douche, or as a disinfectant salve.

SAFETY Avoid goldenseal during pregnancy. Because it stimulates the involuntary muscles of the uterus, it can cause premature contractions.

PURCHASING GOLDENSEAL Look for vivid yellow teas, tinctures, or capsules. If the product looks green, it may contain inactive goldenseal leaf powder. This plant is threatened in the wild, so buy only cultivated goldenseal. If you don't find this information on the label, ask your supplier to contact the manufacturer. Cultivated goldenseal root and seeds for planting are available by mail order.

PART USED Root.

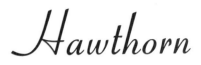

Hawthorn

Crataegus oxycantha; C. laevigata; C. monogyna
ALSO KNOWN AS MAY BLOSSOM; WHITETHORN; HAW

HISTORY AND TRADITIONAL USES   Popular as a quick-growing hedge and ornamental shrub in old England, hawthorn was once known to herbalists simply as a remedy for weak stomachs and edema (swelling). By 1922, herbal doctors began prescribing hawthorn for problems such as cardiac weakness, pain, and palpitations (irregular heartbeat).

HEALING POTENTIAL   Today, herbalists recommend the leaves, white flowers, and red berries of hawthorn without hesitation for long-term cardiovascular improvements. Research shows that when taken for at least six months, this mild herb dilates arteries and as a result, can lower high blood pressure. It also promotes blood circulation, improving poor circulation to the legs and lifting the confusion and forgetfulness that come with inadequate blood supply to the brain. Herbal practice holds that hawthorn also brings more much-needed oxygen to the heart muscle, calms a rapid heartbeat, or normalizes a weak, slow one.

USING HAWTHORN   Hawthorn is often taken as a tea. The leaves and flowers are brewed in just-boiled water, the berries are simmered, or all three are steeped together for up to 30 minutes. Hawthorn may also be prescribed as a tincture (sometimes called an extract).

SAFETY   Have your doctor monitor your heart health if you take hawthorn regularly for more than a few weeks—you may need lower doses of other medicines that you may be taking, such as drugs for high blood pressure. If you have low blood pressure caused by problems with heart valves, don't use hawthorn without a physician's guidance.

PURCHASING HAWTHORN   Hawthorn tea is available at health food stores. Tincture is available by mail order.

PARTS USED   Berries, flowers, and leaves.

Hops

Humulus lupulus
NO OTHER COMMON NAMES

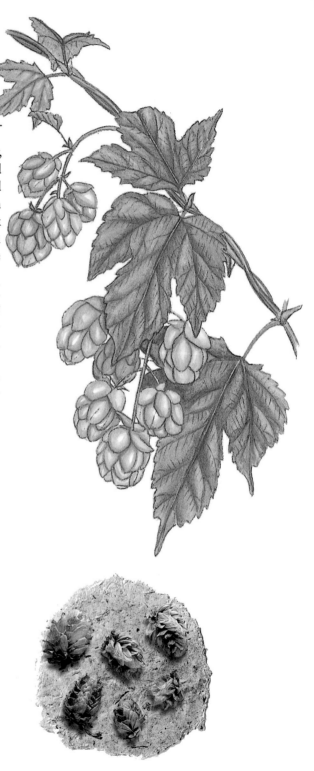

HISTORY AND TRADITIONAL USES Papery, greenish yellow female hops flowers were prescribed in seventeenth-century England to aid digestion and relieve other everyday ailments. In the 1600s, British apothecary Thomas Culpeper noted that a drink made from the seeds started delayed menstruation, an action that hinted at the herb's mildly estrogen-like effect.

In 1787, physicians for mad King George III stuffed the herb into a pillow to promote sleep for their royal patient. Later, hops pillows were recommended as mild sedatives and remedies for insomnia by America's Eclectic doctors.

HEALING POTENTIAL Hidden inside the ripe conelike fruits, or strobiles, of the female hops plant are tiny yellow grains called lupulin that contain the active substances beta-humulene, beta-myrcene, beta-caryophyllene, and farnescene. They help the body secrete bile and digestive juices. These chemicals may also be responsible for as-yet-unexplained sedative powers. Some herbalists believe that hops' antispasmodic action also makes it a good choice for easing stress-related digestion problems, irritable bowel syndrome, and peptic ulcers. And the estrogenic powers of fresh hops make it a good remedy at menopause. Women herbalists recommend it to encourage milk flow in nursing mothers.

USING HOPS The herb is usually taken as a tea or tincture (sometimes called an extract) or in capsules. Hops is also used in baths and in "dream pillows" to induce sleep.

SAFETY Handle hops carefully, as the pollen can cause a skin rash. Avoid using hops during the first trimester of pregnancy and limit to occasional use in the second trimester to avoid the risk of miscarriage.

PART USED Fruit of female plants.

Lady's-Mantle

Alchemilla vulgaris

HISTORY AND TRADITIONAL USES With its gray-green leaves and lacy blooms, lady's-mantle has a long history of use as a "woman's herb" in Europe, where more than 300 different species grow. The plant may have first been associated with women because the leaves resemble a woman's old-fashioned cloak.

In any case, as early as the 1600s, lady's-mantle was used as an aid to conception, a miscarriage preventive, and—of all things—a folk remedy for sagging breasts. The herb was also used to heal wounds and stop excess bleeding, vomiting, and diarrhea—uses that continue to this day.

HEALING POTENTIAL Evidence suggests that tannins in the leaves and flowers make lady's-mantle an effective, astringent remedy for closing and healing wounds and, when taken internally, for bleeding and diarrhea. In its review of scientific literature on lady's-mantle, Commission E, the expert panel that judges the safety and effectiveness of herbal medicines for the German government, recommended it for mild diarrhea that lasts only a few days.

Herbalists believe the astringent properties of lady's-mantle work internally, making it an excellent choice for normalizing heavy periods and bleeding due to fibroid tumors. Herbalists say that lady's-mantle also improves poor uterine tone, eases menopausal hot flashes, and soothes mild menstrual aches and pains. It may also be used during pregnancy to allay morning sickness.

USING LADY'S-MANTLE This herb is taken as a tea or tincture (sometimes called an extract). It's also sometimes applied externally as an herbal wash or poultice.

SAFETY Lady's-mantle is generally regarded as safe.

PARTS USED Leaves, stems, and flowers.

Lavender

Lavandula officinalis; L. angustifolia; L. vera

ALSO KNOWN AS TRUE LAVENDER; GARDEN LAVENDER

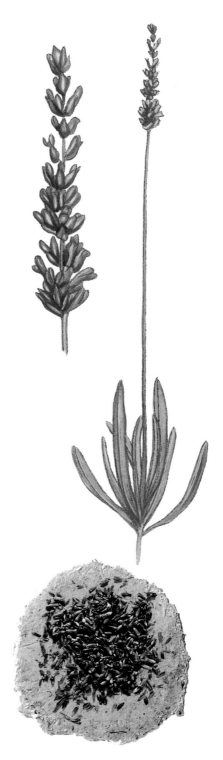

HISTORY AND TRADITIONAL USES Imported from Syria by the ancient Greeks for its fragrance, lavender's scent freshened rooms, perfumes, and baths—in fact, its botanical name, *Lavandula*, comes from the Latin *lavare*, meaning "to wash." As far back as the Middle Ages, this shrubby plant was used as a popular home remedy for stress, hysteria, menopausal problems, headaches, and even palsy, convulsions, and fainting. Even in modern times, lavender is an important ingredient in smelling salts. Traditionally, flatulence, spasms, colic, toothache, sprains, acne, and nausea have also been treated with lavender.

HEALING POTENTIAL Researchers have found that the fragrant, volatile oil in lavender blossoms, which contains more than 100 chemical compounds, does calm the central nervous system. Herbalists consider lavender—often combined with other herbs such as valerian, borage flowers, or lemon balm—a potent remedy for headaches, muscle spasms and cramps, depression, and digestive upsets.

USING LAVENDER Lavender is taken as a tea or tincture (sometimes called an extract) or used externally as an essential oil in baths, facial steams, and massage oils. In stark contrast to its lovely scent, the taste of lavender in tea has been described by herbalists as soapy. To disguise the taste, you may want to add honey to the tea.

SAFETY Lavender is generally regarded as safe.

PURCHASING AND GROWING LAVENDER Lavender tea and oil are sold at health food stores, and tinctures are available by mail order. In the garden, plant lavender in light, well-drained soil. While garden centers and catalogs sell various species, *L. angustifolia* is best for areas with cold, hard winters. Harvest buds when the flowers are about to open.

PARTS USED Flowers.

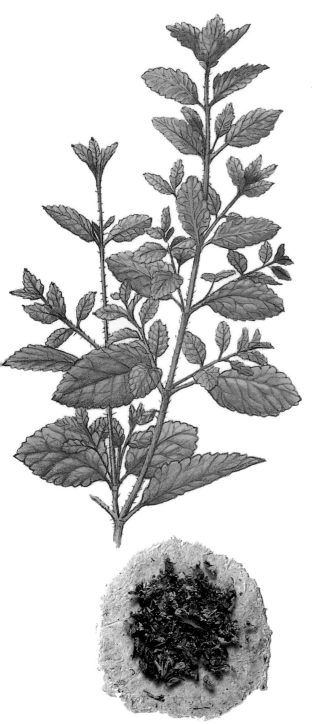

Lemon Balm

Melissa officinalis

HISTORY AND TRADITIONAL USES This nerve-soothing, stomach-settling herb may have originated in southern Europe or even Turkey. Experts can't be certain, because lemon balm now grows and is used in Asia, western Europe, North and South America, and the Middle East. More often a household remedy than a doctor's prescription in times past, lemon balm relieved "weak stomachs," took away "griping pains of the belly," and caused "the mind and heart to become merry," according to seventeenth-century English herbalist Nicholas Culpeper.

Lemon balm was sometimes used to ease the ache (and presumably the crying) of an infant's teething.

HEALING POTENTIAL Today, herbalists recommend the fuzzy, citrus-scented leaves of lemon balm to calm tension; raise the spirits; relieve depression, insomnia, nervousness, and tension headaches; and calm digestive problems, especially when stress is the cause. Research suggests that its antiviral properties help battle herpes outbreaks.

For women, herbalists say that lemon balm may relax uterine spasms that cause painful periods, ease morning sickness, and reduce tension during childbirth. As a tea mixed with nettle, it is said to be an effective aid to allergy relief during pregnancy, when stronger allergy medicines must be avoided. Lemon balm contains essential oils rich in terpenes, substances that are responsible, in part, for its antiviral action.

USING LEMON BALM This herb is usually taken as a tea or used in a calming bath.

SAFETY Lemon balm is generally regarded as safe.

PURCHASING LEMON BALM When buying dried lemon balm at your local health food store for tea, crush a leaf—the herb should smell like mint and lemon.

PARTS USED Leaves.

Licorice

Glycyrrhiza glabra
ALSO KNOWN AS SWEET WOOD

HISTORY AND TRADITIONAL USES   Licorice is a grand old herb. Favored in China for over 5,000 years, its intensely sweet, fibrous root is still prescribed by herbalists for respiratory and digestive problems, and it is frequently used to heighten the effects of other herbs. In seventeenth-century England, licorice was boiled with figs to quiet coughs and chest pains and steeped in teas to relieve constipation and fevers.

Licorice has been found in women's herbal formulas for hundreds of years, perhaps because it contains estrogen-like compounds.

HEALING POTENTIAL   Suck on a slice of dried licorice root, and your tastebuds will quickly encounter this plant's most active compound: glycyrrhizin, a saponin that's 50 times sweeter than sugar. Structured like your body's hormones, glycyrrhizin may have a mild estrogen-like effect, making it valuable for regulating hormones at menopause, according to herbalists and scientists. Researchers also have found that compounds in licorice have anti-inflammatory, anti-allergic, and anti-arthritic actions. It is also used to ease coughs, clear respiratory congestion, soothe the digestive system, and promote elimination.

USING LICORICE   It is usually taken as tea.

SAFETY   Do not use licorice daily for more than four to six weeks. Overuse can lead to water retention, high blood pressure caused by potassium loss, or impaired heart and kidney function. Use this herb with caution if you are at risk for high blood pressure or water retention, and avoid it during pregnancy and while nursing. Do not use licorice if you have been diagnosed with diabetes, high blood pressure, liver or kidney disorders, or low potassium levels.

PURCHASING LICORICE   Licorice root is available at health food stores.

PART USED   Root.

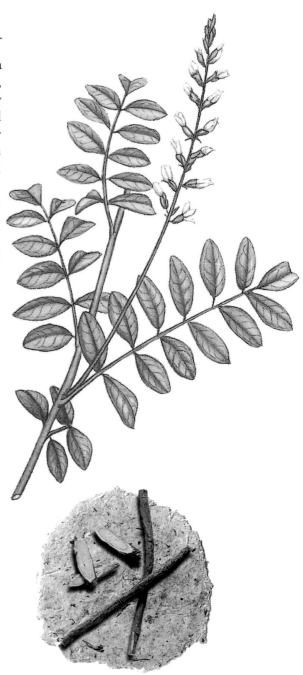

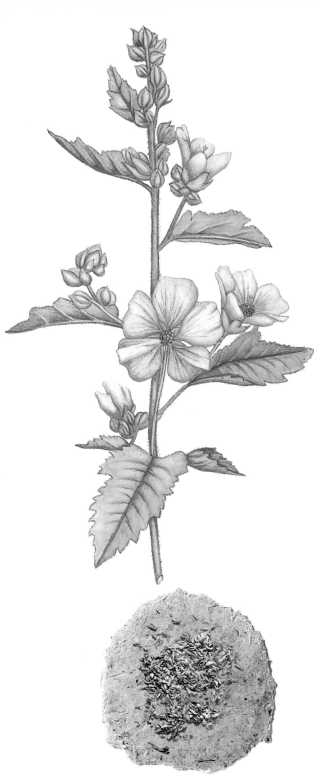

Marshmallow

Althaea officinalis

<small>No other common names</small>

HISTORY AND TRADITIONAL USES Centuries ago, royal dinners in Europe concluded with a trendy dessert called *pate de guimauve*, a spongy mix of sugar, egg whites, and ground marshmallow root. Thus, the marshmallow was born. But its slippery, slightly sweet main ingredient had already been established for thousands of years as a soothing remedy for irritated skin, coughs, sore throats, and wheezing.

Marshmallow poultices were said to give nursing mothers abundant milk; the juice was reported to speed childbirth. More than 2,000 years ago, the Greeks employed marshmallow to ease bladder infections, diarrhea, incontinence, and respiratory problems—the same cures that may have prompted Puritans to grow this European herb in Colonial America.

HEALING POTENTIAL Modern-day marshmallow candy doesn't contain real marshmallow root, but researchers have discovered why this pretty marsh-dwelling plant calms and heals wounded skin and mucous membranes. The root contains a hefty 35 percent mucilage, a slippery, indigestible complex sugar that coats, cools, and moisturizes wounded, inflamed tissue from the throat to the intestines to the urinary tract.

USING MARSHMALLOW Marshmallow is taken as a cold or hot tea or used as a poultice of mashed roots. Some herbalists suggest making a cold infusion to derive the most mucilage from the root.

SAFETY Marshmallow may slow absorption of other medications taken at the same time.

PURCHASING AND GROWING MARSHMALLOW Dried marshmallow root is sold in health food stores. The herb will grow outside a marsh, provided the soil is rich. Plants, which are available by mail order, can be harvested in the fall when the root is three years old.

PART USED Root.

Milk Thistle

Silybum marianum

ALSO KNOWN AS MARY THISTLE; MARIAN THISTLE; LADY'S THISTLE

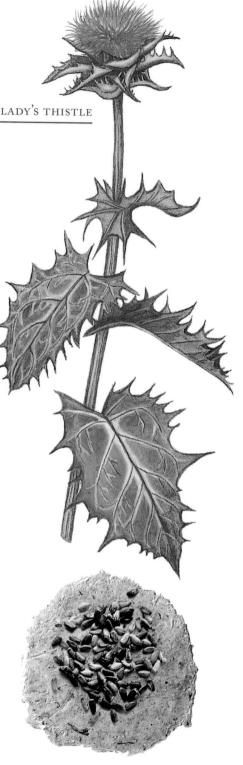

HISTORY AND TRADITIONAL USES Milk thistle is a centuries-old remedy for liver problems. The famous English herbalist Gerard wrote that it is "the best remedy that grows, against all melancholy diseases." (The word *melancholy*, derived from the Greek words *melan*, meaning "black," and *chole*, meaning "bile," was used in the Middle Ages to describe any liver or bile-related disease.)

HEALING POTENTIAL Milk thistle's active ingredient, silymarin, is one of the strongest liver protectors known. Studies in people have shown that it improves cirrhosis, hepatitis, and liver damage caused by toxic chemicals. Silymarin binds to the membranes of liver cells, preventing toxins from doing damage. If the damage is already done, silymarin spurs the liver to speed production of proteins that help heal it.

Research suggests that as an antioxidant, silymarin may be 10 times more potent than vitamin E. It stems the damage caused by free radicals, destructive molecules that damage cells.

USING MILK THISTLE Milk thistle is taken in tea, capsules, tablets, and tinctures (sometimes called extracts). Commercial milk thistle products are usually standardized to contain 70 to 80 percent silymarin. Capsules and tablets of the standardized extract may be your best bet: Some herbalists say that because silymarin doesn't dissolve in water, milk thistle teas are virtually useless. And some point out that you'd need to consume a large amount of an alcohol-based tincture to get an adequate amount of silymarin.

SAFETY Milk thistle is generally regarded as safe.

PURCHASING MILK THISTLE Milk thistle products are sold in health food stores, and dried seeds are available through mail order.

PARTS USED Seeds.

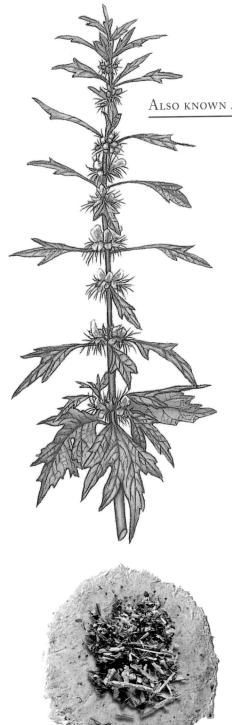

Motherwort

Leonurus cardiaca

ALSO KNOWN AS MOTHER HERB; HEART HEAL; LION'S TAIL; LION'S EAR

HISTORY AND TRADITIONAL USES One old herbal describes motherwort as powerful protection against wicked spirits—and indeed, it has been used for thousands of years to dispel doldrums and anxiety. With its dull green leaves and purplish blooms, this ancient herb "makes mothers joyful and settles the womb, therefore it is called Motherwort," according to seventeenth-century British apothecary Thomas Culpeper. It was called upon to aid women in childbirth, bring on menstruation, and alleviate fainting.

A heart remedy throughout Europe and Asia, bitter-tasting motherwort was used in China to lengthen life. (Legend has it that a daily cup of motherwort tea let one wise man live to see his 300th birthday.) The Greeks and Romans relied on it to cure all manner of physical and emotional problems.

HEALING POTENTIAL Motherwort's leaves and flowers contain leonurine and stachydrine, alkaloids that herbalists say promote menstrual bleeding and the uterine contractions that lead to childbirth. The herb also contains bitter glycosides, mild sedatives and relaxants that may temporarily lower blood pressure.

Herbalists today use motherwort for a wide variety of "women's conditions." It soothes the stress of premenstrual tension and menopausal hot flashes. Evidence shows that it can also restore cardiac health and regulate a rapid heartbeat brought on by anxiety.

USING MOTHERWORT Motherwort is taken as a tea or tincture (sometimes called an extract). If taken for tension relief, it may take about 15 minutes before you feel the effects.

SAFETY Motherwort may stimulate uterine contractions, so don't use it during pregnancy.

PURCHASING MOTHERWORT You can find tinctures and dried motherwort in health food stores.

PARTS USED Leaves, flowers, and stems.

Nettle

Urtica dioica

ALSO KNOWN AS STINGING NETTLE; WILD SPINACH

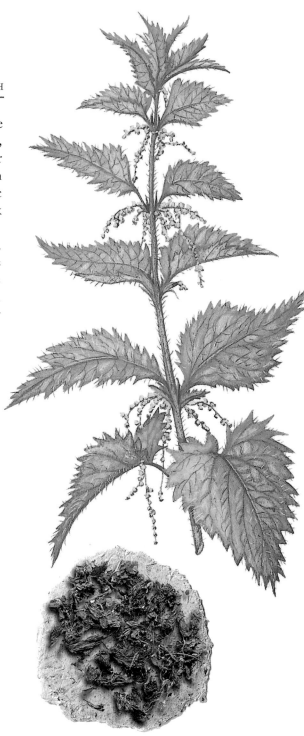

HISTORY AND TRADITIONAL USES Native Americans used nettle to treat ills as varied as coughs, colds, epilepsy, gout, stomachaches, insanity, and hair loss. During and after pregnancy, Native American women relied on this herb as a strengthening tonic that prevented hemorrhaging and encouraged milk flow.

In Europe, nettle gargles were used to ease sore, swollen throats; nettle drinks expelled kidney stones by increasing urination; and nettle leaves and salves healed sores, stopped nosebleeds, and eased gout. In nineteenth-century America, nettle tea was a remedy for diarrhea, dysentery, and hemorrhoids.

HEALING POTENTIAL The stems and dull green leaves of nettle are covered with fine hairs that release irritating chemicals when touched. Fortunately, the dried herb is sting-free. Herbalists use it as a diuretic as well as a remedy for rheumatism, gout, and kidney "gravel" and as an astringent that can stem heavy menstrual periods, stop nosebleeds, and halt bleeding from wounds. Nettle may also alleviate allergies and hay fever. Some forms of nettle may be used externally to soothe bites, stings, and burns. Nettle is often prescribed by women herbalists to replenish iron stores lost during menstruation, menopausal flooding, or childbirth.

USING NETTLE This widely used herb may be taken as a tea or tincture (or extract), freeze-dried in capsules for hay fever, or used as a compress.

SAFETY In some people, allergy symptoms get worse after using nettle, so medical experts recommend taking no more than one dose a day for the first few days.

PURCHASING NETTLE Nettle teas, tinctures, and capsules are available at health food stores.

PARTS USED Leaves and stalks.

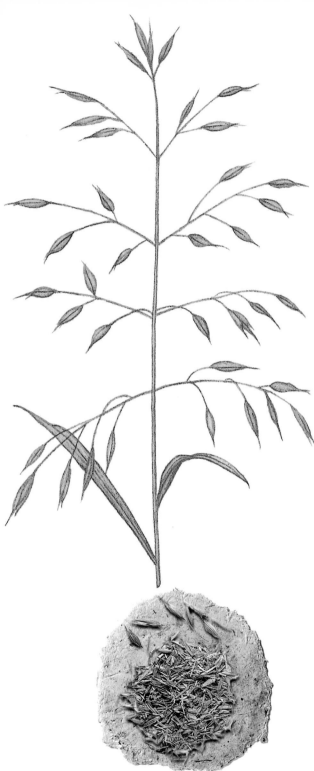

Oatstraw

Avena sativa
ALSO KNOWN AS WILD OATS

HISTORY AND TRADITIONAL USES A traditional staple of northern European diets, oats have been cultivated since at least 100 B.C. While oats were prized as a stomach-satisfying grain, tea brewed from the herb's dried, pale green stems, leaves, and grain husks (or straw) was and still is a common folk remedy for nervous exhaustion and sleeplessness. Historically, a good soak in an oatstraw bath was said to relieve arthritis and rheumatism, among other problems.

In nineteenth-century and early twentieth-century America, the plant ranked among the best restoratives for exhaustion brought on by a fever and for headaches associated with overwork or depression.

HEALING POTENTIAL Herbalists report that tension headaches, insomnia, nervous exhaustion, and that "frazzled" feeling all respond well to oatstraw, which modern herbalists regard as a tonic that can relieve both physical and emotional fatigue as well as depression. Oatstraw contains calcium and silicic acid (a component of silica), reportedly making this herb a good tonic for hair, nails, and bones.

Herbalists say a few cups of oatstraw tea every day can increase strength and energy and foster a feeling of calm. Combined with lemon balm or St.-John's-wort, it may help lessen herpes outbreaks, according to theory. It's also believed that oatstraw may encourage sweating and help remedy colds. In addition, it sometimes may be used to fight yeast infections during pregnancy.

USING OATSTRAW This herb is taken as a tea or tincture (sometimes called an extract) or used as a healing wash for skin conditions.

SAFETY Oatstraw contains gluten, so don't ingest it if you have gluten intolerance (celiac disease).

PURCHASING OATSTRAW Oat tincture and dried oatstraw are available at health food stores.

PARTS USED Stems, leaves, and husks.

Partridgeberry

Mitchella repens

ALSO KNOWN AS SQUAW VINE; DEER BERRY; MOUNTAIN TEA; WINTER CLOVER; HIVE VINE

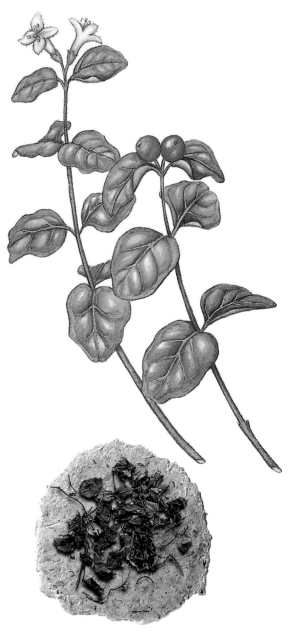

HISTORY AND TRADITIONAL USES Native American women sought this pretty, low-growing herb with shiny, evergreen leaves and brilliant red berries to allay menstrual cramps and soothe sore nipples while nursing, but most of all, they used it to ease childbirth. From the Cherokee to the Iroquois, many native peoples relied on partridgeberry to strengthen the uterus and make labor safer, easier, and faster.

This herbal tradition found its way into American consulting rooms of the nineteenth and early twentieth centuries, where doctors prescribed "mothers' cordial," a uterine tonic made from partridgeberry and other herbs. "It is believed by some to have a salutary influence upon the pregnant woman," one doctor wrote of the herb in 1922, "easing many of the distresses incident to her condition . . . strengthening her for the ordeal of childbirth."

Although it was also prescribed for diarrhea, partridgeberry was believed to have a special affinity for the uterus, functioning as a general "female regulator" to bring on missed menstrual periods, ease cramps, lighten heavy menstrual flow, and stave off miscarriage—uses that continue today.

HEALING POTENTIAL Rich in saponins, partridgeberry is still revered by herbalists as an important female tonic. In combination with red raspberry leaf, another uterine toner, it has been called the perfect pregnancy tonic, priming the womb for childbirth.

USING PARTRIDGEBERRY Partridgeberry can be taken as a tea or tincture (sometimes called an extract).

SAFETY Partridgeberry is generally regarded as safe.

PURCHASING PARTRIDGEBERRY You can purchase mixtures of the dried leaf and stem at health food stores and by mail order.

PARTS USED Leaves, stems, and berries.

Passionflower

Passiflora incarnata

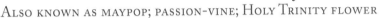

ALSO KNOWN AS MAYPOP; PASSION-VINE; HOLY TRINITY FLOWER

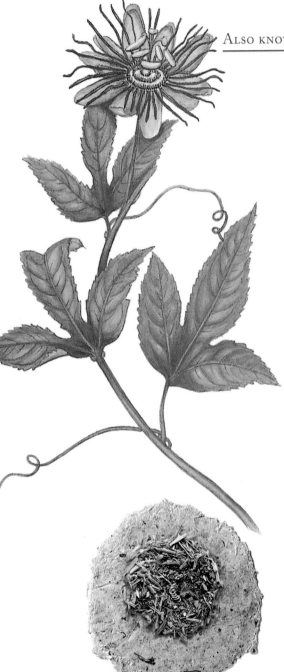

HISTORY AND TRADITIONAL USES Native Americans pounded or boiled the root of this twining vine to make medicine for boils, earaches, and liver problems. The Cherokee consumed passionflower's leaves and sweet yellow fruit as food. The plant's exotic and remarkably intricate flowers reminded Spanish explorers and missionaries of the crown of thorns of Christ's passion—the crucifixion. Hence its name, which refers to spiritual suffering, not to sexual or artistic passion.

Passionflower grows wild in the southern United States, where it's a folk remedy for insomnia and rattled nerves.

HEALING POTENTIAL The flower, vine, and leaves of this showy herb contain alkaloids and flavonoids that, in laboratory studies, have demonstrated sedating effects. Herbalists say that it is one of the best tranquilizing herbs for insomnia, making it a good sleep inducer when nighttime rest is disturbed by anxiety or during menopause. They also recommend passionflower to ease the stress of premenstrual syndrome. It can reportedly calm many stress-related physical problems, such as high blood pressure, headaches, hot flashes, and abdominal pain.

USING PASSIONFLOWER Passionflower is taken as a tea or tincture.

SAFETY While passionflower may be recommended by some herbal practitioners in place of commercial pain relievers during pregnancy, its use should be limited because the herb influences the central nervous system. It is best used in small doses, for up to seven days at a time.

PURCHASING PASSIONFLOWER The dried herb and tincture are available at health food stores and by mail order.

PARTS USED Flowers, leaves, and vine.

Peppermint

Mentha piperita

ALSO KNOWN AS FIELD MINT

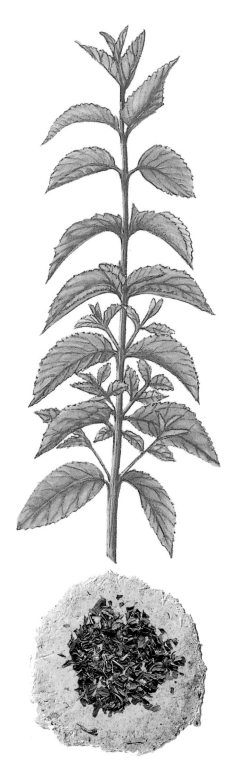

HISTORY AND TRADITIONAL USES With its sharply aromatic scent and handsome, dark green leaves, peppermint's specific stomach-soothing and gas-suppressing powers have a long history. In medieval Europe, mint jellies aided diners in digesting heavy meats at banquets. In the Arab world, mint tea is favored as an after-dinner drink. One seventeenth-century English herbalist praised peppermint as a remedy for "nausea, retchings, and looseness." In North America, the Cherokee took it for vomiting, colic, and gas. At the turn of the century, doctors prescribed peppermint to stop nausea and vomiting, ease stomach cramps, and relieve coughs and headaches.

HEALING POTENTIAL Peppermint leaves contain menthol-rich volatile oils as well as tannins and bitters. As the premier stomach tonic, herbalists use it to counteract nausea and vomiting, promote digestion, calm stomach muscle spasms, relieve flatulence, and ease hiccups. Scientific evidence suggests that it can kill many kinds of microorganisms and may boost mental alertness.

USING PEPPERMINT Peppermint is taken as a tea or tincture (sometimes called an extract). When using fresh peppermint, crush the leaves first.

SAFETY Peppermint is generally regarded as safe.

PURCHASING AND GROWING PEPPERMINT Dried peppermint, teas. tincture, and oils are sold in health food stores. Plant peppermint seeds in rich, moist, well-drained soil in full sun to partial shade. Beware: This herb can quickly overwhelm other garden plants. Barricade the roots by planting seedlings in large bottomless cans sunk into the soil. Harvest just before the flowers open, then dry or freeze the leaves.

PARTS USED Leaves.

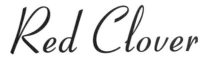

Red Clover

Trifolium pratense

ALSO KNOWN AS PURPLE CLOVER; MEADOW TREFOIL

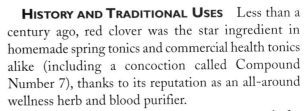

HISTORY AND TRADITIONAL USES Less than a century ago, red clover was the star ingredient in homemade spring tonics and commercial health tonics alike (including a concoction called Compound Number 7), thanks to its reputation as an all-around wellness herb and blood purifier.

The Chinese revered red clover sap as a remedy for colds and influenza. A popular healing plant in England and Germany, it traveled across the Atlantic with colonists and settlers in North and South America, where it grows wild today. The red, sweet-scented flower heads were "adopted" by Iroquois women, who took the herb at menopause, and by the Cherokee and Rappahannock. At the turn of the century, the herb was typically brewed into a strong tea to halt spasmodic coughing. Mennonite communities still rely on it to ease whooping cough and croup.

HEALING POTENTIAL Herbalists report that red clover brings on a normal menstrual cycle, promotes fertility, balances hormones at menopause when menstrual periods are irregular, calms restlessness, soothes coughing, and eases eczema and psoriasis.

The blossoms contain hormonelike substances called estrogenic plant sterols. Red clover also has important vitamins and minerals, including calcium, magnesium, potassium, and vitamins B and C.

USING RED CLOVER For a red clover tea, soak the flowers in cool water overnight to extract the minerals. Tea gets stronger as it soaks.

SAFETY Do not use this herb during pregnancy.

PURCHASING AND GROWING RED CLOVER In health food stores, look for colorful, intact dried flowers—they're the freshest. Or pick wild clover from unsprayed locations, choosing blossoms that are fresh and colorful—a bright, rosy purple.

PARTS USED Flowers.

Red Raspberry

Rubus idaeus

ALSO KNOWN AS BRAMBLE

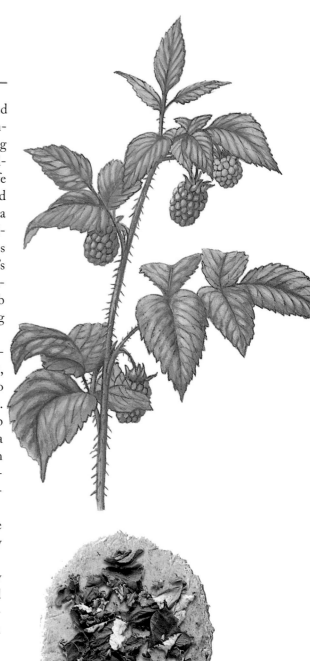

HISTORY AND TRADITIONAL USES Plucked from thorny brambles, raspberry leaves have a centuries-old reputation as a vital, uterus-toning "woman's herb." As the most famous of childbirth allies, it has long been used to encourage quick, safe labor and delivery, speed postpartum recovery, and boost milk production. Cherokee women drank a strong infusion of red raspberry leaves to allay childbirth pains. Native Americans also relied on the leaves to halt diarrhea. At the turn of the century, raspberry's astringent qualities were often deployed against intestinal problems. Doctors also believed that the herb could strengthen feeble uterine contractions during childbirth.

HEALING POTENTIAL Inside this herb's two-tone leaves (forest green on top, silvery white below), researchers have discovered an alkaloid that appears to relax and strengthen pelvic and uterine muscles. Helpful before, during, and after childbirth, this herb may also ease menstrual cramps and maintain a healthy uterus at menopause. It may also help with hormonal changes after a miscarriage, when discontinuing birth control pills or other hormone medications, or after uterine surgery.

Herbalists say that tannins in raspberry help reduce excess menstrual bleeding. It is also used as a fertility promoter.

USING RASPBERRY In pregnancy, raspberry leaves are taken in a warm tea during the second and third trimesters. At other times, herbalists say raspberry can be taken as a tincture (sometimes called an extract) or as a daily tonic tea.

SAFETY Raspberry is generally regarded as safe.

PURCHASING RASPBERRY You can buy dried leaves at health food stores and through mail order.

PARTS USED Leaves.

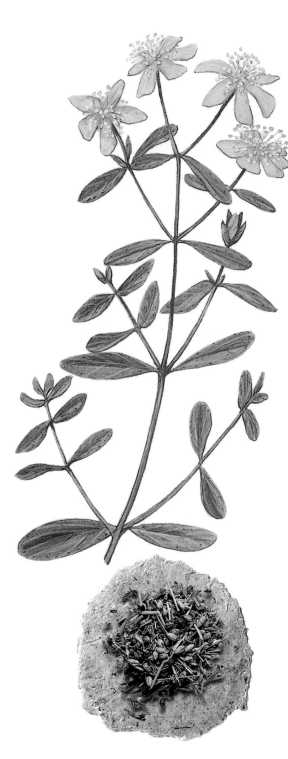

St.-John's-Wort

Hypericum perforatum
ALSO KNOWN AS HYPERICUM; ST.-JOAN'S-WORT

HISTORY AND TRADITIONAL USES The yellow flowers of St.-John's-wort release blood red juice when crushed—juice associated with the blood of St. John the Baptist (or, alternately, the "witches' blood" stirred into ancient love potions). Known as a wound healer since 500 B.C., this old medicinal herb was said to alleviate pain and dispel melancholy and madness. European peasants would gather and burn it on June 24—St. John's Day—to ward off goblins and devils.

At the turn of the century, doctors acknowledged that the plant had "undoubted power over the nervous system" and used it for depression.

HEALING POTENTIAL Researchers have identified at least three substances in this weedy-looking plant that dispel mild depression. Hypericin, for one, protects the brain's natural "feel-good" chemicals, such as serotonin. In studies involving more than 3,000 women and men who used the herb, 80 percent felt improved or totally free from the debilitating blues of depression.

USING ST.-JOHN'S-WORT The herb is widely available in the form of tea, tincture (sometimes called an extract), powder, capsules, tablets, or, for external use on wounds, an oil. When used as an antidepressant, St.-John's-wort products should contain standardized levels of hypericin, as studies show that these work best. It may take two to six weeks or longer to see beneficial results.

SAFETY The herb may cause sun sensitivity. Do not use with other antidepressants without medical approval.

GROWING ST.-JOHN'S-WORT St.-John's-wort grows easily from cuttings or root divisions in full sun to partial shade. Collect the tops of the plants—leaves, stems, and flowers—when the flowers are in bloom.

PARTS USED Leaves, stems, and flowers.

Skullcap

Scutellaria laterifolia

ALSO KNOWN AS MAD-DOG WEED; HELMET FLOWER

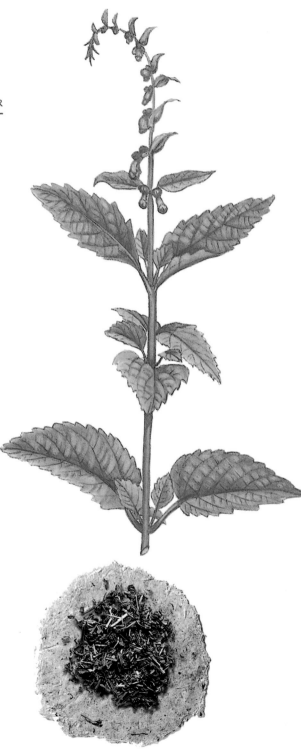

HISTORY AND TRADITIONAL USES With its pointed leaves and delicate blue flowers, skullcap is a native North American medicinal herb found throughout the United States and Canada. Native American women used skullcap to bring on menstrual periods, quiet cramps, soothe breast pain, and ease kidney problems.

By the beginning of the twentieth century, the herb was well-respected as a nerve tonic that dispelled anxiety, restlessness, and nervousness. It was said to calm convulsions, tremors, and hysteria.

HEALING POTENTIAL Herbalists say that skullcap nourishes and revitalizes the nervous system, thanks in part to minerals it supplies, which include calcium, iron, potassium, and magnesium. This plant is a woman's herbal ally during times of stress, easing tension headaches, stress, anxiety, exhaustion, and depression. It's a mild lullaby herb that promotes sleep and won't leave you feeling groggy in the morning. Skullcap may ease premenstrual syndrome and severe menopausal mood changes if taken daily for about three months. It may also help in the withdrawal from tranquilizers or antidepressants.

USING SKULLCAP This herb is taken as a strong tea for insomnia and as a tincture (or extract) for extreme anxiety or premenstrual syndrome.

SAFETY Skullcap is generally regarded as safe. Do not confuse it with Chinese skullcap (*S. baicalensis*), however, which has entirely different properties.

PURCHASING AND GROWING SKULLCAP Good-quality store-bought skullcap should contain tiny bits of the dried, purplish blue flower. Health food stores also carry tinctures. When buying skullcap, check with the source to be sure that it has not been combined with germander, a potentially toxic herb.

PARTS USED Leaves and flowers.

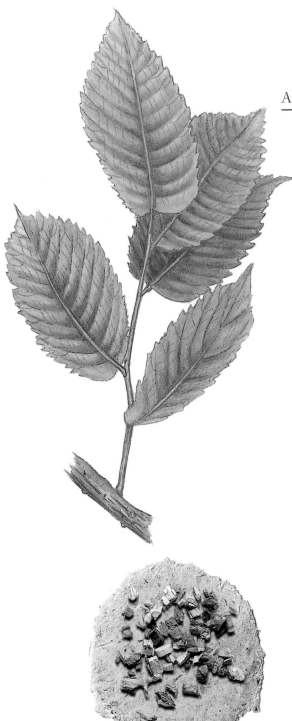

Slippery Elm

Ulmus fulva

ALSO KNOWN AS SWEET ELM; MOOSE ELM; INDIAN ELM

HISTORY AND TRADITIONAL USES Before Dutch elm disease destroyed many of the continent's mature trees, Native Americans relied on the sweet-tasting inner bark to ease childbirth, soothe labor pains, and relieve many other ailments, from diarrhea to dysentery, rheumatism to sore eyes, coughs to sore throats, and wounds to ulcers.

Rich in slick mucilage, slippery elm was widely used at the turn of the century to coat and soothe irritated mucous membranes in the digestive system, mouth, throat, lungs, uterus, kidneys, and bladder. It also cooled hemorrhoids.

HEALING POTENTIAL Today, proponents say that the mucilage in slippery elm bark is still an excellent remedy for bladder infections, diarrhea, peptic ulcers, coughs, colitis, acid stomach, and many more irritations and inflammations of the reproductive, digestive, and respiratory systems as well as of the urinary tract. Externally, homemade slippery elm paste or gel may help heal wounds, soothe inflamed skin, repair a torn perineum after childbirth, and restore vaginal lubrication at menopause.

USING SLIPPERY ELM When made into a beverage, shredded slippery elm bark is bundled together and tied at one end with a long string, then suspended in a glass of cool water for several hours before being consumed. As a healing poultice for cuts, wounds, burns, and skin ulcers, slippery elm is mixed with water or glycerin.

SAFETY Slippery elm is generally regarded as safe.

PURCHASING SLIPPERY ELM Slippery elm bark is harvested from young saplings. You can purchase shredded and powdered slippery elm bark in health food stores and by mail order.

PART USED Inner bark.

Uva-Ursi

Arctostaphylos uva-ursi

ALSO KNOWN AS BEARBERRY; BEAR'S GRAPE; MOUNTAIN BOX

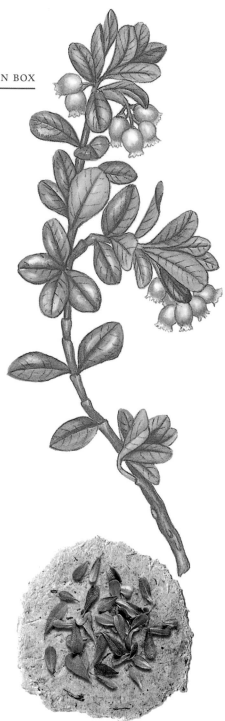

HISTORY AND TRADITIONAL USES Marco Polo and Kublai Khan learned about uva-ursi's healing potential on their treks through Asia. No one knows whether they actually took home this tiny groundcover with its bright red berries that attract bears (hence its Latin name, which means "bear's berry"). But by the thirteenth century, European herbalists considered uva-ursi an important medicinal herb. Over in the New World, naturalists discovered that eating it warded off scurvy. Today, herbal practitioners consider it a highly effective treatment for urinary tract infections.

HEALING POTENTIAL Uva-ursi is a tonic for the urinary system, used for more than 100 years to treat chronic bladder problems. The leaves contain arbutin, an antiseptic that was discovered in 1852. Once in the urinary system, arbutin yields a urinary disinfectant called hydroquinone. Uva-ursi leaves also contain anesthetic properties, which help numb urinary tract pain, and antibiotic properties. Herbalists say that uva-ursi is one of the best herbs to use for cystitis and certain other bladder problems.

USING UVA-URSI Uva-ursi can be taken as a tincture (sometimes called an extract), as a tea, or in capsules.

SAFETY Since uva-ursi leaves contain generous amounts of tannin, a natural compound that can irritate the stomach, don't use it for more than two weeks, and don't use it at all if you have a kidney disorder, as the tannin could cause further damage. Also, don't use it during pregnancy, since it can stimulate the uterus.

PURCHASING UVA-URSI Uva-ursi tincture and capsules are available at most health food stores; dried uva-ursi is available by mail order.

PARTS USED Leaves.

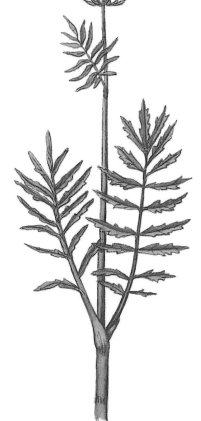

Valerian

Valeriana officinalis

ALSO KNOWN AS ALL HEAL; MOON ROOT; GREAT WILD VALERIAN

HISTORY AND TRADITIONAL USES   Long before Valium, there was valerian. This showy plant with feathery pink blooms has roots so stinky that the Greek physician Dioscorides called it *phu*. But the substance responsible for valerian's dirty-sock aroma has also made it nature's top tranquilizer and sleep aid for more than 1,000 years. Headaches, trembling, palpitations, hysteria, and stress-related digestion problems have been calmed by valerian root. In Traditional Chinese Medicine, valerian also eases backaches, menstrual problems, colds, bruises, and sores.

HEALING POTENTIAL   As an insomnia remedy, valerian shortens the time it takes to fall asleep and reduces middle-of-the-night awakening for many people, without any of the morning-after grogginess that often comes with conventional sleeping pills. It relaxes tense nerves and muscles, so it's used to relieve menstrual cramps and mood swings.

Research indicates that components in valerian attach to the same brain receptors as tranquilizers like diazepam (Valium) but with milder effects—and without causing dependence or addiction.

USING VALERIAN   Valerian can be taken as a tea or tincture (sometimes called an extract) or in tablets or capsules.

SAFETY   If valerian acts as a stimulant, as it does in a few women, stop using it. Also avoid valerian if you're taking other sleep-enhancing or mood-regulating medications such as Valium or amitriptyline (Elavil).

PURCHASING VALERIAN   Good-quality, dried valerian root, available in health food stores and some pharmacies as well as through mail order, is yellow brown and has a bitter taste and penetrating smell. Other products are also sold in health food stores.

PART USED   Root.

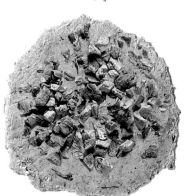

Yarrow

Achillea millefolium

ALSO KNOWN AS NOSEBLEED; MILLEFOIL

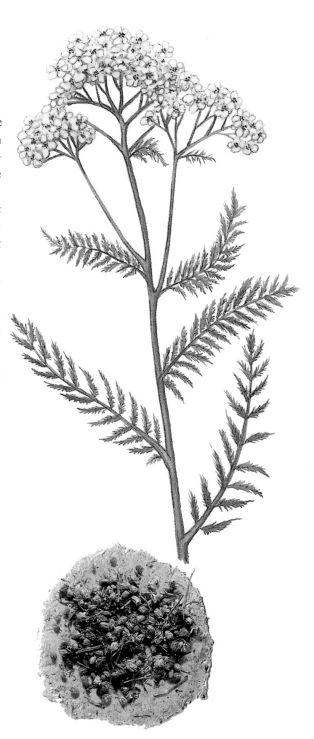

HISTORY AND TRADITIONAL USES Native American women reached for yarrow's feathery green leaves and clusters of tiny white flowers to hasten delayed menstrual periods, soothe breast abscesses, ease childbirth, and expel the placenta after delivery.

Around the turn of the century, America's Eclectic physicians, who combined natural cures with mainstream medicine, prescribed yarrow for urinary tract woes, digestive health, and menstrual problems.

HEALING POTENTIAL This pungent-smelling, all-around healing herb contains more than 120 compounds, including a fever-reducing, anti-inflammatory substance called azulene and others such as flavonoids, coumarins, and lactones. In herbalists' experience, yarrow helps control heavy menstrual bleeding, shrink fibroid tumors, cool menopausal hot flashes, soothe menstrual cramps, and heal bladder infections. Practitioners credit hot yarrow tea with reducing fevers and relieving colds, flu, coughs, and sore throats. Modern herbalists still use yarrow as a wash or poultice to stop bleeding and heal wounds.

USING YARROW This versatile herb is taken as a hot or cold tea, a tincture (sometimes called an extract), or in capsules. It is also used as a poultice or wash. Commission E, the expert panel that judges the safety and effectiveness of herbal medicines for the German government, recommends a hot herbal bath with yarrow to ease menstrual cramps.

SAFETY Yarrow stimulates the uterine muscles, so avoid it during pregnancy. Rarely, handling the flowers causes an allergic skin rash.

PURCHASING YARROW Dried yarrow is sold in health food stores and pharmacies and by mail order. You can also find tea, tincture, and capsules at health food stores.

PARTS USED Flowers, leaves, and stems.

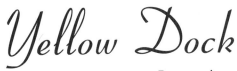

Yellow Dock

Rumex crispus

ALSO KNOWN AS CURLY DOCK; NARROW-LEAVED DOCK

HISTORY AND TRADITIONAL USE Thanks to its long, golden-hued taproot, yellow dock has been cursed by farmers and lawn-proud homeowners as a troublesome intruder but praised by European herbalists, Mennonite housewives, and Arab physicians alike as a cleansing tonic for the bowels, liver, and skin.

Traditionally, itching, jaundice, and edema (swelling) were said to respond to its healing powers, as were poison ivy and snakebite. After European colonists brought yellow dock to America, Native Americans adopted it for other purposes: healing wounds, easing constipation, and purifying the blood.

HEALING POTENTIAL Just how this cleansing herb works remains a mystery to researchers. It contains thiamin, iron, and vitamin C (which assists the absorption of iron), plus compounds called anthraquinone glycosides that stimulate bile production, thereby aiding digestion and nudging a sluggish liver.

A gentle laxative, yellow dock works within hours. Herbalists say that chronic, stubborn skin problems like acne, eczema, psoriasis, and rashes improve with long-term use. And women who feel tired all the time benefit from the herb's energizing minerals.

USING YELLOW DOCK This herb is taken as a tea or tincture (or extract) before meals for best nutrient absorption and at bedtime for overnight constipation relief. It may also be taken in capsules.

SAFETY Do not use this herb during pregnancy. Because yellow dock contains oxalates that can cause kidney stones, you should consult a physician before using it if you have a history of kidney stones.

PURCHASING YELLOW DOCK Dried root is available in health food stores or by mail order; good-quality root is yellow-brown. Tincture, tea, and capsules are also sold in health food stores.

PART USED Root.

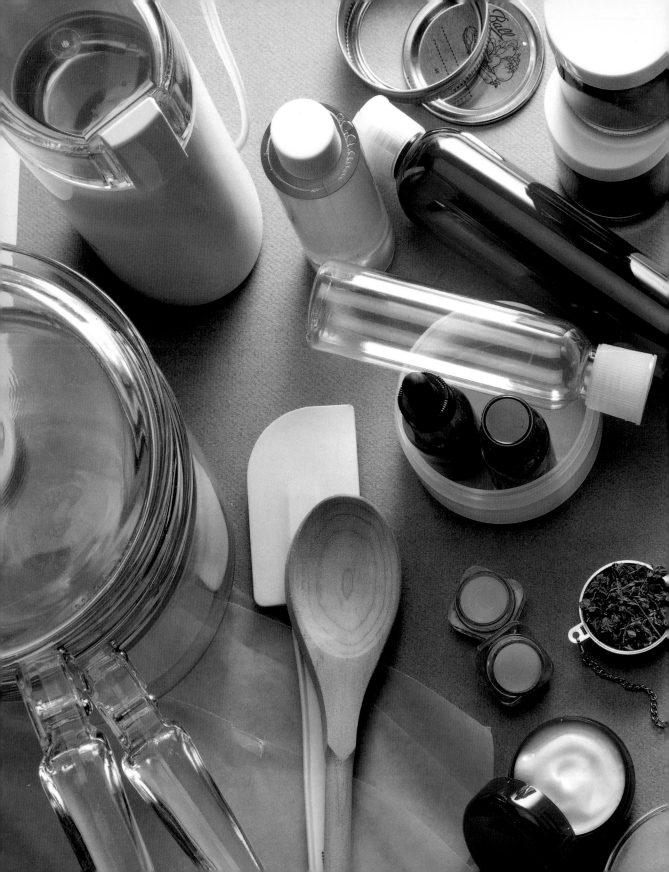

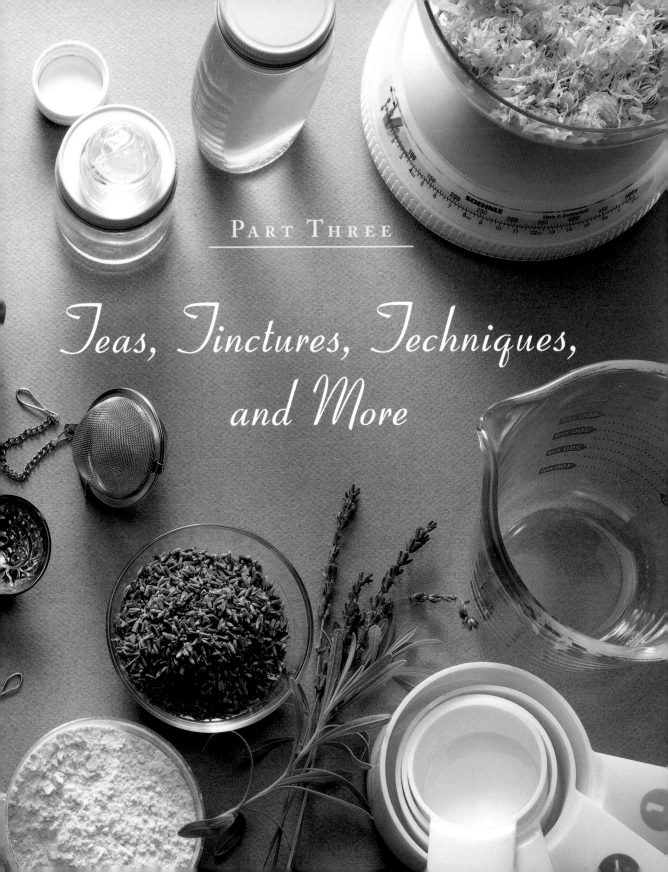

PART THREE

Teas, Tinctures, Techniques, and More

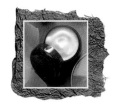

Making Herbal Medicines at Home

Sometimes, using medicinal herbs is a lot like taking vitamins or over-the-counter medications: Swallowing a capsule will do the job. Other herbs work best as tinctures, which are alcohol-based liquids that you can buy or make. And sometimes, an herbal tea, poultice, compress, or bath is just the ticket. Herbalists say that it's well worth the trouble to make these preparations, as homemade versions may be less costly than store-bought products.

Say you're taking chasteberry tincture to relieve hot flashes. Herbalist Susun S. Weed, an herbal educator from Woodstock, New York, and author of the *Wise Woman* series of herbal health books, suggests 30 to 90 drops three times a day for several months or more. A one-ounce bottle of chasteberry tincture from the health food store contains approximately 200 drops— enough for two days or less—and costs

around $10. But for less than $20 or so, you can make up a whole quart of tincture, and it will last for months.

By making your own herbal medicines, you can also tailor-make remedies to suit your needs. Suppose you want to combine damiana and dang gui with chasteberry in a tincture for menopausal symptoms, a remedy recommended by Andrew Weil, M.D., director of the program in integrative medicine at the University of Arizona College of Medicine in Tucson and author of *Spontaneous Healing*. Since you probably won't find that tincture combination available commercially, you would have to purchase tinctures of each of the three ingredients and combine them. For a lot less money, however, you can make the combination yourself. Recipes and techniques for making herbal preparations vary from herbalist to herbalist, but the techniques shown in the chapters that follow are fairly typical.

The ritual of making your own medicines is powerful medicine in itself. "When you make a tea, tincture, or other herbal preparation, you're affirming that you want to get better—and you're putting positive energy into your healing process," says Betzy Bancroft, a professional member of the American Herbalists Guild and manager of Herbalist and Alchemist, an herbal medicine company in Washington, New Jersey.

What's more, making herbal medicines is as easy as making chicken soup—and it can be just as satisfying. Think back to the last time you made chicken soup from scratch. First, you probably made the basic stock. Then you chopped up a few carrots and some onions and celery and tossed them into the pot with the chicken. Maybe you added some basic seasonings, such as salt, some pepper, or some dill or parsley, and placed the pot on the stove to simmer. A couple of hours later, your simple ingredients had turned into a soul-soothing soup, and you felt the comfort of knowing that your own two hands had concocted something far more savory than anything you could ever find in a can. Your kitchen was filled with a familiar, heart-warming aroma. Finally, as you ladled the golden nectar into a bowl, you felt a small but undeniable prick of pleasure and pride at your handiwork.

Equipping Your Herbal Laboratory

You won't need a lot of exotic equipment to make your own herbal remedies. For most, you can press into service standard items that you already have on hand in your kitchen. Here are the basic necessities.

Double boiler. This is useful for making infused oils, creams, and salves.

Coffee grinder. A good coffee bean grinder is invaluable for grinding tough bark, berries, and roots. Models by Krups and Braun have been found to do a particularly good job. Reserve it for herbs, though, so you don't unintentionally end up with herb-flavored coffee (or coffee-flavored herbs).

Blender. To make skin creams, pestos, and other herbal remedies, you'll need a sturdy kitchen blender, preferably with a removable knob in the lid. As with the coffee grinder, it's probably a good idea to have a separate herb blender.

Jars and bottles. If you plan on making your own tinctures, salves, herbal oils, or vinegars, you may want to invest in special jars and bottles, available by mail order. You can buy clear or amber-colored bottles with droppers as well as other vessels that are exactly the right size and shape for your offerings (see "Where to Buy Herbs and Herbal Products" on page 462 for sources). You can also recycle wide-mouth food jars—the kind in which you buy salsa, roasted peppers, or mayonnaise. If you refrigerate your remedies or store them in a dark cabinet, you don't necessarily need dark glass bottles.

Pots and utensils. Don't use aluminum or copper pots for herb preparation. Aluminum leaches into herbal preparations as they cook, and copper destroys the vitamin C content of certain herbs. The best materials for utensils are glass, stainless steel, ceramic, and enamel.

Dried Herbs

HARVESTING, DRYING, AND STORING HERBS RIGHT

Although fresh herbs have great appeal, herbalists agree that drying medicinal plants and storing them carefully extends their shelf life.

A well-stocked health food store or mail-order supply company should carry all the dried herbs you need, including hard-to-grow or hard-to-find herbs like astragalus, blue cohosh, goldenseal, or dang gui. But if you're like a lot of women, once you start using healing herbs, you'll be seduced into growing your own.

Some decide to grow a hardy favorite, such as lemon balm, on the patio. Others, more ambitious, grow a bountiful herb garden that delights their senses for months. Still others, well-trained in the safe collection of wild plants, seek out meadows or a wooded glen that's lush with healing herbs (and blessed with a knowledgeable owner who grants permission for their harvest).

Just as growing healthy herbs is an art, so is knowing how to pick and preserve herbs so that they retain their medicinal value. Happily, it's a simple art that's simply mastered.

Do's and Don'ts for Your Harvest

To gather home-grown or wild herbs, you'll need little more than brown paper grocery bags and a sharp pair of clippers, scissors, or pruning shears. For best results, herbalists offer these tips.

🌿 Snip, don't tear, leaves, flowers, or flowering tops of plants. Ripping off the plant's parts encourages the invasion of disease in the remaining plant.

🌿 To collect leaves, cut the stem just below a leaf. Doing so allows new growth.

🌿 Put harvested herbs in brown paper bags, not plastic. Paper "breathes," while plastic increases the chances of mold.

🌿 Don't collect more than you can use: In one harvest, take just enough to loosely fill half of a paper grocery bag.

🌿 Don't harvest parts of a plant that look wilted, diseased, insect-damaged, or moldy.

🌿 Don't collect herbs growing close to a roadside. They may be contaminated with pollutants from vehicles.

Drying Herbs at Home

Carefully dried and stored, herbs can retain their medicinal value for months. Here's how expert herbalists dry herbs easily.

🌿 Dry-brush the plants with a clean, soft-bristle toothbrush or pastry brush or carefully wash them to remove dirt. Be careful not to overwet the herbs. Thoroughly pat them dry with paper towels or spin them in a salad spinner.

🌿 Thinly slice roots and bulbs.

🌿 Cut large, fleshy leaves (such as mullein and comfrey) in strips to help prevent mold.

The Call of the Wild: Gathering Medicinal Herbs

Gathering herbs in meadows or woodlands can be a great way to add to your botanical medicine chest. Herbalists call the practice of gathering wild herbs wildcrafting. To harvest herbs safely, follow these important guidelines.

Know precisely what you're picking. To the inexperienced eye, many potentially poisonous plants resemble healing herbs or nonmedicinal plants. Angelica, for example, is easily confused with poison hemlock, a plant that's lethal. In the wild, comfrey plants resemble foxglove, the basis for the heart drug digoxin. In his book *The Green Pharmacy*, James A. Duke, Ph.D., a former ethnobotanist with the U.S. Department of Agriculture who specializes in medicinal plants, tells of an elderly couple who thought they were picking comfrey. The consequences were fatal.

Follow a guide. Before you head out to gather wild herbs, arm yourself with education. Dr. Duke recommends that you contact your local botanical garden, university, scouting organization, museum, or hiking club. Ask about classes in the identification of local plants or other programs that teach you how to harvest wild herbs safely.

Don't pick endangered herbs. Herbalists also caution would-be wildcrafters to harvest wild herbs with respect and to learn which herbs are considered endangered. Here's why: Goldenseal's popularity caused it to be seriously overharvested, notes herbalist Rosemary Gladstar, director of the Sage Mountain herbal education center in East Barre, Vermont, in her book *Herbal Healing for Women*. As a result, it is now considered an endangered herb, and Gladstar urges you to buy only cultivated, not wildcrafted, goldenseal.

Other herbs considered to be endangered include American ginseng, helonias, beth root, and echinacea.

Dry the herbs in a warm, shady, airy place. Aim for an ideal drying temperature of 80° to 120°F for roots and bark and 80° to 105°F for leaves and flowers. A warm attic is ideal, as long as there is adequate ventilation. Watch the temperature closely. If it's too low, the herbs will take longer than a week to dry and increase the chance of mold. If it's too high, the herbs can "cook," which destroys volatile chemicals such as essential oils.

Avoid drying herbs in direct sunlight, which bleaches out their flavor and color.

Herbs are perfectly dried when they are crisp and the stems or leaves are still green. Under ideal conditions, herbs take about a week to dry. If they still aren't dry after a week, you may have to finish the process in a dehydrator or a very low oven (140°F) to prevent mold growth. Leave the herbs in the oven or dehydrator only until they are crisp, which should take a few hours. Check them fre-

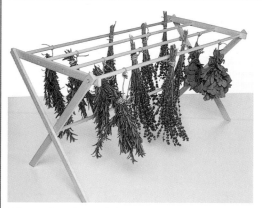

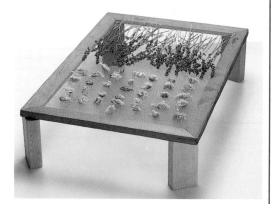

Hang herbs with stems. For herbs like mint, lavender, and chamomile, the stems serve as convenient handles for air-drying. Gather the stem ends of each bunch of herbs into a bundle about as fat around as your finger and bind them with string or rubber bands. Take extra care when using string, because as the herbs dry, the stems shrink, and the bundles may fall apart. If you're lucky enough to have ceiling beams, you can hang the herb bundles from them with thumbtacks or nails. Alternately, you can use a portable clothes rack or a wooden pasta-drying rack.

Screen-dry flowers and leaves. For herb flowers like calendula or tree leaves like ginkgo, screen-drying works better than bundling. Place the herbs in a single layer on clean window screens, flat baskets, wicker trays, or clothes-drying screens. Raise the screens so that air circulates underneath. If necessary, you can put books or blocks under the corners. You can also use trays or even paper towels, as long as you arrange the herbs so that air circulates around them. If you use trays or paper towels, be sure to leave space between the herbs when you arrange them; you may have to turn them over or stir them occasionally to expose all surfaces to the air for even drying.

quently. (Some herbs, such as red clover and alfalfa, retain their color better when dried in a dehydrator.)

Once you've dried the herbs, store them carefully to preserve their potency for as long as possible. They can last as long as a year if you follow these simple directions from expert herbalists.

🍵 Store herbs as whole as possible. They take up less space if they're crumbled, but they tend to lose potency quickly.

🍵 Use brown paper bags or glass jars with tight-fitting lids for storage. Bags are nice because they can be tied with string and stacked away, but jars are better in areas that are damp or bug-infested. Dark glass jars are ideal because they protect the herbs from light.

🍵 Store herbs out of light, heat, and air and away from contaminants like smoke and air fresheners, all of which can sap their healing properties.

Teas and Infusions

A RITUAL THAT HEALS BODY AND SOUL

Made with the fresh or dried leaves and flowers of a particular herb, what we casually refer to as herbal tea is, technically speaking, an infusion. If you've ever brewed tea English-style, using loose tea leaves in a real teapot, you've made an herbal infusion. Like a well-made cup of tea, infusions are warm and soul-soothing.

Brewing an herbal infusion is a time-honored ritual that begins with your choice of

---

Making an Infusion

To make a true herbal infusion, you'll need the following materials.

✓ Fresh or dried loose herbs
✓ Measuring spoons
✓ A glass, ceramic, or plastic infuser, cloth tea bag, or metal tea ball

✓ A teapot
✓ A measuring cup
✓ A kettle or pot

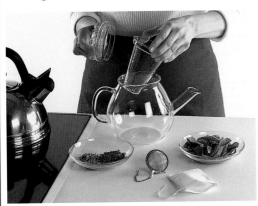

1. Start with fresh or dried. Measure the herbs and put them in an infuser, tea bag, or tea ball, then place it in a teapot, as shown. Or put loose herbs into the pot and strain them out when you pour the tea. Use 2 tablespoons of dried herbs or about a handful of fresh herbs to a pint of water.

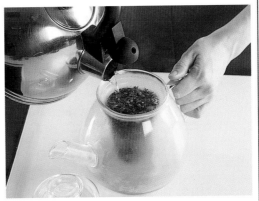

2. Boil, then brew. Place water fresh from the tap or bottle in a kettle or pot and bring it to a boil. When the water boils, remove it from the heat until the bubbles subside, then pour it over the herbs in the teapot, cover, and steep for 10 to 20 minutes. (You can also use a large travel mug with a cover to brew just one cup. The lid prevents the herb's essential oils from leaching out in the steam.)

herb. Why are you making the tea? To ease a cold? To ward off hot flashes? To relax and get a good night's sleep? With your healing intent in mind, you select the appropriate herb or herbs. As you measure what you need, focus on the unique aromas, textures, and colors of the herbs you've chosen. Then spoon the herbs into your teapot and steep them for a while, smelling the fragrance as it wafts through the room. Twenty or so minutes later—ahhh—you're sitting in your favorite chair, sipping the healing brew that you just made for yourself.

Herbalists say that this simple ritual unites a healer (you) and a healing substance (the herb) with a healing intention ("I want to get rid of my cold." "I want these hot flashes to stop." "I want to relax and get a good night's sleep."). The idea is that intention—and the ritual itself—can go a long way toward abetting the body's innate healing process because you're affirming your desire to heal yourself.

Herbal tea bags are ubiquitous these days: You can find scores of popular blends any-where that tea and coffee are sold. But to help ensure the medicinal quality of herbs for treating specific conditions, some herbalists suggest that you buy herbs at a health food store, purchase them from an herbal mail-order company, or grow them yourself.

Herbal Iced Teas

Theoretically, some fresh herbs, especially succulent varieties such as cleavers or those with a high mucilage content such as skull-cap, may extract better in cold infusions. Cold infusions, which are sort of herbal iced teas, use the same proportion of herbs to water as do hot infusions. Pour cold water over the fresh herbs and allow the tea to steep for several hours or overnight in the refrigerator (some herbalists recommend overnight steeping for mineral-containing herbs such as nettle or red raspberry leaf, to extract as many nutrients as possible). Since the water isn't boiled, be sure to use clean, rinsed herbs. If you like, you can add some honey to taste.

Decoctions

GENTLE WAYS TO SIMMER TOUGH HERBS

Tougher herb parts—bark, roots, rhizomes, dried berries, or seeds—need more heat to release the healing power of their constituents than fragile herb parts do. So herbalists use a long, gentle simmering process called a decoction to coax out the plant's medicinal qualities. To make a decoction, simply simmer fibrous plant material slowly in water in a covered pot.

Commonly decocted herbs include cinnamon, black haw bark, and licorice root. You can save very dense, fibrous herbs like cin-

Making a Decoction

Here's what you'll need to make your own herbal decoctions.

- ✓ Fresh or dried herbs
- ✓ A cutting board and knife (if using fresh herbs) or a coffee grinder
- ✓ A glass or stainless steel pot large enough to hold the herb and liquid
- ✓ Pint or quart glass jars
- ✓ A fine-mesh plastic strainer
- ✓ A wooden spoon
- ✓ A coffee filter

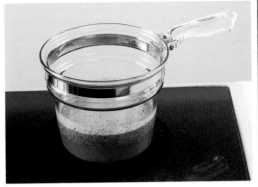

2. Simmer gently. Place the herbs in a pot and add water. Bring to a full, rolling boil, then reduce the heat to the lowest setting and let the decoction simmer gently for 10 to 20 minutes. Keep the pot covered so that the herb's essential oils don't leach out in the escaping steam.

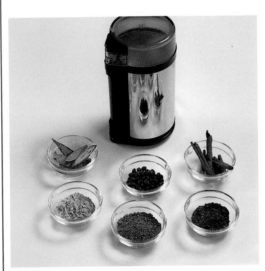

1. Prepare the herbs. To break down the cellular structure and make it easier to extract their maximum medicinal value, herbs for a decoction need to be crushed, chopped, or well-bruised. If you plan to make herbal remedies regularly, consider getting a sturdy coffee bean grinder (such as Krups or Braun) to chop hard, woody herbs easily.

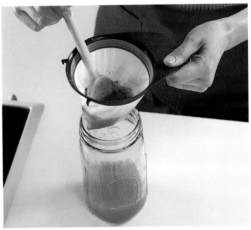

3. Strain the decoction. When the decoction has finished simmering, strain it through a fine-mesh plastic strainer into a glass jar or a mug. Press on the herbs in the strainer with the back of a wooden spoon in order to extract as much liquid as possible. If you've used a fuzzy herb like rose hips, line the strainer with a coffee filter to eliminate any irritating particles.

namon bark and ginger for a second or sometimes even a third use. As long as the decoction's color and aroma are rich and deep, there's healing power left in the herbs. Once the herbs are spent, use them for compost, if you can.

Decoctions use the same water-to-herb proportions as infusions do—about an ounce (by weight) of herb for each pint of water. Use the decoction as it is or follow the recipe for a specific remedy. You can store decoctions for a day or two in covered glass jars in the refrigerator.

Tinctures

HERBAL EXTRACTS OFFER POWER AND CONVENIENCE

Tinctures are highly concentrated liquid herbal extracts, and herbalists rely on them because they are concentrated and convenient. A teaspoon of tincture, for example, provides the same healing power as a cup of tea. In addition, an alcohol-based tincture extracts more of the plant's medicinal constituents than can be delivered in capsules or tea. Tinctures are easy to take, easily portable, and last for years.

For convenience, you can buy tinctures of countless herbs, from agrimony to yucca, at health food stores or through herbal mail-order companies. (In some cases, they may be labeled as "extracts," especially in mail-order catalogs.) But tinctures are also easy to make, and homemade tinctures are far less costly than store-bought products.

Choose Your Medium

Before you make a tincture, you have to choose a menstruum, the solvent that extracts an herb's healing power. You can use alcohol, glycerin, or vinegar, depending on the herb or herbs used and what you're trying to heal. According to herbalists, each has its own intrinsic benefits.

Alcohol. Vodka, brandy, or gin can be used to extract fats, resins, most alkaloids, some volatile oils, and other healing components from herbs. One-hundred-proof vodka or gin assures a 50:50 proportion of alcohol to water, allowing for extraction of both water-soluble and alcohol-soluble chemicals. Brandy is generally lower in proof—around 80. Any alcoholic proof over 50 (that is, 25 percent alcohol) will do nicely, however. Alcohol tinctures last for three to five years.

Glycerin. A very sweet substance found in plants and animals, glycerin doesn't dissolve resinous or oily plant constituents, so it's not as effective a menstruum as alcohol. But for those who must avoid alcohol in any amount or form and for children, glycerin makes an acceptable tincture. Two parts glycerin to one part water is a preferred menstruum ratio. Use only 100 percent pure vegetable glycerin,

Making a Tincture

Here's what you'll need.

- ✓ Fresh or dried herbs
- ✓ A cutting board and knife or a coffee grinder
- ✓ A clean glass jar large enough to hold the desired amount of tincture
- ✓ Menstruum (solvent) of your choice
- ✓ Labels

- ✓ A wire-mesh strainer
- ✓ Cheesecloth, muslin, or a coffee filter
- ✓ A 2-cup glass measuring cup
- ✓ A funnel
- ✓ Dark glass bottles

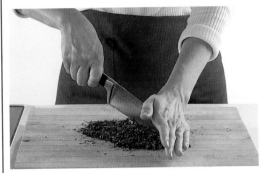

1. Chop the herbs finely. You can cut them by hand, as shown, or in a coffee grinder (such as Krups or Braun). Don't forget to clean fresh herbs first.

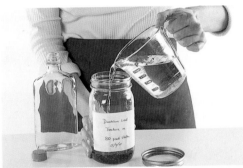

2. Combine. Place 1 part herb to 2 parts liquid in the jar, with 1 to 3 inches of liquid above the herbs. Close it tightly and label with the name of the herb, the menstruum, and the date. Place the jar in a warm, dark place and steep for at least four weeks—the longer, the better. Shake the jar daily and add more liquid if necessary.

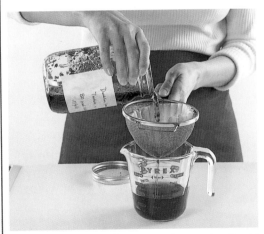

3. Strain the tincture. Pour the liquid through a wire-mesh strainer lined with cheesecloth, muslin, or a coffee filter into a glass measuring cup.

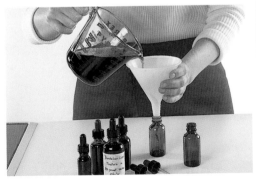

4. Fill the bottles. Using a funnel, carefully pour the tincture into clean, dark bottles (such as amber or cobalt blue). Label them with the type of tincture and the date.

The Right Dose

*I*n recommending herbal tinctures for various purposes, herbalists use three different ways to measure doses. To measure tinctures accurately, follow these guidelines.

By the drop. Most store-bought herbal tinctures come in bottles with droppers that allow you to measure out doses. Herbalists often express tincture doses in three ways: by the drop, half-dropperful, or dropperful. The exact amount of the herb taken this way will vary slightly, depending on the herb itself, the size of the dropper and its bulb, and whether you're using an alcohol or glycerin-based tincture. Droppers are the least precise measuring tool, however, and herbalists prefer more accurate teaspoons and milliliters.

By the teaspoon or tablespoon. Herbalists sometimes recommend taking a dosage of tincture measured in teaspoons or tablespoons. As with cooking or baking, use a standard liquid measuring spoon, not your silverware.

In milliliters. This is the standard medical measurement for herbal tinctures, and some herbalists prefer it because it's more accurate than dropper measurements and more precise than teaspoon measurements. A few herb companies offer droppers marked with milliliters for tincture bottles, or the droppers can be purchased at many drugstores.

Pay attention to what herbalists suggest for a particular remedy. "For many herbs, it doesn't matter whether you're a few drops off in either direction, but other herbs call for precise doses in milliliters," says Tieraona Low Dog, M.D., a family practice physician at the University of New Mexico Hospital, professional member of the American Herbalists Guild, and member of the Alternative Medicine Research Group at the University of New Mexico School of Medicine in Albuquerque.

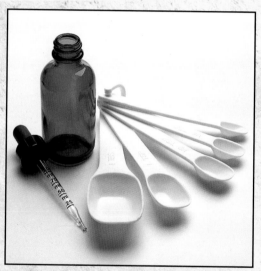

When it comes to measuring tincture dosages, herbalists may recommend drops, teaspoons, or milliliters; it's important to heed their advice.

which is available at health food stores or from mail-order sources (see "Where to Buy Herbs and Herbal Products" on page 462).

Vinegar. A mild acid, vinegar extracts alkaloids, vitamins, and minerals but not plant acids, so it's not as effective a solvent as alcohol. Vinegar tinctures do help maintain the body's acid/alkaline balance, however, and are suitable for everyone. For tonic tinctures that you take regularly over time, vinegar is an excellent menstruum. Use organic apple cider vinegar when possible, and add a little honey for a tincture that can be sipped or slipped onto salads or vegetables. If you use 100 percent vinegar, check that the label says it contains 5 to 7 percent acetic acid. A vinegar tincture will probably last for years when stored in a cool, dark place, but if water is added or the fresh herbs are too moist, the tincture will have a shorter shelf life.

In addition to your solvent of choice, you'll need high-quality herbs. Herbalists say that tincturing preserves a fresh plant's attributes, but good-quality dried herbs work fine, too. You can buy bottles for storing tinctures at kitchen supply stores or from the suppliers in the resource list.

Store the tinctures in a cool, dark place such as a cupboard or closet. Discard a tincture if it begins to ferment or smell spoiled. You can also tell that a tincture has gone bad if it becomes moldy, separates into clear liquid and brown "glop," or crusts around the jar. And always discard a tincture if gases escape when you open it.

Baths

HERBAL SOAKS FOR RELAXATION AND HEALING

To the ancients, bathing was an aromatic art form—and an essential healing tool. The Egyptians perfumed their baths with a substance called Kyphi, which was said to induce spiritual visions and sleepiness. Hippocrates, the great Greek physician who is known as the father of medicine, is credited with writing that "aromatic baths are useful in the treatment of female disorders." In Rome 400 years later, the licentious Emperor Caligula spent dazzling sums of money on his perfumed baths. He believed, according to legend, that frequent fragrant soaks would restore health to his body, which was ravaged by the effects of sexual excess.

Modern-day herbalists, too, tout the benefits of the bath for relaxation and healing. Aside from relieving stress, herbal baths earn high marks for their power to treat hemorrhoids, post-childbirth pain, sore muscles, and various skin problems.

Herbal baths work in three ways. First, the warm bathwater opens your pores, so you absorb the herb's healing constituents. And, suggest herbalists, when you inhale the plant's aromatic volatile oils in a steamy bath, they enter the bloodstream through the lungs.

What's more, inhaling certain oils may signal nerve receptors in the brain to trigger a relaxing response that can ease emotional strain.

Herbalists recommend any of a myriad of herbs for the bath, depending on the condition being treated. Lavender, chamomile, and ylang-ylang make for an especially relaxing bath, for example. (And they smell heavenly, too.) Rosemary also may increase blood circulation to the brain, enhancing alertness.

Three All-Purpose Herbal Baths

There's more to an herbal bath than tossing a handful of dried herbs into a tubful of water. The specific herbs used, as well as the temperature of the water and how long and how often you should soak, vary. Herbal-ists usually recommend that you soak for 15 to 30 minutes, and they suggest one of three types of baths, depending on your needs.

🌿 Hang a muslin bag filled with fresh or dried herbs right under the hot water tap as you fill the tub.

🌿 Add a strong herb tea of your choice to warm or comfortably hot bathwater.

🌿 Add a few drops of your favorite essential oil to the bath. Dilute essential oils in a carrier oil such as grapeseed, almond, or apricot before adding them to the bathwater, especially if you have sensitive skin or are bathing a baby. Add the essential oil to ½ cup of carrier oil and then add it to the bathwater. The oil will make your tub slippery, so use a nonskid bath mat and be careful. If the tub's still slippery after you've finished, give it a once-over with a bathtub cleaning product to prevent falls.

Compresses

HOT AND COLD FIRST-AID

A compress—a cloth soaked in an herbal preparation—is a soothing, simple first-aid treatment for headaches, bruises, backache, menstrual cramps, sore muscles or joints, varicose vein discomfort, wounds, acne, and a host of other problems.

Healing compresses may be applied to the skin wet or dry, hot or cold. Adding an herb or herbs to a compress enhances its healing potential and may accelerate healing, say herbalists, because the medicinal compounds in plants pass through the skin and have in-ternal benefits. How long you apply a compress—or how often—depends on what you're treating. The same is true of temperature. While cool compresses soothe dilated blood vessels and can relieve a headache, for example, for other conditions (like muscle soreness), warm compresses are more effective. (To keep a compress warm, cover it with a hot water bottle wrapped in a towel to protect skin areas not covered by the compress.) Alternating hot and cold compresses may increase circulation, according to herbalists.

Making a Compress

To fashion a compress, here's what you'll need.
- ✓ The appropriate herb infusion, decoction, or diluted tincture
- ✓ A medium to large bowl
- ✓ A soft cloth such as a washcloth

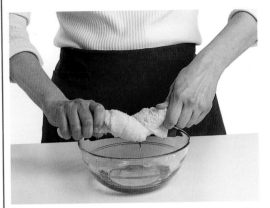

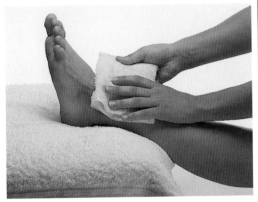

1. Soak a cloth. Place a strong infusion, decoction, or diluted tincture in a bowl and immerse a cloth in it, soaking it thoroughly. Gently wring it out to avoid excess dripping.

2. Apply the compress. Fold the cloth to fit the affected area—ankle, forehead, back, joint, or leg—whatever hurts. Either lie down or loosely tie the compress with rolled cotton gauze to keep it in place. For best results, repeat as needed until you feel better.

Poultices

HERBAL WRAPS THAT WORK

Back in the seventeenth century, herbalist Nicholas Culpeper wrote that "poultices are those kind of things which the Latins call 'cataplasmata'; it is indeed a very fine kind of medicine to ripen sores." Centuries later, American folk doctors and "Dr. Moms" still used poultices to soothe coughs, relieve sore throats, and ease congestion. Right up until the 1940s or so, home recipes for poultices called for ingredients

Here's what you'll need.
- ✓ Herbs for the condition you plan to treat
- ✓ A sharp knife and a cutting board or a blender
- ✓ A small bowl
- ✓ Gauze pads and rolled gauze

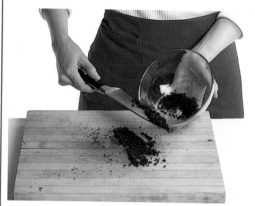

1. Make a paste. Chop fresh herbs with a knife or in a blender, using a little water, if necessary, to dampen the mixture. (The natural moisture in fresh herbs is often all you need, but if you don't have fresh herbs, you can use finely chopped or powdered dried herbs and add a little hot water.)

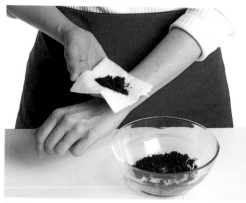

2. Grab the gauze. Place the herb paste on a gauze pad. The herbs should be wet enough so that they feel damp through the gauze but not so wet that moisture drips through it.

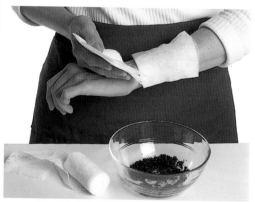

3. Position the poultice. Place it over the affected area and cover with another piece of gauze.

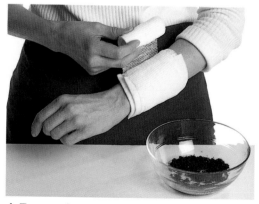

4. Fasten it. Use a larger piece of rolled gauze to tie the poultice lightly in place.

ranging from common to bizarre. Onions fried in vinegar and mixed with flour were said to sweat out a cold overnight. Another odd concoction for colds included kerosene, turpentine, camphor, and vinegar added to flour. Some poultice recipes called for fat from opossums, raccoons, and even skunks. Perhaps the most famous (or infamous) of all the traditional poultices was the mustard plaster.

These days, herbalists use poultices for a range of healing treatments. Modern poultices usually consist of a dampened mixture of chopped or bruised fresh or dried herbs that is held in place on the skin by a wet piece of gauze, sometimes covered by a bandage.

Like poultices of yore, modern poultices are also used to heal wounds and insect bites, relieve chest congestion, decrease joint pain, and increase circulation. Herbalists believe that poultices work because the herb's medicinal components pass through the skin and have internal benefits.

To help wounds heal, herbalists often fashion a poultice of comfrey and plantain. Other natural substances pressed into service for poultices include chickweed leaves for insect bites and bentonite clay for poison ivy. Directions for poultices vary, depending on what you're treating, but the basic guidelines are outlined on the opposite page.

Liniments

A BORN-AGAIN FOLK REMEDY

Take a look at America's brightly checkered era of patent medicines, back at the turn of the century, and you'll find liniments, a favorite remedy of folk healers. In those days, liniments were marketed as panaceas for all sorts of pain. The best-known, Sloan's Liniment, was called The World's Liniment Recommended for Rheumatic Aches and Pains and Sprains and Strains—and it's still sold today. Another best-seller, Dr. Brown's Magic Liniment, was touted as a remedy for

sciatica, lumbago, and neuralgia of the face, stomach, spleen, and ovaries—and painful menstrual cramps.

Herbalists still use liniments in the form of concentrated herbal extracts. Today, they're used externally, usually to treat skin problems or muscle aches and pains. According to herbalists, liniments are absorbed quickly through the skin. Some contain stimulating oils or cayenne to increase circulation at the affected spot.

An herbal liniment that contains cayenne

Making a Liniment

Here are the materials you'll need for a simple herbal liniment.

✓ A knife and cutting board
✓ Herbs for the ailment being treated
✓ A clean quart jar with a tight-fitting lid
✓ Rubbing alcohol
✓ A funnel
✓ A coffee filter
✓ A dark bottle or jar with a tight-fitting lid, large enough for the desired amount of liniment
✓ Labels

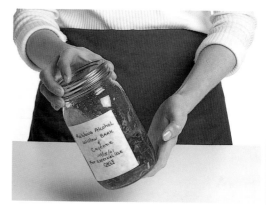

2. Store and shake. Store the jar in a cool, dark place for two to six weeks. Every couple of days, shake or thoroughly swirl the jar to mix the herbs with the alcohol. Herbalists suggest that each time you shake the bottle, you envision your healing intent for the liniment.

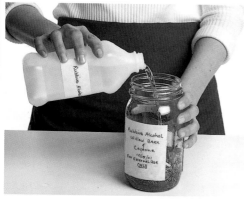

1. Use 1 part herb to 2 parts alcohol. Finely chop fresh or dried herbs and place them in a clean glass jar. Add enough rubbing alcohol to completely cover them. Cover with the lid and immediately label the jar with the ingredients and date and mark it "For external use only."

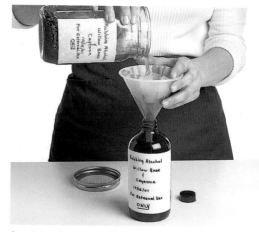

3. Strain and label. Pour the liniment through a funnel lined with a coffee filter into a clean, dry, dark glass bottle or jar. Seal it with the lid, and once again, be sure to label it clearly, as shown.

is capsaicin cream, which is sold in many drugstores for arthritis relief. Usually, however, liniments are homemade.

Unlike tinctures, which are made from vinegar, glycerin, or beverage-grade alcohol, liniments are made with rubbing alcohol, which can be lethal when swallowed. So you should never drink liniment—and be sure that bottled liniment is clearly labeled "For external use only."

As with any medicine, store liniments out of the reach of children.

Infused Oils

MEDICINAL BLENDS FOR RUB-IN RELIEF

Infused, or medicinal, oils are among the most versatile of nature's remedies. Herbalists say that, depending on the ingredients, herb-blended oils can conquer ailments ranging from stomachaches to sunburn. They also serve as exquisite massage oils and insect repellents.

The ancient Romans quite likely made herbal medicinal oils based on olive oil. Nicholas Culpeper, an herbalist practicing in the early seventeenth century, traces olive oil's medicinal use back to Galen, a prolific second-century Roman physician and writer.

You can easily concoct an infused oil using olive oil or another vegetable oil as a base into which you infuse the herbs of your choice. High-quality seed and nut oils also work well. (Don't confuse infused oils with essential oils, which are highly aromatic medicinal oils used in aromatherapy. Essential oils are distilled from huge quantities of plants and can't be made at home without sophisticated equipment.)

Start with the Right Oil

First, choose an oil that meets your needs. For medicinal use, most herbalists prefer top-quality extra-virgin olive oil. Olive oil is relatively stable and doesn't become rancid as quickly as other oils. But a lighter, less aromatic oil like apricot, almond, or grapeseed (available at health food stores) will also do nicely, especially for cosmetic purposes.

Although you can use either fresh or dried herbs, herbalists recommend that if you've never made herbal oils before, you start with dried herbs from a reputable source. The moisture in fresh herbs can promote the growth of mold and ruin the oil. Too much

Making an Infused Oil

You'll need these materials for your homemade medicinal oil.

- ✓ Herbs
- ✓ Oil
- ✓ An enamel, stainless steel, or glass double boiler
- ✓ A wire-mesh strainer
- ✓ Muslin or a coffee filter
- ✓ A bowl large enough to hold the desired amount of oil and herbs

- ✓ A wooden, stainless steel, or plastic spoon
- ✓ A 2-cup glass measuring cup
- ✓ A funnel
- ✓ A bottle large enough to store the amount of oil you've made

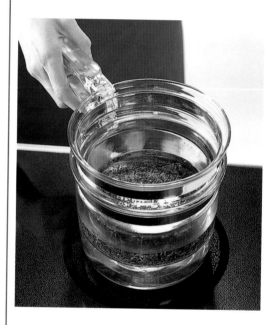

1. Warm it. Place the herbs in the top of a double boiler and cover them with oil. To make approximately 2 cups of infused oil, use 2 cups of dried herbs and 4 cups of olive oil. Make sure that the herbs are completely immersed in the oil.

Fill the bottom of the double boiler about three-quarters full of water and place the top of the pot over it. Set it over *very* low heat, bring to a very slow simmer, and heat slowly for 3 hours. Check the oil frequently; if it starts bubbling and smoking, reduce the heat. Very low heat and long, slow cooking will produce the best-quality oil. *Note:* Overheated oil can cause a fire, so be extremely careful. Follow instructions to the letter, and keep a fire extinguisher handy. *Never* leave the room while making a medicinal oil.

moisture can also promote the growth of the bacteria that cause botulism, a potentially fatal type of food poisoning that can trigger paralyzing symptoms if contaminated oil is ingested.

If you intend to use fresh herbs, herbalists recommend that you reduce the moisture as much as possible to discourage spoilage. Choose herbs that are as healthy and vibrant as possible. Rinse them under cold water to remove dirt, then pat them dry with a towel and place them in a dry, warm, shady spot for several hours or overnight. At this point, the herbs should be drier than when they were

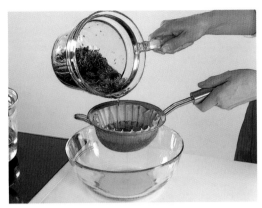

2. Strain it. Line a wire-mesh strainer with clean muslin or a coffee filter. Pour the oil from the top of the double boiler through the strainer into a bowl.

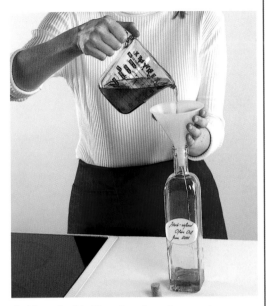

4. Bottle it. Transfer the oil to a glass measuring cup, then pour it through a funnel into a clean, dry bottle, leaving as little air space as possible to discourage spoilage. Seal the bottle with a cork or tight-fitting cap and store.

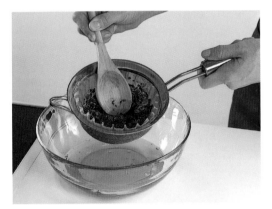

3. Extract it. Press on the herbs in the strainer with the back of a spoon to squeeze out as much oil as possible.

freshly picked. They may look wilted, but they shouldn't be crisp.

Infused oil is rarely ingested, but if there's a chance that yours will be, store it in the refrigerator. If it will be used only topically—as is most often the case—you can simply store it in a cool, dark place. Properly made and stored, medicinal oil should last for several months, especially if stored below 68°F, but not for more than a year. Check it regularly to make certain that it doesn't smell bad. If gas escapes when the oil is opened, it's becoming rancid. If it is spoiled or shows any signs of mold, throw it out.

Syrups and Lozenges

YOUR OWN HONEY-BASED HERBAL SOOTHERS

Like commercial cough medicines and other medicated syrups, herbal syrups are sweet and concentrated. They are decoctions or infusions of herbs that are concentrated via long, slow simmering. And you can make them at home.

Herbalists say that the high sugar content extends a syrup's shelf life and makes some herbs more palatable. Your homemade syrup should keep in the refrigerator for a few weeks without spoiling. The higher the sugar content, the longer it will stay fresh. Discard syrup that smells moldy or releases gas when opened. Lozenges made from syrup should last for several months if stored in a cool place.

You can find some herbal cough syrups and lozenges in health food stores. You can also order herbal syrups from mail-order herb companies. Bottles suitable for syrup are also available by mail order (see "Where to Buy Herbs and Herbal Products" on page 462).

Although you can use any kind of sugar to make a syrup, honey's an excellent choice, especially for cough syrups and others that call for a soothing element. Honey-sweetened syrup also takes less cooking time to thicken.

Since you may not have the energy to make medicinal syrup when you need it the most, you may want to make a batch to have on hand, or at least stock the ingredients. For instructions on making basic infusions and decoctions, see "Teas and Infusions" on page 89 and "Decoctions" on page 90.

Creams

THE NATURAL SECRET TO A YOUNGER-LOOKING COMPLEXION

Women have been enhancing their natural beauty with homemade creams for thousands of years. In 1400 B.C., for example, Queen Thuthu of Egypt was entombed with special little pots to hold her precious creams and oils.

A millennium-and-a-half later, the Roman physician Galen created what may have been history's first recorded face-cream recipe. It consisted of oils, wax, and water—a formula that herbalists rely on to this day.

Like any cream, an herbal cream is an emulsion of two ingredients—oil and water—

(continued on page 106)

Making Syrup and Lozenges

Here's what you'll need.

- ✓ A decoction or infusion for the problem you plan to treat
- ✓ Honey or sugar
- ✓ A glass, ceramic, or stainless steel pan
- ✓ A rubber spatula or wooden spoon
- ✓ A funnel
- ✓ A bottle with a cap
- ✓ Labels
- ✓ Wax paper
- ✓ Plastic wrap

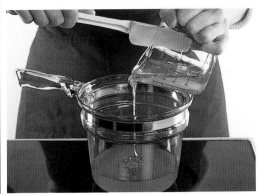

1. Simmer and stir: Place 1 cup of decoction or infusion in a pan and add ½ cup of honey or sugar. Simmer over low heat, stirring occasionally with a spatula or wooden spoon.

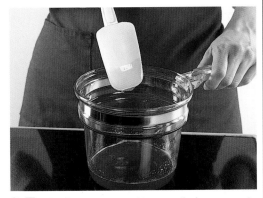

2. Test. Continue cooking until the syrup is thick enough to coat back of the spatula or spoon.

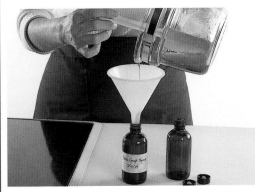

3. Bottle and label. Remove the pan from the heat. When the syrup has cooled to room temperature, pour it through a funnel into a bottle. Cap the bottle, label it with the date and contents, and store it in the refrigerator.

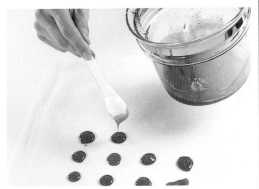

4. Make lozenges. Cook the syrup until very thick (test by dropping a small amount onto wax paper; as it cools, it should harden and hold its form). For each lozenge, drop ½ to 1 teaspoon of syrup onto wax paper. Let cool, wrap individually in plastic, and store in a cool place.

Making a Cream

Here are the materials you'll need to mix your homemade skin cream.

- ✓ A glass or stainless steel (not aluminum) double boiler
- ✓ Oil-based ingredients (see page 108)
- ✓ A rubber spatula or wooden spoon
- ✓ Measuring cups and spoons
- ✓ A food grater
- ✓ A food scale
- ✓ Water-based ingredients (see page 108)
- ✓ A blender
- ✓ Small cream jars
- ✓ Labels

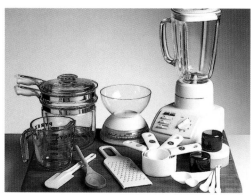

1. Assemble your equipment. Before you begin, gather the necessary materials and wash the utensils in hot, soapy water.

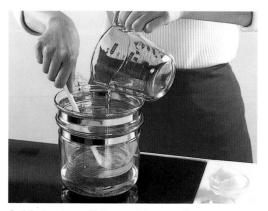

2. Melt the oil-based ingredients. Fill the bottom of a double boiler with water and bring it to a simmer over medium heat. Reduce the heat to low. Grate and measure the beeswax, then place it in the top of the double boiler and set it over the water. Measure the rest of the oil-based ingredients and add them to the pot. Stir gently with a spatula or spoon and warm over low heat just until melted. Pour the mixture into a 2-cup glass measuring cup and let cool to room temperature. The oils should become thick, creamy, semi-solid, and cream-colored. If you're in a hurry, you can chill the mixture in the refrigerator, but be careful that it doesn't get too cold or too hard.

that usually don't mix. (Almond oil mixed with rose water, for example, is an emulsion.) Today's herbalists know, as did the ancients, that natural ingredients like oils, fats, and herbs provide a natural way to moisturize your complexion. And moister skin looks younger, firmer, and plumper. Herbalists point out that making a homemade face cream—sans synthetic ingredients—gives you complete control over what you put on your skin.

Making your own face cream is a lot like making your own mayonnaise, say herbalists. It takes some time to emulsify the ingredients. But what you get is a luscious cream that smells heavenly, glides on smoothly, and moisturizes and nourishes your complexion—at a fraction of the cost of upscale department-store products. (If you're pressed for time, you can buy or order high-quality creams and lotions that contain similar ingredients. Check

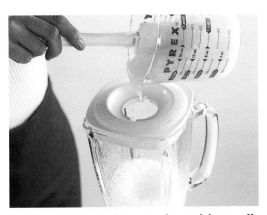

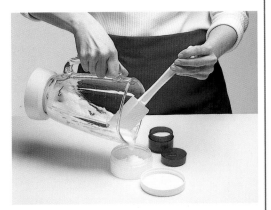

3. Blend oil- and water-based ingredients. Measure the water-based ingredients and place them in a blender. With the blender at the highest speed, slowly spoon the oil-based mixture into the center of the mixture in the blender. When most of the oil mixture has been added, listen to the blender and watch the cream. Continue to blend until the blender "coughs and chokes," the cream is thick and white (resembling buttercream frosting), and there are no water droplets in it. If any liquid remains, carefully blend a second or two longer or transfer to a mixing bowl and beat briefly by hand.

4. Fill the jars. Transfer the cream into clean, dry jars and label them with the ingredients and the date you made the cream. It will keep at room temperature; if you make more than you need, it will keep longer if you store the excess in the refrigerator. Discard the cream if the oils begin to smell sour or rancid or the mixture is moldy.

the shelves of your local health food store or scan the resources in "Where to Buy Herbs and Herbal Products" on page 462.)

As with any other face or body lotion, you can slather herbal cream on your face, neck, or anywhere else on your body to soften and moisturize the skin, say herbalists. And a little bit goes a long way.

The recipe that follows was adapted from one created by herbalist Rosemary Gladstar, director of the Sage Mountain herbal education center in East Barre, Vermont, and author of *Herbal Healing for Women*. Gladstar's recipe is considered the gold standard for face creams, and herbalists frequently use it to teach students how to make top-quality herbal creams. It makes about two cups of cream.

Once you make this concentrated cream, you can customize it to your needs and preferences by changing the fragrance, using different oils, or adapting ingredients to your skin type. If you have allergies to skin-care products or have extra-sensitive skin, try a dab of the cream first in a sensitive, easily monitored spot (the inner forearm, for example) daily for two days, then wait another two days to make sure that you're not sensitive.

You can buy jars or recycle used pimiento jars or face-cream containers by washing them in the dishwasher or by hand in hot, soapy water.

To make your cream, you'll need two kinds of ingredients: Oil-based and water-based. All ingredients must be at room temperature. (For information on where to buy the ingredients listed, see the resource guide.)

Oil-Based Ingredients

🍃 ³/₄ cup almond, apricot, or grapeseed oil. Grapeseed oil is the lightest and least oily choice, and it works well for teenagers or women whose skin tends to be oily.

🍃 ¹/₃ cup coconut oil and/or cocoa butter

🍃 1 teaspoon lanolin (optional; use only if you are not allergic to lanolin or wool)

🍃 ¹/₂ ounce grated beeswax

Water-Based Ingredients

🍃 ²/₃ cup distilled water, distilled rose water, or orange flower water. You can choose one kind of water or mix two or three in any proportion to make ²/₃ cup. If your skin is oily, you can replace part of the water with witch hazel or Queen of Hungary's Water, an herbal astringent that is available by mail order.

🍃 ¹/₃ cup aloe vera gel. Use pure aloe vera gel, available at health food stores. Do not use gel from an aloe plant, as it may introduce mold-producing bacteria.

If you like, you can add a drop or two of your favorite essential oil for fragrance. If you're allergic or highly sensitive to fragrances and usually buy unscented products, you may want to consider leaving out the fragrance. This cream will have a pleasing scent from the coconut oil and/or cocoa butter it contains.

Suppositories

INTERNAL SALVE FOR HARD-TO-REACH AREAS

Making homemade suppositories may not be at the top of your "to do" list. But for some women, herbal suppositories are simple remedies worth considering for chronic problems such as hemorrhoids or vaginal infections.

Any medicated compound that is designed to be slipped into the rectum or vagina constitutes a suppository. Once the suppository is inserted, body heat melts it, allowing the medication to bathe the surrounding tissues.

Making Suppositories

For homemade herbal suppositories, you'll need the following materials.

- ✓ Pure cocoa butter
- ✓ A glass or stainless steel double boiler
- ✓ Finely powdered herbs appropriate for the condition being treated
- ✓ A glass measuring cup
- ✓ A thimble
- ✓ Suppository molds or aluminum foil
- ✓ Scissors

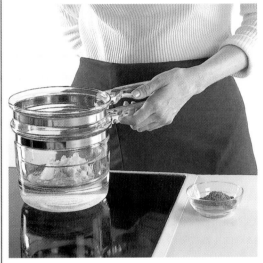

1. Melt the cocoa butter. Melt about an ounce of pure cocoa butter in the top of a double boiler set over hot (not boiling) water. Remove from the heat and stir in powdered herbs.

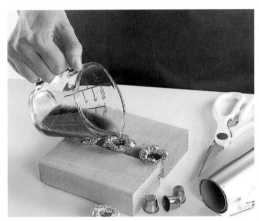

2. Mold into shape. Pour the cocoa butter mixture into a glass measuring cup, then into suppository molds. To make a mold, press a thimble into a sheet of foil, making an indentation about the size of the top two joints of your little finger. Cut away the excess foil around the indentation, leaving a lip at the top so that the mold looks like a small cylinder. To keep it from tipping over when you fill it, place it between two supports, such as two small boards or blocks of wood, as shown. Repeat, making as many molds as you need. After filling, cover the suppositories with foil and put them in the refrigerator to cool and harden. This is a messy process. Be sure to handle the suppositories and molds with clean hands.

Herbal suppositories contain finely powdered herbs blended in a base, such as cocoa butter, that remains solid at room temperature. Unlike medicated suppositories, herbal suppositories are hard to come by in stores, yet taking the time to make them offers clear benefits, say herbalists. Just by changing the herbal formula, for example, vaginal suppositories can be adapted for several different problems, says herbalist Rosemary Gladstar, director of the Sage Mountain herbal education center in East Barre, Vermont, in her book *Herbal Healing for Women*.

Recipes for herbal suppositories range from the simple to the complex and may contain many different herbs. This basic recipe for the classic cocoa-butter-based suppository that herbalists use can be adapted to suit your healing intention by adding appropriate herbs.

If you plan to make lots of suppositories, consider getting ready-made molds. They are difficult to find but are sometimes available at apothecary supply stores in larger cities or at very well stocked herbal mail-order companies. Otherwise, you can make aluminum foil molds that work fine. Always use new aluminum foil, and watch out for tears in the foil that could leak. To store, place them in a clearly labeled container so your kids won't mistake them for Easter candy, and put them in the refrigerator. They'll keep for up to six months.

Salves and Ointments

HERBAL RELIEF FOR TROUBLED SKIN

Medicated ointments (commonly known as salves) are indispensable soothers, used by almost everyone at one time or another for bumps, bites, bruises, burns, and beauty needs. A true ointment forms a separate protective and soothing layer over the skin rather than soaking in as a cream does.

Why take the time to make an herbal salve when you can buy medicated salves at the drugstore? Herbalists offer various reasons—some practical, some philosophical. An herbal salve is yet another way to harness the healing power of herbs. And you can customize it to meet your specific needs. Moreover, a remedy that you make yourself offers the heart and healing touch that mass-produced products lack, says herbalist Rosemary Gladstar, director of the Sage Mountain herbal education center in East Barre, Vermont, in her book *Herbal Healing for Women*.

The base of your herbal salve is an oil infused with the herbs appropriate for the salve's use. (For instructions, see "Infused Oils" on page 101.) Beeswax is added for proper consistency. The proportion is four parts oil to one part beeswax.

If you like scented ointments, you can add fragrance by using a few drops of an essential oil. Two good choices for this are lavender, which is so soothing that you can add as much as you like, and tea tree oil, which has antiseptic and antifungal properties. For salves that will be used on sunlight-exposed skin, steer clear of essential oils made from citrus fruits, including bergamot, cold-pressed lime, bitter orange, and, to a lesser extent, lemon and grape-fruit. These oils can cause skin photosensitivity that could lead to a rash or severe sunburn.

In the event that you don't have the time to whip up your own salve, many herbalists and herb companies offer their own versions for a variety of uses, from first-aid to beauty care. Check the products available at your local health food store or scan the list in "Where to Buy Herbs and Herbal Products" on page 462.

Making a Salve

To set up shop to formulate your own herbal salve, here's what you'll need.

✓ Infused oil
✓ Grated beeswax
✓ Measuring cups
✓ A double boiler
✓ A plate
✓ Short, wide-mouth jars with lids (like half-pint canning jars)
✓ Labels

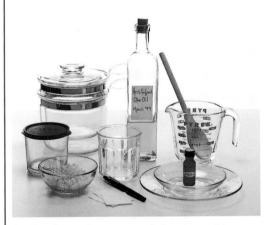

1. Gather the materials. Assemble your equipment, then wash the jars in the dishwasher or by hand in hot, soapy water and dry them thoroughly.

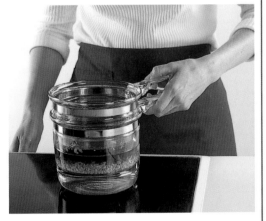

2. Heat very gently. Pour the oil into the top of a double boiler set over hot—not simmering—water and heat just until warm. Slowly add most of the grated beeswax and stir until melted.

(continued)

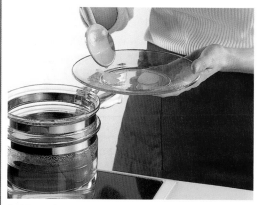

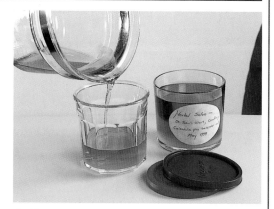

3. Test for consistency. When you've added most of the beeswax, drop a spoonful of the mixture onto a plate and let cool to room temperature. It should be soft enough to scoop from a jar but firm enough to hold together well. If it's too runny, continue to add beeswax until it reaches the desired consistency. Remove from the heat. If desired, add 5 to 20 drops of essential oil.

4. Pour into jars. Carefully pour the hot liquid into jars and cover with lids. Label the jars with the date and contents, then store them in a cool, dark place away from all light. If carefully stored, the salve will keep for at least a year.

Using Herbs Wisely and Safely

FORAGING FOR THE PERFECT REMEDY

Shopping for herbal remedies used to be simple: Stroll to a nearby sunlit meadow or shady forest and gather leaves, flowers, berries, or roots and take them home. Prepare a tea, an ointment, or another remedy or dry the herbal harvest for future use.

How things have changed! While a few women know how to gather wild herbs, most of us are likely to "forage" for convenient, ready-to-use herbal remedies at the local drugstore, supermarket, or health food store, or even in mail-order catalogs. Saunter down the herbal products aisle or peruse a catalog of herb preparations, and you'll quickly discover that hunting for the right herbal remedy these days is no simple errand.

The choices are dazzling, from old-fashioned bulk herbs to suggestively titled tea blends such as Winter Blues, Blossoms of Health, and Wise Woman. You'll find capsules filled with powdered herbs, freeze-dried herbs, and even dried herbal extracts. You may happen upon herbal chewing gums and flavored throat lozenges, eardrops and throat sprays, and salves and solid extracts. Liquid herbal extracts, called tinctures, may claim to be "maximum strength," "supreme" or "double-macerated" (a double-soaking process) and may even come flavored with black cherry, tangerine, lemon-lime, or strawberry. Added to those are alcohol-based tinctures, sweet-and-gentle glycerin extracts, and tablets that melt under your tongue.

You have lots of options but little information. Herbalists have much to say about the power of herbs to remedy and even prevent health problems. But by law, herbal products cannot carry medicinal claims on their labels. Some carry no health information at all. As a result, it can be difficult or impossible to match an herb to your health needs simply by reading labels.

Navigating the Herbal Information Maze

How can you find the right herbal remedy and feel confident that you're taking it in the safest, most effective way? By following sensible, familiar guidelines similar to those that you would rely on when choosing and using over-the-counter medicines for yourself or your family, says Martha Howard, M.D., medical director of Wellness Associates in Chicago. The idea is to match the right herb to your health needs at a dose that provides benefits without unwanted side effects.

"Finding appropriate herbal remedies can seem overwhelming to beginners," says Kath-leen Maier, a physician's assistant, professional member of the American Herbalists Guild (AHG), director of the Dreamtime Center for Herbal Studies in Flint Hill, Virginia, and former advisor on botanical medicine to the National Institutes of Health. "And with so many new products in stores, even women who already use herbs can feel overwhelmed by what they find. In order to feel confident and secure with the remedies you choose, it is best to either work with a practitioner trained in botanical medicine or do your own research."

Yes, using herbal remedies wisely and safely takes some extra effort, a bit more time and thought than it usually takes to run to the drugstore and grab an over-the-counter medicine. Herbal experts say that this extra effort has a big payoff, though, in feelings of pride and accomplishment as well as in the knowledge that you've found a natural, nourishing way to improve your health.

Learning to use medicinal herbs is much like learning to use cooking herbs, notes Mary Wulff-Tilford, an herbalist and professional member of the AHG from Conner, Montana. When you first learned to cook, you probably began slowly, carefully adding measured amounts of oregano to spaghetti sauce or cinnamon to a coffee cake recipe. As you gained experience, you could confidently flavor your cooking with a variety of herbs and spices, experimenting with quantities and combinations to achieve just the right effect.

"Learning to use herbal remedies is exciting and empowering," says Wulff-Tilford. "You start with something simple, and as your knowledge grows, you become braver and more comfortable with herbal remedies. You might start out using an herb like dandelion for water retention and go on to something for a cold or the flu or to help reduce feelings of stress. You build your repertoire and keep on learning. It's a lot of fun."

Labeling Lag

Say that you have a headache, and you're trying to decide between an over-the-counter painkiller like ibuprofen and an herbal remedy like feverfew. The label on a bottle of ibuprofen can say "medicine for body aches and pains." In contrast, the label on a bottle of feverfew, an herb that's often recommended for migraines, might say nothing of the sort.

The labeling is vague because of government regulations. The Food and Drug Administration (FDA) classifies herbal products that have not been through its drug premarket approval process—which means most of them—as dietary supplements, not as drugs, says Judith Foulke, an FDA spokeswoman. "Dietary supplements such as herbal products cannot make druglike claims on their labels," she says. "An herbal product label can include scientifically backed claims about how an herb will change the body's structure or function. But it cannot claim to prevent, cure, or treat a disease."

Vague labeling confuses consumers who are looking for easy-to-understand information about herbal remedies, says Mark Blumenthal, executive director of the American Botanical Council in Austin, Texas. "A label can say that garlic supplements have been shown in clinical studies to lower LDL cholesterol (the bad cholesterol that can promote artery clogging) in the bloodstream," he says. "But it cannot say that regular use of garlic may prevent heart disease." Labels for the popular Chinese botanical dang gui may call it a woman's herb or a feminine tonic for monthly health or say that it supports gynecological health. These are all true but rather vague claims. In practice, dang gui can ease symptoms of PMS. But the label cannot say that, says Michael McGuffin, a trustee for the American Herbal Products Association, a Bethesda, Maryland–based trade organization, and managing editor of the *Botanical Safety Handbook*.

How can you cut through the confusion? "The FDA believes that education is your best tool," Foulke says. That means learning all you can and talking it over with a doctor or other qualified health-care practitioner who has training and experience in using herbs medicinally. (The term *qualified health-care practitioner* is used throughout this book to mean a conventionally trained medical doctor or doctor of osteopathy—M.D. or D.O.—who is also trained in herbal medicine or who consults with a naturopathic physician—N.D.—or other trained herbalist.)

Nail Down a Diagnosis

First, it's important to know that used in the proper doses, herbs are generally very safe. But make sure that you know what condition you're dealing with, advises Dr. Howard. "While it's perfectly fine to treat some problems all by yourself, there are times when you should get a doctor's diagnosis," she says. "Underlying a simple, day-to-day problem could be a serious health issue that you need to be aware of so that you can make an intelligent choice."

If you experience occasional insomnia, for example, one of several herbs could safely lull you into a night of restful slumber. But if you have persistent insomnia, the real cause might be breathing interruptions (sleep apnea) or severe depression, problems that may call for something more than a mild sedative herb, Dr. Howard says. "A doctor's diagnosis can help to determine what's really happening," she says. "Once you've identified the problem, you may still elect to use herbs. You may elect to use herbs even for a serious illness. However, you may want to get medical treatment or use a combination of both." To determine whether or not to seek a medical diagnosis, Dr. Howard offers these guidelines.

Minor or occasional problems? Go for herbs. For small health concerns that come and go, such as the occasional headache or sleepless night, a cold or the flu, a bout of indigestion, a fever under 103°F that lasts less than two days, a case of poison ivy, an insect bite, a short-lived rash, menstrual cramps, or a short period of stress, it's generally safe to use herbs as you would use an over-the-counter medication, Dr. Howard says.

Frequent or troubling problem? Get a doctor's diagnosis. Before treating a persistent health problem on your own, it's important to see a physician to rule out serious illness, Dr. Howard says. "Even a seemingly minor problem like headaches, coughing, or sleeplessness should be checked out if you experience it frequently, if it bothers you for more than a few weeks, or if it is getting steadily, progressively worse," Dr. Howard notes.

As for whom to consult, Dr. Howard suggests getting a diagnosis from a holistic doctor (a doctor who practices medical care that emphasizes the whole person—physical, mental, emotional, and spiritual) or one who is at least open-minded about nutrition and herbs. This could be either an M.D. or a D.O. "These doctors are trained in a Western medical tradition to recognize serious medical problems," she says. "Once you have your diagnosis, you may still elect to try an herbal treatment before opting for drugs or an invasive procedure. The advantage is that you and your doctor will know the real problem you're working on." (Be sure to keep your doctor informed of any herbs that you may be taking. And don't give herbal remedies to children or elderly adults without advice from a qualified health-care practitioner.)

When Herbal Home Remedies Aren't the Answer

While herbal home remedies can be extraordinarily effective, herbalists acknowledge that botanicals can't solve all health problems. "If you have a condition that you'd normally ask your physician to treat, and your intuition tells you not to use over-the-counter drugs, then don't self-medicate with herbs, either," says Chanchal Cabrera, a member of Britain's National Institute of Medical Herbalists (NIMH) and a professional member of the AHG who practices in Vancouver.

The following circumstances call for medical treatment, says Dr. Howard.

Major health conditions. If you have been diagnosed with heart disease, high blood pressure, diabetes, a thyroid condition, cancer, or any other major health condition, or you suspect that you have one of these conditions, and you want to use herbal remedies, work with a doctor who integrates conventional Western medicine with knowledge of herbal healing, suggests Dr. Howard.

You could also find a qualified clinical herbalist who will consult with your physician about integrating herbs into your wellness plan, suggests David Winston, a professional member of the AHG and founder of Herbalist and Alchemist, an herbal medicine company in Washington, New Jersey. (For more information, see "Finding an Herbal Healer You Can Trust" on page 116.)

Finding an Herbal Healer You Can Trust

Consult an herbal practitioner, and you'll learn about more than herbs. Most likely, she will make recommendations about healthy eating, regular physical activity, reducing stress, and even emotional well-being and good sleep habits, says David Winston, a professional member of the American Herbalists Guild and founder of Herbalist and Alchemist, an herbal medicine company in Washington, New Jersey.

"Herbalists try to look at the whole picture of health," he says. "One of our greatest strengths is that we don't hurry. We listen. We talk with our clients about their jobs, their families, and their well-being. Then we try to educate them about ways to live healthier lives." To find an herbal practitioner, he suggests the following steps.

Choose a pro. There's no national licensing process for herbalists, but you can get referrals from several professional organizations, many of whose members are trained in the use of herbs, Winston says. Here's a partial list.

✔ The American Herbalists Guild (AHG). Professional members are peer-reviewed, professional herbalists. Write to the AHG at P. O. Box 70, Roosevelt, UT 84066. They charge a small fee for this request.

✔ The American Association of Naturopathic Physicians (AANP). Members are naturopathic doctors (N.D.), licensed to practice medicine, with degrees from accredited naturopathic colleges. Contact the association at 601 Valley, Suite 105, Seattle, WA 98109. Ask about the fee for their membership list.

✔ The National Commission for Certification for Acupuncture and Oriental Medicine (NCCAOM). This organization can refer you to practitioners of Traditional Chinese Medicine, which combines Chinese herbs with massage and acupuncture. NCCAOM certifies practitioners in acupuncture, Chinese herbology, and Oriental bodywork therapy. For names of members near you, write to NCCAOM at 11 Canal Center Plaza, Suite 300, Alexandria, VA 23314.

Emergencies. Get immediate medical attention, Dr. Howard says, if you have any of the following symptoms.

🐝 A fever of 104°F or higher

🐝 Seizures

🐝 Bleeding that won't stop

🐝 Any rectal bleeding, bleeding from the ear or eye, or bleeding caused by coughing

🐝 A puncture wound, dirty wound, or gaping wound

🐝 Persistent swelling or infection

🐝 A bone fracture

🐝 Chest pain, especially if there's a feeling of pressure or if pain radiates to the left arm, neck, or jaw

🐝 Airway obstructions of any kind

🐝 Breathing difficulties

🐝 Any head injury, even if it seems minor

🐝 Fainting or loss of consciousness

🐝 Vomiting that won't stop

🐝 Severe pain

✔ The American Holistic Medical Association (AHMA). This organization publishes a directory of doctors, dentists, nurses, psychologists, and other health-care practitioners who practice holistic, or integrative, medicine. Write to the AHMA at 6728 Old McLean Village Drive, McLean, VA 22101-3906. Ask about their fee for the membership list.

Ask people you trust for references. If you prefer to scout around on your own, you can try to find a good herbalist the same way you'd go about finding a family doctor, auto mechanic, or other professional: Ask family and friends for referrals. You could also attend classes given by the herbalist or ask your family doctor if she works with an herbalist. Ask prospective herbalists for client references and talk to people they've counseled.

Ask questions. To decide whether or not a prospective herbalist is a good match for you, ask the practitioner about her training and philosophy. Responses may vary from one herbalist to the next. As with evaluating any health-care practitioner, let your intuition and common sense guide you to a practitioner whom you feel you can trust. On the phone or in person, ask the following questions.

✔ Where and how were you trained in herbal medicine?
✔ What is your philosophy about healing and herbal remedies?
✔ How long have you been in practice?
✔ How many people have you treated with herbs?
✔ What is your experience with the kinds of health concerns I have?
✔ How do you treat chronic health problems?
✔ How will you evaluate my needs?

Steer clear of practitioners who want to sell you one particular brand of herbal products, Winston warns. Herbalism shouldn't be a marketing scheme.

Also get medical attention for the following:
🌿 A sore that won't heal
🌿 A mole that changes size or shape
🌿 A newly discovered lump
🌿 A persistent cough that lasts more than three weeks
🌿 Any vision changes (such as partial vision loss or waviness or grayness)
🌿 Persistent dizziness or loss of balance
🌿 Loss of the ability to move or feel an arm or leg
🌿 Redness, swelling, or pain in the calf after sitting for a long time

"All of these symptoms may signal major health problems that need immediate treatment," Dr. Howard notes. "These are not situations to treat at home with herbs."

Pregnancy. Stop using herbs as soon as you know you are pregnant, says Mary Bove, N.D., a naturopathic doctor, midwife, and member of the NIMH who practices at the Brattleboro Naturopathic Clinic in Vermont.

How to Talk to Your Doctor about Herbs

You'd tell your doctor that you took an aspirin for a headache, so why not confide in her about that echinacea you took for your last cold?

"Some people are afraid to talk to their doctors about herbs for fear of negative reactions," says Mary Wulff-Tilford, an herbalist and professional member of the American Herbalists Guild (AHG) from Conner, Montana. But your doctor may surprise you. "Doctors are paying more attention to herbal medicine these days. And they need to know what herbs you're taking, both for their information and for your safety."

Start by telling your doctor about herbs that you're currently taking. Be specific about how much you take, how often, for how long, and what effects you've experienced, suggests David Winston, a professional member of the AHG and founder of Herbalist and Alchemist, an herbal medicine company in Washington, New Jersey. Ask how herbal remedies may affect any medications you take.

Supply your doctor with any written information you may have about the herb or herbs you're using, Wulff-Tilford advises. Above all, be patient and low-key. "By presenting information in a way that's not confrontational, you'll build a better relationship with your doctor," she says.

Dr. Bove and other herbalists suggest avoiding herbs during the first three months of pregnancy and using only gentle, nutritive herbs later in pregnancy. (For more information on safe herbs for the later months of pregnancy, see "Pregnancy" on page 325.)

Since you might not know right away that you are pregnant, you shouldn't take herbs while trying to become pregnant. "Generally, it is best to take only vitamins and no medications or herbs while trying to conceive," says Dr. Howard.

Zero In on the Right Remedy

Once you know what's ailing you, figure out what you need. Botanical remedies have a long history of traditional uses, many of which are supported by scientific research and by healers' own experience. The remedies most often suggested by herbalists often come in specific forms, usually teas and tinctures and sometimes capsules, herbal vinegars, salves, poultices, and even suppositories. It's to your benefit to use the recommended form. When you're choosing among suggested remedies, this expert advice can help.

Tea or tincture? Weigh the benefits. Occasionally, a remedy can be taken as a tea or as a tincture, depending on which you find most convenient. "Teas are nourishing as well as medicinal. They contain some of the vitamins and minerals found in herbs," says Wulff-Tilford. "Tea is also warming, and it is the least expensive way to take herbs for a long period of time."

Tinctures are more convenient than teas (all you have to do is open the bottle), and drop for drop, they are also more potent, she notes. These liquid herbal extracts are often made with alcohol, which can extract some healing compounds that cannot be dissolved in hot water and thus are not present in a cup of tea. Nonalcoholic tinctures, made with glycerin, are also available. Some herbalists use alcohol tinctures straight, but they can be diluted in water, juice, or tea before taking them. Purchased tinctures are more expensive than teas, but if you make your own, they'll cost less to use.

Capsules are widely available and convenient to take, but it's harder to judge quality and freshness, so they're not as highly recommended as teas and tinctures.

Start simply. Begin your journey into the world of healing herbs with simple recipes that use a single herb, herbalists suggest. "That way, you'll know whether it's working. As with prescription drugs, not all herbal medicines work the same on all people, so use one herb at a time until you learn which herbs work for you and which do not," says Douglas Schar, a practicing medical herbalist in London, editor of the *British Journal of Phytotherapy*, and author of *Backyard Medicine Chest*.

As you gain experience, you can try herbal combinations. "Many herbs work together synergistically, which means that combined, they work on a health problem in several different ways," Wulff-Tilford says. "I recommend using combinations of up to four herbs, and I try not to use more than six in a mixture. More than six, and it's really hard to tell which herb is having which effect in your body." (The exceptions are certain multi-herb formulas for tough problems such as endometriosis.)

Learn both names of the herb. "A plant's botanical, or Latin, name is its universal name, the one by which it will be known no matter where you are. But its common name can vary throughout the country and the world," says Dr. Bove.

While most herbal product manufacturers use a standard set of common names that do not vary from product to product or company to company, says McGuffin, knowing botanical names is helpful when buying herbs or discussing them with a health-care practitioner (see "Botanical Names of the Healing Herbs" on page 458).

Leaf? Root? Flower? Every healing herb has one or more parts that are used medicinally, says Schar. Often, the various parts of an herb have the same healing potential; both the leaves and roots of echinacea stimulate immunity, for instance. Occasionally, however, different parts are endowed with different healing properties. Dandelion root improves digestion, for example, while dandelion leaf helps ease water retention, he says. Throughout this book, specific parts of an herb are recommended wherever it is appropriate.

Safety Check

Every woman's health, medical history, and level of sensitivity are different. Just as you would exercise some caution with over-the-counter medicines, women who use herbal remedies are wise to stay alert to the possibility of allergic reactions, herb-drug interactions, and unique, unpleasant side effects, says James A. Duke, Ph.D., a botanical consultant, former ethnobotanist with the U.S. Department of Agriculture, and author of *The Green Pharmacy*, who specializes in medicinal plants. You can minimize the chances of side effects by following this expert advice.

Get acquainted. "Before you take any herb, know its full range of actions," recommends Dr. Bove. Licorice, for example, is known to contain phytoestrogens—plant

Do You Need a Standardized Remedy?

More and more herbal preparations sport the word *standardized* on the label as an indication that the product has been processed to guarantee a significant amount of one or more major active ingredients, says James A. Duke, Ph.D., a botanical consultant, former ethnobotanist with the U.S. Department of Agriculture, and author of *The Green Pharmacy*, who specializes in medicinal plants.

Standardization also means that you will probably pay more for the preparation, Dr. Duke says. But are these chemically controlled products worthwhile? "Standardization compensates for the natural chemical variations found in herbs," he notes. "It takes away any uncertainty over whether you're getting enough of important active ingredients."

Standardization is a good choice when buying herbs such as ginkgo, because it must be processed into a concentrated extract in order to have health benefits, and ginseng, because product checks have shown a wide range of levels of this herb's active constituents, called ginsenosides. But for other herbal products, standardization isn't necessary, says Dr. Duke. "We don't necessarily know which of many active compounds is really doing the trick."

---

substances that simulate the action of the female hormone estrogen. That makes licorice a good herbal ally for some women during menopause. "But licorice can raise blood pressure, so it's the wrong herb for women who have hypertension," says Dr. Bove. Pay attention to cautions about potential side effects of herbal remedies.

Watch for allergic reactions. Just as foods and pollens can cause allergic reactions, so can herbs, Dr. Howard says. "In my experience, allergic responses to herbs are rare, but they do happen. And they can be serious, so knowing how to recognize an allergic reaction and knowing what to do could save your life."

If you have any unusual reaction to an herb, stop taking it immediately. If you have hives or shortness of breath or your throat begins to tighten and close, get emergency medical help fast. If you have a very minor reaction, such as a slight headache or mild digestive discomfort, take a break for a few days, then take a very small amount, such as a few drops of tincture or a few sips of tea, Dr. Howard says. If the symptoms return, stop using the herb. If not, you can use it in small doses, she says.

Don't randomly mix herbs and medicines. "Most mild herbs will not interact with prescription drugs, but we won't have hard-and-fast answers until researchers study each and every herb," says Winston. "Gentle tonic herbs, like mint, lemon balm, chamomile, and nettle, are generally safe."

Just as prescription drugs can sometimes interact unpleasantly or even dangerously with each other and with certain foods, herbs and drugs can interact, too. If you take prescription drugs regularly and want to use herbal remedies, you should first talk with your health-care practitioner or find a qualified herbalist who will consult with your doctor to devise a healing plan, suggest Winston and Dr. Howard.

According to experts, two kinds of reactions can cause problems: those that occur when you combine herbs and drugs that have the same action, and those that occur when you use herbs that strengthen a drug's effect. If you have water retention, for instance, taking an herbal diuretic such as dandelion leaf while you are also taking a diuretic drug could lead to dehydration because both will help your body eliminate excess fluid, says Winston. And sedating herbs like valerian and kava-kava can heighten the effect of sedative-hypnotic drugs like diazepam (Valium) or alprazolam (Xanax), he says.

Dangerous Herbs?

Concerns regarding adverse reactions to herbal products are related to misuse or excessive dosage, says McGuffin. "Taken in the right form at recommended doses for the recommended periods of time, most common herbs are entirely safe for most people," he says. "It's important to remember that we have to respect the plant world: There are poisonous herbs that no one should take, and there are strong herbs that should only be given in tiny quantities, under the care of an expert. But the herbs that people will find in a drugstore or health food store don't usually fall into those categories."

One potentially dangerous yet widely available herb that's received wide attention is ephedra, or ma huang, which is used in some herbal weight-loss aids. A central nervous system stimulant that contains the drug ephedrine, ephedra constricts blood vessels, says Blumenthal. It should not be used by anyone with heart disease, high blood pressure, glaucoma, prostate problems (in men), diabetes, or thyroid problems, he says, and it should never be used by pregnant or nursing women. According to the FDA, products containing ephedra should never be taken for more than seven days. Thus, this herb should not be part of a long-term weight-loss program.

Herbalists say, however, that ephedra does have important medicinal value, and under certain circumstances, they may recommend it to relieve respiratory problems like asthma. (For more information on the use of ephedra, see "Respiratory Problems" on page 341.)

Also, the FDA warns that consumers who have bought laxatives or teas containing plantain should check the manufacturer or distributor and call the FDA's Consumer Hotline (800-FDA-4010) for a list of products suspected of being contaminated with digitalis, a drug that disrupts heart rhythm.

Figure Out the Right Dose

To minimize the chances of unwanted side effects, pay attention to how much of an herb you decide to use. Here's how.

Start small. Doses of herbs are most often given in ranges, not absolutes. An herbalist may suggest, for example, using 15 to 30 drops of an herbal tincture three times a day. Start off with the lowest dose, suggests Wulff-Tilford. Move to a higher dose within the safe range only if you do not experience beneficial effects within a day or two for a sudden problem such as a cold, indigestion, or cramps or within a few weeks or months for a longer-term problem, she says.

Don't overdo it. "Often, less is better," Dr. Howard notes. "Stay within recommended dosage levels for your chosen herbs."

Know when to stop. Follow recommended treatment periods for each herbal remedy. Where suggested, take breaks if you're using a remedy for several weeks or

Herb-Drug Interactions to Watch For

There are hundreds of herbs on the market and hundreds of drugs being prescribed, plus hundreds of over-the-counter medications being sold. Prudence says that you can't randomly mix herbs and drugs without risk.

"Once, the kind of person who took herbal remedies believed in a back-to-nature philosophy and probably wasn't taking any drugs," observes Michael McGuffin, a trustee for the American Herbal Products Association, a Bethesda, Maryland–based trade organization, and managing editor of the *Botanical Safety Handbook*. "Now we have people using prescription medications and wondering how to combine them with herbs."

The best advice? If you're taking a prescription or over-the-counter medication for a condition, don't use an herb that does the same thing, suggests Martha Howard, M.D., medical director of Wellness Associates in Chicago. If you're taking prescription medicines, check with a doctor who practices or is open to integrative medicine before adding herbs to your personal health-care regimen, she says. "You need someone who can monitor you to make sure that the drugs do not interact negatively with the herbs," she notes. "This is vitally important. There's a lot we don't know yet about herb-drug interactions." (Also, be sure to tell your regular doctor about any herbs you take.)

The following table lists some potential interactions, based on what medical researchers know about herbal ingredients and how they could affect the body when combined with some common medications.

Type of Drug	Type of Herb	Possible Effects If Combined
Anti-allergy drugs such as diphenhydramine (Benadryl), hydroxyzine (Vistaril), and astemizole (Hismanal)	Sedative herbs such as passionflower, skullcap, and valerian	Drowsiness caused by antihistamine drugs may be increased
Diuretics such as furosemide (Lasix) and indapamide (Lozol)	Diuretic herbs such as buchu, cornsilk, dandelion, uva-ursi, and yarrow	Diuretic effects may be much stronger, with a risk of abnormally low potassium levels

months. "Give your body time off from medicines," says Wulff-Tilford. "That way, you can see if the herbs have a lasting effect. You also minimize the chances of reactions."

If you have been using an herbal remedy for the recommended period of time and your health condition has not shown signs of improvement, you should consider switching

Type of Drug	Type of Herb	Possible Effects If Combined
Antidepressants such as fluoxetine (Prozac), amitriptyline (Elavil), and imipramine (Tofranil)	Sedative herbs such as passionflower, skullcap, and valerian	The drug's sedative side effects may be increased
	St.-John's-wort	The drug and herb may work against each other
Cardiac glycosides such as digitalis medications like digitoxin (Crystodigin) and digoxin (Lanoxin)	Herbs with ingredients that can affect the cardiovascular system, such as coltsfoot, goldenseal, hawthorn, and motherwort	The drug's effects may be increased
Blood pressure medications such as nifedipine (Adalat), enalapril (Vasotec), and prazosin (Minizide)	Herbs with ingredients that may raise blood pressure, such as licorice	The drug's effects may be lessened
	Diuretic herbs and herbs with ingredients that may lower blood pressure, such as garlic and hawthorn	The drug's effects may be increased or altered
Hypnotic and mild sedative drugs such as flurazepam (Dalmane), diazepam (Valium), and alprazolam (Xanax)	Sedative herbs such as passionflower, skullcap, and valerian	The drug's sedative effects may be increased
Laxative drugs such as psyllium (Cillium), docusate sodium (Colace), and polycarbophil (Fibercon)	Laxative herbs such as aloes, cascara sagrada, plantain, rhubarb, senna, and yellow dock	The drug's effects may be increased

remedies or seek medical help, Wulff-Tilford says. "If your condition has gotten worse, it's time to see a doctor," she says. "If the problem that you're treating is minor, then think about switching to a different herbal remedy. Sometimes we find that one preparation works better than another for a given person."

Keeping Herbs Fresh and Potent

High-quality herbal products are fresh and potent. To get your money's worth, follow this expert advice on purchasing and storing herbal remedies. As with over-the-counter remedies, you should always store herbal remedies out of the reach of children.

Bulk Herbs, Tea Blends, and Tea Bags

Herbs such as burdock, chamomile, and milk thistle are often sold in dried form. Here's how to buy and store them.

Purchasing tips. Check color and aroma. "Do they smell fresh? Do they have vibrant color—green leaves, colored flowers? Dried herbs should look and smell alive," Wulff-Tilford says. "If they're just a brownish dust, don't buy them."

Storage tips. Place dried herbs in airtight glass containers and keep them in a cool, dark place. They will retain potency for up to six months, Wulff-Tilford says.

"The longer you store dried herbs, the less potent they become," notes Dr. Duke. "Light, oxygen, and heat trigger chemical changes that make them lose potency over time."

"It's a good idea to buy dried herbs and tea bags in small quantities—whatever you think you'll use within six months—so you're not left with old herbs that may only be fit for the compost pile," Wulff-Tilford says.

Tinctures

These guidelines will help you find and use good-quality tinctures.

Purchasing tips. Check the origin of the herb and, if possible, of the manufacturer. If information about the origin of the herb is not on the label, you can call the manufac-

turer to find out. "I look for tinctures made with herbs that have been grown organically or harvested ethically from the wild," Wulff-Tilford says. "That way, you're getting a pesticide-free product from a source that's not harming the environment."

Storage tips. Buy alcohol-based tinctures in dark glass bottles and keep them in a cool, dark place. "Alcohol tinctures will keep pretty much indefinitely," Wulff-Tilford says. "There are a few rare exceptions, however. For instance, chemicals in coltsfoot change after two to three years and lose potency. So check the label for any special instructions."

Glycerin-based tinctures, which also come in dark glass bottles, should be refrigerated to prevent spoilage, she says. Less stable than alcohol extracts, these tinctures will stay potent for two to three years.

Capsules and Other Herbal Products

Like over-the-counter medicines, herbal products don't stay potent forever. Here's how to gauge and maintain their effectiveness.

Purchasing tips. Look for an expiration date. "More and more capsules and other types of herbal products carry expiration dates," McGuffin notes. "That's your best gauge of how long to store and use them. If there is no date, I won't use a product that's over two years old. I'll go get a new one if I need it rather than wasting time with something that may not be very strong anymore."

Storage tips. Keep capsules in a closed jar away from heat and sunlight, McGuffin says. "With some exceptions, most carefully stored capsules will remain potent for up to two years," he says. "The active compounds in feverfew break down within a year, for example, while goldenseal remains stable for many years."

Pregnant? Breastfeeding? Heed This

To maintain a healthy pregnancy and to safeguard your child before birth and while nursing, experts advise caution when using medicinal herbs. (For more information on safe use of herbs for these special times, see "Breastfeeding Problems" on page 174 and "Pregnancy" on page 325.)

Pregnancy

Some herbalists and naturopathic physicians recommend completely avoiding the medicinal use of certain herbs during pregnancy. Others recommend using some herbs on a limited basis, especially during the first three months. It's also a good idea to talk to a qualified health-care practitioner—such as a physician with special training in the medicinal actions of herbs—about your concerns before using any herbal home remedies during any stage of pregnancy, even if you don't see them listed here. These herbs are generally safe when used in small quantities to season or prepare food, however.

USE WITH CAUTION

Aniseed	Fennel	Rosemary
Basil	Fenugreek	
Chamomile	Lemongrass	

AVOID INTERNAL USE

Aloe	Bladderwrack	California
Angelica	Bloodroot	poppy
Arnica	Blue cohosh	Chasteberry
Ashwaganda	Boneset	Cinnamon
Barberry	Borage leaf	Coltsfoot
Beth root	Buchu	Comfrey
Black cohosh	Butternut	Dang gui

Elecampane	Lovage	Sarsaparilla
Ephedra	Motherwort	Senna
False unicorn	Mugwort	Shepherd's
root	Myrrh	purse
Feverfew	Oregon grape	Spikenard
Goldenseal	Osha	Turmeric
Guggul	Parsley root	Uva-ursi
Hops	Pleurisy root	Vervain
Horehound	Red clover	Wild indigo
Horse	Rhubarb	Yarrow
chestnut	Sage	Yellow dock
Kava-kava	San qui gin-	
Licorice	seng	

Breastfeeding

To ensure a safe supply of breast milk for your new baby, do not take the following herbs internally in medicinal quantities unless you are directed to do so by an expert qualified in their appropriate use. Using herbs such as basil in cooking is not a problem, however.

Alkanet	Bugleweed	Ephedra
Aloe vera	Cascara	Feverfew
Basil	sagrada	Garlic
Black cohosh	Coltsfoot	Licorice
Bladderwrack	Comfrey	Rhubarb
Borage	Elecampane	Senna

SKIP THESE MILK-FLOW REDUCERS

Parsley, peppermint, and sage, while not dangerous to use while breastfeeding, are counterproductive when consumed in medicinal quantities because they reduce or stop milk flow. Using them as flavoring or in cooking is fine, however.

Your Guide to Safe Use of Herbs

While herbal home remedies are generally safe and cause few, if any, side effects, herbalists are quick to note that botanical medicines should be used cautiously and knowledgeably. Some herbs may cause adverse reactions if you are allergy-prone, have a major health condition, take prescription medication, take an herb for too long, take too much, or use the herb improperly. (For guidelines for using herbs during pregnancy and breastfeeding, see page 125.)

Before you try the remedies in this book, check these safety guidelines, based on the American Herbal Products Association's *Botanical Safety Handbook*—the latest word on herb safety—and on the advice of experienced herbal healers. Then you can enjoy the world of herbal healing with confidence.

Herb	Safety Guidelines and Possible Side Effects
Aloe	May delay wound healing; do not use gel externally after cesarean delivery or other abdominal surgery. Do not ingest the leaf, which is a potentially toxic laxative.
Angelica	Use sparingly and only for short periods of time. Increases sun sensitivity and may cause skin rash; avoid prolonged sun exposure.
Arnica	Do not use on broken skin.
Basil	Do not take large amounts (several cups a day) for extended periods.
Black cohosh	Do not use for more than six months.
Black haw	Do not take without medical supervision if you have a history of kidney stones; contains oxalates, which can cause kidney stones.
Bladderwrack	May reduce gastrointestinal absorption of iron, sodium, and potassium; do not take for more than six weeks. Can aggravate existing acne. Should not be given to children.
Bloodroot	May cause nausea and vomiting in doses higher than 5 to 10 drops of regular-strength tincture more than twice a day. Safe when used in commercial dental products or under the guidance of a trained herbalist.

Herb	Safety Guidelines and Possible Side Effects
Boneset	May cause an allergic reaction in those with allergies or sensitivities, especially to chamomile, feverfew, ragweed, or other members of the daisy family. Can cause vomiting and severe diarrhea in large doses.
California poppy	Do not use with antidepressant MAO inhibitor drugs such as phenelzine sulfate (Nardil) and tranylcypromine (Parnate) unless under medical supervision.
Cayenne	May irritate the gastrointestinal tract if taken on an empty stomach.
Chamomile	Very rarely, can cause an allergic reaction when ingested. People allergic to closely related plants such as ragweed, asters, and chrysanthemums should drink the tea with caution.
Chasteberry	May counteract the effectiveness of birth control pills.
Coleus forskohlii	May enhance the effects of medications for asthma or high blood pressure, with negative results; do not use unless under medical supervision.
Coltsfoot	Do not use for more than one week unless under supervised care.
Comfrey	Do not use topically on deep or infected wounds; can promote surface healing too quickly and not allow healing of underlying tissue.
Dandelion root	If you have gallbladder disease, do not use dandelion preparations without medical approval.
Dang gui	Can increase blood loss; do not use while menstruating, spotting, or bleeding heavily.
Echinacea	Do not use if you have tuberculosis or an autoimmune condition such as lupus or multiple sclerosis. Do not use if allergic to plants in the daisy family such as chamomile and marigold.

(continued)

Your Guide to Safe Use of Herbs—Continued

Herb	Safety Guidelines and Possible Side Effects
Ephedra	Do not use if you have been diagnosed with high blood pressure, glaucoma, heart problems, diabetes, or thyroid disease. Do not use if you are taking asthma medications. May increase the action of prescription drugs. Do not take regularly for more than seven days or exceed a single dose of 8 milligrams.
Eucalyptus	Do not use if you have inflammatory disease of the bile ducts or severe liver disease. May cause nausea, vomiting, and diarrhea in doses higher than 4 grams a day. Do not apply eucalyptus preparations to the face, especially the nose, in infants and young children.
False unicorn root	May cause nausea and vomiting in doses higher than 5 to 15 drops of tincture, ½ cup of infusion, or 3 to 4 cups of tea blend per day.
Fennel	Do not use medicinally for more than six weeks without supervision by a qualified herbalist. Do not give pure fennel oil to infants or children; may cause throat spasms.
Feverfew	Fresh leaves can cause mouth sores in some people if chewed.
Figwort	Do not use if you have a rapid heartbeat.
Gentian	May cause nausea and vomiting in large doses. Do not use if you have high blood pressure, gastric or duodenal ulcers, or gastric irritation and inflammation.
Ginger	May increase bile secretion; if you have gallstones, do not use therapeutic amounts of dried root or powder without guidance from a health-care practitioner. Fresh ginger is safe when used as a spice.
Ginkgo	Do not use with antidepressant MAO inhibitor drugs such as phenelzine sulfate (Nardil) or tranylcypromine (Parnate), aspirin or other nonsteroidal anti-inflammatory medications, or blood-thinning medications such as warfarin (Coumadin). Can cause dermatitis, diarrhea, and vomiting in doses higher than 240 milligrams of concentrated extract (the usual dose is 120 milligrams per day).

Herb	Safety Guidelines and Possible Side Effects
Ginseng	May cause irritability if taken with caffeine or other stimulants. Do not take if you have high blood pressure.
Goldenrod	Do not use if you have a chronic kidney disorder.
Guggul	Rarely, may trigger diarrhea, restlessness, apprehension, or hiccups.
Hawthorn	If you have a cardiovascular condition, do not take hawthorn regularly for more than a few weeks without medical supervision. You may require lower doses of other medications, such as blood pressure drugs. If you have low blood pressure caused by heart valve problems, do not use without medical supervision.
He-shou-wu	May cause gastric distress; do not take if you are experiencing diarrhea.
Hops	Do not take if prone to depression. Rarely, can cause skin rash; handle fresh or dried hops carefully.
Horse chestnut	May interfere with the action of other drugs, especially blood thinners such as warfarin (Coumadin). May irritate the gastrointestinal tract.
Horsetail	Do not use tincture if you have heart or kidney problems. May cause a thiamin deficiency. Do not take more than 2 grams per day of powdered extract or take for prolonged periods.
Kava-kava	Do not take with alcohol or barbiturates. Do not take more than the recommended dose. Use caution when driving or operating equipment; this herb is a muscle relaxant.
Kelp	If you have high blood pressure or heart problems, use only once a day or less.
Licorice	Do not use if you have diabetes, high blood pressure, liver or kidney disorders, or low potassium levels. Do not use daily for more than four to six weeks; overuse can lead to water retention, high blood pressure caused by potassium loss, or impaired heart and kidney function.

(continued)

Your Guide to Safe Use of Herbs—Continued

Herb	Safety Guidelines and Possible Side Effects
Lobelia	Can cause nausea and vomiting in large doses.
Marshmallow	May slow the absorption of other medications taken at the same time.
Myrrh	Can cause diarrhea and irritation of the kidneys. Do not use if you are bleeding for any reason, including heavy menstrual bleeding or breakthrough uterine bleeding.
Nettle	May worsen allergy symptoms; take only one dose a day for the first few days.
Oatstraw	Do not use if you have celiac disease (gluten intolerance); contains gluten, a grain protein.
Parsley	If you have kidney disease, do not use large amounts; increases urine flow in large doses (several cups a day). Safe as a garnish or ingredient in food.
Poke root	Do not take more than 30 drops a day or apply to broken skin without supervision from a qualified herbalist. May cause digestive problems when taken internally.
Reishi mushroom	Rarely, can cause dry mouth or stomach upset when used for more than three months.
Sage	Do not use if you are hypoglycemic or undergoing anticonvulsant therapy. Can increase sedative side effects of some drugs.
St.-John's-wort	Do not use with antidepressants without medical approval. May cause photosensitivity; avoid overexposure to direct sunlight.
Sarsaparilla	May affect the effective dose of prescription medications.
Shepherd's purse	Do not use if you have kidney stones.
Turmeric	Do not use as a home remedy if you have ulcers, gallstones, or bile duct obstruction. Safe as a food herb.

Herb	Safety Guidelines and Possible Side Effects
Uva-ursi	Do not use for more than two weeks without the supervision of a qualified herbalist. Do not use if you have kidney disease; contains tannins, which can cause further kidney damage and irritate the stomach.
Valerian	Do not use with sleep-enhancing or mood-regulating medications such as diazepam (Valium) or amitriptyline (Elavil). If stimulant action occurs, discontinue use. May cause heart palpitations and nervousness in sensitive individuals.
Willow	Do not take if you need to avoid aspirin, especially if you are taking blood-thinning medication such as warfarin (Coumadin); the active ingredient is related to aspirin. May interact with barbiturates or sedatives such as aprobarbital (Amytal) or alprazolam (Xanax). Can cause stomach irritation when consumed with alcohol. Do not give to children under 16 who have any viral infection; may contribute to Reye's syndrome, which affects the brain and liver.
Yarrow	Rarely, handling flowers can cause skin rash.
Yellow dock	If you have a history of kidney stones, do not take without medical supervision; contains oxalates and tannins that may adversely affect this condition.

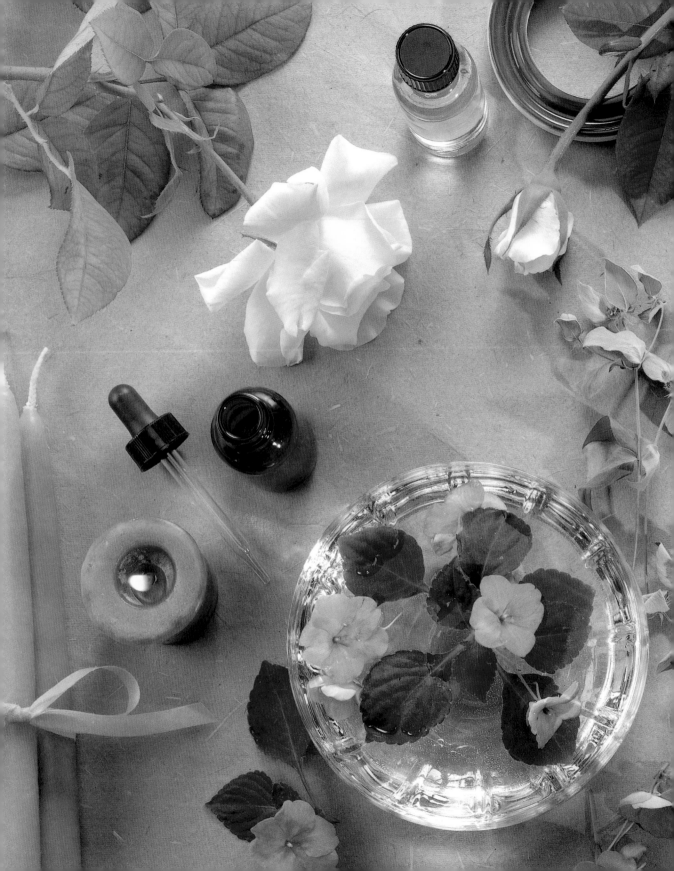

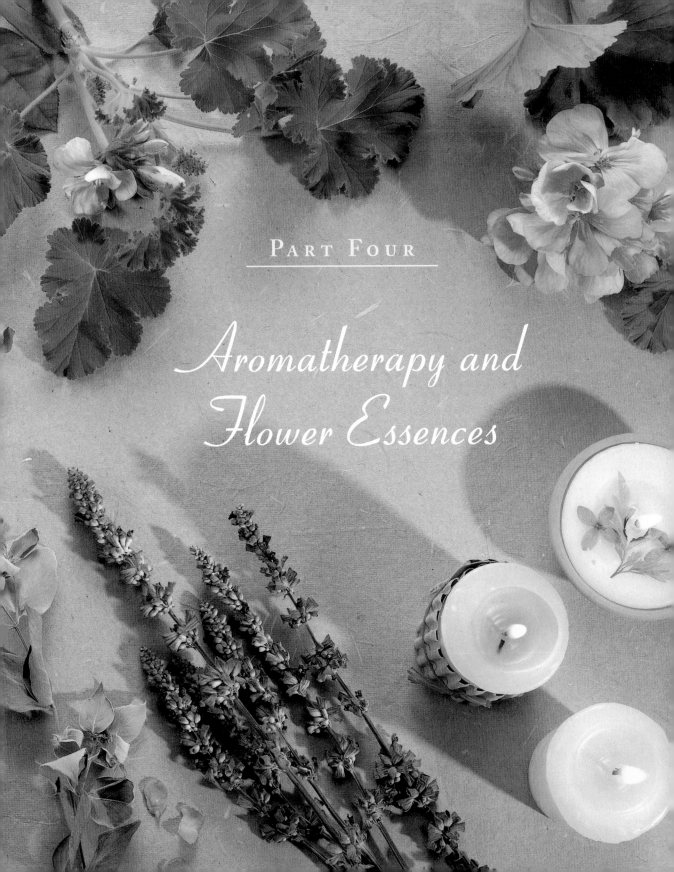

PART FOUR

Aromatherapy and Flower Essences

Aromatherapy

GET IN SYNC WITH SCENTS

I've barely slept in two days! Can you help me?" The voice on the telephone was ragged with fatigue. "I have a business meeting in the morning, and I have jet lag. I'm tired, but my body's not ready for sleep."

Swiftly, aromatherapist Jade Shutes selected a tiny bottle of fragrant essential oil and hurried to meet her weary client.

"I went to my client's hotel and gave her a massage with rose geranium oil," recalls Shutes, who founded the Institute of Dynamic Aromatherapy in Seattle and has diplomas in aromatherapy from England's Raworth College of Natural Medicine and from the International Therapists Examining Board. "Afterward, she had an incredibly restful night's sleep. I think the geranium oil, which was mixed with massage oil, helped restore her body's natural rhythms."

Practitioners claim that when inhaled or applied to the skin, certain aromatic plant-based oils relieve a laundry list of emotional and physical problems. PMS? Sniff lavender. Hot flashes? Take a whiff of clary sage. And so it goes, for menstrual distress, water retention, depression, anxiety, low self-esteem, headaches, infections, skin problems, pain, insomnia, arthritis, colds, high blood pressure, and poor digestion. As a result, drugstore shelves are packed with scented hair-care products. Body lotions claim to deliver aromatherapy-like benefits, and health food stores and catalogs offer blends with alluring names like Inner Woman, Well-Being,

and Tranquillity. You can buy aromatherapy gadgets for your home, your car, and your office, and even to wear as jewelry.

"At one time, the conventional stance was that essential oils do nothing," says Kurt Schnaubelt, Ph.D., founder and scientific director of the Pacific Institute of Aromatherapy, director of Original Swiss Aromatics, both in San Rafael, California, and author of *Advanced Aromatherapy*. "That's changed," he says. A growing body of scientific research is beginning to support aromatherapists' contentions.

At the heart of aromatherapy are natural essential oils—extracts distilled from the flowers, leaves, fruit, bark, resins, and roots of plants. More than 1,000 essential oils exist, ranging from the commonplace like peppermint and cinnamon to exotics such as tea tree from New Zealand, patchouli from Indonesia, and rosewood from India.

Essential oils are potent and complex. "It's not unusual for an essential oil to contain more than 300 different chemical compounds," notes Mindy Green, a professional member of the American Herbalists Guild, faculty member at the Rocky Mountain Center for Botanical Studies and director of education at the Herb Research Foundation, both in Boulder, Colorado, and co-author of *Aromatherapy: A Complete Guide to the Healing Art*. "Oil is so concentrated that an essential oil can be 50 to 100 times stronger than the herb from which it came," she explains. "So you use just a few drops at a time."

Aromatherapy 101: Start with a Soak

The best introduction to aromatherapy is a sensuous bath made fragrant with just one or two versatile, easy-to-find oils, according to Kurt Schnaubelt, Ph.D., founder and scientific director of the Pacific Institute of Aromatherapy, director of Original Swiss Aromatics, both in San Rafael, California, and author of *Advanced Aromatherapy*.

"Start with a scent that you like," suggests Dr. Schnaubelt. "As you gain experience and confidence, you'll gradually learn how to best use aromatherapy."

The best beginner's oils? Try lavender, chamomile, or rose geranium, alone or in any appealing combination. Fill a tub with comfortably warm water. Shake no more than 5 drops of oil (or a mixture such as 2 drops of lavender and 3 of chamomile) into the tub. Swish the water well to disperse the oil, then slide in for a relaxing soak. (Be careful, though; the tub may be slippery.)

As health needs arise, you'll find new uses for your first oils. Herbalists say that lavender oil may prevent scars and stretch marks, soothe insomnia, and alleviate the blues. German chamomile oil, they say, may relieve sore muscles, aching joints, and skin rashes. And preparations using rose geranium oil can reportedly ease premenstrual syndrome and reduce anxiety.

Nose Science

In 1928, French perfumer René-Maurice Gattefoss coined the term *aromatherapy* after the lavender oil that he applied to burns sustained in a laboratory explosion seemed to heal his burned skin. Yet for thousands of years before that, women had been putting fragrance to good use.

Legend has it that Cleopatra drenched the sails of her barge with jasmine, a strong aphrodisiac, before sailing to rendezvous with Marc Antony. He fell for her. In ancient Greece, priestesses hunched over smoldering bay leaves because the fumes were said to induce a pleasant trance. Chinese women carried fans carved from fragrant sandalwood. In the Middle Ages, the abbess and herbalist Hildegard von Bingen spoke highly of fragrant herbs, especially lavender. In India, women preparing for a tantric (Hindu or Buddhist) sexual ritual were anointed with five different essential oils, including patchouli and spikenard, for arousal.

Today, researchers know why scent has such a profound effect on the emotions, especially for women. "We have an immediate response to smells because the same part of our brains—the limbic system—processes both odor and emotions," says Susan Schiffman, Ph.D., a scent researcher and professor of medical psychology at Duke University School of Medicine in Durham, North Carolina. "Aroma and emotions are inseparable."

While women and men seem equally able to detect scents, women are more keenly aware of odors and so may react more strongly to aromatherapy, Dr. Schiffman says. That reaction may vary throughout the menstrual cycle because the female sense of smell rides a monthly roller coaster. It's keenest in midcycle at ovulation, when it increases a thousandfold, and lowest at menstruation.

While it is still not clear whether scent affects us because it directly alters brain chemistry or simply because it triggers memories, researchers and health-care practitioners have documented the effect of aromas on mood, stress levels, and physical health. Here are some of their findings.

🌿 In a study of 56 women ages 45 to 60 at Duke University, Dr. Schiffman found that pleasant floral fragrances eased tension, depression, and confusion for menopausal women.

🌿 In a laboratory experiment with animals, Tokyo researchers found that inhaling chamomile vapors reduced levels of stress hormones in the bloodstream—a finding that seems to support the use of chamomile for menopausal stress.

🌿 Case studies by a nurse in England have found that massages with lavender, bergamot, jasmine, rose geranium, sandalwood, and lemon balm reduced stress and discomfort in women and men who had psoriasis.

🌿 When researchers at Memorial-Sloan Kettering Cancer Center in New York City added vanilla scent to the air during cancer tests for 57 women and men, 63 percent of the participants felt less anxious.

🌿 Scenting the air of a British nursing home with lavender oil helped people sleep just as well as sedative medications had.

🌿 Brain-wave tests show that inhaling the scent of black pepper, rosemary, and basil increases beta waves, indicating a state of heightened awareness. In contrast, lavender and rose produce more alpha and theta waves, which are associated with relaxation

and well-being, according to John Steele, an aromatic consultant, researcher, and founder of Lifetree Aromatix in Sherman Oaks, California.

From the Forest to You

In nature, essential oils help plants attract pollinating insects, repel predators, protect their "turf" against the roots of encroaching plants, and fight disease, says Dr. Schnaubelt. Consequently, nearly all essential oils have antiviral and antibacterial properties.

In aromatherapy, an essential oil might be diluted in water and inhaled using a special device called a diffuser that sprays a cool, scented mist throughout a room. Essential oils are also diluted in so-called carrier oils, such as almond, jojoba, or grapeseed oils, and applied to the skin via massage, body oils, baths, and compresses.

The tiny, easily absorbed molecules in an essential oil, when combined with a neutral

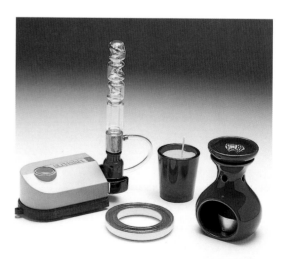

To enjoy the benefits of aromatic essential oils, choose from (from left) an electric diffuser, a lamp ring, a scented candle, or a ceramic diffuser.

carrier oil and rubbed into the skin, quickly make their way to muscles, nerves, and the bloodstream. "These natural oils are perfectly equipped to penetrate the skin," says Dr. Schnaubelt. "So aromatherapy involves the skin as well as the nose. There's nothing else quite like it."

Two Tons of Rose Petals

Plants contain very small quantities of essential oil, so extracting a plant's "lifeblood" can be an elaborate undertaking, says Marcel Lavabre, author of *Aromatherapy Workbook*, president of Aroma Vera, an essential oil company in Los Angeles, and one of the founders of the American Aromatherapy Association. As a result, some oils are quite costly.

It takes 12 pounds of lavender flowers to produce an ounce of lavender essential oil but as many as 125 pounds of rose blossoms to produce an ounce of rarer, more costly rose essential oil. As a result, at this writing, rose oil sells for up to $200 for $1/2$ ounce, compared with $12 for the same amount of French lavender.

Most essential oils are extracted by steam distillation, a process that historians believe was used by the ancient Egyptians. But many citrus scents, such as orange, tangerine, and white grapefruit, are cold-pressed from the oil-rich peel of the fruit. Flowers whose essential oils are too delicate to withstand steam distillation often undergo solvent extraction. The final product is called an absolute; common absolutes include jasmine, orange blossom, and ylang-ylang.

Another aromatherapy product is a hydrosol, or herb-scented water. A by-product of steam distillation, hydrosols are often used in skin care, says Lavabre. Rose water and or-

ange water, two common hydrosols, are also used in cooking.

Aromatherapists insist that only pure, natural essential oils can provide the full range of physical and psychological benefits. "You want the full range of aromatic compounds from the plant," says Steele, who considers essential oils "the lifeblood, or the spirit, of the plant."

Essential oils' natural origins make these extracts especially attractive in our increasingly technological world, says Dr. Schnaubelt. "We feel cut off from nature," he notes. "Not everyone can take a vacation to the Amazon rain forest, but you can go to the health food store and pick up a bottle of wonderful essential oil that transports you to the natural world."

But obtaining high-quality essential oils requires some detective work, notes Steele. Here's his advice.

Ask questions. Call the distributor or manufacturer. Ask about the source of the oils, the distillation process, and whether the plants were grown commercially with fertilizers and pesticides, grown organically, or gathered in the wild, he suggests. "The more a company will tell you, the more you can trust them."

Train your nose. "Compare the same type of oil from several different companies," Steele says. "Start to get a feel for those that really smell like the original plant as opposed to those that just smell like a pale shadow of the original." A genuine essential oil product smells rich, round, and full-bodied, he says, while a synthetic product often smells less complex but more harsh, without the subtle nuances of the true oil.

Avoid impostors. Some fragrances are not available as natural essential oils, adds Green, because they cannot be distilled. They

A Potpourri of Exotic Oils

*C*hoices, choices. With hundreds of essential oils on the market—from rare French jasmine selling for nearly $900 an ounce to Atlas cedarwood, Nepalese spikenard, and beyond—it's tough to decide which to try first when you want something different and exciting. We asked top aromatherapists which unusual or overlooked essential oils they use at home and recommend to women they counsel. Here are their personal favorites.

Red mandarin. This oil has a full-bodied citrus scent—the aromatherapy equivalent of curling up with a good book on a rainy day. "It's like having a warm blanket to comfort you," says Jade Shutes, who founded the Institute of Dynamic Aromatherapy in Seattle and has diplomas in aromatherapy from England's Raworth College of Natural Medicine and from the International Therapists Examining Board.

Helichrysum. Also known as straw-flower, immortelle, or everlasting, helichrysum has a spicy aroma with floral undertones. Practitioners say that it protects and repairs the skin after injury. "Mixed with evening primrose oil and a base oil, helichrysum may prevent bruising and reduce pain, and it may even regenerate tissue, getting rid of scars," says Kurt Schnaubelt, Ph.D., founder and scientific director of the Pacific Institute of Aromatherapy, director of Original Swiss Aromatics, both in San Rafael, California, and author of *Advanced Aromatherapy*.

Carrot seed. This oil has a fruity, uplifting aroma. It improves skin tone, leaving it firmer in appearance. "This is one of my favorite oils because it's so great for the complexion," says Mindy Green, a professional member of the American Herbalists Guild, faculty member at the Rocky Mountain Center for Botanical Medicine and director of education at the Herb Research Foundation, both in Boulder, Colorado. "It's often found in skin-care products, but women overlook it for home use."

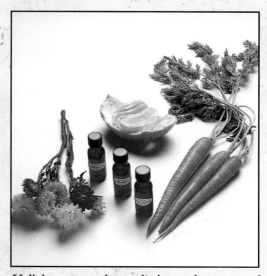

Helichrysum, red mandarin, and carrot seed oils are among herbalists' favorites.

include honeysuckle, lotus, apple blossom, gardenia, and lily of the valley, she says, so if you find these oils on a store shelf, don't buy them. They are synthetics.

Top 10 Essential Oils for Women

While a trained aromatherapist may use as many as 50 to 100 essential oils in her work, you can fill most of your needs with just these 10, recommended especially for women by top aromatherapists. While researchers have documented the effects of essential oils such as lavender and tea tree, the health benefits of others on this list have not been studied as extensively. Aromatherapists and herbalists choose them and recommend them on the basis of years of experience.

Lavender: First-Aid for Body and Soul

If you opt to use just one essential oil, make it lavender. A medicine chest in a bottle, it's one of the safest and most widely used oils in aromatherapy. Lavender may help relieve depression, insomnia, headaches, and exhaustion, creating a feeling that's serene and focused. Evidence suggests that it fights vaginal infections, menstrual cramps, and sore muscles.

Lavender is one of the very few essential oils that can be applied directly to the skin, undiluted. It has a reputation for healing burns, skin infections, and sun damage. All this, wrapped in a sweet floral scent. "When in doubt," notes Green, "use lavender."

A small study in Britain showed that a massage with lavender oil helped ease the discomfort that can follow breast cancer treatment. And when a few drops are sprinkled on your pillow at night, it promotes sleep. "If you're anxious, you can put a dab on a handkerchief or tissue and sniff it once in a while to feel soothed," says Shutes. "Mixed with other oils, it's a great remedy for PMS."

Chamomile: Blue-Hued Calm

Fans of chamomile tea may be surprised by this essential oil. Made from the same tiny, daisylike flowers of German chamomile that are used in the hot drink, chamomile oil is bright cobalt blue, thanks to the presence of a compound called chamazulene. And it has a pungent odor. "Chamomile is good for migraines and PMS. The chamazulene helps reduce inflammation and puffiness," says Green. "Like the tea, it also calms frayed nerves."

Inhaled, chamomile has been used by aromatherapists to alleviate anxiety and depression at menopause. Science is beginning to substantiate that use: In Tokyo, a group of researchers found that chamomile vapors can reduce stress hormones in the blood.

Geranium: Righting the Body's Natural Balance

Distilled from the fragrant leaves of the rose geranium (not the common geranium found on many windowsills), this sweet, rose-and-citrus-scented oil is used by herbalists and aromatherapists to ease fluid retention and menstrual cramps. In skin creams and lotions, aromatherapists use rose geranium to treat acne, eczema, and inflamed and infected wounds. It is even said to delay wrinkles.

"I use it for balancing menstrual irregularities and hormonal irregularities whenever the body's natural balance is thrown off-kilter," says Shutes. "It's great in the bath or in massage oil."

Clary Sage: Well-Being by the Droplet

Distilled from the plant's velvety leaves and purplish blooms, clary sage oil has a winelike aroma and, according to Green, the power to convert depression, PMS, and post-partum depression into feelings of well-being and even elation. It cools hot flashes, quiets menstrual cramps, and prompts intense dreams, too, she says.

"We use it in a PMS blend with geranium, lavender, and a dash of bergamot," says Shutes. "Mixed in a massage oil, you rub it on your abdomen and lower back. I used it for six months and no longer have a problem with menstrual pain or emotional turmoil before my period."

Aromatherapists caution that women with breast cysts and uterine fibroids should avoid long-term use of this essential oil, however, because it has an estrogen-like effect on the body.

Tea Tree: Gentle on Your Skin

With its spicy, eucalyptus-like scent, tea tree (sometimes called ti tree) oil probably won't find a place in your perfume collection. But it may play a starring role in your medicine cabinet. Studies show that this Australian oil effectively fights both fungal and bacterial infections, including the bacteria found in acne blemishes. Aromatherapists recommend tea tree oil for fighting infections of all sorts, from yeast infections to sinus infections and from vaginal infections to lung infections.

Yet tea tree oil is unusually gentle. Unlike most essential oils, if diluted, it can be applied directly to small areas of the skin for short periods of time. Jeanne Rose, an aroma herbalist from San Francisco and author of *The World of Aromatherapy* and *Herbs and Aromatherapy for the Reproductive System*, suggests dabbing it right on acne blemishes.

Grapefruit: A Tangy Pick-Me-Up

Spritzed into the air to cool hot flashes, stirred into a hot bath to relieve menstrual cramps, or inhaled as a depression-fighting scent, grapefruit oil is a brisk refresher. In one small Japanese study, people with depression who inhaled citrus scents were able to discontinue or drastically reduce doses of antidepressant medications.

"Grapefruit is a good example of the variety in essential oils," says Rose. "There are actually several types. I like the bite of white grapefruit oil, but for relieving hot flashes, I sometimes prefer the warmth of pink grapefruit oil. It's nice to know that if your desires change, you can try various options."

Bergamot: The All-Around Remedy

Pressed from the zest of small, inedible fruits grown in Italy, bergamot is the familiar taste in Earl Grey tea, and, says Green, it's a good remedy for water retention, yeast infections, and depression. This oil may even help control compulsive behaviors associated with eating disorders, she notes. An Italian study of bergamot suggests that this essential oil calms the nervous system.

Among the compounds in bergamot oil is dipentene, a chemical that, in nature, helps plants attract pollinating insects and repel germs that cause infection. Dipentene can act as a sedative, among other actions. Bergamot

A Buyer's Guide to Quality Oils

The search for a high-quality essential oil begins with the label, says Mindy Green, director of education at the Herb Research Foundation and co-author of *Aromatherapy: A Complete Guide to the Healing Art*. Even before you twist off the cap and sniff the fragrance, use these clues to track down quality extracts.

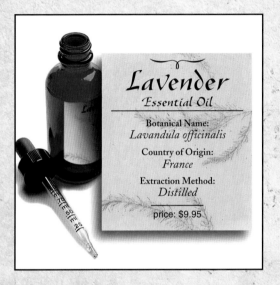

The words "pure plant essential oil." If the label says "essence oil," "fragrance oil," or "perfume oil," it's not a true essential oil.

The plant's botanical name. Latin botanical names are the surest way to identify plants—and the source of essential oils—accurately.

Country of origin. Plants grown in different parts of the world have different characteristics that reflect different growing conditions, and therefore, so do their essential oils. If you like a particular oil from a particular manufacturer, knowing where the plant was grown (such as lavender from France) may help ensure that you'll get what you expect when you buy another bottle.

Extraction method. Was it distilled? Most are. A good manufacturer may indicate the method of extraction on the label or box. Other extraction methods are cold pressing, which is commonly used for citrus oils, and solvent extraction. Solvent-extracted oils are called absolutes.

Price. Beware of uniformly priced oils. Production costs and yield of different essential oils vary widely; normally, their commercial prices reflect that. Given the choice between a $5 bottle and a $10 bottle of a specific oil, the $10 one will probably be of higher quality.

Type of bottle. The bottle should be amber or blue glass or have a dark carrying case to protect the oil from deterioration caused by ultraviolet light.

A dropper. Set in the neck of the bottle for easy use, a dropper also prevents oxidation and evaporation.

---

also contains linalool, a second compound that can fight infection. Another compound, bergapten, may cause a photosensitizing reaction when skin is exposed to the sun. If you plan to use homemade skin-care products that contain bergamot when you will be exposed to the sun, Green suggests buying bergapten-free essential oil.

Ylang-Ylang: Sensuous and Sexy

Exotic and heady, the sweet odor of ylang-ylang is an aphrodisiac for both women and men, according to Rose.

The intense fragrance of this essential oil, which is extracted from a plant whose name means "the flower of flowers," heightens the senses, according to aromatherapists. In small amounts, such as 10 to 12 drops in an ounce of massage oil, this flowery oil has an anecdotal reputation as an aphrodisiac, says Green. But beware, she notes: In concentrations stronger than that, its intensely sweet smell may produce headaches and nausea.

Rose: Irrepressibly Feminine

Intensely floral and totally romantic, oil of rose may very well be the essential oil of love. Green and other herbalists say that rose oil can heal relationship conflicts, "open" the heart, spark sexual desire, and rejuvenate the complexion. "It's the universal female tonic," she notes.

Adding rose oil to a bath is not only soothing and relaxing; according to Rose, it can also counteract heavy menstrual bleeding. The catch? Rose oil is one of the costliest essential oils you can buy. At this writing, ⅛ ounce—less than 25 drops—sells for more than $50.

Breathe in the sweet aroma of rose, and you may ease the pain of loneliness, rejection, or a broken heart, says Green, who counts rose among her top essential oils for women.

Marjoram: The Hard-Working Healer

In a study in Scotland, researchers found that essential oil of marjoram inhibits the growth of some bacteria and fungi. Diluted and applied to the skin, Green says that this oil helps heal bruises and burns as well as easing menstrual cramps and even constipation when applied to the affected areas of the body.

Dilute, Dilute, Dilute

Don't let their yummy, fruit-and-flower aromas fool you; essential oils are concentrated chemicals that can cause burning and irritation if applied full-strength to the skin, says Green. "Dilution is probably the number one rule for using essential oils," she says. "A little is all you need."

Just how little? Most of the time, 10 to 12 drops of essential oil in an ounce of massage oil or unscented body lotion—a proportion known as a 2 percent solution—is just right, Green says. "There is no need to go beyond a 3 percent solution—that is, 15 to 18 drops per ounce of carrier oil—for any purpose," she notes. She recommends a 1 percent solution—5 to 6 drops per ounce of carrier oil—for the elderly, pregnant women (only after the first trimester), and those with health concerns.

Safe dilutions recommended by Green for other uses include baths, 3 to 15 drops; compresses, 5 drops per pint of water; inhalants, 3 to 5 drops in a two-quart bowl of boiled water that has been allowed to cool for one minute before you breathe the steam; foot baths, 10 to 20 drops per one- to two-gallon basin of water; fragrant body water, 5 to 10 drops in four ounces of water (shake well before using).

The exception is lavender, which can be applied full-strength to spot areas for burns, insect bites, pimples, and other skin problems, Green says.

A wide variety of carrier oils can be used to dilute essential oils. How to choose? Rose recommends vegetable oils such as grapeseed, olive, hazelnut, avocado, or sweet almond for massage. "For body oils, a heavier-feeling oil like olive or sunflower oil works well for people with darker complexions, while a lighter oil like almond is good for those with fairer skin, which doesn't absorb the heavier oils as readily," she says. "Jojoba is great for scalp treatments. Experiment until you find the oil that works best for you."

Aromatherapists also offer these tips for using essential oils safely and wisely.

Celebrate diversity. Enjoy a variety of oils, Shutes suggests. Alternate favorite oils and blends, and don't use the same one for more than two weeks as a whole-body massage oil or body lotion. One exception: You can safely use the same oils on your complexion for longer periods of time, notes Green, because your face is only a small part of the total surface area of your body. But keep essential oils away from your eyes, she adds, because they can sting.

Practice safe sunning. Avoid essential oils that cause sun sensitivity for at least seven hours before going out into the sun, Shutes says. Among the most powerful photosensitizing oils are bergamot, cold-pressed lime, neroli, and to a lesser extent, lemon and grapefruit. Use these oils at night or indoors, suggests Green. Other phototoxic essential oils include angelica root, cumin, ginger, lovage, and verbena.

Guard sensitive spots. Keep essential oils that inflame mucous membranes away from the genitals, ears, mouth, and nose, suggests Green. These include allspice, cinnamon, clove, oregano, savory, spearmint, and thyme, among others.

Don't get irritated. Avoid essential oils that are known skin irritants, even when diluted. These are cinnamon, clove, dwarf pine, oregano, savory, and thyme. Other potentially irritating essential oils include basil, cedar-wood, eucalyptus, ginger, lemon, parsley, and peppermint.

Take the patch test. If you have sensitive skin or allergies or you are uncertain about using a particular oil, first do a patch test to gauge your sensitivity, Shutes suggests. Dab a 2 percent solution of the oil in question (diluted with a carrier oil, as described above) on your inner arm or on the back of your neck at the hairline. Over the next 12 hours, notice whether any redness or itching develops. If it does, use a weaker dilution or choose another oil, Green suggests.

Do not take internally. As little as a few drops to $\frac{1}{2}$ teaspoon or less of some essential oils can be toxic if swallowed, says Green, so limit their use to massage, inhalation, and other external uses.

Store oils as you would medicines. Keep aromatherapy products, including essential oils, out of the reach of children, Green says.

Proceed with caution. If you have heart disease, high blood pressure, asthma, epilepsy, or cancer, use essential oils with extreme caution and only after consulting your health-care practitioner, says Green. "Chemical constituents in various oils could exacerbate a health problem by affecting the nervous system, thinning the blood, stressing the kidneys, irritating hypersensitive airways, or acting like a hormone in your body," she notes.

Be very cautious with essential oils if you are pregnant, especially during the first trimester, Green recommends. Avoid them throughout your pregnancy if you are prone to miscarriage. In weak dilution, the following oils are generally considered safe for healthy pregnant women after the first trimester, she says: Lavender, chamomile, ylang-ylang, rose, neroli, rose geranium, sandalwood, spearmint, frankincense, and tan-

What to Do When You've Overdone It

Don't let their sublime aromas fool you: All essential oils pack a potent chemical punch. Practitioners agree that if you use too much, you may develop a rash, feel a burning sensation on your skin, get a headache, or even feel nauseated. Drip or splatter even a droplet in your eyes, and it's sure to sting. Swallow anywhere from a few drops to ½ teaspoon of one by mistake, and it could be toxic.

Here's how to undo the discomfort—and even save your life—when you've overdone it, according to Jade Shutes, who founded the Institute of Dynamic Aromatherapy in Seattle and has diplomas in aromatherapy from England's Raworth College of Natural Medicine and from the International Therapists Examining Board.

If your skin is irritated: Place a few drops of a plain oil (anything from sweet almond oil to olive oil from your kitchen will do) on the inflamed area and allow it to soak into your skin. Leave the skin uncovered and exposed to the air for at least a half-hour. If a rash develops that doesn't clear up in two to three days, seek medical attention.

If you get an essential oil in your eye: Place a small drop of any plain oil in your eye; this will absorb the irritating essential oil. Then draw the oil out of your eye with a tissue or cloth. Rinse with water if your eye still feels sore. Immediately seek medical help if your eye is red and inflamed or if your vision is blurred.

If you've inhaled an essential oil and feel sick: If you feel nauseated, confused, disoriented, or unsteady, or you have a headache, open a window or leave the room and breathe fresh air. You should begin to improve immediately, although some residual symptoms may last for several hours. If your symptoms progressively worsen, especially after you've been breathing clean air for a while, get medical attention.

If you've swallowed an essential oil by mistake: Immediately call 911, your local emergency number, or your local poison control center. You should not induce vomiting; just rinse your mouth with water to remove any oil.

gerine oils. Consult your health-care practitioner before use.

Don't confuse your nose. When using essential oils for their therapeutic benefits, avoid competing fragrances such as air fresheners, heavy perfumes, scented skin-care products, and strong-smelling cleaning products, Green suggests. "Ideally, a therapeutic aromatherapy bath should be taken after you've had a shower," she says. "Don't combine it with scented soaps, shampoos, or conditioners."

Buy what you like. If a scent doesn't appeal to you, you won't derive that essential oil's aromatic/psychological benefits, notes Rose. "It may still penetrate your skin and have some therapeutic effect, but it won't have the psychological and emotional effects you want," she says. "For that, pick another oil with similar effects and a scent that you find pleasing."

Flower Essences

FLORAL THERAPY FOR EMOTIONAL HURTS

The notion that flowers can heal emotional pain isn't all that hard to grasp. We send flowers to console someone who's lost a loved one. We plaster our homes with flowered wallpaper, wear flowered frocks, and plant flowers to beautify our yards and walkways.

Flower essences take floral therapy one step further.

First, a perfect flower is floated in pure spring water in a glass or crystal bowl. Then the bowl is placed on the ground near the plant. After a few hours in the sun, the flower is carefully removed from the water with a small twig. Healers believe that the plant's "energetic imprint"—its emotional healing power, if you will—is transferred to the water. The water is then added to a little dropper bottle half-full of brandy, *et voilá!* A healing flower essence is born.

To use a flower essence, available in health food stores, you simply trickle a few drops on your tongue or sip a small glass of water to which a few drops have been added. They are used for emotional, not physical, problems, depending on what's bothering you.

"Flower essences can shift emotional or spiritual patterns that people may be stuck in," says Gail Ulrich, an herbalist and founder/director of the Blazing Star Herbal School in Shelburne Falls, Massachusetts. "For example, morning glory's flower essence helps to prompt the qualities of alertness and awakening. It etherically conveys the concept of arising with a cheerful outlook on the day,"

says Ulrich. The theory of how morning glory and all flower essences work stems directly from the plants' characters.

"The morning glory's flower opens up beautifully bright with the sun's first light, and it closes tightly in the evening," says Ulrich. "That makes it the right flower essence for someone who hates waking up in the morning," she notes.

"Traditionally, healers treat physical problems with physical remedies, whether they're herbs, pharmaceuticals, surgery, or other treatments," says Ulrich. "But we use flower essences to treat underlying emotional patterns with the unseen energy of flowers." Healers like Ulrich believe that when those underlying emotional patterns are out of whack, the door to illness swings open.

The Origin of Flower Essences

The first flower essences were created some 70 years ago when a respected British immunologist, bacteriologist, and pathologist by the name of Edward Bach, M.D., became soured on his era's medical establishment. Dr. Bach felt that doctors focused on easing symptoms at the expense of curing the underlying causes of disease. And, in his opinion, diseases sprang from emotional discord. He believed that distress emanating from fear, anxiety, panic, impatience, and intolerance sapped the body's ability to fight

(continued on page 148)

Flower Power

THE BACH 12

Call British physician Edward Bach, M.D., the originator of flower power. Back in the 1930s—30 years before the peace-love-and-granola era of the 1960s—Dr. Bach generated his system of healing with flower essences (many of which are herbs).

Dr. Bach believed that emotional and mental harmony conquer suffering. He also believed that flower essences treat a variety of emotional problems, hence preventing or easing the disease process. He said that the healing power of flower essences was divinely revealed to him, and he called the first dozen essences he identified The Twelve Healers.

Before his untimely death at the age of 50, Dr. Bach discovered 26 additional flower essences, including buttercup, calendula, California poppy, calla lily, chamomile, chaparral, cherry plum, crab apple, elm, heather, holly, honeysuckle, larch, mustard, oak, olive, pine, red chestnut, star of Bethlehem, sweet chestnut, vinifera vine, walnut, white chestnut, wild oat, wild rose, and willow.

Here are the original Bach 12.

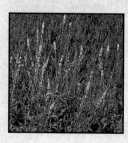

Agrimony. An herb and member of the rose family; for cheerful, peaceful people who loathe discord and whose jovial exterior covers inner torment, sometimes resulting in problems with drugs or alcohol.

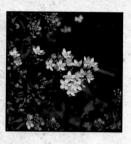

Centaury. An Old World herb related to gentian flowers; for good-natured caregivers who are overanxious to serve others and who could become servants rather than willing helpers.

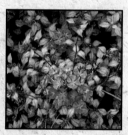

Cerato. A flowering shrub; for those who lack confidence and have trouble making decisions and people who are constantly seeking advice and are often misguided.

Chicory. Chicory is used as a food, a coffee substitute, and an herbal medicine. Its flowers are azure blue. For those whose concern for children and others can be excessive, who continually correct perceived problems, and who need their loved ones to be close by.

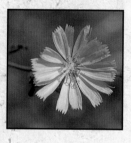

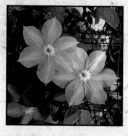

Clematis. A woody climbing vine with fragrant, greenish-white flowers; for dreamy, drowsy, disinterested-in-life people who are quiet, unhappy, and live more in the future than the present.

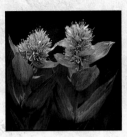

Gentian. A large perennial flowering herb; for the easily discouraged and for people disheartened and doubt-filled over any small setback.

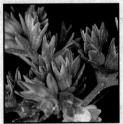

Scleranthus. A flowering herb; for those torn between two choices and for people who keep their problems to themselves.

Impatiens. A garden annual commonly used as a bedding plant; for people who are doers—quick in thought and action and likely to be impatient when they're sick or when others are slow.

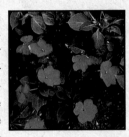

Vervain. A profuse garden flower, usually a deep blue; for those with the courage of their convictions, who are convinced of their rightness, and who have a need to convert those around them to their own views.

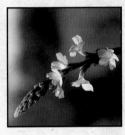

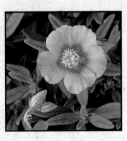

Mimulus (monkey flower). An annual or perennial flowering herb; for fear of the dark, accidents, pain, loneliness, or poverty—or just everyday life, especially for people who keep their fear to themselves.

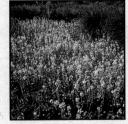

Water violet. A flowering herb; for those who in health or illness like to be alone, who are independent, talented, capable, clever, calm, and self-reliant.

Rockrose. A woody herb; for accidents, shock, sudden illnesses, and extreme terror. Can be applied to the lips if someone has lost consciousness due to an accident.

disease. His philosophy: Cure the distress, and you prevent or even cure the disease.

Ending his medical career at its height, Dr. Bach began seeking remedies to restore emotional well-being. He spent the rest of his brief life—he died at age 50—intuiting which flowers, trees, and plants could help people close "the path to the invasion of illness."

Dr. Bach chose 38 flowers, plants, and trees whose "essences" are now known to the world as the Bach Flower Remedies.

Giving Ease
to Emotional Discord

Each of the 38 Bach Flower Remedies is used to ease an emotional condition. The common garden impatiens, for instance, is "for those who think and act quickly and so want everything done without delay. They are often happier working or being alone so that they can go at their own speed, for they are often impatient or irritated by others who do things more slowly." The impatiens plant, as most gardeners know, gets "impatient" when not watered regularly—just one or two hot, dry afternoons, and it's wilting for the watering can.

During the 1970s, two healers, Patricia Kaminski and Richard Katz, founded the Flower Essence Society (FES). In addition to developing new flower essences, the FES trains practitioners. To date, approximately 60,000 professionals around the world are affiliated with FES, and about 3,000 have taken the FES training, says Kaminski, who is now the director of FES in Nevada City, California.

Interestingly, while Dr. Bach's remedies reflect the downtrodden Depression-era spirit of England in the 1930s, the essences developed by Kaminski and Katz reflect the age-of-Aquarius spirit that dawned in 1970s California, says Kaminski. Among other ac-

tions, FES remedies are said to enhance spiritual development and help remove blocks to creativity and sexual enjoyment. The California poppy, for example, is recommended for those who seek "spiritual highs outside of themselves or are attracted to the glamour and brightness of psychedelic drugs, charismatic teachers, or occult rituals."

Flower essences have sprung up in many far-flung corners of the world, too, including Alaska, Australia, Hawaii, Scotland, the Himalayas, Africa, and the Amazon.

Power of Suggestion?

So, do flower essences work? And if so, how?

"Flowers have traditionally held a sacred place in many healing traditions," says Kaminski. "For weddings or funerals, to cheer sick people, or when you want to send a special message to a loved one, you don't use a plant's roots, you use flowers—lots and lots of them."

Anyone looking for science to explain how flower essences evoke these emotional healing responses, however, is likely to be disappointed, says Anne McIntyre, a member of Britain's National Institute of Medical Herbalists (NIMH), a medical herbalist in practice in Oxfordshire, England, and author of *Flower Power*, which explores the healing power of flowers. No traditional scientific studies exist to back up claims that flower essences help people achieve emotional balance—or anything else, for that matter.

And, says Kaminski, there's a very good reason for the dearth of research. "When you test a remedy for colds, for example, you test a random group of people who all have pretty much identical physical symptoms, like coughs and runny noses," she explains. "You give half of them a remedy, and the other half get a sugar pill. Under those circumstances, it's easy to see what works and what doesn't."

But that model doesn't work for flower essences, says Kaminsky. First of all, flower essence healers don't treat physical symptoms. They focus on the person as a whole, and only after conducting a lengthy history to determine that person's individual emotional pattern do they determine which flower essence is the most appropriate emotional balancer, she notes.

McIntyre concurs. "Flower essences fall into the category of things that can't be computed scientifically. Science will only give you one dimension. Flower essences touch us in ways far beyond the physical into the realms of the emotional, mental, and spiritual. "

McIntyre says that she was once skeptical about the notion of healing emotional upsets with little more than "flower water." "I first and foremost am involved with plants. I grow hundreds in the gardens of our home and use many of these in our clinic, where we make all of our own medicines," she explains. "But I've now come to understand that the relationship between using herbs as herbal medicine, as aromatherapy, as homeopathy, and as flower essences is a very close one. The healing effects of the flower essence of a particular plant are generally in keeping with the herbal use of that plant, and even with its use in aromatherapy."

The closest science has come to testing flower essences in anything resembling a medically acceptable trial involves the use of Dr. Bach's Rescue Remedy, a five-flower combination that's said to relieve stress. Jeffrey Cram, Ph.D., a psychologist with the Sierra Health Institute, an integrated health-care practice in Nevada City, California, studied a group of 24 people. To 12 of them, he administered a placebo (fake) version of Rescue Remedy. The other 12 people got the real Rescue Remedy. Neither group knew if they were being given the real remedy.

Dr. Cram hooked the participants to biofeedback machines to measure the stress produced at key energy sites throughout the body. He then gave all 24 people a stress-provoking serial-arithmetic test.

"All 12 people who got the placebo responded to the test with raised stress levels at the energy sites at the heart and throat. Those sites, or chakras, are said to govern calmness," Dr. Cram says. "The 12 people who got the real Rescue Remedy did not register stress at those sites, indicating that they were calmer and better able to detach themselves from the stress induced by the tests."

Why Healers Use Flower Essences

Healers give different reasons for using flower essences in their practices.

"I find that they're very effective when I'm working with someone who has trouble dealing with a blocked emotion or an emotional wall," says Chanchal Cabrera, a member of the NIMH and a professional member of the American Herbalists Guild who practices in Vancouver. "I use the full set of essences to mix up specific remedies for a particular need, and I find that it helps people deal with issues that they may have been avoiding for a long, long time."

"I think of flower essences as a gentle nudge that helps people connect to their own healing," says Dr. Cram. "I believe there's tremendous power in the ritual of using the essences. When you choose a specific flower essence, one with the attributes said to ease your specific state of mind, you're encouraging change and growth, in the same way that watering a newly planted seed encourages growth."

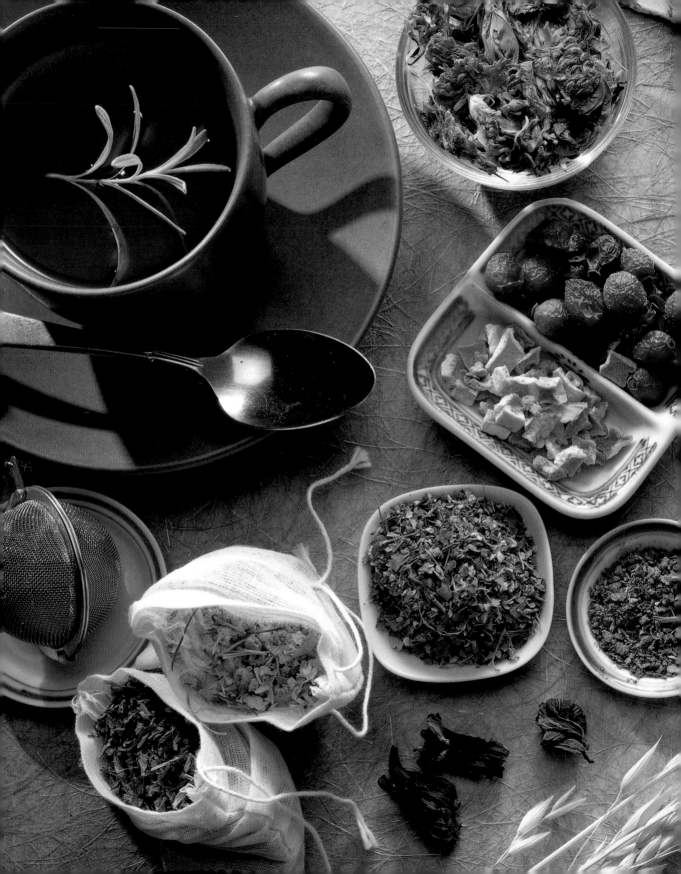

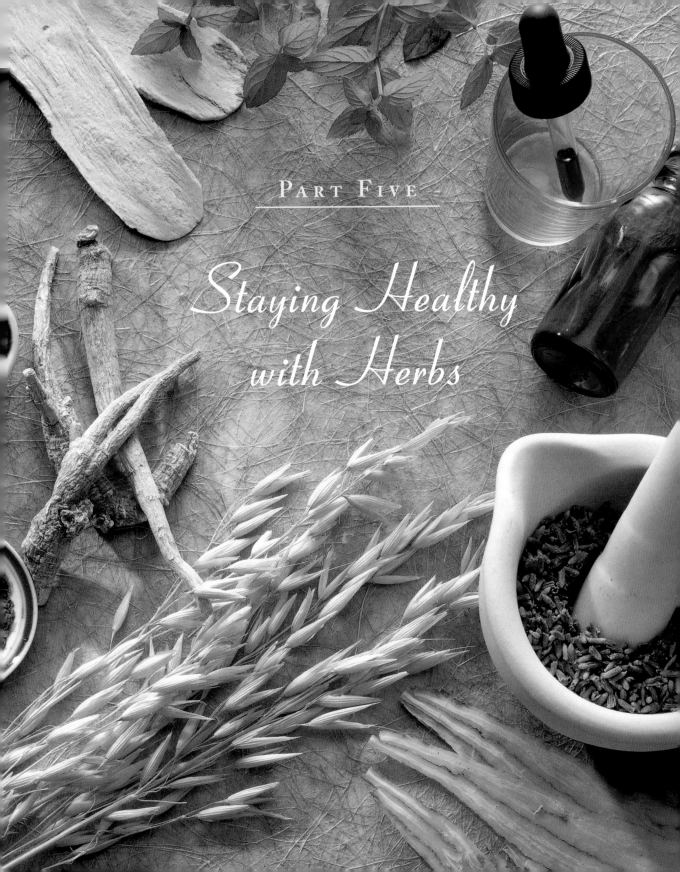

PART FIVE

Staying Healthy
with Herbs

Herbal Tonics

Preventive Medicine from Nature

If you think that an herbal tonic is a natural alternative to a cocktail made with gin or vodka, think again. In fact, you might say that an herbal tonic is the exact opposite of a gin-and-tonic: It's an ancient way of helping your body operate at a healthy peak of efficiency.

Tonics may benefit your health in much the same way that exercise or vitamins do. Herbalists consider tonic herbs to be nourishing, supportive, and restorative. They claim that used appropriately over time, tonic herbs will produce lasting benefits with no dramatic side effects.

"Herbal tonics are a basic concept of Traditional Chinese Medicine—a concept that doesn't currently exist in Western medicine," says David Winston, a professional member of the American Herbalists Guild (AHG) and founder of Herbalist and Alchemist, an herbal medicine company in Washington, New Jersey, where he maintains one of America's largest private herb libraries.

"At one time, at least some American doctors—known as Eclectics—did recognize the value of tonics," says Winston.

"The Eclectics practiced holistic medicine and believed in treating the causes of disease rather than just the symptoms," says Douglas Schar, a practicing medical herbalist in London, editor of the *British Journal of Phytotherapy*, and author of *Backyard Medicine Chest*. "They understood and relied on the healing power of tonic herbs to stimulate vibrant health," he adds.

Not a Quick Fix

Dozens of herbs qualify as tonics. The most familiar are garlic, a classic ingredient in Mediterranean cooking, and ginseng, a time-honored restorative from Asia.

There are two kinds of tonics, says Schar. The first gently improves general health and well-being. The second improves the functioning of a system, such as the respiratory tract or reproductive system. Both types of tonics act slowly and take time to manifest themselves, he says. "Tonic plants slowly undo the unhealthy things that we do to our bodies," says Schar.

The key word here is *slowly*. Using tonics takes patience.

"People want quick fixes, but tonics work slowly and imperceptibly," says Schar. "We're used to downing a cup of coffee and getting that immediate zip, but that's not how tonics work," he notes.

Take garlic, one of the tonics for general well-being, for example. It reduces blood pressure and cholesterol, thus helping to prevent the formation of plaque in the arteries that can lead to heart damage, Schar notes. "But arterial plaque doesn't form overnight—it accumulates over years. And garlic can't cure it overnight, either. No herb or medicine can. So we should start taking garlic now, while we're young," he says.

What's more, tonics work best as part of an overall program of good health, notes Schar. "If you ignore the other known risk factors for heart disease—eating steak seven days a week, working under stress, exercising little, if at all, and so forth—all the garlic in the world won't make you healthy. Tonics work, but they aren't miracle workers. "

Multiple Benefits

Technically speaking, tonic herbs are categorically known as adaptogen plants. That simply means that the herb helps the body adapt to or cope with whatever occurs. To qualify as an adaptogen, an herb has to meet three criteria, says Schar.

"First, it must help the body adapt to various circumstances. As an example, garlic has long been used to help people adapt to high altitudes and to prevent altitude sickness. Another adaptive feature of garlic is its ability to help a person who is working around a lot of sickness avoid getting sick. Schoolteachers and bus drivers are constantly exposed to other people's germs. Garlic's built-in antibiotic helps their bodies deal with this bacterial pollution."

Second, to be considered an adaptogenic plant, an herb must support all major body systems, says Schar. "Garlic improves the functioning of the digestive, respiratory, and cardiovascular systems. It would be fair to say that garlic supports most of the systems critical to life," he says.

Last, but not least, an adaptogenic herb must be perfectly safe to take for long periods of time. "Garlic was eaten as a food by the Israelites while they built the Egyptian pyramids. We know that garlic is safe to use for extended periods of time," notes Schar.

Another good example of an adaptogenic herb is maitake, a medicinal mushroom used in Asia to support vigorous health, says Schar.

"Maitake is used to treat rheumatoid arthritis, a condition in which the immune system is overactive and overzealous," Schar notes. "Yet it's also used as a therapy for AIDS, a disease in which the immune system is dangerously suppressed. In other words, maitake works on either an underactive or an overactive immune system. The dual nature of these herbs confounds people."

Qi Tonics: The Stress Busters

Herbalists like Schar and Winston also separate tonics into two categories—general well-being strengtheners (called qi tonics) and system-specific tonics.

Qi (pronounced *chee*) tonics—from Traditional Chinese Medicine—stimulate the life force. "These tonics activate kinetic energy, the energy that causes the blood to flow and the heart to beat. This is the energy that the Chinese refer to as qi, or 'that which is always in motion,'" says Winston.

"We may not know what the life force is, but we sure know when it's gone," says Schar. "View a dead body, and you know instantly that the person isn't sleeping—the life force has disappeared. Similarly, we may not know what qi is, but we all understand what it's like to be too exhausted to get off the couch to answer the phone," Schar adds.

Ginseng is the best known, most widely used, and most available of all the qi tonics, says Schar. And its popularity crosses cultural borders, not to mention prairies and oceans. "The Chinese have used one type of ginseng for thousands of years. And in this country, at a time when transcontinentental communication was virtually nonexistent, Native Americans used another type of ginseng in the same ways as the Chinese did—as an energy-boosting tonic," he notes.

(continued on page 158)

Your Customized Herbal Tonic

"Herbal tonics really shine in two key areas: Preventing disease and improving subtle problems—those times when you don't feel quite right, but your doctor cannot find anything in particular that's wrong," says herbalist Betzy Bancroft, a professional member of the American Herbalists Guild and manager of Herbalist and Alchemist, an herbal medicine company in Washington, New Jersey.

The most effective herbal tonics are combination formulas customized to meet a woman's special health needs, Bancroft says. "When a professional herbalist suggests herbs to clients, each individual is given a unique formula or remedy."

You can use some of the same common sense that herbalists use to formulate a simple tonic of two to five herbs, based on your individual needs. You can brew a tonic from dried herbs, making them into a tea flavored with orange peel, fruity hibiscus, or spices. Or for convenience, you can take your tonic as a tincture (also known as an alcohol- or glycerin-based extract) added to juice or other beverages as needed.

To create your own personalized formula for better health, Bancroft offers these guidelines.

Identify Your Inherited Health Needs

First, think about health concerns that run in your family. Are you worried that you'll face heart disease, high blood pressure, or other health problems? If your doctor says that you're basically healthy but your elders are subject to heart trouble, for example, then taking a heart tonic may head off future trouble. Then think about your own day-to-day health concerns—perhaps you feel run-down or catch colds and flu easily. Or perhaps stress leaves you depleted. Again, if your doctor says that there's no underlying health problem that needs medical attention, tonic herbs can help bolster and nourish your health so that you can better withstand the onslaughts of a busy lifestyle.

Use your goals to determine which body system to nourish with herbs. "Focus on the one body system that seems to be the weak link or the most problematic," says Bancroft. Then consult the table on the opposite page to select the one or two major tonic herbs that best address your concerns.

Add an Herbal Helper or Two

Next, identify the personal health goal that's most important to you. Do you feel tired all the time? Catch colds easily? Maybe your digestion isn't quite right. If you catch a cold every few weeks, you'll want to boost your resistance to infection. Or maybe a bout with the flu has left you wiped out. If you're tired all the time, you'll probably want to replenish your reserves. Feel gassy after eating certain foods? Maybe your digestive system needs help from herbs.

Major Tonic Herbs

Herb	Body Functions Helped	Potential Benefit
Astragalus	Respiration	Strengthens immune system
Chasteberry	Reproduction	Balances female hormones
Dandelion	Liver function; digestion	Stimulates flow of digestive juices
Dang gui	Reproduction	Promotes uterine function and circulation
Ginger	Digestion; reproduction	Stimulates digestion and relieves menstrual cramps
Ginkgo	Circulation	Promotes circulation and sharpens memory
Lady's-mantle	Reproduction	Improves muscle tone of uterus
Lemon balm	Nerves	Calms and lifts mood
Milk thistle	Liver function	Protects liver from damage
Motherwort	Nerves; circulation	Relaxes heart and calms nerves
Nettle	Kidney function	Enhances kidney function
Oatstraw	Nerves	"Nourishes" nervous system
Red raspberry	Reproduction	Improves muscle tone of uterus
Skullcap	Nerves	Relieves tension
St.-John's-wort	Nerves	Relaxes and lifts mood
Yarrow	Reproduction	Improves muscle tone of uterus

Added to your primary herbs of choice, other "helper" herbs can address additional problems, says Bancroft. These herbs include nerve soothers (important for any woman who feels overwrought or exhausted), stress relievers (to help the body adapt to stress and remain resilient), gentle cleansing herbs (which help if you feel sluggish), and digestive herbs (to promote the way your body processes food and absorbs nutrients). Choose one or two from the list on page 156, based on your needs.

Make Tonics a Habit

You can sip your wellness formula as a daily tea or take it as a convenient tincture, dropped into warm water or juice, Bancroft says. "Personally, I recommend using wellness formulas as teas, sipped throughout the day from breakfast to bedtime," she says. But if you prefer the ease of taking a tincture, that's fine, too. "The most important thing is to take the herbs on a very regular basis by making them a part of your lifestyle. A busy woman

(continued)

Your Customized Herbal Tonic—
Continued

could make up a day's supply of her tea in a thermos in the morning," says Bancroft.

Making a Tonic Tea

Mix equal parts of your chosen herbs. Add a teaspoon of mixed dried herbs (or 1 tablespoon of fresh herbs) per 8 ounces of hot water. Gently simmer woody herbs like cramp bark, yellow dock, or dang gui for 20 minutes, then turn off the heat and add leafy or flowering herbs such as chamomile, oatstraw, or nettle. Steep for 15 to 20 minutes, then strain.

"Always begin with small amounts of the tea—½ cup or so—to make sure an herb is well-tolerated by your system," she suggests. Stop if you notice any adverse side effects. If you experience no side effects, increase to 2 or 3 cups a day.

To flavor your tea, Bancroft suggests adding lemon verbena or dried organic peel for a citrusy flavor, cardamom or cloves for a spicy taste, rose hips or hibiscus for a fruity taste, linden flower for sweetness, or spearmint for a cool mint tone. Use a pinch or so per cup of tea.

Making a Tonic Tincture

Mix equal parts of your chosen herbs in tincture or extract form. To determine the right dosage, look for a ratio on the tincture bottle, such as 1:1 or 1:5, which represents the concentration of herb to liquid. The concentrations of most pur-

Herbal Assistants

Herb	Potential Benefit
Black haw bark	Relaxes muscle tension; relieves menstrual cramps
Burdock	Soothes skin; fights infections
Calendula	Acts as "cleanser" for immune system; soothes skin; fights infections
Chamomile	Aids digestion; fights infections
Cinnamon	Relaxes nervous system; fights infections
Cramp bark	Relaxes muscle tension; relieves menstrual cramps
Ginseng	Eases stress; improves physical strength and endurance
Lavender	Relaxes nervous system, relieves gas
Marshmallow	Soothes inflamed mucous membranes throughout body
Peppermint	Promotes digestion
Red clover	Soothes skin; promotes fertility
Yellow dock	Promotes digestion; improves liver function

chased tinctures range from 1:2 to 1:5, with 1:2 being stronger.

Start with ½ dropperful (about 10 drops) of tonic three times day, diluted in warm water, tea, or fruit juice, suggests Bancroft. "Pay attention to your reaction. If you're sensitive, test each herb tincture individually before combining them. If you have no adverse reaction after a week, increase the dose to 2 to 4 dropperfuls three times a day. Dilute the tincture to your taste," she says. "Grapefruit juice is especially good for masking flavors."

Here are some additional tips.

Don't assume that more is better. "These herbs work slowly but diligently to improve health. You're looking for slow, steady improvement, not an overnight transformation," says Bancroft.

Time it right. "If improving digestion is one of your goals, the best time to take your formula is 15 to 20 minutes before each meal, to prime the digestive system," says Bancroft. "Or to balance energy levels or hormone levels, try to take your formula at very regular intervals so that the amount of herbal compounds in your bloodstream remains relatively constant."

Take short breaks. "Some women stop taking herbs during the first week of their menstrual cycles," Bancroft says. "Others just stop for a few days once a month. This periodic use of herbs, called pulsing, is a practice followed by some herbalists for a long time. Some feel that it makes the herbs work more effectively."

Top off your tonic, then quit. Once you're feeling better, continue taking the formula for about another three weeks as insurance, then stop. Then you can continue taking a maintenance dose, select a new wellness goal, or take a break from using tonic herbs. It can sometimes take months to feel better, in which case you may need more than three weeks' worth of insurance. There is no standard, says Bancroft, because the time is proportional to how long it takes to heal.

Decide on your next goal. "Once you've been on an herbal formula long enough to really feel like it has done its work, you have some choices," Bancroft says. "If there are other areas of your health that you would like to improve, repeat the same process with herbs chosen for new goals. If you want to maintain the vitality and wellness you have achieved, continue taking the same mixture, but take it less often—for example, have one dose a day for a week, then stop for a month, then have one dose a day for another week," she says.

Check herb quality. If you don't notice signs of improvement after using your herbal wellness formula for two to three months, the problem could be poor herb quality. "Look for better-quality herbs," Bancroft suggests. Or you may need professional help in choosing a wellness goal and selecting the right herbs to address it. "Remember, herbs have a lot to offer," Bancroft says. "Don't be afraid to keep trying." (For more information about buying high-quality herbs and finding a qualified practitioner, see "Using Herbs Wisely and Safely" on page 112.)

Scientists first studied ginseng in the 1960s and identified it as an adaptogen. Now herbalists recognize a number of herbs as having similar properties. In addition to Korean ginseng, there's American ginseng and Siberian ginseng. Although Siberian ginseng is only distantly related to the other two herbs, herbalists say that it has similar actions and often group them together.

Astragalus, schisandra, ashwaganda, codonopsis, and gotu kola are also considered adaptogenic herbs. According to practitioners of herbal medicine, these herbs can increase the body's resistance to stress, which also helps increase resistance to disease.

Herbal Tune-Ups, Organ by Organ

Other tonic herbs improve the functioning of specific systems, says Schar. They work slowly to rejuvenate an organ system and help reinvigorate a system following an illness or acute stress. Herbalists frequently speak of "balance" when referring to system-specific tonics because they believe that these herbs help your body normalize itself. Here are a few examples of herbs that act as tonics for specific systems. (For more information about the healing potential of these herbs, see the specific entries in part 2.)

Dang gui. This herb is famed among practitioners as a uterine tonic because they say it has both stimulating and relaxing properties. Herbalists rely on this Chinese herb, a member of the angelica family, for its ability to ease a variety of menstrual problems, including irregular or painful menstrual periods, as well as other complaints.

Hawthorn. There's plenty of science behind hawthorn's positive tonic benefits for the cardiovascular system. In Germany, where herbs are regulated by Commission E, an expert panel that judges the safety and effectiveness of herbal medicines for the German government, hawthorn has been approved as a preventive herb against heart disease. Its actions include regulating the heartbeat and strengthening the force of the heart's muscular contractions.

Licorice. As a specific herbal medicine, licorice is useful for treating inflammatory conditions of the digestive and respiratory systems, like peptic ulcers and asthma, according to herbalists. But licorice, one of the most widely used plants by the world's traditional herbal practitioners, also has tonic properties similar to those of ginseng and is recommended for use following times of extreme stress or illness. Many herbalists believe that adding licorice helps herbal formulas work better.

Oatstraw. A supreme tonic for the nervous system, oatstraw contains saponins known as avenacosides. Although there's little in the way of science to back up its effects, herbalists say that oatstraw is useful as a long-term tonic during times of stress and that it helps you make slow, sustained progress against stress-related disorders like shingles, herpes, and chronic depression.

Taking Tonics Wisely

Although tonic herbs are gentle and generally suitable for long-term use, some people can have reactions to them, says David Edelberg, M.D., founder of the American WholeHealth Centers in Boston, Chicago, Denver, and Bethesda, Maryland, and section chief of holistic medicine at Illinois Masonic Medical Center and Grant Hospital, both in Chicago.

"You're never going to know exactly what action an herb will have on a person until she uses it," says Dr. Edelberg. "Generally, the side effects with tonic herbs are much milder and take much longer to emerge, so many herbalists suggest taking a break from time to time when you take tonics." After using tonics for two months, Dr. Edelberg suggests taking two weeks off.

If you do experience anything unusual while taking a tonic herb or herbs, you should either lower the dose, change herbs, or consult a qualified health-care practitioner, he says. Specifically, he offers these guidelines.

Allergic? Start small—very small. If you're sensitive to drugs, foods, dust, perfume, and other allergens, or if you are generally sensitive to various chemicals in the environment, start with a minute dose of the tonic herb at first, Dr. Edelberg recommends. And for highly allergic people, it's probably best to use one herb at a time rather than combinations, at least at first.

Watch for side effects. "Side effects may not materialize for a long time," says Dr. Edelberg. When he recommends a tonic herb or herbal formula, he gives people a range of symptoms to look for, including the following.

Skin rash. Developing a rash is an extremely common reaction with both herbs and conventional medications. The body is quickly saying no to the substance, explains Dr. Edelberg. Stop taking it immediately and don't ever rechallenge yourself. Usually the rash subsides by itself, and most people take an antihistamine, such as Benadryl, for itching, he says. However, if you're feeling sick, having shortness of breath, or the rash is not subsiding, see your doctor.

Low-grade nausea. "Your stomach may just feel 'not quite right,'" says Dr. Edelberg. If the feeling persists for more than two days, discontinue the tonic, he recommends.

Loose stools. You may feel no discomfort, and the problem may go away within a dose or two. If the loose stools become diarrhea or continue for more than a few days, take it seriously. Consider taking a lower dose of the herb or changing the formula, Dr. Edelberg suggests.

Headache. This is very rare, says Dr. Edelberg, but some people do experience low-grade or front-of-the-head headaches from herbs. Again, consider lowering the amount of herbs or changing the formula, Dr. Edelberg advises.

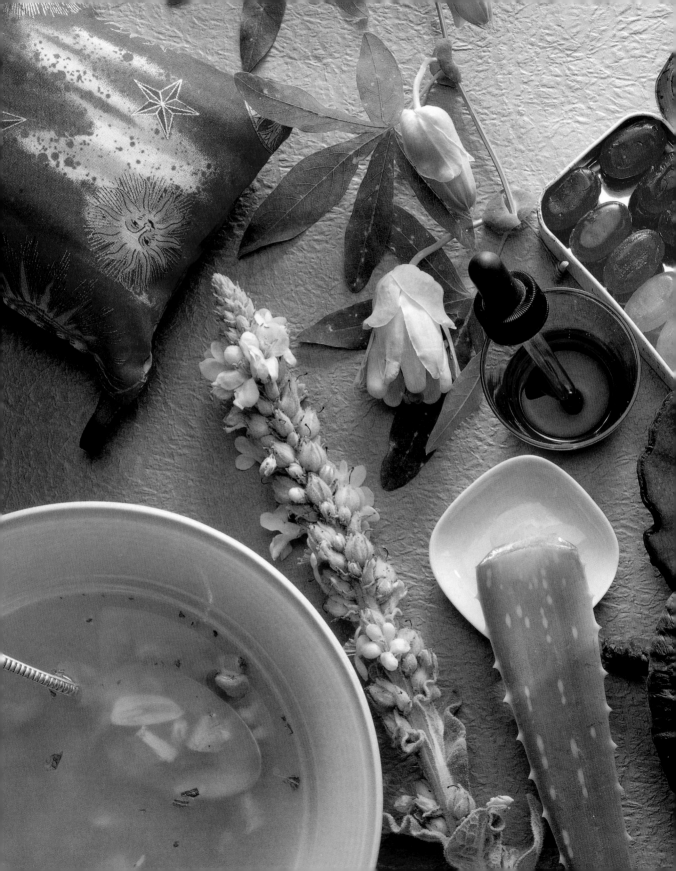

PART SIX

The Healing Power of Herbs

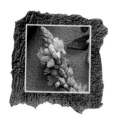

An A-to-Z Guide to Common Problems

Use herbs, and you follow in the footsteps of such illustrious healers as Hippocrates and Pliny the Elder. Back before the Roman Empire, those physicians knew, for example, that licorice could quell a cough. Now science knows that a substance in licorice called glycyrrhizin thins whatever gunk is clogging up your lungs, giving you the productive cough that speeds recovery.

Mediterranean cultures have been touting the ancient plant chamomile as a cure for stomach ailments for thousands of years. And it turns out that there's good reason to embrace the herb: A light blue oil within the chamomile plant causes the smooth muscles of the stomach to relax, says Varro E. Tyler, Ph.D., professor emeritus of pharmacognosy at the Purdue University School of Pharmacy and Pharmacal Sciences in West Lafayette, Indiana, and author of *Herbs of Choice.*

Need a mood boost? St.-John's-wort has been so effective that it's been approved for the treatment of depression, anxiety, and nervousness by Commission E, the expert panel that judges the safety and effectiveness of herbal medicines for the German government and is the German equivalent of our Food and Drug Administration. Even the conservative and highly prestigious *British Medical Journal* attests to the herb's effectiveness. St.-John's-wort appears to affect various neurotransmitters that maintain good spirits, says Dr. Tyler.

And so it goes. In the following pages, you'll find herbalists' "prescriptions" for over 60 everyday conditions, from the miseries of altitude sickness to the annoyance of water retention.

That said, a few caveats are in order. Never try to diagnose a medical condition yourself. And even if you've already seen a doctor about a particular problem, don't use an herbal therapy in place of your prescribed treatment without discussing the change with your doctor. This is especially true if you have a chronic illness such as high blood pressure or diabetes. Some herbs can make it possible to lower the dosage of certain prescription drugs, but this can only be done with careful supervision.

Be extra-careful with heart medications. "Hawthorn, for example, an herb that's commonly recommended as a heart tonic, may increase the effect of digitalis-based medicines," advises Betzy Bancroft, a professional member of the American Herbalists Guild and manager of Herbalist and Alchemist, an herbal medicine company in Washington, New Jersey. So taking both the drug and the medicine can cause serious problems.

Don't try herbal remedies when you're pregnant or nursing. It's also best not to give herbal remedies to children under age 2. For other children under age 16 or people over age 65, seek the advice of a qualified health-care practitioner. She may advise you to adjust the dosage.

And use common sense: If an herb disagrees with you in any way or you develop new symptoms after taking it, stop using it and see your doctor immediately.

Altitude Sickness

HEAD IT OFF AT THE PASS

 ike water, oxygen is one of those things that we take for granted—until the supply wanes.

This is exactly what happens as we rise in altitude. As we climb high above sea level, the oxygen molecules become less dense, and the less oxygen we breathe, the lower our blood oxygen level. At 16,000 feet above sea level, your blood contains a third less oxygen than it would if you were on a raft on the Pacific. Lack of sufficiently oxygenated blood affects the heart, lungs, and nervous system. At 8,000 to 10,000 feet above sea level, symptoms include headache, fatigue, nausea, dizziness, breathlessness, and vomiting. If you go higher than that, potentially life-threatening swelling of the lungs and brain can occur.

Altitude sickness can strike anyone who ventures toward the sky—young or old, man or woman, fit or not-so-fit. Its domain is anyplace where you can almost touch the clouds, from the ski resorts of Aspen, Colorado, to the 29,028-foot-high summit of Mount Everest in Nepal. Folks who live at sea level—the very bottom of the "ocean" of air—and travel to high elevations are two to three times more likely to experience altitude sickness than mountain dwellers, says Benjamin Honigman, M.D., medical director for emergency medical services and trauma at the University of Colorado Health Sciences Center in Denver.

Altitude-Adjustment "Musts"

Herbs can go a long way toward helping your body cope with the physical stresses of high altitude, but a few other steps are also in order. To keep altitude sickness from laying you low, follow these simple rules, says Benjamin Honigman, M.D., medical director for emergency medical services and trauma at the University of Colorado Health Sciences Center in Denver.

✔ Rest a day or so after arriving to help you get used to the altitude.
✔ Don't ascend more than 1,000 feet a day if you're at 12,000 feet or more.
✔ Drink two to three times more water than usual to replenish your body fluids. Aim for one to two quarts a day.
✔ Avoid heavy food, smoking, caffeinated beverages, and alcohol, all of which can make symptoms worse.

Natural Ways to Cope

Most of us are more likely to ski the Rockies than to scale Mount Everest, so priority one is to prevent the mild to moderate symptoms of altitude sickness that are typically experienced at less-than-extreme elevation. Herbalists living in the high country of Colorado say that herbs can help. The ones they recommend contain substances that, taken several days before traveling to higher elevations, help the body adapt to stress and reduce altitude-related symptoms such as headache, nausea, and vomiting.

Adapt with Siberian ginseng. Soviet cosmonauts use it when they blast into space. But Siberian ginseng can help us earthbound folks cope with high altitudes as well, says Brigitte Mars, a professional member of the American Herbalists Guild who teaches at the Rocky Mountain School of Botanical Medicine in Boulder, Colorado.

Siberian ginseng isn't the same as Korean ginseng, which is considered true ginseng, but they share certain properties. Like the Korean type, Siberian ginseng is an adaptogen—that is, it works by helping to increase the body's resistance to stress, "particularly environmental stress," says Mars. (An old-fashioned word for an adaptogen is *tonic*.)

Take Siberian ginseng capsules, available at most drugstores and health food stores, beginning two to three days before your trip, advises Mars. Different brands vary in potency and concentration, however, so follow the dosage instructions on the label, says Mars. The average brand has a dosage of two capsules three times a day, she says.

Quell queasiness with ginger. Ginger is the herb most likely to keep your stomach calm at high altitudes, says Mars. This spicy herb has already been shown in clinical tests to ease motion sickness. Substances called gingerols and shogaols are responsible for its ability to soothe nausea and prevent vomiting.

The recommended dosage is four 500-milligram capsules a day—two in the morning and two in the evening. Start taking the ginger two or three days before your trip, says

Mars. You'll find ginger capsules in health food stores and some drugstores.

Head off headaches with ginkgo. This herb helps the lungs and brain use oxygen more efficiently, says Mars, which is important when you're 10,000 feet above sea level.

Studies have shown that a standardized extract of ginkgo leaves increases the flexibility of blood vessels in the brain, which improves circulation, says ethnobotanist Rob McCaleb, president and founder of the Herb Research Foundation in Boulder, Colorado. Ginkgo also thins the blood, which tends to thicken at high altitudes. The resultant rush of oxygen-rich blood to the brain can help reduce the headaches, dizziness, and confusion that often accompany altitude sickness, says Mars.

Start taking ginkgo capsules several days before your trip, says Mars. Follow the dosage instructions on the label; the usual dose is 120 milligrams a day.

Anemia

IRON-BOOSTING HERBS TO RESTORE YOUR VERVE

The word *anemia* is derived from the Greek *anaimia*, meaning "bloodlessness." And aptly so. Simply put, anemia is the medical term for a decrease in the number of red blood cells or a reduction in hemoglobin, the oxygen-carrying protein in red blood cells. When hemoglobin plummets, oxygen becomes less available to your body's cells.

Several types of anemia can occur, for various reasons. But iron-deficiency anemia is the most common type, affecting nearly 3.5 million American women. Because 95 percent of your body's chemical reactions depend on adequate oxygen, anemia's impact can be profound. It can leave a woman weak and weary—so weak and weary that even simple activities like folding laundry can seem like burdensome chores. It can leave her looking washed-out and pale. At its worst, anemia can wreak havoc with a woman's digestion, including causing abdominal pain and diarrhea.

Diets deficient in iron can lead to anemia. Other risk factors include heavy menstrual bleeding or other blood loss, pregnancy, and breastfeeding, since iron is lost in blood, shunted to a growing fetus, or passed off in breast milk.

Herbs versus Supplements

If you walk into your physician's office with iron-deficiency anemia, you'll probably walk out with a prescription for iron supplements in the form of ferrous sulfate. An herbalist, however, is likely to take a different tack. For one thing, herbalists and other experts question how well inorganic iron supplements like ferrous sulfate (from chemical rather than plant or animal sources) are absorbed by the body. They also point out that iron supplements may cause side effects, including constipation. What's more, evidence suggests that high levels of iron taken for an extended period of time may fuel the formation of free radicals, oxygen-stealing molecules that contribute to diseases such as colon cancer and heart disease.

"There are questions about toxicity and whether inorganic iron aggravates the condition it's supposed to cure," says Cascade Anderson Geller, an herbal educator and consulting herbal practitioner from Portland, Oregon, who teaches herbal medicine to health-care professionals.

Instead of prescribing iron supplements, an herbalist may tell you to eat more leafy, dark greens and other iron-rich foods. And she may suggest some herbal remedies.

Team up with dandelion.   "Dandelion is a great herbal ally for treating anemia," says Ryan Drum, Ph.D., a professional member of the American Herbalists Guild (AHG) and lecturer at Dominion Herbal College in British Columbia.

"Dandelion is a good source of iron and magnesium, which may help your body utilize iron better," says Dr. Drum. "But dandelion also seems to pamper the liver, and it enhances the production of bile, an essential substance that helps your body absorb nutrients."

Make a dandy salad dressing.   "Turn a dandelion into a delicious salad dressing," suggests Dr. Drum. Cut the dandelion leaves off right at the crown of the plant, rinse thoroughly to remove any dirt, and toss a few handfuls into a blender. Add some oil and vinegar (use the same proportions as for your

favorite salad dressing), then season to taste with your choice of herbs and spices. Blend until the dandelion is pureed. Pour freely over a salad of dark, leafy greens like kale, spinach, and parsley. (Make sure, however, that the dandelion you pick comes from a pesticide-free yard.)

Disguise some yellow dock.   "Yellow dock root banishes anemia quickly," says Dr. Drum. But, he adds, its bitter taste can be a challenge to conceal. So try this: Grate 3 to 5 grams (about 1 teaspoon) of dried yellow dock root and add it to dishes flavored with curry, ginger, or cumin. The spices will completely cancel out the herb's bitterness, he says. Another option is to fill two or three "00" size gelatin capsules with grated yellow dock root and take daily. Or simply take commercially made capsules according to label directions. "In my experience, you can end anemia in about a month by taking yellow dock regularly," says Dr. Drum.

Look to the sea(weed).   "The iron in seaweed is easily assimilated," says Dr. Drum, who has harvested and sold seaweed for years. "Use dried, powdered, unrinsed seaweed (available at health food stores), not granular kelp or other rinsed seaweed products. Put it in a jar or bowl on your dining table and sprinkle it freely on food. Aim to add 3 to 5 grams (about 1 teaspoon, or to taste) of seaweed to your meals daily," he recommends.

Use nettle to sting anemia.   "Nettle contains iron," says Corinne Martin, a professional member of the AHG who practices in Bridgeton, Maine. Take $1/4$ to $1/2$ teaspoon (about 30 to 60 drops) of nettle tincture (also called an extract) four times a day, she suggests. Or make a strong nettle infusion: Toss a handful of dried nettle into a quart jar or place the herbs in a reusable cotton tea bag (available by mail order; see "Where to Buy Herbs and Herbal Products" on page 462) and put it in the jar. Nearly fill the jar with boiling water and let steep overnight at room temperature. You don't have to refrigerate it. In the morning, strain the infusion or remove the tea bag, pressing on the solids in the strainer or on the tea bag to extract as much liquid as possible. Add a dropperful of yellow dock tincture to the infusion and drink freely throughout the day.

As you notice improvement over a two- to three-month period, you can decrease the number of daily doses until you feel better, says Martin. If you don't notice improvement in that time period, consult a qualified health-care practitioner.

Herbalists note that it's a good idea when using any herb for the first time to start with one dose the first day and work up to the suggested dose gradually, especially if you tend to have allergies. In some people, taking more than one dose of nettle a day may worsen allergy symptoms.

Brew a blood-building vinegar. Geller offers a vinegar recipe that "tastes delicious and helps boost your iron, too," she says. Soak a handful of yellow dock root and nettle—fresh or dried—in a quart of red or white wine vinegar or apple cider vinegar. Make sure the herbs are completely submerged, and shake periodically. There's no need to refrigerate. After a week to 10 days, strain out the herbs, pressing well to extract as much liquid as possible. You can store the vinegar unrefrigerated in a jar or bottle for a year or longer. Use it on salads or vegetables or in cooking, Geller suggests.

Enjoy a fruit compote. "I like to use a lot of dried fruits to treat anemia because combined, they're high in iron, and they taste so good," says Geller. Put 1 ounce (about ¼ cup) each of dried figs, dates, mangoes, pears, and prunes in a saucepan. Add water to just cover the fruit and simmer until soft, about 5 to 10 minutes Add the juice of a lemon just before you're ready to drink the juice and eat the fruit; the lemon will help you absorb the minerals in the fruit, says Geller.

Arthritis

HERBAL PAINKILLERS TO EASE ACHY JOINTS

Picture the rusty Tin Man in *The Wizard of Oz*. Those creaky, crackly, frozen joints and that herky-jerky walk probably weren't created as the perfect visual metaphor for arthritis. But as metaphors go, it's pretty accurate. If the Tin Man had been female, the image would have been even more on point.

More than a hundred forms of arthritis exist. Degenerative joint disease (osteoarthritis) is commonly called the wear-and-tear arthritis because it occurs when the cartilage within the joints breaks down. The cause of rheumatoid arthritis, another common form, is unknown, but experts speculate that it may occur when the immune system attacks normal joint tissues.

"Two to three times as many women as men get rheumatoid arthritis, and osteoarthritis tends to be a woman's problem, too," says Douglas Schar, a practicing medical herbalist in London, editor of the *British Journal of Phytotherapy*, and author of *Backyard Medicine Chest*. Osteoarthritis is actually two to three times more common in women than in men.

"The mainstream approach to treating arthritis is to rely on drugs like steroids, nonsteroidal anti-inflammatory drugs, and sometimes surgery," says Eugene Zampieron, N.D., a naturopathic doctor, professional member of the American Herbalists Guild (AHG) from Woodbury, Connecticut, and co-author of *The Definitive Guide to Arthritis*. "Steroids and surgery can have serious complications," he notes.

Tea, Bath, or Massage?

"Herbal medicine has some wonderful answers for arthritis pain," says Margi Flint, a professional member of the AHG from Marblehead, Massachusetts, who teaches herbal approaches to health at Tufts University School of Medicine in Boston and is a practicing herbalist at AtlantiCare Hospital in Lynn, Massachusetts. "Taking a hot herbal bath or getting a massage with medicinal oils can go a long way toward easing pain and stiffness. When a woman with arthritis consults me, I ask her which treatment she would prefer, baths or massage. Then I make up an anti-arthritis formula just for her—an infusion for the bath, bath salts, or massage oil. When I make her something that she likes to use, she's more likely to stick with the program."

No matter which type of arthritis makes you ache and creak, herbalists offer these remedies for the pain and stiffness.

Sip some white willow bark tea. "Aspirin was discovered more than 100 years ago by a German chemist who studied white willow bark's pain-relieving properties," says Schar. But white willow bark has an edge over aspirin—it doesn't cause stomach irritation as aspirin can, adds Schar. It may not be the best-tasting beverage, but a strong cup of white willow bark tea will do wonders to relieve the inflammation in a sore joint, he notes.

To make the tea, steep 1 teaspoon of white willow bark in a cup of boiling water, covered, for 15 minutes. Strain out the bark and drink a cup three times a day.

Mix up an herbal rubdown. "A medicated rub made with pure essential oils can ease inflammation and joint pain," says Schar. "Here's my favorite: Get a small jar of petroleum jelly and discard 1 tablespoon. To the jar, add 20 drops of essential oil of lemon and 20 drops of essential oil of sandalwood. Mix the oils well into the petroleum jelly and apply a dab to the sore joint four times a day."

Infuse yourself with some burdock and dandelion. "Herbalists know that if you stimulate liver function and improve the flow of bile, it helps to improve arthritis," says Schar. "Old medical books say that arthritis is caused by improper elimination of waste. While we don't know whether that's true scientifically, we do know that people feel that their arthritis improves when they use herbs like dandelion and burdock, which stimulate liver and kidney function."

For tea, boil 1 teaspoon each of dried dandelion root and dried burdock root in 3 cups of water for 5 minutes, then sip it throughout

Nettle Cuts Need for Arthritis Drug

If you've ever walked through a meadow or weeded a brushy backyard patch, you've probably experienced the welt-raising sting of common stinging nettle. Now, a scientific encounter with nettle suggests that the weedy plant may be able to boost the painkilling ability of a drug taken to relieve arthritis pain.

Scientists at the University of Frankfurt, the University of Dusseldorf, and St. Elisabeth's Clinic in Straubing, Germany, studied 40 people with sudden, severe episodes of arthritis. Half the people were given 200 milligrams of diclofenac (Cataflam), a non-steroidal anti-inflammatory drug (NSAID) used for arthritis pain. The others were given 50 milligrams of diclofenac and 50 grams of stewed nettle leaves. (Heating or drying nettle removes the sting.) In other words, the second group took considerably less medication.

People in both groups experienced considerably less pain and stiffness. The researchers noted a previous study in which people with arthritis were able to cut their doses of NSAIDs in half by taking 1,340 milligrams of dried, powdered nettle. The next step, they say, is to find out whether stinging nettle can ease acute attacks of arthritis on its own, without the use of drugs. But until researchers learn more, please check with your doctor before trying to cut back on the amount of medication you take.

the day. Drink it daily until you notice some improvement. Be prepared, though—the tea tastes bitter. You can add a little honey to make it more palatable, Schar says.

Try agrimony. "Known as a traditional medicine for what people used to call rheumatism, agrimony is a great herb for reducing pain and inflammation," says Flint. Herbal textbooks recommend taking one to three drops of tincture (also called an extract) one to three times a day as needed for pain.

Rub on black cohosh oil or cream. "I like to make an infused oil with black cohosh leaves, which you can pick from the plant without sacrificing the root, so it regenerates," says Flint. "Black cohosh holds an affinity for women in their menopausal years, when arthritis typically develops." (Black co-hosh should not be used for more than six months.)

Flint sees symbolic connections between black cohosh and women entering their mature years. "When you look at black cohosh in the spring, it is all curled up within itself, looking like an arthritic limb," Flint says. "Then it opens and straightens to wave its beautiful white flowers atop the fairy wand. It's a wonderful signature for the changes in menopause as we turn white and learn to straighten and wave in the wind."

Traditionally, Native Americans used black cohosh for rheumatism; American colonists used it for similarly painful conditions such as lumbago, a type of back pain.

"You can also make the oil with dried black cohosh leaves or root," says Flint. "Infused black cohosh oil makes a wonderful cream with the addition of a drop or two of a warming essential oil like eucalyptus or ginger, which help ease pain." Follow the directions for making face cream on page 104, substituting the infused black cohosh oil and adding the essential oil of your choice. (To make your own infused oil, follow the directions in "Infused Oils" on page 101. Some infused oils are also available by mail order; see "Where to Buy Herbs and Herbal Products" on page 462) Whether you use the oil or the cream, rub it on the painful area once or twice a day, advises Flint.

Bathe in black cohosh. Add a few tablespoons of black cohosh infused oil to a tub of hot water, suggests Flint. The combination of the heat and the herbal oil will help relieve pain, she says.

Concoct your own bath salts. "To ¼ cup of sea salt, add 1 tablespoon of either St.-John's-wort infused oil or black cohosh infused oil," says Flint. Used externally, St.-John's-wort helps reduce inflammation. Fill a tub with hot water and add the bath salts. "The salt absorbs the oil, and when the water dissolves the salt, the oil floats on top of the water," says Flint. "The combination helps remineralize your body and coats it with the therapeutic oil." Be careful getting out of the tub, though—the oil may make it slippery.

Athlete's Foot

DITCH THE ITCH WITH TEA TREE OIL AND GARLIC

*L*ike microscopic banditos, the tiny fungi responsible for athlete's foot discomfort hide out in some unsavory, hard-to-reach locales—the warm, moist layers of skin on your feet, your nails, and even your scalp.

Once they've moved in, these fungal bad guys raise a ruckus in the form of itching, peeling, cracking skin. Evicting them can be a tough job—over-the-counter and even prescription medicines can have a hard time penetrating to their dead-skin headquarters. Herbal remedies, however, are able to penetrate to the netherworld where fungal infec-tions hide out, says Lisa Murray-Doran, N.D., a naturopathic doctor and instructor at the Canadian College of Naturopathic Medicine in Toronto.

Relief in Five Days or Less

Dr. Murray-Doran uses topical herbal remedies. But she doesn't stop with surface cures. According to naturopathic wisdom, fungal infections may be a sign that your immune system isn't working all that well—a red flag that you should be looking deeper, she says. "I advocate adding immune-enhancing herbs for anyone with this problem," she says. (For more information on strengthening your immune system, see "Low Immunity" on page 276.)

To start quelling the itch right now, try these fungus stoppers. If your rash gets worse, see a dermatologist. What you thought was fungus may actually be an allergy.

Fend off fungus with tea tree oil. "I've known people who've had athlete's foot for years—with itching, cracking skin and infected nails—who've used everything they can find at the drugstore, to no avail. But after using tea tree oil, they've experienced big improvements," Dr. Murray-Doran says.

Mix an antifungal soak by diluting 5 to 7 drops of tea tree essential oil in 4 ounces of warm water in a tub large enough to accommodate your feet. Double the recipe if you need more water to cover the affected area. Soak once a day for 20 minutes. "In five days, the fungus should be gone," Dr. Murray-Doran says. "If you have a very stubborn fungal infection, you can soak up to three times a day. It's safe. You can't overdo it."

After each soak, dry the affected area well with a clean towel. "And then put that towel in the laundry immediately," Dr. Murray-Doran says. "Don't reuse it, because it could spread the fungus." Put on clean cotton socks. "Your feet need to breathe and stay dry," she says. "Fungi love damp. You want to discourage them."

For nail fungus, follow the same routine, Dr. Murray-Doran suggests, or try using undiluted tea tree oil directly on affected nails. Dip a cotton swab in the oil and apply to the top of the nail, then cover with a bandage.

A traditional remedy, tea tree has been shown by researchers to be as effective as an over-the-counter fungal remedy for toenails infected with athlete's foot fungus. Anyone with sensitive skin should dilute the oil, using about 7 drops of the essential oil to 3 drops of vegetable oil, to avoid skin irritation. Undiluted tea tree oil is toxic when applied to the skin, and it should be kept out of the reach of children.

Stir in garlic. For more fungus-fighting power, add 4 to 6 drops of garlic essential oil to the above formula, Dr. Murray-Doran suggests. Garlic is a traditional antifungal remedy, and its fungus-fighting abilities have been backed by laboratory studies.

Or you can concoct a simple garlic foot bath, suggests Paul Bergner, clinical director of the Rocky Mountain Center for Botanical Studies in Boulder, Colorado, editor of *Medical Herbalism*, and author of *The Healing Power of Garlic* and *The Healing Power of Echinacea and Goldenseal and Other Immune System Herbs*. Puree 6 garlic cloves in a blender or food processor. Fill a small tub with enough comfortably hot water to cover your feet, then add the garlic and soak for 15 minutes.

"Garlic is an old, old remedy with scientifically proven antifungal action," Bergner notes. "I've seen cases of athlete's foot clear up in two to three days with a garlic foot bath. The advantage of a warm foot bath is that the hot water softens the skin, which allows the garlic to penetrate better."

You may want to stay clear of loved ones, though. Not only can a garlic bath make your feet odoriferous but the offending compounds can travel through the bloodstream to your lungs, giving your breath that pungent smell. And don't apply garlic directly to the skin, as it can cause irritation.

Promote healing with calendula. After using an antifungal soak for three days, add calendula to your routine, Dr. Murray-Doran suggests. Research suggests that calendula petals, used traditionally to heal wounds, help promote the growth of new skin cells.

After soaking and drying your feet, apply a light calendula cream or salve or rinse your tootsies with warm calendula tea. Make a calendula foot wash by adding 1 to 2 teaspoons of dried calendula flowers to a cup of boiling water, then steep for 10 to 15 minutes. Strain, if necessary, and cool. Use the calendula cream or rinse three times a day. "It's perfect for the stage when the fungus has died off, but you still have cracked skin because healing is slow," Dr. Murray-Doran says.

Stay dry all day with lavender. You can fend off fungus all day by sprinkling on some lavender, which Dr. Murray-Doran says can help discourage fungus growth. Grind ¼ cup of lavender flowers in a coffee grinder or food processor, then mix with ½ cup of powdered bentonite clay. Sprinkle it onto your clean, dry feet or into your clean cotton socks. "The clay helps keep your feet dry, and in my experience, the lavender works as a mild antifungal agent," she says. "And it smells nice."

Bad Breath

BANISH HALITOSIS WITH AROMATIC BOTANICALS

At a meal's end, an Indian restaurant might offer fennel seeds for the after-dinner chewing pleasure of diners. At an elegant Persian dinner, guests could find bowls of fresh, fragrant coriander, parsley, spearmint, and tarragon to nibble between courses. And what American hash house, pizzeria, or coffee shop would neglect to keep its bowl of after-dinner mints full to the brim?

After-dinner mints may seem like a culinary cliché, but the fact is that mint is a terrific breath scrubber, and not just because it's so minty fresh. The aromatic oil and menthol in peppermint help kill germs, which frequently are the bad guys behind bad breath.

A Personal Purification Strategy

Germs aren't the only cause of halitosis, say herbalists. "I look to a person's diet when bad breath's a problem," says Ellen Hopman, a professional member of the American Herbalists Guild who practices in Amherst, Massachusetts. "I often recommend more fruits and vegetables, and especially green juices. Watercress and parsley, for example, are loaded with chlorophyll and seem to purify the breath," she notes.

A bad tooth can also put out some pretty revolting odors. "Whenever anyone comes to see me complaining of bad breath, I send them straight to the dentist," says Douglas Schar, a practicing medical herbalist in London, editor of the *British Journal of Phytotherapy*, and author of *Backyard Medicine Chest*. "Once any dental problem is ruled out, herbal medicine has much to offer a person suffering from compost-pile breath."

Another leading cause of bad breath is bad gums. Periodontal disease occurs when bacteria wedge themselves down in the spaces between teeth and gums. Bacterial colonies form, and their waste products produce a distinctly offensive odor.

Finally, chronic bad breath can be a sign of other, more serious conditions, including liver and kidney problems or diabetes. So if your breath has people keeping their distance on a regular basis, consult a qualified healthcare practitioner. For freshen-me-now relief, read on.

Juice up some greens. Toss a few handfuls of parsley, alone or with watercress, in a juicer, then sip some juice whenever you suspect that your breath needs freshening. "Parsley contains chlorophyll, which is a known breath deodorizer," says Hopman.

Eat your garnish. Don't pass up that piece of parsley decorating your dinner plate—it can K.O. bad breath in the same way juicing it can. Nibble a few sprigs of fresh parsley whenever you're in need of a little extra breath refreshment, suggests Hopman.

Chew on some cardamom. Cardamom, a popular spice in Arabian cuisine, is rich in cineole, a potent antiseptic that kills bad-breath bacteria, says James A. Duke, Ph.D., a botanical consultant, former ethnobotanist with the U.S. Department of Agriculture, and author of *The Green Pharmacy*, who specializes in medicinal plants. You can buy whole cardamom at health food stores, specialty herb shops, and some supermarkets. To freshen bad breath, discard the pods and chew on a few seeds, then (discreetly) spit them out when you're finished.

Drink some peppermint tea. The aromatic oil that gives peppermint its distinctive flavor and smell is a potent antiseptic that can kill germs that cause bad breath. Drink a cup of peppermint tea whenever you feel the need.

Make your own gargle. Combine tinctures (also called extracts) of sage, calendula, and myrrh gum (available at health food stores) in equal proportions. Gargle four times a day for as long as it takes to clear up the problem, suggests Schar. "This mix has the added advantage of increasing the strength of the gums, which we know are often at the root of bad-smelling breath," he adds. Be sure to keep the gargle in a tightly sealed jar at room temperature.

Herbal Wisdom
Personal Use Led to a Career

"It was my own struggle with eczema, asthma, and allergies that eventually led me to herbs. It is my goal to educate the public to the practical applications of herbal medicine. This is important to women because they are the major household caregivers and are more intuitively in tune with the natural cycles of nature and healing ways of herbs."

—*Daniel Gagnon, medical herbalist*

Breastfeeding Problems

HERBAL SUPPORT FOR NURSING MOTHERS

Nursing sounds so simple, so natural: Your breasts make milk. Your new baby needs milk. Put the two together and . . . usually, you get mother-and-child bliss.

But sometimes nature needs a nudge. Perhaps your milk isn't coming in as quickly as your hungry newborn would like. Perhaps there's too much of a good thing, and your breasts are uncomfortably full. Or maybe your nipples are feeling a little worse for wear. That's where these gentle herbal remedies, safe for nursing moms *and* their babies, come in.

Insufficient Milk

If your breasts don't seem to produce enough milk to satisfy your baby, or if you're pumping breast milk and are concerned that the supply won't keep pace with the demand, herbal healers suggest turning to traditional botanicals that help boost milk production.

Known as galactagogues—from *gala*, the Greek word for milk—these herbs have been used by nursing mothers around the world for hundreds if not thousands of years.

Sip a calming infusion. "This tea can help a new mother relax, overcoming one of the biggest obstacles to milk letdown, which is stress," says Aviva Romm, a certified professional midwife, herbalist, and professional member of the American Herbalists Guild who practices in Bloomfield Hills, Michigan, and is author of *The Natural Pregnancy Book* and *Natural Healing for Babies and Children*. "At the same time, it helps build your milk supply."

Combine 1 part each of chamomile and oatstraw, $\frac{1}{2}$ part each of lavender and nettle, and a pinch of fennel for each cup of tea you'll make from the mix. Brew by steeping 1 teaspoon of the blend in a cup of boiling water for 15 minutes, then strain and sip. "You can have anywhere from a cup to a quart a day," Romm notes. (Commission E, the expert panel that judges the safety and effectiveness of herbal medicines for the German government, advises that fennel not be used for a prolonged time without direction from a qualified herbalist.)

Research suggests that chamomile, oatstraw, and lavender reverse the effects of stress and nervous exhaustion and calm the nervous system. Both nettle and fennel are traditional lactation-promoting herbs. As a bonus, chamomile and fennel can also relieve or prevent colic in infants. "That's a nice little quality to pass on to your baby," notes Romm.

Enjoy an ancient mother's helper. Goat's rue, nettle, crushed fennel seeds or aniseed, and milk thistle or blessed thistle are all traditional lactation promoters that are still recommended by herbal healers today. "They're good to use if you aren't making enough milk or if you want to make more milk because you're pumping breast milk for

Blessed Thistle:
Mother's Little Herbal Helper

With its prickly leaves and thorny, yellow flower, blessed thistle seems like a plant that's shouting to be left alone. But this low-growing herb, also called holy thistle or spotted thistle, is a useful remedy for nursing mothers who hope to increase milk production, herbalists say.

Blessed thistle promotes blood flow to the mammary glands; by bringing in more oxygen and nutrients via the blood, it enables a woman's breasts to produce more milk, according to herbalist Rosemary Gladstar, director of the Sage Mountain herbal education center in East Barre, Vermont, in her book *Herbal Healing for Women*. Dried, bulk blessed thistle is available at health food stores and by mail order (see "Where to Buy Herbs and Herbal Products" on page 462).

One caution: Do not start using blessed thistle until after your baby is born. Herbalists advise against using this herb during pregnancy because it could cause uterine bleeding.

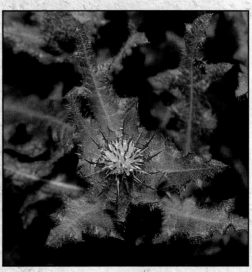

Herbalist Rosemary Gladstar suggests combining bitter-tasting blessed thistle with fennel or other good-tasting herbs to make a more pleasant tea.

your baby," says Mary Bove, N.D., a naturopathic physician, midwife, and member of Britain's National Institute of Medical Herbalists who practices at the Brattleboro Naturopathic Clinic in Vermont.

Choose one of the herbs listed above or blend equal parts of two of them. Make a tea with 1 teaspoon of the herb or herb blend per cup of boiling water. Steep for 15 minutes, then strain. Dr. Bove recommends one to three cups a day.

Cracked, Sore Nipples

Perhaps your baby's a champion nurser—she latches onto your breast easily, drinks happily, then falls into peaceful slumber. But ouch! All that clamping and sucking have left you with painful, cracked, and even bleeding nipples.

What to do? First, let your nipples air-dry, and (if practical) expose them to sunlight for a few minutes. Both seem to promote healing, say natural healing experts. Also, have your baby checked for thrush, a mouth infection that can cause nipple problems for a nursing mother. Then try one of these herbal salves and gels. "And always remember to wash *any* herbal product off your breasts completely with mild soap and warm water before your baby nurses," says Romm.

Soothe with calendula. Pharmacological studies show that compounds in calendula encourage the growth of healthy new skin and may prevent infection. A cream or ointment rich in skin-healing calendula can gently promote the recovery of cracked, sore nipples, Romm says. "This is my favorite remedy," she notes. "It's effective yet mild."

Smooth on aloe vera. Research shows that aloe vera gel promotes wound healing and eases pain. Snip a leaf from that aloe plant on your windowsill, slit it open lengthwise, and scrape out the cool, clear gel within. Apply this soothing, healing natural remedy to sore nipples, Romm suggests. "Before breastfeeding, thoroughly wash off the gel," she adds. "Aloe vera gel has a very bitter flavor that your baby will not enjoy." Plus, it's not good for the baby to ingest aloe.

Engorged Breasts

Sometimes, especially in the first few days after childbirth, a nursing mom's breasts produce more milk than a new baby needs. If your breasts become warm, swollen, hard, and painful, they are engorged, says Lisa Murray-Doran, N.D., a naturopathic doctor and instructor at the Canadian College of Naturopathic Medicine in Toronto.

If engorgement is not reduced quickly, milk ducts inside your breasts can become blocked, leading to more pain and swelling and to an infection called mastitis. Consult your health-care practitioner if you have signs of mastitis—a fever, flulike symptoms, and tender, red skin on one or both breasts—or if nursing leaves your breasts red, hot, swollen, and painful.

To reduce engorgement, continue to nurse your baby, says Dr. Murray-Doran. To express extra fluid when your milk is first coming in, massage your breasts in a comfortably hot shower. Prevention is the best treatment, she says. Don't allow your breasts to become engorged—express the milk, nurse often, and be aware of the consequences. You can also try these botanical remedies.

Soothe with a potato-ginger poultice. This traditional remedy cools and soothes warm, engorged breasts. Grate a medium-size white potato and a little fresh gingerroot (about 1 teaspoon); apply this poultice to your breasts and cover with an old clean towel. Keep the poultice in place until it becomes warm, then remove it and apply fresh potato-ginger mixture, Dr. Bove suggests. Repeat until your breasts feel comfortable.

Alternate with chamomile tea bags. Another soothing strategy is to alternate between potato-ginger poultices and cool, wet chamomile tea bags, suggests Dr. Bove. Place a moist tea bag that has been soaked in cool water over each nipple and keep them in place until they grow warm. (In Europe, chamomile is used on the skin to soothe and help heal inflammations and irritations.)

Breast Pain, Lumps, and Tenderness

Soothing Strategies to Ease the Discomfort

For most women who menstruate, breast discomfort waxes and wanes with each monthly cycle. When levels of the female hormone estrogen are highest, which they are just before and during menstruation, your breasts may swell and ache. Tiny milk glands inside one or both breasts morph into fluid-filled cysts. These changes are quite normal, although finding a lumpy spot or a painful area can be a scary discovery.

If you perform a monthly breast self-exam as health-care practitioners recommend, you will be more likely to know if any lumpiness or discomfort is normal and cyclical or if, indeed, you have a new lump that needs special attention. Any new lump should be evaluated by your doctor as soon as possible.

The consistent breast lumpiness that you may feel month after month is sometimes called fibrocystic disease, although it's not really a disease. It's caused by many small fluid-filled sacs and strands of fibrous tissue, and it's very common.

If, as is usually the case, the lumpiness is not cause for serious medical concern and is simply tied to your menstrual cycle, herbalists have much to offer that can bring relief, diminish the problem, and help prevent an unwelcome return.

Where should you begin? Herbal healers suggest that women with lumpy, tender breasts cut back on or eliminate coffee (caffeinated and decaffeinated), colas, black tea, and chocolate. These foods contain methylxanthines, which are substances that may contribute to the discomfort. You should also limit your consumption of animal fats, which seem to boost estrogen levels, and focus on organic whole grains, fruits, and vegetables as much as possible. This mealtime strategy will boost dietary fiber, which helps normalize estrogen levels, and shield you from farmyard crop sprays and animal feeds that can introduce estrogen-like chemicals into your body.

"These steps alone can help ease the discomfort of fibrocystic breasts in two to three months," notes Jill Stansbury, N.D., a naturopathic physician, director of the Battleground Naturopathic Family Practice in Battleground, Washington, and chairman of the botanical medicine department at the National College of Naturopathic Medicine in Portland, Oregon.

An Herbal Relief Package

Beyond what dietary measures can do, herbalists note that herbs can improve breast discomfort in three ways: first, by correcting hormone imbalances; second, by stimulating sluggish lymphatic flow associated with infection-fighting nodes in the vicinity of the breasts; and third, by helping the liver and bowels work properly so that your body breaks down and eliminates hormones as it should, Dr. Stansbury says. "Herbally, we may have more finesse for handling cysts than conventional medicine has," she says. "An herbalist will look at why your breasts are producing cysts and try to correct the underlying problem." Here's what they might recommend.

Supplement with evening primrose oil. This golden oil is an anti-inflammatory that has the ability to soothe pain and help shrink lumps. To reduce harmless but bothersome lumps, Dr. Stansbury suggests taking one or two capsules (either 500 or 1,000 milligrams; she prefers 1,000 milligrams) of evening primrose oil three times a day for several months. Evening primrose and other plant oils—such as flax and borage—supply essential fatty acids. Incorporating these oils into your diet can eventually reduce the need to take them as supplements, according to Dr. Stansbury.

Spell relief p-i-n-e. Native Americans applied poultices made with pine to their skin to relieve pain and inflammation. To try a modern version of this time-honored remedy yourself, wash your breasts with pine-tar soap or rub on a pine-based salve, suggests Ellen Kamhi, R.N., Ph.D., of Oyster Bay, New York, an herbalist, professional member of the American Herbalists Guild, and host of the nationally syndicated radio show *Natural Alternatives.*

You can also make your own pine salve, Dr. Kamhi suggests. (Follow the directions for making a salve in "Salves and Ointments" on page 111.) Start with olive oil infused with a

large handful of pesticide-free white pine needles gathered from your own yard or from a local wooded area (if you are certain that the trees have not been treated with chemicals). "I think pine stimulates circulation and in that way helps relieve lumpiness," Dr. Kamhi says.

Warm and soothe with castor oil. Herbalists recommend old-fashioned castor oil packs for reducing the pain and inflammation of lumpy breasts. Castor oil has been employed for hundreds of years in India, Egypt, and China as an external remedy for sores and abscesses. "It has been used historically as a drawing agent and to stimulate healing," Dr. Stansbury says. "It works, although we don't really know chemically why it does."

To make a castor oil pack, sprinkle 2 ounces of castor oil on a piece of flannel that's wide enough and long enough to cover both breasts, say herbalists, or you can rub the castor oil directly onto your breasts. Cover with plastic wrap and a thin towel. Keep the pack warm with a heating pad set on low or a hot water bottle. Bundle yourself up in a warm robe or just get under the bedcovers to hold the wrap in place, suggests Dr. Stansbury. This wrap will soothe your breasts with warmth for about 45 minutes, she says.

You can relieve sore breasts with this pack once a week or more often as needed, says Kamhi.

"Making a castor oil pack can seem like a big production, but once women try it, they find that it feels really good, and they adopt it as a regular routine," according to Dr. Stansbury.

Ease lumpiness with poke oil. Poke is an herb used traditionally for breast problems. Herbalists say that it can help the lym-

Cleavers: The Cleansing Herb

Call it goosegrass or gripgrass, hedge-burs, or even stickywillie—this common weed is revered by herbal experts as an important cleansing herb that perks up a sluggish lymphatic system. The lymphatic system ushers illness-causing substances out of your body. In the face of disease or other assaults, lymph nodes near your breasts may swell or become inflamed, causing discomfort.

Leave it to cleavers to ease swollen lymph nodes and help relieve monthly breast discomfort and lumpiness. Although it is yet to be widely studied by modern science, the plant's stem, juicy leaves, and tiny flowers are all used as herbal medicine. "Cleavers is a safe herb for stimulating the elimination of toxins from the body by moving lymph and stimulating the kidneys," says Jill Stansbury, N.D., a naturopathic physician, director of the Battleground Naturopathic Family Practice in Battleground, Washington, and chairman of the botanical medicine depart-

ment at the National College of Naturopathic Medicine in Portland, Oregon.

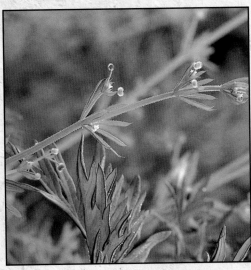

Cleavers can help clear toxins from your system. But herbalists also suggest using the juice from freshly crushed leaves as a quick outdoor medicine to stop bleeding from cuts and speed healing.

phatic system function properly, an action that Dr. Stansbury says will help reduce inflammation and breast tenderness. Look for poke oil in health food stores or mail-order catalogs.

To make a poke oil pack, apply a few drops of the oil to lumpy, tender breasts, massage it into the skin, then cover with plastic wrap and a thin towel. Place a heating pad set on low or a hot water bottle on top. Keep the pack in place for 15 to 30 minutes, then wash your breasts with soap and cool water. Use a

pack once or twice daily for at least a month to see results, Dr. Stansbury says. When your breast discomfort is gone, you can stop the treatment.

One caution: Do not take more than 30 drops of poke a day or apply it to broken skin without an herbalist's guidance. This herb contains compounds that, when taken internally, could cause digestive problems and, in larger doses, could even be fatal. "But poke is safe to use externally," Dr. Stansbury notes. "It works especially well for squishy rather than hard breast lumps." Make sure that you're using poke oil made from the root, however, as the berry juices can be toxic even when applied to the skin.

Brew a digestion-improving tea. "I've found in my practice that breast problems are often a sign of poor liver function," says Dr. Stansbury. Herbalists believe that the same bitter roots that stimulate digestion and support liver function can ease breast pain and lumpiness by normalizing levels of circulating hormones in your body. "When the liver is working properly, it removes hormones from the bloodstream so they can be eliminated," says Dr. Stansbury.

Help your liver with this tea: Combine equal parts of dandelion root, burdock root, Oregon grape root and yellow dock root; then, for flavor, add equal parts of licorice, fennel seed, organic dried orange peel, dried gingerroot, and broken pieces of cinnamon sticks. To brew the tea, gently simmer 1 teaspoon of the herb mixture in a cup of boiling water for 15 minutes. Strain and enjoy three or more cups a day, Dr. Stansbury suggests.

"This is a rich, hearty tea that we drink instead of coffee in my office," Dr. Stansbury says. "We actually brew it in our coffeemaker, putting herbs in the basket instead of ground coffee. Simmering the herbs would be even better, as you would get more of the chemical constituents. I suggest keeping this mixture on hand for regular use. It's good for all-around liver support and menstrual cycle irregularities."

Burdock has been used traditionally as a mild laxative. Research suggests that bitter compounds in dandelion root stimulate bile and improve digestion. Oregon grape contains a bitter-tasting compound called berberine and has been used traditionally as a

digestive aid that supports liver function by improving bile flow. Yellow dock also stimulates bile flow.

Or try a breast-friendly tincture mix. Herbs that help the lymphatic system work optimally by moving fluid through your body rather than letting it gather in swollen lymph nodes can help ease breast lumpiness, Dr. Stansbury says. "Your breasts are surrounded by lymphatic tissue," she says. "Promoting good lymph flow can help ease lumpiness and tenderness."

Combine equal parts of tinctures (also called extracts) of rosemary, cleavers, sarsaparilla, and milk thistle. Take $1/4$ to $1/2$ teaspoon three to five times a day until lumps subside, Dr. Stansbury suggests.

Herbal experts consider cleavers to be a good plant remedy for improving the function of the lymph system. It promotes lymphatic flow and also acts as a kidney tonic, helping to regulate water and electrolytes. Rosemary, according to Dr. Stansbury, may help act as a drying agent to improve fluid-filled cysts, and it also has a mild hormone-balancing effect.

Sarsaparilla is thought to contain weakly estrogenic substances that can help tender, lumpy breasts by crowding out the body's stronger natural estrogens at estrogen-receptor sites, she says. "The effect is a weaker response than to more potent natural hormones." Research shows that milk thistle helps protect liver cells from damage and helps build new cells. "Women who take milk thistle often see breast improvements within two menstrual cycles," according to Dr. Stansbury.

Ease the ache with black cohosh. Black cohosh is a traditional pain reliever for everything from arthritis and rheumatism to menstrual pain and difficult childbirth. Studies show that this herb is a mild sedative and has anti-inflammatory action.

"When a woman feels dense, heavy, aching pains in her breasts above and beyond normal breast tenderness, black cohosh is the herb to use," Dr. Stansbury says. She suggests taking a dropperful of black cohosh tincture in tea, juice, or warm water three or four times a day every day for several months until symptoms subside. You can usually use less each month, she says, and eventually discontinue it altogether.

Do not use black cohosh if you suspect that you may be pregnant, because it stimulates the uterus and can cause premature contractions. Do not use this herb while nursing.

Bruises

BANISH BLACK-AND-BLUE BLOTCHES

Bruises add insult to injury, telegraphing to the world in bold black-and-blue—and sometimes, in every color in the crayon box—that there's been a collision: between shin and coffee table, hip and the stairway banister, shoulder and car door.

The result of these collisions? Broken circulatory vessels that leak blood beneath the surface of the skin, causing pain, swelling, and that embarrassing, hard-to-hide discoloration.

Herbs to the Rescue

Left alone, a bruise will heal in a few weeks. But herbal healers say that you can speed the process—or minimize damage in the first place—with these botanical measures.

Apply arnica, pronto. A traditional bruise buster and the first choice of many herbalists for soothing black-and-blue spots, arnica has been shown by researchers to contain a substance called helenalin, which has anti-inflammatory actions. Commission E, the expert panel that judges the safety and effectiveness of herbal medicines for the German government, concurs that this herb is helpful for treating bruises.

Applied to unbroken skin at the point of impact, arnica can lessen or even help prevent the discoloration and swelling of a bruise, says Lisa Murray-Doran, N.D., a naturopathic doctor and instructor at the Canadian College of Naturopathic Medicine in Toronto. "Important advice to remember about this powerful herb is that arnica is toxic if taken internally or if absorbed into the bloodstream by contact with scratched, cut, bleeding, or otherwise broken skin," she says. "So use it only on unbroken skin." Also, people with very sensitive skin should not use arnica because the oils can be irritating.

Arnica: The First-Aid Herb

*B*ruised shin from a run-in with an open file drawer? Sore calf muscles, courtesy of an all-day hike? Arnica, a tall, flower-bearing plant also known as mountain tobacco and mountain daisy, can relieve such everyday aches, pains, bumps, and bang-ups.

According to the Eclectics—turn-of-the-century practitioners who teamed man-made drugs with healing plants—arnica "gives grateful relief to sore muscles that have undergone much strain and exertion."

Modern-day research indicates that arnica really does work. Clinical studies show, for example, that one of the active ingredients in arnica, helenalin, relieves pain and reduces swelling.

You can buy arnica creams, gels, and ointments wherever herbal products are sold, and arnica plants are available by mail order (see "Where to Buy Herbs and Herbal Products" on page 462). If you have sensitive skin, use these products with cau-

tion. In some people, arnica may leave skin red, itchy, and inflamed. To be safe, use arnica preparations on unbroken skin only, and discontinue use at the first sign of a reaction.

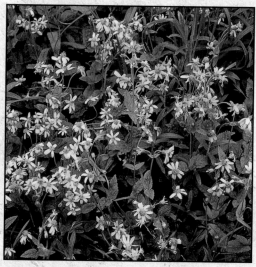

Native Americans rubbed mashed arnica flowers on bruises.

(Don't confuse the herb with homeopathic remedies using arnica, which are extremely dilute and therefore safe.)

If you've banged your shin, fallen, or otherwise set the scene for a painful purple shiner, apply arnica cream, salve, or a compress to the spot, Dr. Murray-Doran suggests. To make a compress, add 60 drops of arnica tincture (also called an extract) to a cup of warm water. Soak a cloth in it, then lay it on your skin. Hold the compress in place with

a dry cloth tied over it, she says. "Leave it in place for 20 minutes to an hour, until the wet cloth dries," Dr. Murray-Doran says. "If you do this soon enough after getting bumped, you may not see a bruise at all."

You can also use arnica gel, says herbalist Sharleen Andrews-Miller, a faculty member at the National College of Naturopathic Medicine in Portland, Oregon, and associate medicinary director at the college's public clinic.

Parsley Cubes for the Black-and-Blues

Parsley has a traditional reputation for dispelling black-and-blue marks. Ice can prevent swelling. Combine the two in parsley-packed ice cubes, and you have an instant bruise remedy that you can stock ahead of time in your freezer, says herbalist Sharleen Andrews-Miller, a faculty member at the National College of Naturopathic Medicine in Portland, Oregon, and associate medicinary director at the college's public clinic.

"Just whirl a handful of parsley and about ¼ cup of water in a blender or food processor until it looks like slush. Then fill ice cube trays half-full," she suggests. "Apply to bruised spots as needed, wrapped in gauze or thin cloth. Parsley ice cubes also work well for cooling minor burns." Discard them after use.

"As a bonus, you can grab a parsley cube out of the freezer when you're cooking and you need a little parsley in a soup or sauce," adds Andrews-Miller.

Use an arnica compress and ice. You can also alternate between an arnica compress and an ice pack on bruised skin, suggests Leslie Gardner, an herbalist in Sebastopol, California, professional member of the American Herbalists Guild, and staff member at the California School of Herbal Studies in Forestville. You can make a compress by steeping the fresh herb in hot water, straining it, and then soaking the cloth. "I would alternate the two for one to four hours, then rub arnica cream or oil into the bruised area," she says.

Make a poultice with comfrey or calendula. Concoct an herbal poultice by rehydrating a tablespoon of dried herbs in an equal amount of warm water or by crushing fresh comfrey leaves or calendula petals, Dr. Murray-Doran suggests.

Comfrey, a traditional skin remedy dating back to ancient Greece, contains a substance called allantoin, which prompts tissue repair even below the surface of the skin, and rosmarinic acid, which reduces swelling. While herbalists caution against taking comfrey internally without guidance due to the plant's concentration of potentially dangerous pyrrolizidine alkaloids, applying comfrey externally to a bruise does not pose a threat, Dr. Murray-Doran says.

Calendula's sunny yellow and orange flowers have a long-standing reputation as antiseptic wound healers for bruises and other skin ailments. This herb has potent abilities to repair damage to the skin caused by sunburn, according to herbalists.

"Apply this poultice directly to bruised skin and hold it in place with an adhesive strip, or use gauze and tape for a larger area. Leave it in place for three to four hours, and you should see swelling, pain, and discoloration reduced. Or, if you apply the poultice as soon as you're injured, it may keep the area from looking and feeling bruised," advises Dr. Murray-Doran.

Burns and Scalds

SAVE SINGED SKIN WITH CALENDULA PLUS

*B*lame home cooking, hot curling irons, and microwaved edibles. One-and-a-half million of us are burned each year, most frequently in accidents at home.

The good news? Most burns and scalds are minor and can be treated safely without a trip to the emergency room. And by stocking a few herbal remedies, such as an aloe plant on the windowsill, you can turn your kitchen into a burn-treatment center, says Lisa Murray-Doran, N.D., a naturopathic doctor and instructor at the Canadian College of Naturopathic Medicine in Toronto.

Cool, Protect, and Heal

A few ground rules about singed skin: Burns that simply look red or blister a little are safe to handle at home. You should seek medical help, however. if the burn causes great pain, is larger than the palm of your hand, or is on your face, hand, foot, or genitals. The same goes for a burn that is painless or looks white or charred, Dr. Murray-Doran says. "That's a third-degree burn, and there will be deep skin damage," she notes.

Begin any at-home burn treatment by cooling the spot completely, she says. Run cold water over the area for at least five minutes and continue for as long as it takes to ease the pain and take heat out of the area. Then gently pat the burn dry and proceed

with these herbal burn and scald soothers that reduce pain, protect against infection, and promote healing.

Apply an herbal compress. "Once you're beyond the initial cooling-down, you can apply an herbal compress that will help healing begin and protect the burn from infection," says Sharol Tilgner, N.D., a naturopathic physician, professional member of the American Herbalists Guild, and president of Wise Woman Herbals in Creswell, Oregon.

Combine 1 teaspoon each of calendula, St.-John's-wort, echinacea, and Oregon grape root tinctures (also called extracts) in $\frac{1}{4}$ cup of very cold water. Soak a clean cloth in the mixture and apply it to the burn, Dr. Tilgner suggests. You can apply this compress a few times a day, she adds. Traditional skin healers, these herbs have all demonstrated antibacterial or immune-stimulating activity in laboratory studies.

Start healing with aloe. Herbalists' top recommendation for burn relief? "Plain, raw aloe vera gel," Dr. Tilgner. "It stops the pain and keeps burned tissues moist, which is important for healing."

If you have an aloe plant, cut off an outer leaf, then slit it open lengthwise. Squeeze or scrape out the gel and smear it on the burn, Dr. Tilgner suggests. Apply several times a day until the burn is healed. Or you can cut open an aloe leaf and lay it gel-side down on top of the burned area, then cover it with a

A Saintly Burn Soother

You thought St.-John's-wort was just a depression lifter? Look again. In one study, the blood red oil made from this herb's small yellow blossoms healed first-degree burns in 48 hours and mended second-degree burns three times faster than conventional treatments did, with less scarring. "The oil also eases the pain that can come with nerve damage in a burn," notes Lisa Murray-Doran, N.D., a naturopathic doctor and instructor at the Canadian College of Naturopathic Medicine in Toronto.

To make your own St.-John's-wort oil, put 1 cup of fresh yellow flowers in a quart jar and cover with olive oil. Close with a tight-fitting lid. Place the jar in a sunny window or a warm spot and shake it daily. The oil will turn red. After two to three weeks, strain out the flowers and store the oil in a dark, cool place. To use the oil, thoroughly cool the burned area of skin with cold water, dry the area carefully, and dab on the oil. Reapply two or three times a day, as needed.

bandage to hold the leaf in place, Dr. Tilgner says.

If you don't have a plant, or you have a small one and need more gel than it can provide, you can purchase aloe vera gel at health food stores, says Sharleen Andrews-Miller, a faculty member at the National College of Naturopathic Medicine in Portland, Oregon, and associate medicinary director at the college's public clinic.

"The beauty of aloe gel is that it won't hold heat in a burn the way creamy or oily salves and ointments can," notes Dr. Murray-Doran. Research suggests that this clear, cool gel protects skin from infection and penetrates injured tissue, easing pain, reducing swelling, and dilating capillaries, which increases blood flow to the burned area and brings in more of the body's own skin-fixing substances. In one small study, researchers in Thailand found that burns treated with aloe vera gel healed in an average of about 12 days, compared with 18 days for burns treated with plain petroleum jelly.

Later, rub on a calendula-and-comfrey salve. Once a minor burn is healing, a calendula-and-comfrey salve will help the skin heal with less scarring, Dr. Murray-Doran says. Both herbs have traditional reputations as skin menders. Comfrey contains a substance called allantoin that prompts rapid tissue repair, and researchers suspect that compounds in calendula called triterpenes prompt the growth of new cells.

But do not use comfrey on deep burns or on burns that show signs of infection, such as redness, puffiness, or oozing, Dr. Murray-Doran cautions. Comfrey promotes such quick cell regeneration that the surface of the burn could heal, leaving infected or damaged skin underneath.

Caffeine Addiction

NATURAL BREWS TO EASE THE CAFFEINE-WEAN

Call it a Coffee Renaissance. Whether you're an urbanite, a suburbanite, or even a rural-ite, you're probably just a hop, skip, and a jump away from some exotic, dark brown brew with a sexy Italian name.

As a social drink, coffee is steeped in tradition. Coffee breaks are like oases in the landscape of office life. And as a morning pick-me-up or a work or study aid, coffee has its merits. Research indicates that coffee (like cola drinks and tea) may help you concentrate when you're on deadline for certain kinds of tasks. But for some people, drinking too much coffee too often can lead to indigestion, sleep problems, diarrhea, and other discomforts.

The Black Sheep of the Herb Family

The dictionary defines coffee as "a beverage made by percolation, infusion, or decoction from the roasted and ground seeds of the *Coffea arabica* plant." Sounds like an herb—and it is, but one that's not entirely benevolent. For example, caffeine is a methylxanthine, a substance linked to fibrocystic breast disease (harmless but worrisome breast lumps) in some women. Research also indicates that caffeine raises blood pressure and heart rate, causing hot flashes in menopausal women. Anxiety, jitters, heart palpitations, and headaches can be caffeine-related, too. Since caffeine makes material move through the bowel more quickly than normal, it can contribute to irritable bowel syndrome. Studies show that drinking three cups of coffee a day may make it difficult for women to conceive. And for pregnant women, the more coffee you drink, the higher your risk of miscarriage. Women who drink four cups a day may have three times the miscarriage risk of those who down only one or two cups.

Black tea ("a beverage prepared from leaves by infusion with boiling water," according to the dictionary) comes from the shrub *Camellia sinensis*. Tea, like coffee, contains caffeine. So do regular cola and some other soft drinks, chocolate, and some painkilling medications (such as some menstrual cramp remedies).

How much caffeine is too much? That depends on you and your personal sensitivity to it. Some women may find that breast problems improve when they cut back to just a cup or two a day, while even that's too much for other women. For most women, say experts, no more than a 5-ounce cup or two of coffee a day is about right. FYI: An 8-ounce mug of tea or a 12-ounce can of soda has about as much caffeine as a 5-ounce cup of joe.

Jilt the Java Juice

Many women think about giving up caffeine but worry about losing the zip they need to get through the day. Don't. After a few short weeks of using these energizing herbal remedies, you may find that you have more get-up-and-go than ever.

Ease off slowly. To prevent withdrawal headaches (not unusual in coffee drinkers who try to quit), gradually replace caffeine by diluting your caffeinated coffee with decaf or water over a couple of weeks, suggests Douglas Schar, a practicing medical herbalist in London, editor of the *British Journal of Phytotherapy*, and author of *Backyard Medicine Chest*. But people abuse stimulants like coffee and tea because they need energy, he says, so an even better way to gradually decrease your caffeine consumption and increase your energy is to drink coffee sold as "Cajun blend." That's 50 percent coffee and 50 percent chicory, and it can be found in supermarkets everywhere.

Chicory is an ancient herb long used to stimulate the liver into heightened action, explains Schar. "The liver governs the release of energy into the circulation, so a properly functioning liver means that you will have the energy you need to get through your day. I recommend using a 50-50 Cajun blend for three months, then switching to a 50-50 blend of Cajun and decaf coffees, further reducing your caffeine consumption," he says. "After three months, your final step would be to use a 50-50 blend of chicory and decaf. This way you get the coffee flavor you like without the caffeine and the energy herb chicory at the same time."

Try green tea. Green tea comes from the same plant as black tea does. The difference is in the processing: Black tea is partially dried, crushed, and allowed to oxidize in heat—an alcohol-free fermentation process. Green tea is simply steamed, rolled, and dried. Depending on how long it's steeped, a cup of green tea contains from 40 to 100 milligrams of caffeine, so don't let it steep too long, or you'll get as much caffeine as you would in a cup of coffee. But green tea also has good-for-you plant substances, including a hefty 300 to 400 milligrams of polyphenols, depending on the brew. One of these, identified as EGCG, is found in no other plant and is one of the most powerful antioxidants ever discovered—stronger than vitamins E and C. (Antioxidants cancel out the harmful effects of free radicals, maverick substances created either in the normal course of metabolism or as an upshot of exposure to cigarette smoke or pollutants.) Several studies suggest that green tea may have some cancer-protective benefits.

Substitute nutritious herbal infusions. "Some of my favorite herbs for infusions in-

---

Herbal Wisdom
Antidotes to Civilization

"For two-thirds of the people on Earth, traditional medicine is herbal medicine. Nature is not an alternative; it surrounds us. As such, herbalists are less interested in a quick symptom fix than in an integrated lifestyle to support long-term health, providing realistic goals for self-improvement, self-reliance, and interconnectedness to one's world.

"Herbal medicine is the answer for the malaise of a global culture divided from its natural source. Where urban stress clashes with life's goal of Grace, and where rural job losses threaten self-worth and natural beauty . . . these are the ills for which only a return to Life's wholeness is the relevant prescription."

—*Amanda McQuade Crawford, herbalist, teacher, and author*

clude peppermint, nettle, red clover blossom, and oatstraw," says Susun S. Weed, an herbalist and herbal educator from Woodstock, New York, and author of the *Wise Woman* series of herbal health books. Red clover has a rich, earthy flavor that you just might find as satisfying as coffee, and peppermint will "get you going," giving you an energizing lift and stimulating the bowels, notes Weed. As a bonus, nettle has lots of iron, oatstraw is said to increase strength and energy and promote a feeling of calm, and red clover is recognized as an herb that may help prevent cancer. (For directions on making herbal infusions, see "Teas and Infusions" on page 89.)

Try a caffeine-free energy booster. The steady drip, drip, drip of stress saps your energy and can exhaust you, says Schar. "Drinking coffee to boost your energy only makes matters worse, because you're stimulating yourself when your body really needs to take it easy," he notes. Here's an energy-building tonic that helps your body adapt to stress and will also help make it easier for you to quit coffee: Blend equal parts of chicory root, dandelion root, and milk thistle seed. Use 1 tablespoon per cup of boiling water. Available in health food stores, all of these plants have a stimulating effect on the liver, boosting energy.

Canker Sores

HERBS THAT OUST THE OUCH

On life's sliding scale of health problems, a canker sore is a pretty petty annoyance for most women, ranking way below a gallbladder attack or kidney stones. But still, there it is, snuggled into the darkest recesses of your mouth, daring you to eat or drink anything it doesn't like (which is practically everything). Allow even a little slosh of a vinegary salad dressing to touch the little bugger and E-e-e-k! Your tiny canker sore lets you know it exists, big time.

Don't confuse canker sores with cold sores; they are two completely different problems. Canker sores, also known as mouth ulcers, are single or clustered ulcers that are white in the center and surrounded by fairly even red borders. They can crop up anywhere inside your mouth, and they may be caused by lots of things, including stress, nutritional deficiencies, trauma such as biting your tongue, bacteria, and irritation from highly acidic or salty foods. Cold sores, or fever blisters, on the other hand, occur outside the mouth, on the lips, and are an unwelcome gift from the herpes simplex type 1 virus. (You can read about cold sores in "Herpes" on page 256.) As health problems go, canker sores are run of the mill. As many as one out of five people get them on a recurrent basis.

The Natural Plan of Attack

Most canker sores will heal themselves within a week or so, but if you'd like to speed things along, try these natural tactics.

Precede herbs with C and zinc. "Since canker sores usually indicate a vitamin C deficiency, the first thing I tell people is to take 1,000 to 3,000 milligrams of vitamin C daily, along with a 50-milligram chewable zinc tablet, which speeds healing," says Claudia Wingo, R.N., a member of the National Herbalists Association of Australia. Be aware, however, that excess vitamin C may cause diarrhea in some people. And you should only take zinc supplements in excess of 15 milligrams a day for few days.

Swish with echinacea. Add a dropperful or two of echinacea tincture (also called an extract) to a glass of water and rinse your mouth two or three times a day, herbalists suggest.

Make your own mouthwash. In one study, licorice was shown to heal canker sores in just three days, and chamomile and calendula are known for their healing properties. Wingo makes a mouthwash of equal parts of dried licorice root, chamomile, and calendula flowers. Blend the dried herbs together and follow the directions in "Teas and Infusions" on page 89. Swish the tea around in your mouth for several minutes three times a day, then spit it out.

Grab some grapefruit. While eating fresh grapefruit may be torture if you have a canker sore, grapefruit extract may actually help.

Natural grapefruit seed extract works wonders for bacterial infections of the mouth such as canker sores, says Wingo. Dab some right on the sore a few times a day or add five drops to a glass of water and swish the solution around in your mouth three times a day, she suggests. "It's very bitter," Wingo says, "but it really works." Grapefruit seed extract is available in health food stores.

Cervical Changes and Genital Warts

HERBALISTS' OPTIONS

What does the phrase "sexually transmitted disease" bring to mind? AIDS, most certainly. Herpes, most likely. And baby boomers and their elders will probably recall, with a slight shudder, the dangers of syphilis and gonorrhea.

But these days, one of the most common sexually transmitted diseases is none of these. It is the human papillomavirus (HPV), a nearly symptomless virus that causes cervical changes and genital warts.

If the cells of the cervix are affected, HPV can cause cervical changes (dysplasia) or cervical cancer. "If the virus affects the external anal or genital region or the inside of the vaginal wall or the surface of the cervix, it causes a genital wart," adds naturopathic physician Tori Hudson, N.D., professor at the National College of Naturopathic Medicine and director of A Woman's Time, a women's health clinic, both in Portland, Oregon.

HPV is transmitted sexually, and these days, transmission occurs at alarming rates, notes Dr. Hudson. "Something like 20 to 50 percent of sexually active adults carry HPV, but less than 5 percent show any symptoms, such as having abnormal Pap smears or visible genital warts," she says. Studies show that about 70 to 90 percent of the male partners of HPV-infected women also carry the virus.

Since cervical dysplasia often has no telltale symptoms, it can be detected only by having a Pap smear, a painless procedure that your gynecologist, naturopath, or certified midwife can perform in about five minutes. The Pap smear alerts women early to abnormal changes in the cells of the cervix, the tube-shaped structure that connects the vagina to the uterus. Despite the fact that these changing cervical cells resemble cancer cells, dysplasia is *not* cancer, although it can become a cancerous condition if not detected and treated in time.

On the other hand, genital warts may occasionally be seen or felt, says Dr. Hudson. "An external genital wart may look like a little bump or nodule on your anus or genitals, and sometimes it itches," says Dr. Hudson. "But the flat, symptom-free warts that hide on the cervical surface or the vulvar or vaginal walls are more trouble than visible ones, because they're usually caused by the most virulent strains of HPV," she notes.

What might predispose a woman to having cervical changes or genital warts? There are several risk factors, including:

🌿 Becoming sexually active prior to the age of 18. The younger you are when you start having intercourse without a condom, the more at risk you are for acquiring the virus.

🌿 Having multiple male sex partners (more than three in a lifetime).

🌿 Smoking cigarettes.

🌿 Poor nutrition.

Not a Do-It-Yourself Treatment

Treating yourself for genital warts and cervical changes is risky business, say experts in botanical medicine and women's health. Prompt treatment should be sought from an experienced health-care practitioner. "Cervical dysplasia is not a condition that you should try to treat on your own, under any circumstances," says Lisa Alschuler, N.D., a naturopathic physician and chair of the department of botanical medicine at Bastyr University in Bothell, Washington. "Herbal alternatives to conventional medical treatment exist. But success depends on the severity of your dysplasia and upon close supervision by a highly experienced practitioner."

"I've had good experience treating all severities of dysplasia and genital warts with an herbal protocol I developed," says Dr. Hudson. "I've been able to prevent the progression of the disease, reverse the dysplasia, and prevent recurrence."

Dr. Hudson steps in with herbal therapy when a conventional physician might take a wait-and-see approach. "When a woman's Pap smear is only mildly abnormal, her doctor might advise her to come back and have another test in three months or so," she says. "Instead of having a woman come back, potentially allowing the disease to progress even a little, I take action to try halt its progress early on."

"But don't be naïve," she warns emphatically. "If your doctor tells you that your dysplasia is at a stage that requires a colposcopy—examination of the cervical and vaginal tissues under magnification—and biopsy, it's a no-brainer: Have the procedure." These days, several simple techniques are used to remove the precancerous cells, including freezing away abnormal tissue or cutting it out with a looplike device under local anesthesia.

Removing the precancerous cells is necessary to determine the extent and severity of the dysplasia. "Once we know what we're dealing with, we can determine what treatment is best for you. You may be a candidate for the naturopathic approach or one of the conventional treatments, or a combination of the two," explains Dr. Hudson.

"I've seen very sad cases where women have ignored their doctors' warnings to be fully diagnosed and then treated for dysplasia because they believed that 'natural is better' than conventional medicine. Natural may be effective in most cases, but it's very important to determine the appropriate treatment and then follow up and monitor the results. When women refuse the biopsy and/or treatments and go it alone, and their disease pro-

gresses, the results are usually tragic," says Dr. Hudson.

A Naturopathic Approach

If you seek help from an experienced naturopath like Dr. Hudson or Dr. Alschuler, you're likely to find that the doctor employs a three-pronged treatment for cervical changes and genital warts. Here's what to expect.

Topical applications. "The topical application treatment is specific to the degree of abnormality. In some cases, it involves a nightly vitamin A suppository, alternating with an herbal-vitamin C suppository for four weeks. Other cases require the practitioner to apply an enzyme paste and then two different botanical compounds as 'washes' onto the cervix. A vitamin A suppository follows this. The treatment is done twice weekly for three to five weeks, depending on the degree of dysplasia," says Dr. Hudson.

Nutritional support. It's important to shore up your internal defenses when your body is fighting off HPV, says Dr. Hudson. And according to one study, your chances of having severe dysplasia increase three times if your blood levels of beta-carotene are low. In addition, other studies have linked vitamin C and cervical dysplasia: Low vitamin C intake is considered a risk factor for the disease.

"While a woman is under my care, I prescribe 150,000 to 200,000 units of beta-carotene a day, six grams of vitamin C, and a special herbal tincture (also called an extract) that consists of immune system stimulants like echinacea, arbor vitae (commonly called thuja), goldenseal, and osha," says Dr. Hudson (Thuja should be used only with the guidance of a health-care practitioner. For cervical dysplasia, nutrients in such high amounts are best left to the discretion of a trained health professional and not taken indiscriminately on your own.)

Folic acid (a B vitamin) is another essential weapon in the anti-dysplasia arsenal, says Dr. Hudson. In controlled clinical studies, daily folic acid supplements have improved or normalized the Pap smears of some women with mild to moderate dysplasia. Dr. Hudson recommends taking 10 milligrams a day for three months, followed by 2.5 milligrams daily for one year (amounts that exceed the level that consumers can take safely on their own).

Lifestyle support. You can enhance your immune system's ability to check the growth of HPV by adopting a few commonsense health habits, says Dr. Hudson.

- Exercise regularly.
- Eat a sensible, low-fat diet that's high in fruits and vegetables, especially yellow and orange ones.
- Keep stress in check.
- Don't smoke.
- Use a condom (if you have the virus, your partner probably also has it, even if he doesn't have genital warts).

Cuts and Scrapes

Speed Healing with Herbal First-Aid

Sometimes, the world bristles with skin-ripping hazards: Knives that neatly slice a bit of fingertip along with the dinner vegetables. Razors that scrape away more than leg hair. Slippery parking lots that tear stockings—and knees—ragged.

Happily, your skin's prepared for these everyday emergencies. Once skin is broken, your body immediately sends expert repair crews to the scene to protect against infection and rebuild broken cell layers, says Sharol Tilgner, N.D., a naturopathic physician, professional member of the American Herbalists Guild (AHG), and president of Wise Woman Herbals in Creswell, Oregon.

Conventional treatments for cuts and scrapes aim to help the body's natural defense and reconstruction efforts with soaps, ointments, and bandages. Some go a step further by fighting bacteria, protecting sensitive, unhealed skin, and even prompting the birth of lots of healthy new skin cells. Herbal treatments do the same; what's more, you'll find some of these herbal helpers in your kitchen cabinet or growing in your flower garden.

Nature's Antiseptics

The key to healing cuts and scrapes fast is to be prepared and act quickly. Here's how.

Wash and protect with a handy herbal antiseptic. The first step in wound care? Cleaning and guarding broken skin from infection with antiseptic herbs, says Sharleen Andrews-Miller, a faculty member at the National College of Naturophathic Medicine in

Backyard Medicine: A Field Guide

There's a first-aid kit growing in your own lawn—in the form of common plants (or weeds) that have been used for centuries to help heal minor emergencies, including cuts, scrapes, and insect bites and stings, says Steven Foster, medicinal plant specialist from Fayetteville, Arkansas, and author of *Herbs for Your Health* and *Forest Pharmacy*. "If you find yourself outdoors without any ready-made remedies handy, just look around. You'll find plants that are antiseptic, that stop bleeding, and that can be used as bandages, too—provided they come from a spot that you're certain has not been sprayed with chemical pesticides or weed killers," Foster says. Here's a visual guide to the most easily found outdoor remedies.

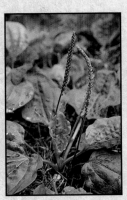

Plantain. Use plantain to clean and disinfect cuts and scrapes as well as insect bites and stings. "Just squish the leaves between two rocks or rub them in your hands until the juice comes out. Then rub it on the affected area," says Lisa Murray-Doran, N.D., a naturopathic doctor and instructor at the Canadian College of Naturopathic Medicine in Toronto.

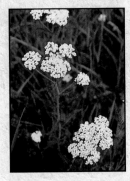

Yarrow. "Yarrow is an amazing first-aid plant. It helps stop bleeding really fast and is also an antiseptic," says 7Song, a professional member of the American Herbalists Guild and director of the Northeast School of Botanical Medicine in Ithaca, New York. "Just crush the leaves and flowers and pack them into a cut or scrape. You can wash the leaves and flowers out of the cut later with water or with a tea made with the yarrow." To make a tea, infuse the yarrow in boiled water for 15 minutes, keeping it covered, he recommends. Let it cool before applying to the skin. It is rare, but some people develop an allergic skin rash after handling yarrow flowers, so be careful if you've never used yarrow before.

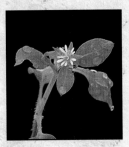

Chickweed. This herb has a traditional reputation for easing itching and healing skin troubles. Chew the leaves well or rub them together in your hands until they're juicy, then place the wet leaves on a bite or sting.

A Flax "Tweezer" for Tough Splinters

Stuck with an impossible-to-remove splinter? Try this flax poultice, suggests Sharol Tilgner, N.D., a naturopathic physician, professional member of the American Herbalists Guild, and president of Wise Woman Herbals in Creswell, Oregon. Grind a small amount of flaxseed in a food processor, mix in just enough water to form a paste, and put it over the splinter.

Bandage the area and let the poultice dry out completely. "Reapply a new poultice every day, covered with a new bandage," she suggests. "I've had luck using this to draw out glass and wood splinters. The longest I've had to use the flax continuously was for a week, but it worked. Flax seems to open the skin and suck out the splinter."

Portland, Oregon, and associate medicinary director at the college's public clinic. She suggests stirring together this easy herbal antiseptic formula in advance, so it's ready when you need it. Mix ½ ounce each of the following tinctures (also called extracts): calendula, echinacea, St.-John's-wort, and Oregon grape root. Store the mixture in a two-ounce dark glass bottle with a dropper in the lid. "This mixture has a shelf life of about a year," she notes. "I keep some at home and also carry it in my first-aid kit." Research shows that calendula and echinacea may have antimicrobial powers.

To use the mixture, mix equal parts of the antiseptic and sterile water (such as distilled water or filtered tap water) and use the liquid to wash cuts and scrapes, she says.

If you have access to fresh calendula petals, substitute ½ ounce of fresh calendula "succus," or juice, for the calendula tincture, Andrews-Miller suggests. Whirl the petals in a food processor with a little alcohol (such as grain alcohol or vodka), then strain and press out the juice.

Soothe scrapes with witch hazel. Scrape your knee on gravel? Scratch yourself on a prickly thorn bush? Cleanse and help mend ragged cuts with witch hazel, suggests 7Song, a professional member of the AHG and director of the Northeast School of Botanical Medicine in Ithaca, New York. "It soothes the tissue, draws together the ragged edges, and helps protect opened skin from infection," he says.

This native American shrub was used by the Cherokee, Chippewa, Mohegan, and Iroquois for scrapes, cuts, and other skin problems. Research shows that witch hazel's bark, leaves, and twigs are rich in tannins, making it an excellent astringent that can soothe and protect inflamed, red, itching skin.

But avoid distilled witch hazel water from the drugstore, 7Song says. "Use witch hazel tincture diluted with water," he suggests. "The tincture contains astringent tannins that prompt proteins in the skin to form a protective layer over a cut." Apply it with cotton swabs or a clean cloth, he says.

Clean up with myrrh. Dissolved in water, this biblical botanical—a gift to the infant Jesus from one of the Three Wise

Men—fights infection and eases the pain of cuts and scrapes, says Lisa Murray-Doran, N.D., a naturopathic physician and instructor at the Canadian College of Naturopathic Medicine in Toronto. Used for centuries as an astringent, myrrh is a reddish-brown resin that flows from the bark of a species of shrubs and small trees native to northeastern Africa and southwestern Asia. Laboratory research suggests that myrrh may have antimicrobial activity.

"I would dissolve a teaspoon of myrrh powder in a cup of warm water and use that liquid to wash out a cut right away," she says. Myrrh powder is available in health food stores and by mail order (see "Where to Buy Herbs and Herbal Products" on page 462).

Disinfect with tea tree oil. For a quicker antiseptic wash, splash 4 to 6 drops of tea tree oil into $\frac{1}{4}$ cup of water, Dr. Murray-Doran suggests. Popularized in Australia in the 1920s and 1930s as an infection fighter for external problems from dirty wounds to athlete's foot, tea tree oil has been shown by research to fend off bacteria.

Try the "picnic" remedy. Chop or crush a clove of garlic into a cup of wine, let stand for a minute or two, then use the liquid to wash a cut or scrape, suggests Paul Bergner, clinical director of the Rocky Mountain Center for Botanical Studies in Boulder, Colorado, editor of *Medical Herbalism* and author of *The Healing Power of Garlic* and *The*

Herbal Wisdom
An Art, Not a Science

"Herbalism was an art long before it was a science. That's why herbal remedies sometimes don't always have formulas with exact measurements or have one-size-fits-all dosages. We tailor medicines to fit the individual people we treat."

—*Lisa Murray-Doran, N.D., instructor at the Canadian College of Naturopathic Medicine*

Healing Power of Echinacea and Goldenseal and Other Immune System Herbs. Garlic's antibacterial powers, first recognized by the French microbiologist Louis Pasteur in the mid-1800s, have been used since the days of the Egyptian pharaohs. "The alcohol in the wine will help release infection-fighting constituents in the chopped garlic," Bergner notes. "You could also take garlic internally to help fend off minor infections in cuts and scrapes. Try blending three garlic cloves with a pint of carrot juice in a blender and drinking it three times a day."

Quiet wound pain with St.-John's-wort. An infused oil of St.-John's-wort "is better than aspirin" for soothing scraped skin and raw nerves, Dr. Murray-Doran says. Used traditionally for cuts with nerve damage, St.-John's-wort is recommended for wounds by Commission E, the expert panel that judges the safety and effectiveness of herbal medicines for the German government.

"Dip a cotton swab in the oil and apply directly to the cut," Dr. Murray-Doran suggests. Look for St.-John's-wort oil in health food stores and mail-order catalogs, or make

(continued on page 198)

Mother Nature's First-Aid Kit

Stocked in your kitchen or medicine cabinet or stowed in your suitcase when vacation time rolls around, herbal first-aid remedies can be at least as effective as conventional ointments and painkillers for those inevitable cuts, scrapes, and other minor skin problems, says Jenny McFeely, a member of Britain's National Institute of Medical Herbalists and a professional member of the American Herbalists Guild, who teaches courses on herbalism through her Herbal Healing and Research Center in Scottsdale, Arizona.

Here are the basics that you'll need to stock a small, portable first-aid kit, as recommended by McFeely and Sharleen Andrews-Miller, a faculty member at the National College of Naturopathic Medicine in Portland, Oregon, and associate medicinary director at the college's public clinic.

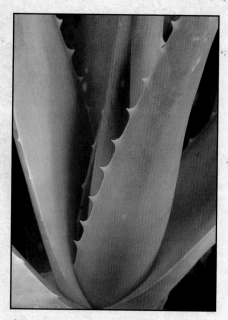

Aloe: skin soother. Keep a plant on a sunny windowsill. Use the gel inside leaves for burns and sunburn.

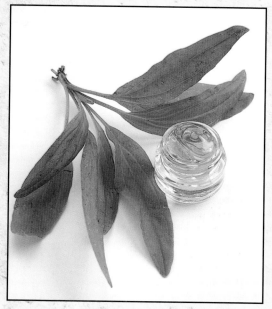

Arnica: bruise fixer. Spread arnica gel on bruised areas to ease pain, swelling, and discoloration. (Shelf life: one to two years.)

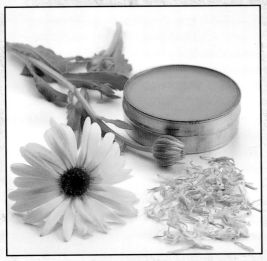

Calendula: disinfectant wound healer.
Use calendula salve for cuts and scrapes or dried calendula petals brewed into a tea (steep for 10 to 20 minutes) to wash wounds. (Shelf life of salve: at least one year.)

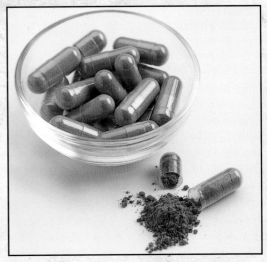

Goldenseal: infection solver. Good for skin infections. Open a capsule and sprinkle the powder onto an infected cut. If an infection doesn't show signs of improvement within a week, see a doctor. (Shelf life: one year.)

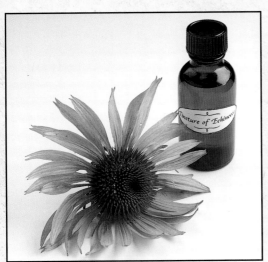

Echinacea: antiseptic skin wash. Dilute equal parts of echinacea tincture and distilled or filtered water as an antiseptic wash for skin infections. (Shelf life: one to two years.)

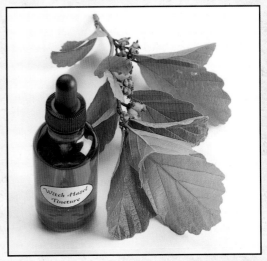

Witch hazel: skin healer. Protects broken skin from infection and has a very cooling effect on hot, inflamed areas. Dab diluted tincture on external hemorrhoids or acne, using a cotton swab. (Shelf life: several years.)

your own with fresh flowers and olive oil, following the directions in "A Saintly Burn Soother" on page 185.

Stop bleeding with shepherd's purse. Heavy, uncontrolled bleeding from a wound requires a trip to the emergency room. But a tincture (also called an extract) of shepherd's purse taken internally can slow (or stop) oozing blood until you are able get medical help, says Dr. Murray-Doran. "Drink 40 drops every five minutes in enough warm water to get the tincture down, until the bleeding halts," she suggests. "Shepherd's purse is better than any other herb for stopping bleeding and is an old, old remedy for this." It is still used today by herbalists and naturopaths, she says.

Apply an herbal skin mender—liberally. Once a wound is clean and disinfected, apply calendula cream, suggests Dr. Murray-Doran. "Gob it on," she says. "Then cover lightly with a bandage so you don't get the cream all over the place."

Studies suggest that preparations made from calendula petals may help speed healing of surgical incisions and slow-healing wounds. Researchers have found that calendula extracts can decrease swelling and increase wound-healing activity that produces new skin cells. An antiseptic that can help stop bleeding, calendula was used to heal bullet wounds on America's western frontier in the 1880s.

"There's an old saying that 'Where there's calendula, there's no need for a surgeon,'" notes Bergner. "That comes from a time when infected wounds could lead to limb amputations. This is a great wound-healing herb."

Look for calendula cream in health food stores or mail-order catalogs, or make your own, Dr. Murray-Doran says. First, make a calendula-infused oil, following the directions in "Infused Oils" on page 101. Then use this oil to make a salve, using the technique described in "Salves and Ointments" on page 110. You can also apply the oil directly to cleaned cuts. "It's especially good for healing cuts that have a ragged ugliness to them," 7Song says.

Consider comfrey—carefully. Herbalists are quick to note that comfrey can mend broken skin quickly—so quickly that this herb must be handled with care. "You have to remember that comfrey is not a disinfectant. What it does best is soothe and cause skin cells to proliferate," notes 7Song. "If there's any infection in the cut, comfrey may heal the top layers of skin right over it, driving infection deeper into skin tissues."

Herbalists suggest using comfrey only on shallow, clean, uninfected cuts and scrapes. Select a comfrey ointment that's dark green, which is usually a sign that the product contains an effective amount of the herb, suggests herbalist Jenny McFeely, a member of Britain's National Institute of Medical Herbalists and a professional member of the AHG, who teaches courses on herbalism through her Herbal Healing and Research Center in Scottsdale, Arizona.

If you have comfrey growing in your backyard, use a blender or food processor to combine comfrey root with enough water to form a paste. "Soak the wound in it, or make a poultice by gobbing the comfrey root slurry on the cut and covering it with a bandage," Dr. Tilgner says. "Change this poultice every few hours."

Research shows that comfrey contains a substance called allantoin, which prompts tissue repair, as well as rosmarinic acid, which reduces swelling. While herbalists caution against taking comfrey internally without guidance because of the plant's concentration of potentially liver-damaging pyrrolizidine alkaloids, external use of this wound-healing botanical does not pose a threat, Dr. Murray-Doran says. "These alkaloids are not absorbed through the skin," she says.

Fight infection with echinacea. As extra "health insurance" against infection, boost your immune response by taking echinacea, suggests 7Song. "When I'm giving someone first-aid care, I usually suggest taking herbs with antimicrobial properties when applying external disinfectants," he says. "You don't want an infection to get started, or to spread if there already is one. This is where echinacea is in its prime—for promoting the body's infection-fighting abilities early on to head off a problem."

If infection is setting in, take one to two dropperfuls of echinacea tincture (also called an extract) every hour until the symptoms (such as redness and swelling), begin to wane, 7Song suggests. If the wound does not begin to heal within a week, see a doctor.

Used traditionally by Native Americans, echinacea seems to work by stimulating infection-gobbling white blood cells to work harder.

Consider an echinacea wash. Echinacea has been shown to help wound healing through its anti-inflammatory properties.

Mix 1 part echinacea tincture with 3 parts water, apply it to the cut, and cover with a gauze bandage. Reapply every two hours. "When applied to the skin, echinacea seems to fight infections by strengthening a gelatin-like barrier between skin cells that acts as one of the body's defenses against bacteria," notes Bergner.

Keep your cool with Rescue Remedy. If the circumstances that caused the cut or scrape leave you emotionally shaken, regain your composure by taking a few drops of Rescue Remedy under your tongue or in a glass of water, suggests Andrews-Miller. A mixture of flower essences in an alcohol-and-water base, Rescue Remedy is said to restore calm feelings.

Andrews-Miller suggests adding 3 to 5 drops of this commercially prepared remedy, available at health food stores and by mail, to your herbal antiseptic mix. She also recommends keeping a bottle in your first-aid kit or glove compartment.

Dental Health

TEAS—AND MORE—FOR CAVITIES AND TOOTHACHES

When it comes to healthy teeth, herbalists are in perfect accord with the dental establishment. Before your herbalist even mentions herbs, she'll probably echo your dentist by reminding you to brush and floss and schedule checkups every six months.

But beyond this basic wisdom, herbalists do have a few ideas of their own for healthy teeth. They'll tell you that some herbs can ac-

Bloodroot: Just What the Dentist Ordered

One of spring's earliest-to-bloom wildflowers, the beautiful bloodroot bears lovely, single white blossoms, often tinted with rose or purple. But its exotic root gives the plant its name. Reddish brown and covered with long orange fibers, the root is blood red inside, and when cut open, it exudes an orange-colored juice.

Native Americans knew bloodroot best as the dye plant they called *musquaspenne*. They introduced it to Virginia's first colonists, and from there early botanical physicians adopted its use.

Bloodroot contains an alkaloid called sanguinarine, which chemically binds to dental plaque and keeps it from sticking to teeth. Today, bloodroot is an ingredient in some toothpastes and mouthwashes. But its ability to prevent plaque and stave off periodontal disease was apparently unknown to the nineteenth-century physicians who popularized the plant. These doctors, known as the Eclectics, used bloodroot as a remedy for coughs and pneumonia, hepatitis, headaches, circulatory problems, and cancer.

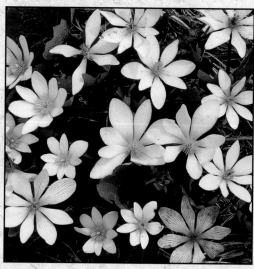

A substance in bloodroot called sanguinarine helps keep dental plaque from sticking to teeth.

tually reduce tooth decay. And they'll offer potent herbal treatments to quell toothache pain until you can get to the dentist's office.

Cavity Fighters from Nature

Herbal experts offer this advice for maintaining a healthy smile.

Take tea and see no cavities. "The very best herb for preventing cavities is *Camellia sinensis*," says Memory Elvin-Lewis, Ph.D., professor of microbiology and ethnobotany in biomedicine at Washington University in St. Louis, Missouri. Dr. Elvin-Lewis has expertise in ethnodentistry, the study of botanical dental treatments.

Never heard of *Camellia sinensis* ? Sure you have—it's just plain tea, green or black, the kind that fills tea bags everywhere. "Tea has plenty of soluble fluoride, which is essential for healthy teeth. In addition, it's rich in tannins, which prevent plaque from forming on the surfaces of teeth," says Dr. Elvin-Lewis. Green tea, which is processed differently from black tea, may contain even more fluoride than the black variety, and it has the extra advantage of being a potent antioxidant, Dr. Elvin-Lewis adds. Four or so cups of tea a day will give you all the fluoride your teeth need, she notes; iced tea and decaffeinated tea also count.

Brew yourself a strong infusion. "To prevent the loss of tooth enamel, which can lead to decay, I believe in drinking mineral-rich herbal infusions every day," says Susun S. Weed, an herbalist and herbal educator from Woodstock, New York, and author of the *Wise Woman* series of herbal health books. "I use only one herb at a time and vary them to mine a broad spectrum of natural minerals. I particularly like nettle, red clover blossoms, oatstraw, or comfrey leaf," says Weed.

To make a tooth-nourishing infusion, place 1 ounce (by weight) of dried (not fresh) herb in a quart jar. "I add a heaping tablespoon of dried horsetail, because it contributes to tooth strength," says Weed. Fill the jar to the top with boiling water. Steep at least 4 hours or overnight. Strain out the herbs, pressing them to release all the liquid. Add honey or salt to taste and drink at room temperature, over ice, or reheated. "I drink a cup or two a day," says Weed.

Sweeten with a bit of licorice. Licorice is not only a natural sugar-free sweetener, it also contains glycyrrhizin, a bacteria killer, and indole, a powerful decay-preventive, says James A. Duke, Ph.D., a botanical consultant, former ethnobotanist with the U.S. Department of Agriculture, and author of *The Green Pharmacy*, who specializes in medicinal plants. To sweeten with licorice, add a little of the dried root to your tea blend before brewing.

Substitute stevia. Stevia is a naturally sweet herb that hails from Paraguay. It's as sweet as sugar but lacks both calories and decay-promoting potential, and you can buy it as a tea. Simply add a pinch to any beverage that you want to sweeten, suggests Dr. Duke.

Add bloodroot to your toothbrush. You'll find bloodroot listed among the ingredients in some toothpastes and mouthwashes; it contains a compound called sanguinarine, which studies show reduces the amount of dental plaque deposited on teeth in as little as eight days. "It doesn't taste very good, but it works," notes Weed. "I use one drop of bloodroot tincture (also called an extract) on my toothbrush and then brush from the gumline to the tooth," she adds.

Bloodroot is safe when used in commercial dental products or under the guidance of a trained herbalist, says Varro E. Tyler, Ph.D., professor emeritus of pharmacognosy at the Purdue University School of Pharmacy and Pharmacal Sciences in West Lafayette, Indiana, in his book *Herbs of Choice*, but don't try to use it on your own.

Herbal Toothache Relief

Once you have a toothache, it's hard to ignore. You can try chewing with teeth other than the painful one but—ouch!—sooner or later, you'll miss and send a jolt of pain screaming up your nerve endings. The only real solution for toothache pain, herbalists agree, is to see your dentist. But until you can get into her chair, try one of these botanical pain relievers.

Stun tooth pain with cloves. Rub a drop of essential oil of clove directly on an aching tooth, suggests Ellen Kamhi, R.N., Ph.D., of Oyster Bay, New York, an herbalist, professional member of the American Herbalists

Cloves: Kill the Pain (and Germs, Too)

Most of us use cloves to flavor foods, from holiday hams to homemade pickles. But this fragrant, spicy herb—actually the dried buds of a tree thought to be native to southeast Asia—is good medicine, too. In China, it is a traditional remedy for nausea and diarrhea.

Clove bud oil contains from 60 to 90 percent eugenol, a potent antimicrobial. Eugenol has been shown to kill a variety of bacteria, fungi, and viruses, including the ringworm that causes athlete's foot and the herpes simplex virus.

Eugenol also deadens pain, which explains why oil of cloves is a time-honored remedy for toothache. Place a drop of clove oil directly on the aching tooth, recommends James A. Duke, Ph.D., a botanical consultant, former ethnobotanist with the U.S. Department of Agriculture, and author of *The Green Pharmacy*, who specializes in medicinal plants.

In a pinch, you can make your own clove oil, experts say. Steep ¼ teaspoon of crushed whole cloves in 3 tablespoons of heated vegetable oil for 5 minutes. Strain the oil and apply. Don't use this remedy for long, though. Clove oil is a powerful irritant and can damage the gums if applied for too long or too often.

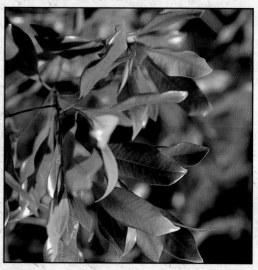

Eugenol, the main chemical in clove oil, kills bacteria, fungi, and viruses.

Guild, and host of the nationally syndicated radio show *Natural Alternatives*. "If you don't have oil of clove handy, just wiggle a whole clove, pointed end down, next to the tooth," she adds. The oil has the official endorsement of the Food and Drug Administration (FDA) as being safe. A scientific committee reporting to the FDA commented that oil of clove was "effective for temporary use on a tooth with throbbing pain," says Dr. Duke. It's widely available at health food stores.

Irritate the pain away. Although it may sound a little masochistic, applying the red-hot heat of cayenne pepper to your tooth can actually ease pain. The principle is called counterirritation, says Dr. Duke. When you temporarily irritate a tooth's surface, toothache pain diminishes. What's more, red pepper contains aspirin-like pain-relieving chemicals called salicylates. Mix a little powdered cayenne in enough water to form a gooey paste, then take a cotton ball, dip it in the paste, and apply it directly to the tooth without touching the gum. If it hurts too much, rinse your mouth and try a different remedy, recommends Dr. Duke.

Open sesame. According to Dr. Duke, sesame contains at least seven pain-relieving compounds. Boil 1 part sesame seed with 3 parts water until the liquid is reduced by half. Cool the resulting decoction and apply it directly to the tooth. Fourth-century Chinese healers used this, and it works, says Dr. Duke.

Digestive Problems

A POTPOURRI OF HERBAL CURES

Hundreds of years ago, when Galileo suggested that the planets revolved around the sun, not the Earth, people thought he'd lost his mind. Years later, of course, everyone realized that he was right.

Today, herbalists who think that the digestive system involves more organs than just the stomach and intestines can identify with Galileo and his misunderstood solar system. The digestive system, they say, consists of more interconnected organs than many of us usually consider. And, they say, those interconnected organs work together in harmony only when your "life force" is properly balanced.

Like most people, you probably assume that the stomach is our digestive gatekeeper. We blame it for just about all of our digestive ills. All manner of digestive system disruptions—such as heartburn, gas, indigestion, diarrhea, constipation, nausea, and vomiting—can be blamed on stomach trouble. Yet, according to herbalists, the stomach usually plays second fiddle to numerous more crucial digestive organs, such as the liver, gallbladder, pancreas, and kidneys—and even the brain, which is linked with the digestive organs via the vagus nerve, a long nerve that connects with the esophagus, stomach, small intestine, pancreas, and colon.

To a Western doctor, such notions might sound preposterous. But herbalists operate on the principle that no bodily organ works without assistance.

Digestive Teamwork

To get an idea of how these organs are interrelated, follow some food through the body. Let's say you're eating an apple. You bite into the apple, and digestion begins as the teeth grind and crush it, releasing saliva from three special glands in the mouth. The saliva lubricates the apple for ease of swallowing, and it contains enzymes, like ptyalin, that begin to break it down. Then you swallow. The chewed-up apple slides down your esophagus and into your stomach. There, three layers of muscle contract every 20 seconds, pulverizing the apple. Meanwhile, the stomach secretes bacteria-destroying hydrochloric acid. Your apple is now a creamy paste called chyme, which is sent by muscle contractions into the small intestine.

Once the apple exits the stomach, your pancreas, liver, and gallbladder secrete important bile and enzymes into your small intestine. Without those secretions, your pasty apple would never break down into digestible molecules. As muscle contractions push it through several feet of intestine, the intestinal walls absorb usable nutrients. The non-nutritive portion—water and fiber—keeps going and eventually enters the large intestine, or colon, which absorbs water from what's left of the apple and sends the remains down to the rectum and back to the outside world.

Along the way, a number of things can go wrong, say herbalists. Sometimes, we blame digestive problems on what, or how much, we ate. But maybe the liver failed to supply enough bile. Even your brain gets involved, throwing digestion into turmoil if you're frightened or worried.

Conversely, if your digestive system is on the fritz, you're not going to feel your best emotionally. Heartburn, constipation, or gas may leave you grumpy or irritable.

"Digestion is integral and essential to good health," says Janet Zand, O.M.D., a doctor of Oriental medicine, professional member of the American Herbalists Guild (AHG), and co-founder of Zand Herbal Formulas in Boulder, Colorado. "In Traditional Chinese Medicine, not only do you have physiological digestive symptoms when digestion is weak, you also have mental symptoms. People who have weak digestion also have a tendency to obsess. Their obsession, the Chinese say, further weakens their digestive systems. In holistic medicine, the emotional, mental, physical, and spiritual are all interconnected," explains Dr. Zand. "If your digestion is impaired, your immunity and other functions will also be impaired."

Herbs for the Fire in Your Belly

Besides those many acids, muscle contractions, and enzymes, herbalists also believe that your digestive tract houses an energy. Different herbalists call this energy different things, from fire to chi to vital force, all words that describe that invisible aspect of digestion that can, if properly balanced, make everything run smoothly.

"Ayurvedic medicine, a healing system that originated in India, regards food as our most important medicine," explains David Frawley, O.M.D., a doctor of Oriental medicine, professional member of the AHG, director of the American Institute of Vedic Studies in Santa Fe, New Mexico, and author of *The Yoga of Herbs* and *Ayurvedic Healing*. "But it's not just a question of what we eat, it's whether we are digesting what we eat. Many people blame food for problems that are really caused by weak digestive fire. If they increased their digestive fire, they could handle more types of food."

Herbalists believe that like prescription and over-the-counter drugs, herbs can suppress symptoms such as diarrhea, gas, and nausea. Unlike medication, however, herbs can also balance that fire just mentioned. They head to the site of your problem, healing the ill health that triggers your symptoms and providing a more lasting fix, says Robyn Klein, a professional member of the AHG in Bozeman, Montana. If you consult an herbalist for diarrhea, for example, she

For Better Digestion, Support Your Liver

*I*f you entered your liver in a contest for underappreciated bodily organs, this three-pound organ would win, hands down. And when it comes to digestion, you might think that your stomach and intestines do all the work. But your liver plays a larger role in digestion than you might guess.

Responsible for more than 500 functions, your liver sees all the blood that leaves the stomach and intestines. It stores glycogen, the energy source that our cells need. The liver detoxifies the blood and rids your body of poisonous substances. And it secretes bile that aids in fat digestion.

"The liver is a filter, and it manufactures 2,000 different kinds of enzymes that are necessary in body functions," says Gayle Eversole, R.N., Ph.D., a nurse practitioner, medical herbalist, and professional member of the American Herbalists Guild (AHG) in Everett, Washington. "For women, the liver is important because it deactivates estrogen so it can be recycled. A lot of women get digestive disorders and menstrual cycle problems because their livers are congested."

PMS and menopausal symptoms of indigestion are often related to liver congestion, Dr. Eversole notes, as are fibroid tumors, breast tenderness, and other difficulties. Diet and lifestyle changes are a necessary part of healing with herbs, she adds.

Any imbalance in this delicate process can show up in the oddest of places. "When people have liver imbalances, they get frontal headaches and sinus pain. They may awake in the morning with a coated tongue and filmy teeth. When they eat fat, they keep burping it up because it takes such a long time to digest," says Daniel Gagnon, a professional member of the AHG, executive director of the Botanical Research and Education Institute, and owner of Herbs, Etc., in Santa Fe, New Mexico.

If you consult an herbalist for excess acid, indigestion, or even gas, don't be surprised if she discusses your liver. She'll probably suggest herbs such as barberry, elderflower, and peppermint, which herbalists say cleanse this important organ.

won't just give you an herb to dry up diarrhea. She'll also give you an herb to counteract whatever triggered the diarrhea, such as nervous tension or low levels of beneficial intestinal bacteria.

"Herbs are particularly good at solving problems in the digestive tract," says Klein. "Mucous membrane tissue lines everything from your mouth to your anus. And herbs come directly in contact with this mucous membrane. Some herbs, such as slippery elm, marshmallow root, and psyllium, are used specifically to soothe the mucous membrane layer."

Because digestive herbs are gentle, side effects are minimal. "Herbs are foods, and as such they are 'digested' by the body, with their medicinal components acting slowly and thereby reducing the side effects that most people associate with drugs," says Gayle

Eversole, R.N., Ph.D., a nurse practitioner, medical herbalist, and professional member of the AHG in Everett, Washington.

On the downside, because herbs lack the strength of prescription or over-the-counter drugs, your symptoms may take longer to be resolved. "It took you 35 years to get where you are, and it may take you a year or two to get where you should be," says Dr. Eversole. So even though you might feel better when you start to take digestive herbs, you ought to continue your herbal routine to ensure resolution of your problem, she says. In general, if you're using an herb for the first time, she recommends taking it for six days, followed by one day off; then for six weeks, followed by a week off; then for six months, followed by a month off. "That will make you aware of the changes your body is making toward healing," says Dr. Eversole. This schedule covers seven months, she explains. At the end of that time, you will have an idea whether you need to repeat the schedule. She emphasizes that herbs are for healing, not just the temporary relief of symptoms.

Wonder Herbs for Your Tummy

As you read the tips throughout this chapter, you'll hear about peppermint, chamomile, and ginger over and over again. That's because, to herbal practitioners, those three herbs can solve just about every problem in your digestive tract. "Drugs usually have only one or maybe two—sometimes three—uses," says Daniel Gagnon, professional member of the AHG, executive director of the Botanical Research and Education Institute and owner of Herbs, Etc., in Santa Fe, New Mexico. "Herbs have a multitude of factors and compounds, and the body can use those different compounds in different areas. That's the beauty of herbs," he says.

Peppermint's menthol-rich oils, tannins, and bitters traditionally have been used for just about all digestive distresses, from gas to nausea to indigestion. Herbalists say that the gingerols and shogaols found in ginger can suppress nausea, vomiting, and motion sickness. Ginger also stimulates saliva flow and digestive activity, which eases pain from gas and diarrhea. And it warms the body, opening your pores and helping you sweat out a fever. "It is an incredible herb," says Gagnon.

Finally, chamomile has earned fame as the gentlest herb with the most uses. "During a class at the National College of Phytotherapy in Albuquerque, my students and I were trying to come up with different mental images for various herbs," says Gagnon. "When we got to chamomile, the image my students created was an all-terrain vehicle with nice, soft seats. Like an all-terrain vehicle, chamomile can go just about anywhere, but it's a smooth ride. It can go from nice roads to terrain that's really rough and full of mud and branches, and it's still able to provide a lot of comfort."

When treating digestive ailments, herbalists also often turn to a class of herbs called bitters. Bitter herbs like gentian, barberry, fenugreek, and angelica lubricate your digestive system. "Bitters send the signal to the brain and by reflex action also to the stomach and the intestine that we are about to receive food, and therefore they should start secreting juices," says Gagnon. Because angelica causes uterine contractions, however, do not use it during pregnancy.

In addition to herbal solutions for specific health concerns such as heartburn, gas, and constipation, herbalists advocate taking certain herbs to improve the overall health of

Bitter Herbs Sweeten Digestion

The French start their meals with an apéritif for a good reason—the highly flavored little drink really does juice up the appetite.

"An apéritif usually has bitters," says French-Canadian Daniel Gagnon, a professional member of the American Herbalists Guild (AHG), executive director of the Botanical Research and Education Institute, and owner of Herbs, Etc., in Santa Fe, New Mexico. "Many apéritifs contain Angostura bitters. The bitter taste gets the salivary glands going. It helps the stomach start secreting juices. The bitterness sends the signal to the brain to get the whole digestive tract—the liver, the pancreas, and the intestines—on the lookout for incoming food. It's like a sneak preview."

Herbal practitioners say that when your tongue gets a dose of Angostura's natural bitterness, your tastebuds tell your brain to tell your gastrointestinal system to release the hormone gastrin, which increases gastric acid, bile flow, and numerous other secretions all along your digestive tract.

Just about any bitter-tasting herb will provide the same benefit, say herbalists. In beer, the flowering bitter herb hops prompts a similar reaction. Gentian ranks as perhaps the most effective bitter digestive herb. The problem is, it's so bitter, few people can stand it. "But it's very effective, especially for people who have difficulty digesting fat," says Janet Zand, O.M.D., a doctor of Oriental medicine, professional member of the AHG, and co-founder of Zand Herbal Formulas in Boulder, Colorado.

Other bitter herbs include milk thistle, dandelion, artichoke, and beet leaf.

Here are some ways to use bitters to aid digestion.

✔ Start each meal with a small salad that contains bitter, dark leafy greens such as arugula. Flavor the salad with lemon juice.

✔ Have ½ cup of gentian tea or hops tea 15 to 20 minutes before meals. To make the tea, use 1 teaspoon of grated gentian root or 1 heaping tablespoon of hops per cup of boiling water.

✔ If you overeat at a restaurant, ask for a shot of Angostura bitters. Pour the shot into a glass of water to dilute it. The bitter taste will speed digestion. "Yes, it's bitter. But in a half-hour, you'll feel so much better that you'll be contemplating a second piece of pie," says Gagnon.

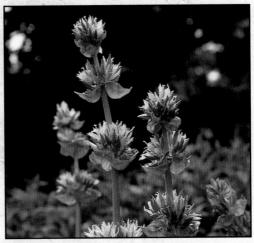

In Europe, people take gentian after a big meal.

your digestive tract and to prevent problems before they occur. Here's what they suggest.

Use cayenne and garlic generously. These herbal antibiotics will kill off germs that can cause problems as benign as the stomach flu and as serious as dysentery, says Dr. Eversole. These herbs also kill the *Helicobacter pylori* bacteria, which are responsible for many cases of ulcers. Flavor your food with either or both often. When handling hot peppers, wear latex or plastic gloves and avoid touching your eyes or nose.

Taste six times. The typical American diet centers on sweet or salty food. We often miserably lack four other very important tastes—bitter, pungent, astringent, and sour, says Dr. Frawley. Making sure our largest meal of the day provides a little of all six tastes could go a long way toward helping our digestive systems do their jobs, he says.

"You can get some sour simply by having some lemon," says Dr. Frawley. "And bitter comes from using spices like fenugreek or turmeric. Or you could start the meal with a salad made with bitter greens, which also will give you the astringent taste. So will cabbage. And for spicy, use cayenne, mustard, or horseradish. Ayurvedic medicine holds that as long as you get all six tastes, you'll be doing your digestive system some good. It helps stimulate bodily processes for the tongue to get those tastes."

Add fibrous foods and herbs to your diet. "The mucous membrane between your mouth and your anus massages and churns your food," says Klein. "You need to exercise those tissues by providing fiber. The tissue needs a chance to stretch and grab onto something and smush it." To add fiber, eat more produce and whole grains as well as fibrous herbs such as slippery elm and psyllium, a powdered seed sold as a remedy for constipation. (But be careful: Taking psyllium without adequate water may cause it to swell and block your throat or esophagus and may cause choking.)

"Slippery elm is slippery," Klein explains. It has a bland, slightly sweet taste and a very slimy texture when it sits in water for a minute. Because not too many people like this texture, she suggests that you put the powder (1 teaspoon) into ½ cup of warm water, then chug it. If you add a bit of honey or mix some other herbs with it, it can be quite a pleasant tea, she adds.

Step up to the water cooler. Herbs won't work if your body is dehydrated, says Dr. Eversole. "Drinking coffee or black tea isn't the same as drinking water," she says. "Neither is drinking juice. I tell people to drink eight, eight-ounce glasses of distilled water a day." Distilled water helps remove toxins and protects the thyroid from interference from chlorination and fluoridation, which displace iodine from receptor sites in the thyroid gland and interfere with metabolism and digestion, Dr. Eversole explains. Ice water and very hot water are harmful to digestive enzymes, and you should avoid drinking water or other fluids with food to prevent dilution of enzymatic processes. Drink at least 30 minutes before or after eating, not during meals, she suggests.

Heartburn

Heartburn strikes most often an hour after eating, especially after the largest meal of the day or after eating sugary, high-fat foods. That's because a large amount of food or fatty, sugary foods can decrease pressure on the sphincter that holds highly corrosive acid in the stomach. This allows the acid to creep up and irritate the esophagus, a process known as reflux, which feels like a fire in your chest.

If you're like most people with heartburn, you've probably consumed your share of over-the-counter antacids, which stop the burn temporarily. But repetitive use of antacids can actually worsen esophagus problems. So can stress.

Herbalists offer herbal solutions and also suggest that you avoid fatty or sugary foods, cut back on coffee, and drink a lot of water. "That's inexpensive and immediate," Dr. Eversole says.

To further calm your digestive system, bring it into balance, and greatly reduce repetitive bouts with heartburn, consider these herbal strategies.

Soothe with chamomile. A mild sedative, chamomile has an anti-inflammatory effect on the mucous membranes, says Corinne Martin, a professional member of the AHG who practices in Bridgeton, Maine. To make chamomile tea, add 1 full tablespoon of whole dried chamomile flowers to 1 cup of hot water and steep for 15 minutes. Strain and drink. If you prefer to use fresh chamomile flowers, that's fine, too, says Martin. Just be sure to double the amount of herbs used. To prevent heartburn recurrence, make a habit of drinking chamomile often throughout the day, she says.

Speed digestion with turmeric. Bitter herbs stimulate the flow of digestive juices, moving food along and preventing acid buildup. So spice up your food with the bitter herb turmeric, which is the base of most Indian curries, says Dr. Frawley. "Turmeric is good for digestion and also helps build the blood. It's a very good spice for women to have in their diets because it also eases men-

struation," he says. If simply flavoring your food isn't enough to stop the burn, he suggests taking two or three turmeric capsules (½ to 1 gram), which are available at health food stores, before a meal.

Eat licorice before meals. A natural antacid, licorice root can prevent heartburn if you take it before a meal, says Dr. Frawley. He suggests taking two or three licorice capsules (½ to 1 gram), which are available at health food stores, before meals.

Sip meadowsweet for relief. Used on a regular basis, this leafy plant acts like a natural antacid to prevent heartburn and acid stomach. To make meadowsweet tea, add 1 tablespoon of the herb (available at health food stores) to 1 cup of hot water and steep for 10 to 15 minutes. Strain and drink one to two cups a day, says Gagnon.

Use dandelion for digestive balance. If you drink generous amounts of coffee to provide the energy needed to accomplish 6,000 tasks in a single day, you're a doer. Practitioners of Traditional Chinese Medicine, who categorize people as one of five different elements—wood, fire, water, earth, and metal—might say that you have a wood constitution or wood imbalance, says Darlena LaOrange-Theocharides, a licensed acupuncturist in Soquel, California, professional member of the AHG, and author of *Herbal Healing Secrets of the Orient*. And many wood types are notorious for excess stomach acid and heartburn, she says.

If you rely on coffee to fuel your drive, she suggests that you first pare down your coffee consumption to a cup a day (three cups a week is a great goal to shoot for). Then eat steamed dandelion greens or a dandelion green salad before your largest meal of the day. The bitter flavor will speed digestion and lower acidity. Flavor the raw or steamed leaves with lemon juice and olive oil, says LaOrange-Theocharides. You can find fresh dandelion in the spring in supermarkets or on lawns. Look for the notched leaves that grow before the plant flowers. If you pick your own, make sure it's from a lawn that hasn't been sprayed with chemical weed killers or fertilizers.

Gas

Aging isn't kind to your digestive system. A natural age-related loss of digestive enzymes lets food sit around longer in your intestine, and it's the fermentation of this slowly moving food that causes gas buildup. Toss in a diet high in sugars and starch—cakes, cookies, pies, and baked goods—and you've got some serious complaints.

To remedy the situation, first cut back on sugar and starches, which feed yeast in the body and create gas. Then, to rid your body of any remaining gas, herbalists suggest that you turn to the following herbs to decrease your bloat without increasing flatulence.

Start with chamomile. Here's yet another use for this wonder tummy herb: Chamomile relieves flatulence by mildly sedating and soothing the digestive tract. To make a soothing tea, add 1 full tablespoon of whole dried flowers to 1 cup of hot water and steep for 15 minutes, says Martin. If you prefer to use fresh chamomile, that's okay, too, Martin adds. Just double the amount: If the recipe calls for 1 teaspoon of dried herbs, use 2 teaspoons of fresh. Drink the tea often throughout the day.

Destress with peppermint. Stress can trigger a gas attack. Fortunately, the smell of peppermint tea will calm your nerves as the active ingredient you sip travels to the gastrointestinal tract. "Peppermint works well for the entire GI tract and digestive function because it helps to re-establish the digestive enzymes," says Dr. Eversole. "It also relaxes the nerves in the digestive tract."

You'll get the best results by growing your own peppermint and using the fresh or dried leaves to make tea. But store-bought peppermint tea also will help, Dr. Eversole says. Have a cup in the morning and a cup at night, or more often. Use 1 tablespoon of whole dried leaves (2 tablespoons of fresh leaves) or a tea bag per cup of hot water and steep for 10 minutes. Sip slowly and smell the tea as you relax. Experiencing sight, smell, sense, and taste—all the things we forget about in our busy lives—is the holistic aspect of healing with herbs, she adds.

Counteract gas-producing foods. You have probably learned to evade gas by cutting back on foods like beans, milk, and cheese, which are notorious for producing it. The problem is, beans and low-fat dairy products are excellent sources of protein, calcium, and other nutrients that are critical for women. You can still eat those foods and avoid gas by having anti-gas spices along with them, says Dr. Frawley. The spices will help your body digest the food. Flavor beans with cumin. Have ginger with milk and cayenne with cheese. Vary the amount according to your tastes.

Chew fennel after meals. Aromatic herbs such as fennel, a perennial plant that produces aromatic seeds, can help the body absorb gas in the intestine. "That's why when you go to Indian restaurants, you see a little bowl of fennel seeds on the table," says Gagnon. "Indians are smart. That country is very crowded."

Start by flavoring your food with fennel and other aromatic spices such as cardamom seeds, basil, and mint. If you're not accustomed to eating highly seasoned food, you may need to give yourself some time to tolerate such flavors, so slowly increase the amount of seasoning you use in your cooking, says Dr. Frawley.

If you're eating as much spice as you can and still have excessive gas, try two or three capsules ($\frac{1}{2}$ to 1 gram) of any of those spices after your meal, says Dr. Frawley. Or chew a teaspoon of raw fennel seeds after meals. They are available at health food stores, most supermarkets, and some gourmet shops.

Warm with ginger. If along with having excess gas you also feel tired and cold, often get sinus infections, and have dry skin or clammy hands, you may have a metal constitution or imbalance, according to the five-element theory of Traditional Chinese Medicine. "Metal types frequently need to lubricate and warm the body," says LaOrange-Theocharides. So incorporate warming herbs such as ginger and garlic into your daily diet, along with foods that contain healthful oils, such as seeds, nuts, and avocado. Often, that will solve the problem, she says.

Indigestion

In the dictionary, *indigestion* is defined as exactly what the word says: the inability to digest. But we've misused the word over the years. Usually when we say we have indigestion, we mean that our stomachs ache, we feel acidic, and we're so full we wish we hadn't eaten the whole thing.

Excess stomach acid may clear up easily with a simple diet adjustment. Avoid relying heavily on foods such as meats, tomato sauce, orange juice, and other acidic foods. To re-establish the acid-alkaline balance in your system, switch to nonacidic fruits and vegetables, says LaOrange-Theocharides. If the problem persists or it's hard to change your diet, herbs can also balance the acid-alkaline levels, she says. Some that can assist include cardamom, fennel seeds, cumin, coriander, rosemary, peppermint, and hawthorn berries. Be prepared, however, as many of these are an acquired taste.

Digest better with gentian. A bitter herb, gentian root increases the flow of digestive juices, which help break down food. The body absorbs gentian extract (also known as a tincture) more quickly than other forms of the herb. Put 10 to 20 drops of extract in $\frac{1}{2}$ cup of water and drink it 15 to 20 minutes before meals, says Gagnon. Or grind up the root and use 1 teaspoon per cup of hot water for tea. Steep for 10 minutes, then strain and drink $\frac{1}{2}$ cup before each meal, Gagnon advises. Gentian extract is available at health food stores or by mail order (see "Where to Buy Herbs and Herbal Products" on page 462).

Try barberry. Like gentian, the bitter herb barberry will juice up your system and help you to digest more easily. Try 10 to 20 drops of barberry extract (available at health food stores or by mail order) diluted in about 4 ounces of water 15 to 20 minutes before meals, says Gagnon.

Calm your nerves with peppermint. Peppermint settles indigestion for the same reason that it dispels gas—it calms the nerves in your digestive system, Dr. Eversole explains. While you'll get best results by growing your own and using the fresh or dried leaves to make tea, store-bought teas can also help, says Dr. Eversole. To make tea,

A Five-Herb Apéritif for Indigestion

Remember the old vegetable juice commercial where people slapped themselves on the head and exclaimed: "I coulda had a V8!" Perhaps a more appropriate line, especially if they were searching for a before-meal drink, would have been "I shoulda had a BH3!" That's "B" for bitter and "H" for herb—three of them.

The bitter herbs—gentian, barberry, and angelica—combine beautifully to make the following apéritif, or premeal digestive aid. Add cardamom and fennel; although they're not bitters, both help dispel gas and make this tea more palatable, says Daniel Gagnon, professional member of the American Herbalists Guild, executive director of the Botanical Research and Education Institute, and owner of Herbs, Etc., in Santa Fe, New Mexico. Sipped a half-hour before meals, the drink will prime your system for an incoming meal, helping you to digest your food without distress.

Drink ½ cup a half-hour before lunch and the rest before dinner. This drink can be taken cold or warm, to your taste, but not ice cold. Gagnon warns that adding ice to the drink will suppress digestion, just the opposite of the goal you are trying to achieve.

Here's the recipe.

1	ounce dried gentian root, ground and sifted
½	ounce dried barberry, ground and sifted
½	ounce dried angelica, ground and sifted
¼	ounce crushed dried fennel seeds
¼	ounce crushed dried cardamom seeds

Combine the ingredients, put them in a glass container with a tight-fitting lid, and store in a cool location (a kitchen cupboard will do fine, Gagnon says). Then, to make a day's worth of apéritif, add 1 teaspoon of the herb mix to 1 cup of boiling water. Cover and simmer for 15 minutes. Allow the drink to cool and then strain the herbs from the liquid.

Makes enough for 20 cups

---

use 1 tablespoon of whole dried leaves (2 tablespoons of fresh) or one tea bag per cup of hot water and steep for 10 minutes. Relax by sipping slowly. Have a cup in the morning and a cup at night, or more often.

Settle down with chamomile. It will come as no surprise that chamomile, a mildly sedating anti-inflammatory herb, can also prevent indigestion. To make tea, add 1 full tablespoon of whole dried flowers to 1 cup of hot water, steep for 15 minutes, and then strain. Have tea often throughout the day to prevent indigestion, says Martin.

Or make a chamomile infusion by filling a quart jar three-quarters full with dried chamomile flowers. Add boiling water until the mixture reaches an inch from the top. Cover the jar and let stand at room temperature overnight. In the morning, strain out the herb and drink the infusion ¼ cup at a time, or as needed to relieve symptoms. Label it and store in your refrigerator for two to three days, says Patricia Howell, a professional member of the AHG in Atlanta.

Drink half a beer. If you like an occasional beer, you're familiar with the taste of hops, the slightly bitter flowering herb that's used in brewing. (Malt, on the other hand, sweetens beer.) Gagnon says a "hoppy" beer such as India Pale Ale might be all you need to get your digestion back on track.

"My grandfather lived to be almost 100 years old," says Gagnon. "Every day before lunch and dinner, he would have half a beer. The bitterness of the beer would get his digestive juices flowing. Now you've heard it from an herbalist: You have permission to drink half a beer twice a day."

More than half a bottle, however, and the alcohol will depress your digestive system, says Gagnon. If you don't like beer or if you need to avoid even small amounts of alcoholic beverages for any reason, you can make hops tea by using a heaping tablespoon of the dried herb per cup of hot water, Gagnon says.

Have fennel for dessert. In India, people traditionally chew fennel after meals to ward off indigestion, says Dr. Frawley. The naturally bitter taste gets the digestive juices flowing. Try chewing a teaspoon after each meal.

Grate some ginger. Generally, people with indigestion have cold hands and feet, says Dr. Eversole. "Those people are cold in the body and in digestion," she explains. Enter ginger, one of the most effective warming herbs. For best results, buy organic gingerroot, grate it, and mix 1 teaspoon to 1 tablespoon in a cup of hot water. Steep for 10 to 15 minutes and then strain (or use a tea ball). You can also buy and use premade

ginger teas, she says. For convenience, Dr. Eversole suggests using premade teas during the week and homemade on weekends. Drink a cup in the morning and one in the evening, before or after your meal.

Diarrhea

Diarrhea is a symptom, not a disease. Before treating diarrhea, you must determine from whence the problem comes. If it is a symptom of your body ridding itself of a bad oyster, for example, it might be better to let nature take its course. If it is a chronic condition, well, that's another situation. If diarrhea lasts more than two days or if you see blood in your stool, are experiencing severe cramping, or have a fever, nausea, vomiting, or signs of dehydration such as excessive thirst, dry lips, and reduced urination, see your doctor immediately.

Before turning to herbs, however, first take a look at your eating habits and stress levels. "Most people I see with problematic bowel movements have problematic lives. They do not have an eating schedule, and when and if they eat, they eat whatever they can lay their hands on," says Douglas Schar, a practicing medical herbalist in London, editor of the *British Journal of Phytotherapy*, and author of *Backyard Medicine Chest*. "If you have chronic diarrhea, the first thing to do is to put yourself on an eating schedule and stick to it—say, breakfast at 7:00 A.M., lunch at noon, and dinner at 6:00 P.M. When you eat, fill your plate with fruit and vegetables. People with high-fiber diets rarely have problems with bowel movements. If you don't correct your eating habits, you can forget having normal bowel movements. No medicine, herbal or otherwise, is going to do you a bit of good," he says.

If after changing your diet, you still have problems or you need a more immediate solution, herbal practitioners support turning to any of the following herbs.

Restore lost nutrients. The herbs alfalfa, nettle, raspberry leaves, and red clover will restore electrolyte minerals such as potassium, chloride, and sodium lost due to diarrhea. Such nutrients also help the body regulate the flow of water across mucous membranes, helping to solidify your stool, says Gagnon. Make a tea from one or all of the herbs, using a total of up to a tablespoon of dried herbs per cup. Steep for 10 to 15 minutes and strain the tea before you drink it. Have a cup twice a day until your symptoms subside, he recommends. You can drink a cup of this brew up to five times a day, according to Gagnon.

In an emergency, use cinnamon tea. If your diarrhea is so copious or frequent that you risk dehydration and you need to quickly dry up the flow, prepare some cinnamon tea. Cinnamon is a natural astringent and will dry up your bowel. "If you find yourself in a crisis situation, cinnamon tea will stop diarrhea quite quickly," says Schar. Mix a tablespoon of dried powdered cinnamon bark into a cup of hot water. Steep for 10 to 15 minutes.

Add bulk with slippery elm. Naturally fibrous, the bark from the slippery elm tree will rebuild your delicate mucous membranes as well as supply a multivitamin's worth of nutrients, which are sorely needed with diarrhea, says Dr. Eversole.

You can take slippery elm in capsule or powder form. Mix a teaspoon of the powder with a small amount of applesauce or cottage cheese, says Martin, and eat some four times

a day until your symptoms are relieved. That means that you will consume four teaspoons of slippery elm daily, she says.

Solidify with psyllium. Another natural fiber source, psyllium husks help ease both diarrhea and constipation symptoms by adding bulk to the stool. You can find psyllium at most supermarkets, drugstores, and health food stores. "The most commonly found brand is Metamucil," says Schar. Follow the package instructions and take it with at least six ounces of water.

Try a bayberry infusion. According to herbal practice, bayberry leaves (available at health food stores) act as an astringent on your intestinal membranes, slightly drying up the runs. Make an infusion by mixing a tablespoon of dried leaves into a cup of boiling water, says Gagnon. Cover and simmer for 15 minutes. Then remove the pan from the heat and strain the herbs from the liquid. Drink ½ cup and put the remaining liquid in a glass jar to drink later. Have ½ cup every two to three hours for up to three days.

Make chamomile a habit. "Replace your beverage of choice with chamomile tea and your whole digestive tract will thank you," says Schar. "You can drink as much of this tea as you want, but have at least six cups per day." Mix a tablespoon of dried flowers with a cup of hot water and let it steep for 15 minutes. You can also use store-bought tea bags.

Use chasteberry for monthly stool irregularities. Ever notice that you get loose stools or constipation around the time of menstruation? Hormone fluctuations can affect the bowels, says Schar, and chasteberry works especially well at clearing up digestive upsets caused by this hormone irregularity. Take 10 drops of chasteberry tincture (also called an extract) every morning during your

Slippery Elm Cereal Stops Diarrhea

An herb called slippery elm doesn't sound like a cure for diarrhea, yet the naturally fibrous bark from the slippery elm tree packs numerous bowel-healing benefits, according to herbal practitioners. Originally used by Native Americans to make canoes and wigwams, slippery elm also has medicinal properties. It solidifies bowel movements, rebuilds mucous membranes, and provides needed nutrition.

"Slippery elm heals as it nourishes you," says Gayle Eversole, Ph.D., a medical herbalist and professional member of the American Herbalists Guild in Everett, Washington. "It's delicious. It's healthy. And it's so nutritious. When consumed as a hot cereal, it's also a food. If you're debilitated with extreme diarrhea, slippery elm will replenish your system." Preparing the cereal takes work, but it's worth it, says Dr. Eversole. You should make it fresh each time, she says.

- 3 ounces slippery elm powder
- 8 ounces hot water
  Cinnamon, maple syrup, or unpasteurized honey

Place the slippery elm powder in a small saucepan and add the water a little at a time, stirring with each addition, just as you would if you were making oatmeal. (For a thicker consistency, use less water.) Heat on low for 7 minutes while beating the slippery elm and water into a paste. Add cinnamon, maple syrup, or honey to taste.

Makes 1 to 2 servings

---

cycle. (Some herbal experts say that chasteberry may counteract the effectiveness of birth control pills, while others say it seems to have no effect.)

Quaff some rice. To bind your stool, boil 1 cup of white rice in 6 cups of water for $\frac{1}{2}$ hour. Strain the rice from the water and let the water cool, then drink it, says Martin. Drink 3 to 4 cups throughout the day, she recommends. The starches in the rice water are binding, Martin explains, and will help ease your diarrhea.

Warm up to teas. If you feel normal but have loose stools, you have what Chinese doctors call "cold" diarrhea. ("Hot" diarrhea smells foul and comes urgently, with severe cramps.) "It usually indicates that there's a weakness in the whole digestive tract," says Howell. Herbs such as ginger, basil, and angelica will warm up this cold digestive tract, she says. You can make a tea from any of those herbs. Mix 1 tablespoon into a cup of hot water and let it steep for at least 10 minutes. Drink three times a day.

Constipation

Constipation means different things to different people—everything from stools that are too hard, too small, or too difficult to pass to those that are too infrequent or incomplete. No matter how you look at it, however, our various definitions all add up to the same thing—"unsatisfactory defecation," in medical terms.

To create regular, easy-to-pass stools, first make some dietary changes. "Many women with constipation eat a tremendous amount of cheese and processed bread and few fresh fruits and vegetables," says Schar. Also, as with diarrhea, putting yourself on a regular meal schedule will help ensure regularity. "The body operates on a time clock. So if you're not eating on a regular basis, you won't be eliminating on a regular basis," he says.

To cure constipation, herbalists and traditional Western doctors alike look to fiber first. Found in raw fruits, vegetables, beans, and whole-grain cereals or bran flakes, fiber increases stool mass and decreases transit time.

Martin suggests that in addition to changing your diet and trying the following herbal remedies, you should also get more exercise, drink lots of water, and massage your belly each morning. If your symptoms are severe and are coupled with pain, cramping, and/or blood in the stool, see your doctor immediately. Also see your doctor if your constipation alternates with bouts of diarrhea.

Start with flaxseed. Naturally high in fiber, flax contains acids that reduce inflammation of the mucous membranes in your intestines and balance hormones, says Dr. Eversole.

Pour 2 tablespoons of seeds (available at health food stores) into an 8-ounce glass of room-temperature water and let stand for 15 minutes. (It's crucial that you take the flax with at least 8 ounces of water, otherwise it will cause obstruction in the digestive tract.) The flaxseed will become "nice and squishy" and gelatin-like, says Martin. Drink a glass of the seed mixture at night. The next morning, don't just take a shower, grab a cup of coffee, and run out the door, Martin cautions. You must allow adequate time for a bowel movement.

You can also sprinkle a teaspoon to a tablespoon of ground flaxseed on hot cereal or on salads, says Dr. Eversole. Flax is very light-sensitive and becomes rancid quickly, so buy it in small amounts and try to use it within a few weeks, she suggests. Store flax in the refrigerator to prevent rancidity.

Consider psyllium. As an alternative to flaxseed, you can buy fibrous psyllium husks at supermarkets, drugstores, or health food stores. Flax and psyllium husks are equally able to move stool along. Although some say that psyllium can make you feel bloated, says Dr. Eversole, it is more palatable than flaxseed.

If you opt for psyllium, take 1 tablespoon of the powder every morning, and your stool will pass more readily, says Schar.

Look to dandelion for relief. The bitterness of this weed can stimulate contractions of the colon and move stools along, says Howell. Use between 1 and 3 dropperfuls of dandelion root tincture in ¼ cup of water. (A dropperful is roughly 15 drops.) Then drink it slowly by holding each mouthful for about a minute. The bitter taste will stimulate bile flow. Drink it three times a day, says Howell.

Reserve licorice tea for tough jobs. When all else fails, licorice will come to the rescue. "Licorice root tea will loosen the bowels in obstinate constipation," says Schar. "If you consume licorice tea and prunes before going to bed, you will have no problem moving your bowels in the morning." To make the tea, boil a tablespoon of licorice root for 30 minutes in a cup of water. Strain the tea before drinking, and let it cool slightly.

Irritable Bowel Syndrome

If you have either constipation or diarrhea accompanied by severe bloating and gas, and a medical doctor has diagnosed irritable bowel syndrome (IBS), get a second opinion before considering herbal remedies. "There's a chance you might have something else," says Lois Johnson, M.D., a physician in private practice in Sebastopol, California, and a professional member of the AHG.

Many people go to medical doctors complaining of the typical IBS symptoms, and when various examinations reveal no abnormalities, doctors can too quickly agree on IBS as the problem. "Doctors usually diagnose patients with IBS when they can't figure out what's wrong with their digestive tracts," Dr. Johnson says. "I never treat IBS until I'm really sure that we haven't missed a cause."

Dr. Johnson advises finding a physician who practices holistic medicine—that is, both conventional medicine and alternative therapy—and requesting a few often-overlooked tests.

Stool analysis. Your doctor may have already asked for a stool sample and found nothing odd. Ask your doctor whether she checked your stool for deficiencies in normal flora. "Usually, doctors only look for pathogens," says Dr. Johnson. Make sure that she has your stool thoroughly analyzed for parasites as well.

Blood test or fast. Often, people who think they have IBS really have a problem with sensitivity to food, usually to gluten, a substance found in various grains. Your doctor can do a blood test, or you can find out yourself by not eating wheat, rye, barley, or oats for a month, says Dr. Johnson. If your symptoms disappear, it's food sensitivity, not IBS.

Supplement review. If you are taking a lot of supplements, tell your doctor which ones and why. Sometimes high amounts of some vitamins or minerals can cause IBS-like symptoms, says Dr. Johnson.

"Occasionally, I do find someone who exhausts all of those possibilities," she says. And that's where herbs come in. Because IBS is strongly linked to nervousness and poor sleep, some of the following herbal suggestions are intended simply to calm you.

Relieve gas with peppermint oil. Peppermint oil slows intestinal contractions and relieves the painful gas that plagues people with IBS. For best results, buy enteric-coated capsules instead of soft gelatin capsules. The hard coating will prevent the oil from being released in the stomach instead of the colon, where it will relax spasms, says Dr. Johnson.

Look for coated peppermint oil capsules with 0.2 milliliters of oil at health food stores. An herbalist will suggest taking two capsules two to three times a day between meals, says Dr. Eversole.

"On days when you're feeling particularly miserable, you can also massage peppermint essential oil, mixed with jojoba or even olive oil, directly onto your abdomen," says Dr. Johnson.

Mix meadowsweet with ginger and fennel. All three herbs will help dispel gas, says Dr. Johnson. The meadowsweet can also harden your stools if your symptoms include diarrhea. You can make a tea with any one or a combination of those herbs according to your tastes. The total amount of herb should not exceed 1 tablespoon per cup of water. "Carry the tea around in a bottle and sip it all day long," she says.

Chase cramps with wild yam. The extract from this root (available at health food stores) can decrease the spasms in your gut, stopping diarrhea and soothing cramping and bloating. Take two dropperfuls of the tincture three times a day, says Dr. Johnson.

De-stress with chamomile. This soothing herb, a standby for digestive grief, can reduce the stress that aggravates your IBS, says Howell. "Since 98 percent of digestive upset is connected to the nervous system, chamomile works very well," she says.

Take a quart jar and fill it three-quarters full with dried chamomile flowers, says Howell. Pour in boiling water until it reaches one inch from the top of the jar. Let stand, covered, at room temperature overnight. In the morning, strain the herb from the liquid and drink ¼ cup. You can store the rest in the refrigerator for two to three days. Drink ¼ cup a day.

Regulate your system with slippery elm. If your symptoms include constipation or diarrhea, slippery elm can improve regularity, says Howell. Put a heaping teaspoon of dried slippery elm bark in a cup and add warm water a little at a time, mixing to form a paste. Continue to add water and dilute the paste until it forms a watery tea. Drink once a day.

Nausea and Vomiting

Like diarrhea, vomiting is your body's way of getting rid of something that it doesn't want sticking around inside, so in many cases, you're better off throwing up than suppressing a retch. In fact, throwing up will probably make you feel better, especially if you have the flu, says Dr. Johnson.

That said, herbs can soothe the unsettled, nauseated feeling that can accompany vomiting. And the following remedies, herbalists say, can heal the problem that's making your body eject what you've eaten.

Treat yourself gingerly. Not only is ginger the best herb to calm nausea, it is also one of the easiest herbs to find. No matter where you are in the world, you can find a grocery store than sells gingerroot. "You can use ginger in any form—liquid extract, capsule, tablet, or grated fresh root," says Gagnon. Some people don't like the taste of fresh ginger, which can be rather strong when taken alone. Also, if you feel nauseated, you'll only be able to stomach pleasant-tasting food. To make it more appealing, you can mix fresh grated ginger with honey or sugar, says Gagnon. Take two capsules, about 1 tablespoon of grated fresh ginger, or 60 drops of extract (also known as tincture), he says.

Take an herbal bath. If you are vomiting, you might throw up any herbs you swallow, even ginger. So let herbs soak through your pores instead. "You'll absorb enough through the skin to actually help you," says Gagnon. Mix a tablespoon of fresh ginger or a teaspoon to a tablespoon of powdered ginger in a quart of hot water. Let the water cool so you don't scald yourself, then soak your hands or feet in the ginger bath until the vomiting subsides, Gagnon recommends. Or place the same amount of ginger in a muslin bag in your tub. Draw a bath and soak. If you have the flu, the ginger packs an added benefit. "The ginger will open up the pores of your skin, getting you to sweat freely and break that fever," says Gagnon.

Mix yarrow with elderflower. If you have the flu, drink yarrow and elderflower tea while you soak in a ginger bath, suggests Gagnon. While the ginger calms nausea, the other two herbs reduce fever and boost immunity. Make a cup of hot yarrow and elderflower tea by mixing ½ tablespoon of each herb in a cup of hot water. Cover and steep for 5 minutes. As your tea steeps, head to the bathroom and draw your ginger bath, described above. Then head back to the kitchen, strain the herb from the tea, take your mug with you to the bathroom, and soak in your ginger bath as you sip the tea. After finishing your tea and bath, get into bed with lots of covers, says Gagnon.

Pair cinnamon with ginger. If food poisoning or the flu has double-whammied you with vomiting and diarrhea, make a ginger-cinnamon tea, says Schar. The ginger will stop your nausea, while the naturally astringent cinnamon dries up your stool. Mix 1 teaspoon of dried cinnamon with ½ teaspoon of grated fresh ginger and add them to a cup of boiling water, suggests Schar. Steep for 10 to 15 minutes, then strain and drink.

Press meadowsweet into service. This pleasant-tasting wildflower acts as an anti-inflammatory, calming your system and reducing nausea. Safe for use during pregnancy, meadowsweet's mild astringent properties can also slow diarrhea if you're dealing with

Herbal Wisdom
Science Backs Up Traditional Use

"In most traditional societies, it was the women who gathered the edible and medicinal wild plants. Throughout history, the knowledge of using medicinal plants was usually passed down from grandmother to granddaughter. Today, much of this accumulated wisdom has been validated by modern scientific studies. For example, German research confirms the estrogenic benefits of the Native American medicinal plant black cohosh for conditions associated with menopause."

—*Mark Blumenthal, executive director, American Botanical Council*

flu, says Dr. Johnson. Make a tea with a tablespoon of the dried herb per cup of boiling water. Steep for 5 to 10 minutes before straining out the herb, then take tiny sips, says Dr. Johnson. If you like the taste of rosemary, you can add a little of that as well. Another natural astringent, with a pleasing taste and smell, rosemary will help make the tea more appealing.

Add taste to black horehound. While not one of the tastiest herbs, the powder made from this tree's root can work wonders, says Dr. Johnson. You'll want to mix this bitter herb with something more appealing, such as cinnamon, fennel, chamomile, or rosemary, to make it more palatable. Such herbs will also decrease any gas that may accompany your nausea, she says. Use a total of 1 tablespoon of both herbs per cup and steep for 5 to 10 minutes. Strain and drink the tea slowly in small sips throughout the day.

Out of ginger? Substitute peppermint. Although not as effective as ginger, peppermint can decrease nausea in a pinch, says

Gagnon. Pour hot water into a cup with a tablespoon of fresh peppermint leaves. Let stand, covered, for 5 minutes to keep the oils from escaping. Then strain and drink.

Make an encore with chamomile. A runner-up to both ginger and peppermint, chamomile can also help soothe nausea by calming the nerves in the stomach, says Gagnon. Mix a tablespoon of dried flowers with hot water and cover the cup with a saucer. Let stand for 5 minutes, then strain and drink.

Ear Infections

AN EARFUL OF HERBAL RELIEF

As an adult, your chances of coming down with a throbbing ear infection are slimmer than they were when you were a kid, but you still aren't immune. Adults usually get infections when viruses or bacteria block the eustacian tube, which runs from the throat to the inner ear, and prevent mucus and other secretions from draining out of the middle ear. Because adults' eustacian tubes are larger and less likely to get blocked than children's, adults are less likely to get chronic, or recurrent, ear infections.

Acute ear infections—that is, sudden, severe infections—are potentially quite dangerous. The pressure that builds in the eardrum from the infection can cause the eardrum to burst, leading to permanent hearing loss in some cases. See a doctor if your ear pain is severe or is accompanied by drainage, discharge, or a fever of 102°F, or if it persists despite treatment. See a doctor immediately if you have a sudden change in hearing, become dizzy, have an inability to concentrate, or notice weakness in your facial muscles on the same side as the affected ear.

The Herbal Route to Clear Ears

To help stop ear infections, physicians usually prescribe antibiotics. To relieve pain, they generally recommend acetaminophen or aspirin for adults. The problem is that ear infections often recur . . . and recur . . . and recur. Herbs may help before, during, and after an infection.

Herbalists first recommend herbs that help numb the pain as well as kill the bacteria or virus that is causing the infection. Then, to avoid subsequent infections, with round after round of antibiotics and painkillers, they can suggest herbs to strengthen your immune system to prevent ear infections from coming back.

"Don't forget to take a look at diet also," adds Janis Gruska, N.D., a naturopathic physician, professor of clinical medicine, and department chair of naturopathic medicine at the Southwest College of Naturopathic Medicine and Health Sciences in Tempe, Arizona. "Lots of times, just by eliminating common foods that cause allergies, such as dairy, wheat, and corn, you can cut the incidence of ear infection in half," she says. "Then you can use herbs to support the immune system as well as to help treat ear infections that do occur."

Here's what Dr. Gruska and other herbal medicine professionals recommend. The oils and tinctures (also called extracts) described below are available at health food stores. Be aware that the products identified as oils are different from products identified as essential oils.

Mix a little mullein. "My favorite herb to treat earaches is mullein flower oil," says Feather Jones, a professional member of the American Herbalists Guild (AHG) and director of the Rocky Mountain Center for Botanical Studies in Boulder, Colorado. "Keep a vial of the oil in the refrigerator. When needed, take the filled dropper and warm it by holding it in your hand for about 30 seconds, so you aren't putting ice-cold drops in your ear. Then place two or three drops in the troubled ear. Cover the ear with a little wad of cotton to keep the oil from running out," says Jones. "Mullein oil is anti-microbial, so it will help kill the bacteria causing the infection. But it will also help loosen up any hard wax in the ear, so the oil can get where it needs to go and the ear can heal more quickly." You can apply more drops every six to eight hours as needed.

Kill bacteria with garlic. Prepared, commercially available garlic oil is also good for ear infections, says Jones, because it works like an antibiotic. "Garlic will also migrate past the eardrum and will help prevent further infection," says Daniel Gagnon, a professional member of the AHG, executive director of the Botanical Research and Education Institute, and owner of Herbs, Etc. in Santa Fe, New Mexico.

"Ideally, I like eardrops that combine garlic

oil and mullein oil, which are available commercially," says Gagnon. "Together, they not only reduce pain and decrease the bacteria causing the infection, they also help establish the proper pH balance in the ear, which is important when you're fighting infection and recurring infection," he says. Apply four drops in the affected ear, then reapply every four to six hours as needed. Just remember to use fresh cotton with each application, he says.

Numb pain with St.-John's-wort. "To help soothe really sore ears, I recommend using St.-John's-wort oil," says Jones. "St.-John's-wort is a neural anti-inflammatory, so it is very effective in soothing inflammation around the nerves of the ear canal and stopping the pain. Plus, it's a good antiviral herb. The best way to use it is by mixing a solution of one-half St.-John's-wort and one-half mullein flower oil." As with other oils, add about three drops to the affected ear, cover with a cotton ball, and reapply every six to eight hours as necessary.

Make a tea tree antiseptic. "Because it is a good antiseptic oil, tea tree oil is useful for fighting both bacterial and viral infections," adds Jones.

You can make your own by mixing a few drops of tea tree essential oil with a little vegetable oil and applying them as you would other eardrops, suggests James A. Duke, Ph.D., a botanical consultant, former ethnobotanist with the U.S. Department of Agriculture, and author of *The Green Pharmacy*, who specializes in medicinal plants.

"I use 5 drops of tea tree oil mixed well with 1 tablespoon of olive oil," Jones says.

Because tea tree oil is strong, you should discontinue use if you experience any irritation, cautions Dr. Duke.

Stay infection-free with echinacea and astragalus. "In the case of chronic ear in-

Eardrops: Proceed with Caution

Applied into the ear canal, some herb oils and essential oils can often be helpful in relieving pain and speeding the healing of an ear infection. But they should not be used as eardrops if your doctor has told you that your eardrum has burst, says David Edel-berg, M.D., founder of the American Whole-Health Centers in Boston, Chicago, Denver, and Bethesda, Maryland, and section chief of holistic medicine at Illinois Masonic Medical Center and Grant Hospital, both in Chicago. So check with your doctor.

fections, I recommend supporting and strengthening the immune system to prevent recurrence," says Dr. Gruska. She especially recommends tinctures of echinacea and astragalus, since echinacea is a good immune system stimulant and astragalus is helpful for keeping the immune system strong over the long term. Take both of these tinctures by mouth.

"I usually recommend taking echinacea tincture at the first sign of trouble," adds Gagnon. "As soon as you feel a little tender-ness or soreness or feel that you're getting sick, start taking one dropperful every hour while you have symptoms. That will help rev up your immune system so you can knock out whatever is causing the infection.

"For long-term prevention, I recommend using astragalus tincture in cycles," he says. "Take 15 to 30 drops twice a day for a month, take a couple of weeks off, and then start again. This will help build your body's natural resistance so that you'll be less likely to get sick again."

Eczema

NATURAL CALM FOR OVERREACTIVE SKIN

Sensitivity can be a many-splen-dored thing: Who'd want to miss the velvety feel of a rose petal or the cool excitement of slipping into a clear mountain lake? But when skin is exquisitely sensitive—to everything from scratchy clothing and temperature extremes to emotional stress and allergens or irritants—tactile experiences aren't always pleasant. The result can be dermatitis, a rash that can be red, itchy, and in extreme cases, come with hives and blisters.

If your skin overreacts on a regular basis with a pink, scaly rash that itches intensely, you may have a form of dermatitis, also known as eczema, especially if your skin becomes thick and painfully cracked in areas. Eczema is often a hereditary condition. Allergies, stress, and even temperature changes can trigger outbreaks. Conventional medical treatments for eczema include a wide array of drugs—cortisone and tar treatments, antihistamines to stop the itch, and sedatives for scratch-free sleep. Herbal healers recommend a different course.

"Most cases of eczema that I've seen turn out to be reactions to common foods like dairy products and wheat, so the first thing I do is recommend a special diet," says Lisa Murray-Doran, N.D., a naturopathic physician and instructor at the Canadian College of Naturopathic Medicine in Toronto. "Then I use soothing herbal creams to help skin heal." Other herbal healers add botanical remedies that help the body process toxins that may be provoking eczema flare-ups.

Herbal Skin Soothers

Herbal healers recommend these calming creams, pastes, and baths for eczema.

Draw on chamomile. Naturopathic doctors say that creams or salves containing chamomile can work as well as—or better than—cortisone cream for relieving itching and inflammation.

Research shows that chamomile contains anti-inflammatory substances, including azulene and bisabolol, that reduce the allergic reaction that prompts the development of eczema. "If you don't have chamomile cream on hand, you could make a strong chamomile tea with 1 tablespoon of dried herb in a cup of boiling water," says Sherry Briskey, N.D.,

a naturopathic physician and chair of the botanical medicine department at Southwest College of Naturopathic Medicine and Health Sciences in Tempe, Arizona. "Let it steep for 15 minutes or more, then strain and cool. Dip a clean piece of gauze in the tea and apply it to the rashy area. Leave the gauze in place for 20 minutes to an hour, changing it when it gets dry and warm. You can use this remedy three times a day until the lesion dries and the inflammation decreases."

Soothe and heal with slippery elm. "Slippery elm contains mucilage, which moisturizes and calms the skin and can help healing," says Dr. Briskey.

Combine slippery elm powder with enough water to make a thin paste, then apply to itchy, inflamed rashes, she suggests. Use whatever water temperature feels soothing to you, and leave the paste on for up to an hour, or until it dries. Then rinse it off gently with water and pat your skin dry. You can repeat this three times a day, she says.

Control infection with goldenseal. Native Americans relieved eczema with goldenseal. Researchers have found that in laboratory studies, berberine, a substance that gives goldenseal its bitter taste and yellow color, kills many forms of bacteria on contact. It may be able to kill bacteria on your skin, too, when applied to wounds. If your dermatitis becomes infected, make an antimicrobial wash by combining 1 part goldenseal tincture (also called an extract) with 3 parts warm water. Soak a clean cloth in the liquid and apply it to the rash for 15 to 20 minutes at a time, changing the cloth as needed when it cools off, Dr. Briskey suggests. Reapply the wash four or five times a day.

Signs of infection include redness, heat in the skin around the dermatitis, and sores that have pus around them. If your skin looks in-

Flaxseed: Worth a Try for Eczema, Too

A slender, flower-bearing plant, flax has been cultivated since at least 5000 B.C. The health benefits of its seeds have been known for almost as long. Flaxseed has been found in Egyptian tombs, and the eighth-century French king Charlemagne passed laws requiring his subjects to eat the seeds to stay healthy.

Today, flaxseed is used mostly as a safe, natural remedy for constipation. The seeds contain mucilage, a gummy type of fiber that absorbs a large amount of fluid in the bowel. This makes the seeds swell, adding bulk to the stool.

Flaxseed may also be helpful in healing eczema because it is rich in essential fatty acids, which can help prevent eczema rashes.

"You can put the ground seeds in muffins or sprinkle them on cereal," says Sherry Briskey, N.D., a naturopathic physician and chair of the botanical medicine department at Southwest College of Naturopathic Medicine and Health Sciences in Tempe, Arizona. "It's best to grind only the amount of seeds you will use at one time. The oil can be used on salads or vegetables. It goes rancid quickly, so buy it from a health food store that keeps the oil in the refrigerator, and refrigerate it at home."

Take two teaspoons of flaxseed oil or one to two teaspoons of crushed flaxseed every day. To avoid gas, cramps, or bloating, drink eight full glasses of water a day. You'll probably have to take flaxseed for at least three months before you notice a difference in your skin.

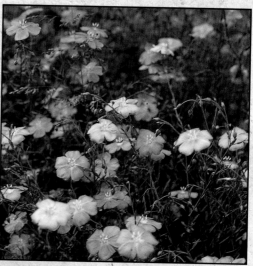

Nutty-tasting flaxseed and flaxseed oil can relieve the inflammation of skin conditions.

fected, see a doctor before attempting to treat the infection on your own, says Dr. Briskey.

Ease itching with oatmeal. Colloidal oatmeal—sold commercially as Aveeno—can soothe an itchy rash, Dr. Murray-Doran notes. Add it to a tub of comfortably warm water and soak. After you dry off, immediately apply a moisturizer or herbal cream, she suggests.

Herbs for Inner Healing

For itchy, rashy eczema, herbal experts also recommend the following botanical strategies that work inside your body to help turn down the volume on overreactive skin.

Try ginkgo. "People with eczema often have allergies," Dr. Briskey explains. "Ginkgo can help decrease that hypersensitivity. When allergic reactions are reduced, you get less redness and itching." In one study, compounds in ginkgo blocked allergic skin reactions.

Look for a standardized ginkgo extract that contains 24 percent ginkgo flavonoid glycosides—the herb's active constituents—Dr. Briskey suggests. Take 40 to 80 milligrams in capsule form (30 to 60 drops of liquid extract) three times a day for three to four months, she recommends.

Add evening primrose oil. Evening primrose oil is rich in essential fatty acids, which help the body produce anti-inflammatory compounds that prevent eczema's red, swollen rashes, says Dr. Murray-Doran.

"The capsules vary in the amount of evening primrose oil they contain, so follow the dosage directions on the package," Dr. Murray-Doran says. "This is a long-term therapy that should be continued for at least three months before you can expect a big change in your skin."

Bolster your liver with burdock and other herbs. Herbs that help the digestive system and the liver can help eczema, too, Dr. Briskey says. "As a naturopathic doctor, I see a problem when the digestive system doesn't metabolize foods properly and when the liver doesn't fully convert toxins to be excreted. These toxins and metabolic by-products end up being excreted through the skin as waste," she says. "When the body reacts to the toxins in the skin, eczema can result."

She suggests yellow dock, red clover, sarsaparilla, dandelion, and burdock for eczema. "Choose two or three to take as tinctures," she says. "Use 30 to 60 drops in a cup of warm water two to three times a day for at least two to three months. If you also eliminate aggravating foods from your diet, you should see some improvement."

Yellow dock, burdock, and red clover have reputations in folk medicine for treating some skin problems. An old-time liver tonic, dandelion has been shown to enhance the flow of bile from the liver, improving liver function. In one study, sarsaparilla prevented bacterial bits called endotoxins from leaving the intestines. Dr. Briskey says that when endotoxins circulate in the bloodstream, they can aggravate skin conditions like eczema.

Endometriosis

HERBAL OPTIONS FOR AN ELUSIVE PROBLEM

Call it menstruation gone mad: heavy on the bleeding, heavy on the pain—with side orders, perhaps, of disrupted sleep, depression, fatigue, and infertility. In fact, endometriosis is thought to cause up to 40 percent of all cases of infertility in the United States.

Go to a medically trained physician, and she will likely suggest hormone therapy, which may lessen the painful inflammation but won't cure the problem, says Amanda McQuade Crawford, a practicing herbalist in Ojai, California, professional member of the American Herbalists Guild (AHG), member of Britain's National Institute of Medical Herbalists, president of the American College of Integrative Medicine in Albuquerque, and author of *Herbal Remedies for Women*. Furthermore, hormones can have side effects, which for some women can be potentially as troubling as the endometriosis itself.

Surgery to remove the endometrial lesions is sometimes suggested, and so is hysterectomy, which removes the uterus and ovaries. But neither of these procedures is a guaranteed cure, McQuade Crawford notes.

Herbal treatments for endometriosis are available as an alternative, although even herbalists are likely to tell you that herbs alone aren't always a cure, either. But here's the good news: Combine herbal therapy with some lifestyle changes, and it's possible to alleviate most of the disease's troubling symptoms—and eventually, even the disease itself—safely and without side effects, herbalists say.

Endometriosis Explained

Endometriosis occurs when endometrial tissue from the lining of the uterus migrates outside the uterus. The wayward tissue can grow almost anywhere—on the ovaries, bowel, bladder, or even the lungs.

Misplaced endometrial tissue behaves just like normal endometrial tissue does, bleeding in response to monthly hormonal stimulation. So each month, at the site of the misplaced tissue, blood gets trapped and becomes encapsulated, possibly forming dark brown lesions known as chocolate cysts. These lesions can cause cell destruction, in-

tense pain, and many other problems, notes McQuade Crawford.

In decades past, doctors thought that they knew what caused endometriosis, a problem that was once considered rare. The most popular theories blamed delaying pregnancy in favor of a career, being sexually active and prone to sexually transmitted diseases, or having abortions or other surgery on reproductive organs. Treatments were pegged to theoretical (but ultimately incorrect) causes.

"The first advice that a physician was likely to offer a woman with endometriosis was 'go home and have a baby,'" notes McQuade Crawford.

An Environmental Link?

Happily, medical opinions have changed. But sadly, endometriosis isn't so rare any more. It's estimated that between 10 and 15 percent of American women are affected.

Once a problem of older, childless women, endometriosis is now seen in women of all ages, including teenagers. Most commonly, it is found in women between the ages of 25 and 40, and it may subside after menopause.

Although no one knows for sure what triggers endometriosis, theories still abound. Heredity and stress may be factors. Many herbalists believe that the rise in endometriosis is linked to a rise in environmental pollution, specifically to highly toxic substances like dioxin (used in some pesticides), chlorine (often found in water and household products), and industrial pollutants such as PCBs (polychorinated biphenyls). Although the U.S. manufacture of PCBs was halted in 1977, they are still kicking around in the environment. Herbalists call these and other environmental pollutants endo-disrupters. Simply put, herbalists believe that they interfere with the endocrine system, which is responsible for hormone regulation. In concert with the nervous system, the endocrine system helps control all of your body's major functions.

Researchers suspect that a faulty endocrine or immune system is linked to endometriosis. And researchers from Dartmouth Medical School in Hanover, New Hampshire, have connected environmental dioxin with endometriosis.

"Endometriosis is considered a hyperestrogenic disease," says herbalist Rosemary Gladstar, director of the Sage Mountain herbal education center in East Barre, Vermont, and author of *Herbal Healing for Women*. "That means it's produced by an oversecretion of estrogen. I believe that the abusive use of hormones that are used in raising beef, dairy cattle, and chickens could very well stimulate the overproduction of these hormones in our own bodies."

On a positive note, taking a few simple steps can help lessen your exposure to substances that may cause or exacerbate endometriosis. And there are some excellent herbal therapies to ease the pain, lessen the bleeding, and relieve the depression it can cause. Expert herbalists recommend that you try one remedy at a time, starting with herbs for immediate relief.

For Immediate Relief

For the pain caused by endometriosis, herbalists offer the following options.

Try a tea. "When I see a woman with severe endometriosis, one of the first things I do is try to ease her pain," says Kathleen Maier, a physician's assistant, professional member of the AHG, director of the Dreamtime Center for Herbal Studies in Flint Hill,

Virginia, and former advisor on botanical medicine to the National Institutes of Health. "This tea combines relaxing herbs like passionflower, damiana, and skullcap, which eases pain, with nourishing, mineral-rich alfalfa leaf, nettle, and red raspberry leaf, which balances hormones." Blend equal parts of each dried herb and infuse 1 tablespoon per 8-ounce cup of freshly boiled water; steep for a minimum of an hour in a covered container. "When dealing with nourishing herbs, I prefer using a tablespoon. It will yield a stronger infusion than the usual teaspoon that is generally recommended," explains Maier. She suggests drinking a cup three times a day.

Blend an herbal pain eraser. To make a simple tincture formula that's very effective, Maier says, blend equal parts of cramp bark, kava-kava, California poppy, and passionflower tinctures (also called extracts) in a four-ounce bottle. She recommends taking one teaspoon three times a day, or as needed for pain. Cramp bark and kava-kava help relax the muscles and ease pain; California poppy and passionflower relax the tension that contributes to muscle pain, says Maier.

Relieve body-bending cramps. "If your cramps are really excruciating, try this tincture formula," advises Ellen Kamhi, R.N., Ph.D., of Oyster Bay, New York, an herbalist, professional member of the AHG, and host of the nationally syndicated radio show *Natural Alternatives*. Use tinctures of Jamaican dogwood, kava-kava, white willow bark, and valerian. Dr. Kamhi recommends taking 10 drops of each tincture two hours before bedtime and again right before you go to bed. Valerian can act as a stimulant in some women, so omit it from the mixture if you react this way.

Jamaican dogwood has traditionally been

used for menstrual cramps and for insomnia due to nervous tension or muscle pain. Kava-kava is an antispasmodic, and white willow contains salicin, the compound from which aspirin was derived.

If you try this tincture formula, don't exceed the recommended dose and use only as needed, not on an ongoing basis. Use only before bedtime or when you'll be home all day, as it can make you drowsy. It should not be used when driving. This formula is not recommended during pregnancy or when breastfeeding, warns Dr. Kamhi.

Grind up some flax. "Essential fatty acids (EFAs) are important for women who have endometriosis because they help control inflammation," says Maier.

"The easiest, least expensive way to add EFAs to your diet is to buy a pound of flaxseed at a health food store. Because flaxseed goes rancid quickly, store it in the freezer and grind up small batches at a time, using a coffee grinder," suggests Maier. "Use about a tablespoon a day, sprinkled over cereal or in soups or stews."

Try a mushroom tonic. The stress of endometriosis can take its toll on other body functions, especially the adrenal glands, which produce and regulate hormones, notes Maier. "That kind of chronic stress can affect the immune system, so I use an immune-strengthening formula of reishi mushrooms and herbs added to a favorite soup," she says.

If soup doesn't work for you, you can try combining an ounce each of astragalus, Siberian ginseng, and reishi mushroom tinctures and take a teaspoon three times a day, suggests Maier. Studies show that astragalus increases the body's antiviral compounds, Siberian ginseng stimulates the immune system and boosts energy, and reishi improves blood flow to the heart. You can use this tonic along with any of the other remedies suggested in this chapter.

Sit in a sitz. "Warming treatments are helpful, and so is aromatherapy," says Mc-Quade Crawford. Try adding three drops each of the pure essential oils of rose geranium, clary sage, and cypress to a nice hot sitz bath (several inches of water in the tub), she suggests.

Geranium is said to ease anxiety and depression, clary sage is used for easing pain and tension, and cypress is recommended for fatigue and mood swings, according to Valerie Ann Worwood, a British aromatherapist and author of *The Fragrant Mind*.

You can also use the essential oils for aromatherapy inhalation, McQuade Crawford says (see "Aromatherapy" on page 134 for directions).

Soak up some castor oil. "Castor oil packs are incredibly useful for just about anything that hurts," says Dr. Kamhi, "and I've seen cases of endometriosis respond phenomenally well." Here's what to do: Take a piece of undyed wool flannel and soak it in castor oil. Place the flannel over the area of the abdomen that's painful and cover with a piece of clear plastic, then with a towel, and finally with a heating pad or hot water bottle heated to a comfortably warm temperature. Leave the pack on for about an hour. "I believe the packs work by helping to shrink the misplaced endometrial tissue," says Dr. Kamhi.

For Long-Term Relief

To beat endometriosis over the long haul, other herbalists offer slightly more ambitious approaches.

"The goal of herbal therapy includes adding nutrient-rich herbs to the diet, which

Herbal Formulas for Endometriosis

Because endometriosis is a complex condition influenced by factors that ebb and flow during the menstrual cycle, herbal treatment is somewhat involved. It's always best when it is tailored to hormonal shifts that occur at ovulation.

These two herbal formulas combine specific herbs that perform specific functions in specific proportions, and they are taken at specific times. They were designed for women with endometriosis by Amanda McQuade Crawford, a practicing herbalist in Ojai, California, professional member of the American Herbalists Guild, member of Britain's National Institute of Medical Herbalists, president of the American College of Integrative Medicine in Albuquerque, and author of *Herbal Remedies for Women.* She suggests that you try the remedies for up to three months. If you don't experience relief within that time, switch to conventional medicine.

Premenstrual Formula

This mixture uses tinctures of six herbs: chasteberry seed (to help normalize hormones), cramp bark (to ease muscle pain), yarrow flower (to tone the bowel wall and improve digestion), skullcap (to reduce tension and help ease pain), wild yam root (to ease depression and pain linked to hormonal changes), and cinnamon bark (to dilate blood vessels and improve circulation). You'll find these tinctures in health food stores. You'll also need a small funnel and a bottle large enough to hold the mixture—a little more than eight ounces.

✓ 1 ounce chasteberry seed tincture
✓ 2 ounces cramp bark tincture
✓ 2 ounces yarrow flower tincture
✓ 2 ounces skullcap tincture
✓ 1 ounce wild yam root tincture
✓ 2 teaspoons cinnamon bark tincture

Using a funnel, pour the tinctures into the bottle. McQuade Crawford suggests taking one teaspoon diluted in eight ounces of water four times a day, from ovulation (about midcycle) through the end of your period.

Postmenstrual Formula

The second formula also uses chasteberry and wild yam root tinctures, combined with tinctures of five other herbs: blue cohosh root (to stimulate tissue health when there's scarring), sarsaparilla root (an immune-system tonic and hormone balancer), milk thistle seed (to aid hormone metabolism and enhance liver function), partridgeberry (to help shrink benign growths), and valerian root (the "queen" of herbal painkillers)

✓ 2 ounces chasteberry seed tincture
✓ 1 ounce blue cohosh root tincture
✓ 1 ounce sarsaparilla root tincture
✓ 2 ounces milk thistle seed tincture
✓ 1 ounce partridgeberry tincture
✓ 2 ounces wild yam tincture
✓ 1 ounce (or more if needed for pain) valerian root tincture

Combine the tinctures as instructed in the previous formula. McQuade Crawford suggests taking one teaspoon of this mixture diluted in eight ounces of water four times a day, from the time your period ends until ovulation (about midcycle).

provide building materials for cell nuclei so that tissue damaged by endometrial lesions can be repaired," says McQuade Crawford. "I also use herbs that support liver function to help clear toxins, and I add herbs to help boost the body's immune system, which improves its ability to scavenge misplaced endometrial tissue." (To use any of her formulas, see "Herbal Formulas for Endometriosis" on page 229.)

Since the symptoms of endometriosis vary so widely from woman to woman, herbalists will tell you to consult an expert health-care practitioner if your symptoms don't respond to natural remedies in one to three months. They will also tell you to be patient: Herbal formulas take a minimum of three months to have a lasting benefit on the symptoms of endometriosis.

McQuade Crawford says that the herbal formulas she prescribes should begin to ease pain within the first few days. "It's absolutely normal to expect a successful treatment to last from six months to one year," she says. "Long-term herbal self-care encourages women to adopt healthy habits for life—and it only takes 15 minutes every three days to make a big pitcher of tea or a few weeks of shaking a jar of mixed herbs to make an affordable tincture that will last for several months."

Lifestyle Changes Help, Too

For optimum relief, herbalists suggest a cleanup program for better uterine ecology. Here are their suggestions.

Enact a tampon taboo. "Tampons are bleached white with chlorine, and so are most sanitary napkins," says McQuade Crawford. "Studies show that chlorinated compounds can cause a number of problems, such as endocrine system disruption, reproductive problems, infertility, and cancer. I tell women to avoid using tampons, at least until they have been free of the symptoms of endometriosis for at least six months," she advises. Unbleached, unscented, nondeodorant cotton pads are available at many health food stores, she notes.

Watch what you drink. McQuade Crawford believes that caffeine and alcohol could be risk factors for endometriosis. "I recommend that women limit coffee to no more than a cup or two a day and limit alcohol to a glass or two of wine or beer or one mixed drink a few times a week," she advises.

Lighten up on red meat. Lowering your intake of animal protein and animal fat can decrease harmful levels of "foreign" estrogen in your body, McQuade Crawford says. If you must eat animal products, she suggests that you scout out organic meats, raised without pesticides or hormones.

Go organic. "One of the first things I do is put women who have endometriosis on a completely organic diet," declares Dr. Kamhi. "But I also recommend steps that go beyond diet. I recommend 86-ing all the toxic chemicals in your life, like those in cleaning products and even shampoos and antiperspirants. A good health food store will have excellent, toxin-free organic alternatives for everything from cosmetics to cleaning supplies," she says.

Say no to plastics. "When a woman with endometriosis comes in to see me, I always tell her to avoid using milk, juice, or bottled water that comes in plastic containers," says Maier, "and to look for glass bottles instead." Plastics are considered by herbalists to be endo-disruptors, and it is suspected that the chemical additives in plastic containers can leach into liquids and foods.

Fever

You run a fever for the same reason that you thoroughly cook a Thanksgiving turkey—to kill all the organisms that would otherwise make you sick. When a virus or bacterium invades your body, your immune system responds like an oven, turning up its internal temperature as a natural defense mechanism against infection or inflammation. You don't want the fever to burn too high, though, or you risk damaging healthy cells. Any fever that's higher than 103°F or that lasts longer than 48 hours requires prompt medical attention. But according to medical experts, you do want to let fever run its course so that you can kill the infectious organisms and get well.

"Suppress your fever, and you suppress your body's ability to fight the invader," says Roy Upton of Soquel, California, vice president of the American Herbalists Guild (AHG). Instead, you should apply a cool cloth to your forehead frequently to keep your fever from burning too hot, especially around your head, where it can cause brain damage if unchecked. And take herbs that promote sweating to allow the fever to run its course more quickly and effectively, says Upton.

"Be patient: Since herbs don't suppress a fever in the same way that aspirin or other over-the-counter medicines do, you aren't necessarily going to feel better right away," says Feather Jones, a professional member of the AHG and director of the Rocky Mountain Center for Botanical Studies in Boulder,

Colorado. "In fact, herbal treatments may make you feel temporarily worse," she says. They'll hasten the process so your fever "spikes" more quickly, and you can go through that period called "flush," when you sweat buckets—but you'll feel a whole lot better when it's through, she says.

Ride It Out with Herbs

Here are the herbs that practitioners say best ease you through a bout with fever.

Break a fever with boneset. Used by the Cherokee people for more than 3,000 years, the bitter herb boneset was traditionally used for "break-bone fever, the kind of fever where your bones just ache and feel hot," says David Winston, a professional member of the AHG and founder of Herbalist and Alchemist, an herbal medicine company in Washington, New Jersey. Boneset works by stimulating the activity of macrophages, special white blood cells that destroy disease-causing microorganisms. It also stimulates your body's immune response to viral and bacterial infection, says Winston, who is also trained in Cherokee medicine.

"The only problem with boneset is that it tastes terrible," says Daniel Gagnon, a professional member of the AHG, executive director of the Botanical Research and Education Institute, and owner of Herbs, Etc., in Santa Fe, New Mexico. So while it is effective as a tea, you'll need to add something sweet to make it palatable, he says.

Three-Herb Fever Tea

Ask herbalists what they recommend for a fever, and they'll usually name some combination of elderflower, yarrow, and peppermint. This recipe, which blends three powerful sweat-inducing herbs, is as old as the hills and is still a favorite today, says Feather Jones, a professional member of the American Herbalists Guild and executive director of the Rocky Mountain Center for Botanical Studies in Boulder, Colorado. "Use it as a medicinal tea, and it will help break a fever fast," she says. Drink this tea until you start to sweat, which usually occurs after you drink a cup or two.

1   **part elderflower**
1   **part yarrow**
1   **part peppermint**
2   **cups water**
    Honey

Combine equal parts of the three dried herbs so they add up to about ¼ ounce of blended herbs and put the mixture in a pint canning jar. Boil the water and pour it into the jar over the herbs. Put the lid on and let stand for 3 or 4 hours. Strain and add honey to taste.

Makes 2 cups

"Use 1 tablespoon of boneset per cup of boiling water and let it steep for 10 minutes, then add honey to taste. Or you can add a little peppermint tea to the boneset, if you prefer," he says. Drink it three times a day.

If the taste still doesn't suit you, use ¼ to ½ teaspoon of boneset tincture (also called an extract) up to three times a day, Winston adds. Boneset is available from mail-order suppliers (see "Where to Buy Herbs and Herbal Products" on page 462).

If you are prone to allergies/hypersensitivities, particularly to chamomile, feverfew, ragweed, or other members of the daisy family, you may also have an allergic reaction to boneset.

Ease it with elderflower. "Elderflower is good for opening pores and inducing sweat to break a fever," says Jones. Plus, the extract from these tiny flowers contains compounds that help break up and clear out excess mucus and inflammation that usually accompany fever due to colds and flu.

To make a tea out of dried elderflowers, pour a cup of boiling water over 2 teaspoons of the herb and allow it to infuse, covered, for 15 to 20 minutes. Drink it three times a day as needed, says Winston. For extra effectiveness, you can also combine elderflower with peppermint or yarrow. Make the mix of herbs equivalent to 2 teaspoons, with elderflower as the largest portion, he says.

Say yes to yarrow. "Yarrow is another excellent herb for fever," says Jones. "It contains volatile oils that open your pores and cause profuse sweating to assist in breaking a fever."

You can make a tea by using 1 tablespoon of the herb per cup of boiling water and steeping it in a covered container for 10 minutes, says Upton.

If you want to take yarrow therapy even one step further, Gagnon recommends sipping a cup of hot yarrow tea as you sit in a warm bath to which you have added a few drops of yarrow tincture. "A hot cup and a hot bath, and you'll open up those pores and sweat that ailment out of your system. After 15 minutes, get out of the bath, dry yourself off, and go to a warm bed, where you will keep sweating the fever out," he adds.

Drink a diaphoretic. For fevers that are associated with colds and flu (but not due to other infections), Upton recommends spicy or pungent herbs known as diaphoretics, including peppermint, yarrow, elderflower, lemon balm, chamomile, lemon verbena, lemongrass (also known as fever grass in the West Indies), gingerroot, sage, thyme, rosemary, or basil.

"Most commonly consumed as teas, diaphoretics stimulate circulation by dilating the blood vessels. Plus, they have a subsequent relaxing effect that causes the pores to open, thus allowing heat to dissipate. Allowing the heat to escape minimizes the chances of fever building to dangerous levels, and it also helps to rapidly reduce a high fever," he explains. They're safe and effective and include some common spices that you probably have right in your kitchen, says Upton.

"Most of these, with the exception of sage and yarrow, are pleasant-tasting. And even yarrow isn't too bad," Upton says. To make fever-reducing teas, prepare all of the herbs mentioned as infusions, which means that they are steeped, not boiled, he says. "Use 1 tablespoon of herb per cup of boiled water, steep in a covered vessel for 10 minutes, add honey for palatability, and drink it hot. Drink it until your pores open and you start to sweat, which usually takes 20 to 25 minutes.

Profuse sweating should bring your fever down to a bearable temperature (from 102° or 103°F to around 100°F) but still allows the fever to do its work stimulating the system to fight infection," Upton explains.

"Once you start to sweat," he adds, "be sure to cover yourself with a blanket to prevent getting chilled. If your fever shoots up again, drink more tea to restart the sweating process."

Bathe your feet. If the taste of diaphoretics isn't exactly your cup of tea, you can treat fever by using these stimulating teas in a footbath instead, says Upton. "Make a hot footbath with plenty of diaphoretic herbal tea—enough to cover your feet," he says. "Let it cool just enough so that you don't scald yourself. Then wrap yourself in a sheet or a blanket and immerse your feet in the steaming tea for 10 to 15 minutes. Sweating will usually start within that time, or soon after," says Upton.

Make it wane with willow. If you have a high fever that leaves you achy—the kind that you'd normally try to reduce with aspirin—willow bark extract could be the perfect herbal alternative, according to herbal practitioners. This bitter extract contains compounds called phenolic glycoside salicins that produce salicylic acid, a pain-inhibiting and inflammation-reducing chemical in your body. Salicin is the same active compound used to create aspirin, so you can use willow bark extract to manage a fever much as you would aspirin. "That's what I do," says James A. Duke, Ph.D., a botanical consultant, former ethnobotanist with the U.S. Department of Agriculture, and author of *The Green Pharmacy*, who specializes in medicinal plants.

Varro E. Tyler, Ph.D., professor emeritus of pharmacognosy at the Purdue University

Feverfew: Better Known for Headaches

You're scanning the health food stores searching for something to soothe your fever. Fennel . . . fenugreek . . . *feverfew*. That sounds like it would work, right? Wrong.

Since ancient times, people erroneously claimed that the name feverfew comes from the Latin *febrifugia*, or "driver out of fevers." In fact, the actual name was featherfoil, given to the plant by folks in the Middle Ages because of its feathery borders. Featherfoil became featherfew, which became feverfew, and an herbal misnomer was born.

"Feverfew is useful as a remedy for migraine headaches," says David Winston, a professional member of the American Herbalists Guild and founder of Herbalist and Alchemist, an herbal medicine company in Washington, New Jersey. "It may be on some of the books as a fever remedy, but I don't know any herbalist who uses it for fevers," he adds.

School of Pharmacy and Pharmacal Sciences in West Lafayette, Indiana, and author of *Herbs of Choice*, recommends willow bark extract capsules.

Gagnon suggests taking three or four 200-milligram capsules of willow bark extract a day, but make sure that the label says it's standardized to 15 percent salicin,. Take it each day until the fever is reduced. Standardized formulas are available at health food stores and some pharmacies.

"Willow works well for bringing down a fever. It may just take a little longer than aspirin," says Tieraona Low Dog, M.D., a family practice physician at the University of New Mexico Hospital, professional member of the AHG, and member of the Alternative Medicine Research Group at the University of New Mexico School of Medicine in Albuquerque. She usually prescribes three to five milliliters of liquid willow bark extract, purchased in a 1:3 plant/fluid ratio (the label should state the ratio). Take it in water or juice every three hours until the fever subsides, she says.

Willow should not be taken with aspirin. Also, since willow contains compounds similar to aspirin, don't take it if you need to avoid aspirin because of ulcers, asthma, diabetes, gout, hemophilia (a blood thrombin deficiency), or kidney or liver disease or if you're taking a blood thinner such as warfarin (Coumadin). Mixing willow bark with alcohol can irritate your stomach. It may also interact with barbiturates or sedatives such as aprobarbital (Amytal) or alprazolam (Xanax). Never give willow to children under 16 who have any viral condition, as they run the risk of contracting Reye's syndrome, a serious condition that affects the brain and liver.

Ease it with echinacea. Finally, whenever you have an inflammatory or infectious condition that commonly triggers fever, you want to take echinacea, says Ed Smith, a professional member of the AHG and founder of Herb Pharm in Williams, Oregon. "Echinacea is a great add-on therapy for virtually any inflammatory condition because it stimulates the disease-fighting white blood cells in the immune system," says Smith.

Gagnon suggests taking 30 to 50 drops of liquid echinacea extract in water, juice, or herbal tea every two hours until fever subsides. As always, it's a good idea to check with your health-care practitioner before using herbs as an adjunct to other treatments that she may have prescribed. If you don't feel better within a week, if you are getting worse, or if your condition has you worried, see your health-care practitioner, he says.

Gum Problems

HERBS THAT NIP PROBLEMS IN THE BUD

Call gum disease a major crisis of the mouth. For many people, gum disease, which can range from minor gingivitis to severe periodontitis, is practically a fact of life. By the age of 13, 63 percent of the population will have some form of gum disease.

Gingivitis sets in when plaque, a soft, sticky bacterial deposit, builds up at or below the gum line. Daily brushing and flossing remove fresh plaque quite nicely. But if plaque isn't removed daily, it hardens into a cement-like substance called calculus or tartar, inflaming the gum tissue. As the tissues become more inflamed with gritty tartar—and infected by bacteria—this leads to a more serious condition called periodontitis. Unless you do something to stop this progression, your gum tissues recede and your teeth work themselves loose from your jaw.

Take Care of Your Gums—Now

Gum disease is common but not inevitable. And like so many health conditions, it's a lot easier to prevent than to treat.

"The treatment for periodontal disease can be both expensive and painful," says Andrew Weil, M.D., director of the program in integrative medicine at the University of Arizona College of Medicine in Tucson and author of *Spontaneous Healing*. "But fortunately, most gum disease can be prevented by not smoking, eating a good diet, and practicing basic steps of good oral hygiene," Dr. Weil adds. To him, good oral hygiene includes the use of herbs to kill the germs implicated in gingivitis.

"In my experience, it takes at least six months of herbal therapy and good hygiene to reverse periodontal disease," says Susun S. Weed, an herbalist and herbal educator from Woodstock, New York, and author of the *Wise Woman* series of herbal health books. "I've learned something else through personal experience," she adds. "If your romantic partner has gum disease, you're at high risk, too. The bacteria that cause it are highly contagious. They pass back and forth between your mouths when you kiss," Weed notes.

How do you know if you have a gum problem? Ask your dentist. You may also notice the early warning signs: bad breath and gums that bleed easily when you brush, floss, or eat. If these symptoms sound familiar, there's no need to worry. According to herbalists, the following time-tested remedies are effective.

Herbalize your water jet. Your dentist may have already recommended the use of a dental hygiene device (such as Water Pik) that uses a high-speed water jet to help remove food particles and plaque. Weed suggests taking its healing power even further. She adds two to four drops of tincture (also called an extract) of bloodroot or echinacea to the water reservoir of her machine and then uses the device as directed.

Bloodroot was used by Native Americans as an oral antiseptic, and studies show that it can help reduce plaque deposits in as little as eight days. Bloodroot is safe when used in commercial dental products or under the guidance of a trained herbalist, says Varro E. Tyler, Ph.D., professor emeritus of pharmacognosy at the Purdue University School of Pharmacy and Pharmacal Sciences in West Lafayette, Indiana, in his book *Herbs of Choice*. It may cause nausea and vomiting if ingested. Bloodroot is not considered a safe herb to use during pregnancy.

Stop gum disease with echinacea. "Echinacea is a great oral antibacterial," says Weed. "Cover your entire gum line with echinacea tincture right before bedtime and leave it on overnight," she advises.

Have a cuppa chamomile. Chamomile tea is useful against gingivitis because it reduces inflammation and kills germs, says James A. Duke, Ph.D., a botanical consultant, former ethnobotanist with the U.S. Department of Agriculture, and author of *The Green Pharmacy*, who specializes in medicinal plants. Infuse 2 teaspoons of the herb in a cup of water that has reached a boil and steep for 5 to 10 minutes. Drink a cup after meals, Dr. Duke suggests.

Make a goldenseal mouth rinse. "Use this rinse two or three times a day as an herbal disinfectant," advises Dr. Weil. To 1 cup warm water, add ¼ teaspoon of salt and ½ teaspoon, or the contents of one capsule, of goldenseal root powder. The herb will not completely dissolve. Swish the rinse around in your mouth for a minute or so, then spit it out.

Tap the power of an ancient gum powder. A thousand years ago, the Arabian medical wizard, Avicenna, penned the million-word *As-Qanum*, a medical book that was highly regarded for its uncanny accuracy. And he created an herbal concoction of myrrh, cayenne, goldenseal, and aloe that heals inflamed gums.

"Although this concoction tastes horrible, it's really effective for killing bacteria and healing inflamed gums quickly," says Ellen Hopman, a professional member of the American Herbalists Guild (AHG) who practices near Amherst, Massachusetts. "The myrrh disinfects and the cayenne will stimulate circulation, which helps the gums heal," she says. "The goldenseal kills the bacteria, and the aloe is healing and soothing."

To make Avicenna's gum powder, use equal parts of powdered myrrh, cayenne, and goldenseal root. You can break open a capsule of each or buy the powders at an herb store and blend them in a jar, which you can then store, tightly closed, in a cool, dark place for up to six months. To use the powder, place the herb blend on one side of a saucer and a small dollop of aloe vera gel

Myrrh: A Balm for Sore Gums

In biblical times, myrrh was a prized ingredient in incense and perfumes, and the Middle Eastern air was heavy with its sweet, warm scent. But since antiquity, myrrh has also been known as an all-purpose healer.

Myrrh is a blend of volatile oils, gum, and resin, the liquid exuded by thick, bushy shrubs native to northeastern Africa and southwestern Asia. As the resin dries, it solidifies and is dissolved in tinctures and oils.

The essential oil, which is distilled from the resin, can be used to make a chest rub that helps get rid of thick phlegm caused by severe colds and bronchitis, says Penelope Ody, Ph.D., a member of Britain's National Institute of Medical Herbalists, in her book *The Complete Medicinal Herbal*. To make the rub, mix ¼ teaspoon of the essential oil with 1 tablespoon of almond or sunflower oils. Apply as needed.

Myrrh tincture or essential oil can be found in some health food stores or by mail order (see "Where to Buy Herbs and Herbal Products" on page 462).

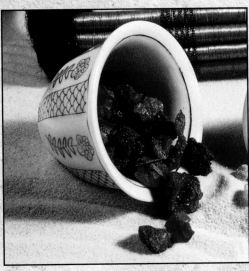

Herbalists consider myrrh a potent antiseptic. In Germany and other European countries, people dab tincture of myrrh on canker sores or other inflammations of the mouth, such as gingivitis.

on the other side. (If you have an aloe plant on hand, break open a leaf and use the fresh gel, or get pure aloe vera gel from a health food store.) Dip your toothbrush in the gel, then in the powdered mixture, and apply it directly to your gums, says Hopman. (This is not a tasty blend, so be sure to avoid your tongue.) Leave it on for about a minute, then rinse your mouth well with water. If your symptoms persist for more than a week or two, see your dentist. You should avoid myrrh during pregnancy, however.

Use a bit of bitter medicine for healthy gums. "Although this isn't entirely an herbal formula, it's a remarkable gum healer," says Ellen Kamhi, R.N., Ph.D., of Oyster Bay, New York, an herbalist, professional member of the AHG, and host of the nationally syndicated radio show *Natural Alternatives*.

First, brush your teeth and gums thoroughly with baking soda. Swish some hydrogen peroxide in your mouth, then floss your teeth. Break open a capsule each of powdered goldenseal root, myrrh, and coenzyme Q10 and put the powder on a small plate. Using a cotton swab, mix in enough aloe vera gel to make a paste, then apply the paste to your gums. ("This paste tastes very bitter," warns Dr. Kamhi.) It's best to leave this mixture on the gums—no rinsing is required.

Coenzyme Q10 is a naturally occurring molecule that's essential for tissue health. A deficiency of coenzyme Q10 has been linked to periodontal disease, and research has shown that it accelerates the healing and repair of periodontal tissue. Coenzyme Q10 capsules are available in health food stores.

Headaches

HERBS FOR BRAIN PAIN

Okay, so technically, head pain doesn't come from your brain. But if you have a headache, it can sure feel that way.

People who experience headaches use various adjectives to describe their pain, from aching, throbbing, pulsing, and pounding to searing and excruciating. Generally, headaches are categorized as tension or muscle-contraction headaches, vascular headaches (namely, migraines), or sinus headaches. If your head hurts, you've probably already tried the usual headache remedies, such as aspirin. Maybe they don't work, or maybe you're worried about side effects—especially if headaches are part of your daily (or monthly) life.

What's Going On in That Head of Yours?

To an herbalist, there's no such thing as a garden-variety headache. And you'll probably never hear your herbalist utter the words, "Take two aspirin and call me in the morning," either. On the contrary, your herbalist will take your headaches very seriously, especially if they're chronic.

"There are a lot of different types of headaches," says David Winston, a professional member of the American Herbalists Guild (AHG) and founder of Herbalist and Alchemist, an herbal medicine company in Washington, New Jersey. "Unless you understand the *cause* of your headaches, you'll never be able to cure them permanently," he says.

Food allergies, spinal or cervical (neck) injuries, muscle tension, stress, and even constipation are a few of the diverse players in the headache game. Medical doctors, too, will take those causes into consideration. And they'll also run a battery of tests to rule out brain tumors or other life-threatening problems. If all of your tests say that there's nothing wrong, but you still hurt, the herbal approach may help by going beyond the textbook approach.

"From the perspective of Traditional Chinese Medicine—a major influence on herbalism—the causes of headaches are myriad," says Winston. "A headache can be caused by what the Chinese call liver stagnation, or liver fire rising, which is often implicated in migraines. In general, a headache is simply a signal that your body isn't functioning as it should be."

Most of us have heard the phrase, "banging your head against a wall," the cliché for going nowhere. "Sometimes, headaches happen when you bang your head against a wall in a spiritual, emotional, or even a physical sense," explains Winston.

When it comes to headache treatment, herbalists also take a different approach from that of most conventional physicians. "Western medicine deals with treating the discomfort headaches cause, but herbalists deal with treating the causes of chronic headaches," says Winston. "Easing the pain is as important to herbalists as it is to conventional physicians, but you have to know what's causing a headache before you know which herbs will cure it."

Here's a good illustration. "A woman consulted me about her migraines, which she'd been having for 15 years or so," recalls Winston. "Her diet was atrocious, and she was incredibly constipated—she only had a bowel movement once every five or six days. 'My doctor said that's normal for me,' she told me. So one of the first things we did was regulate her bowel function, and as soon as we did, her migraines disappeared.

"The next thing I knew, she sent her friend in to see me—a woman with the exact same symptoms—and with treatment, her friend's migraines disappeared, too, for the first time in 50 years! All it took was six months of an improved diet and herbs to stimulate digestion and normalize elimination."

Clearly, herbalists believe that there's more to curing a headache than curing the pain it causes. "Most herbalists are interested in treating the whole person and correcting underlying imbalances," says Winston. "These can even be life issues such as a bad job, family stress, or a destructive relationship. I believe it is necessary to consider these kinds of underlying factors and attempt to help the person make changes. Otherwise, I would only be treating the person's symptoms rather than healing them."

Here's a closer look at each kind of headache and the herbs that may relieve them.

Migraines

The most hellish of headaches, migraines typically begin early in the day and reach peak intensity within an hour or so—and they can last from several hours to several days.

"Migraines are classified as either common, classic, or complicated, " says Tieraona Low Dog, M.D., a family practice physician at the University of New Mexico Hospital, professional member of the AHG, and member of the Alternative Medicine Research Group at the University of New Mexico School of Medicine in Albuquerque. While not all people with migraines have all of these complaints, these head-blasters can cause certain nastily distinctive symptoms: severe pounding or throbbing pain, exquisite sensitivity to light and sound, nausea, vomiting, and loss of appetite.

Of the three types, approximately 85 percent of all migraines are considered common. That means that the headache hits out of the blue with none of the warning signs that typify classical migraines. Before the pain of a classical migraine begins, there's usually a 15- to 30-minute segue of symptoms that signal its onset, including auras of blurred vision or bright spots, disturbed thinking, fatigue, and numbness or tingling on one side of the body. Finally, if these warning symptoms morph into the migraine pain and co-exist with it, you're having a "complicated" migraine.

For women, hormones play a role in migraines. "Sixty percent of women's migraines occur during the luteal phase—that is, late in your cycle when estrogen is at its lowest ebb," says Dr. Low Dog. "This is especially true for women who take birth control pills. Their migraines tend to hit during the part of the cycle when estrogen is not taken."

Herbalists often treat women's migraines based on this theory: Estrogen maintains the vasomotor tone, meaning that it helps to regulate the constriction of blood vessels. When estrogen is low, the blood vessels dilate, or widen, and the circulation surges that result may cause migraines in susceptible women, suggests Dr. Low Dog. "Herbs with estrogen-like properties, such as dang gui and black cohosh, can be very helpful for women whose migraines occur in the late luteal phase."

Herbal treatment for migraines depends on your specific headache symptoms, explains Winston. One kind of headache feels like your head's about to explode. Applying a cool pack seems to help. Other migraines grip your head like a steel band. They tend to feel better when heat's applied, says Dr. Low Dog.

It's important to differentiate what your specific migraine symptoms are, because different herbal treatments are used for each kind, Winston notes.

Head Off Migraines Herbally

If you've ever had a migraine, you'll be first on your feet to applaud the notion of prevention. Here are some suggestions.

Take feverfew tincture or capsules daily. If your migraines are the type that feel as if the top of your head is about to explode, the herb feverfew may help, say Winston and other herbalists. Research demonstrates that small amounts of feverfew can prevent migraines, according to Winston. The herb contains parthenolide, a substance that, along with other constituents of the plant, may maintain levels of serotonin, a nerve messenger, within blood platelets. Serotonin helps to reduce pain.

Herbalists disagree on how to best take feverfew. "Although many experts recommend that you use feverfew extract standardized to 0.2 percent parthenolide, one study used more—a standardization of 0.6 percent parthenolide—and it didn't work at all against migraines," reports Winston. Maybe it didn't work because amounts of other chemicals besides parthenolide were also different, and many active ingredients in feverfew play a role in relieving migraines, he explains. Subsequent studies reported that feverfew is most effective when whole raw leaves are used, he says.

Chewing fresh feverfew leaves—one a day—is one option, says Lisa Alschuler, N.D., a naturopathic physician and chair of the department of botanical medicine at Bastyr University in Bothell, Washington. "But that can cause mouth ulcers in some people. So instead, I recommend taking $\frac{1}{2}$ teaspoon daily of feverfew tincture (also called an extract) made from the whole leaf (the bottle usually indicates if it is from whole leaves) or 500 milligrams in capsule form once a day," she says.

Have a feverfew sandwich. "I put a feverfew leaf between two slices of white bread and eat it like a sandwich," says Corinne Martin, a professional member of the AHG who practices in Bridgeton, Maine. "I believe the bread helps prevent mouth sores—it works for me!" The bread may act as a barrier to protect sensitive mucous membranes.

Sip some rosemary. "A good herbal preventive for some vasoconstrictive migraines is rosemary," says Dr. Alschuler. "Like ginkgo, it helps keep blood vessels dilated." Try sipping one cup of rosemary infusion daily. Use 1 teaspoon of herb per cup, Dr. Alschuler advises. (For directions on preparing infusions, see "Teas and Infusions" on page 89.)

Grab ginkgo and go. As an alternative to the rosemary tea, try ginkgo. This herb improves blood supply to the brain, helps maintain vascular tone, and keeps the blood vessels from leaking inflammatory chemicals, according to herbalists. Therefore, it helps prevent the initial vasoconstriction and ischemia (blood deficiency) that can occur in classical migraines, says Dr. Low Dog. Ginkgolides, substances present in the plant, also block inflammation and allergic responses, which can contribute to headaches, she says. In one study, ginkgo reduced headaches in 80 percent of the people who took it, most of whom were having migraines regularly. They had tried everything possible

for their headaches, but nothing worked until they tried ginkgo.

For migraine prevention, Dr. Alschuler recommends taking ginkgo in standardized extract capsules, 40 milligrams per capsule. two or three times a day.

Ginkgo has been shown to have potentially harmful interactions with some pharmaceutical drugs (MAO inhibitors), and should never be used with aspirin or other nonsteroidal anti-inflammatory medicines.

Make ginger part of your plan. "Ginger inhibits a substance called thromboxane A2, which prevents the release of substances that make blood vessels dilate," says Dr. Low Dog. In other words, it can help keep blood flowing on an even keel, which is essential in migraine prevention. Ginger is tasty and versatile: To prevent migraines, you can grate fresh ginger into juice, nosh on Japanese pickled ginger (available at health food stores), use fresh or powdered ginger when you cook, or nibble a piece or two of crystallized ginger candy every day, suggests Dr. Low Dog.

Herbal Wisdom
Nature's Prescription for Wellness

"Herbal medicine can be effective as part of a holistic health-care plan for treating a wide variety of women's health concerns. By providing essential trace nutrients and by subtly influencing the metabolism and all cellular functions, herbs gently show the body how to be healthier and better balanced, and encourage healing to occur."

—*Chanchal Cabrera, herbalist and teacher*

Try nature's aspirin. One of the active ingredients in aspirin is acetylsalicylic acid, which is a chemical derivative of salicin, a natural pain-relieving agent. Salicin is found in several members of the plant kingdom, including willow bark. "Unless you're allergic to aspirin, using tinctures of these herbs is worth a try," says Ellen Kamhi, R.N., Ph.D., of Oyster Bay, New York, an herbalist, professional member of the AHG, and host of the nationally syndicated radio show *Natural Alternatives*. "And unlike feverfew, which you need to take all the time to head off migraines, willow bark is effective during an attack."

Using willow for pain relief can eliminate the stomach upset associated with uncoated aspirin because it passes through the stomach before it turns into its pain-relieving form, explains Dr. Low Dog. Take three to five milliliters of willow bark extract every two hours until the migraine backs off, she advises.

Do not take willow with aspirin. Also, since it has compounds similar to aspirin, don't take it if you need to avoid aspirin because of ulcers, asthma, diabetes, gout, hemophilia (a blood thrombin deficiency), or kidney or liver disease or if you are taking a blood thinner such as warfarin (Coumadin). Mixing willow bark with alcohol can irritate your stomach. It may also interact with barbiturates or sedatives such as aprobarbital (Amytal) or alprazolam (Xanax).

Consider biofeedback. Some nonherbal strategies may help, too. "I often refer women to a biofeedback therapist," says Martin. "Biofeedback can actually change your circulation by teaching you to relax the blood vessels, which relieves migraine pain," she adds. "I remember one woman with migraines who was taught to warm up her hands, and her headache went away. Raising the temperature of her hands required her to command her body to dilate blood vessels; the blood vessels throughout her body were affected, including the ones causing discomfort in her head."

Keep a headache diary. It helps to log your activities and headache symptoms to find out whether certain foods, such as chocolate, cured meats, cheeses, and alcohol, or other triggers set off your migraines, says Winston.

Get professional help. If your migraines are intense and unrelenting, if your headaches differ from your "normal" migraine, or if they are accompanied by vomiting or a stiff neck and fever, seek help from your physician to rule out any major problems. In addition, a qualified professional herbalist may be of tremendous help, suggests Winston. "There are many powerful herbs that can help migraines, but they belong in the hands of an experienced, well-trained herbalist who will create a treatment plan that specifically meets your needs."

Tension Headache

Something like 80 percent of the American population knows firsthand what a tension headache feels like, says Dr. Low Dog. These headaches can occur at any time, usually when you're tired or stressed, with pain that lasts from several hours to even several weeks. Although the intensity can vary, the pain is pretty standard: It's a persistent, nonthrobbing, dull ache. If you unconsciously contract your head and neck muscles in response to stress, you might find that your scalp is unusually tender or that your neck and shoulder muscles are especially tight. Over time, chronically tense muscles stimulate pain receptors and slow blood flow to the head. The result: A headache.

Not surprisingly, relaxation therapies like massage, deep-breathing exercises, yoga, and exercise are highly recommended to relieve tension and muscle-contraction headaches, says Dr. Low Dog. In tough cases, she recommends acupuncture or neuromuscular therapy to quiet deep-seated muscle spasms. For helpful herbal remedies, read on.

Kick back with a cup of tea. "A lot of nice, mild, relaxing herbs work really well to relax away simple tension headaches," says Winston. "Tension headaches usually go away when you slow down, relax, and take some deep breaths. The healing ritual of preparing an herbal tea is very helpful because it forces you to slow down, take it easy, and focus on something else for a little while. So when a headache strikes, brew yourself a pot of either chamomile, linden flower, lemon balm, or passionflower tea and sip to your heart's delight."

Try a tension-taming tincture. "If stress and tension set off your headaches, tincture of fresh milky oats is an excellent relaxant," notes Winston. (Milky oats come from a specific part of the oat plant and are harvested at a specific stage in the plant's growth, Winston explains. So don't think that you will get the same effect from products marked just oats, oatstraw, or wild oats, which may have different active ingredients.) The Eclectics, physicians who practiced a combination of conventional and botanical medicine over 100 years ago, used oats to relieve nervous headaches. Take five milliliters or one teaspoon of fresh milky oat tincture three times a day, either directly or in water, advises Winston. The tincture is available through mail order (see "Where to Buy Herbs and Herbal Products" on page 462).

Blend a triple-herb sedative. Thanks to valerian's highly complex biochemical makeup, it's an excellent anti-anxiety herb, says Dr. Low Dog. In addition, it contains valerenic acid, which directly relaxes muscles and muscle spasms. The dried root of kava-kava reduces muscle spasms, eases pain, and enhances your sense of well-being—attributes that have been demonstrated clinically but which science can't quite explain. Historically, black cohosh was used for all kinds of rheumatic aches and pains, and it has an incredible ability to ease muscle spasms and reduce inflammation, she says. Together, tinctures of these herbs can erase the pain of muscle-contraction headaches quickly, Dr. Low Dog says. Combine 40 milliliters of valerian root tincture, 40 milliliters of kava-kava root tincture, and 20 milliliters of black cohosh root tincture. She recommends taking 3 to 5 milliliters of the combination three times a day as needed for headache pain.

Do not exceed the recommended dose of kava-kava. It should not be taken simultaneously with alcohol or barbiturates, since it is a mild sedative; use caution when driving or operating other equipment. If valerian has a stimulating rather than a relaxing effect on you, as it does in a few women, stop taking it. Also avoid valerian if you're taking other sleep-enhancing or mood-regulating medications such as diazepam (Valium) or amitriptyline (Elavil.).

Sinus Pain and Pressure

If your head hurts because the hollows around your eyes, nose, and ears are infected

Eyebright: The Eye, Ear, Nose, and Throat Herb

*I*f you have a cold or sore throat along with a headache, you might want to add eyebright to your repertoire of herbal remedies. Eyebright was a pretty popular herb 500 years or so ago. Not only was it reputed to cure "all evils of the eye," it was also brewed into eyebright ale sometime during the reign of the first Queen Elizabeth. On top of that, it was an ingredient in a British herbal tobacco blend "smoked most usefully for chronic bronchial colds," and it was even heralded as a sight restorer for people in their (very) golden years.

Today, herbalists consider this tiny-flowered, grasslike, British and European native to be an excellent remedy for problems of the mucous membranes. It combines antiinflammatory powers with an astringent action, and it has the power to dry up congestion and runny noses. It is also used externally as an eye compress for stinging, inflamed, or weepy eyes and also to heal conjunctivitis.

Eyebright can be consumed as an infusion, used as a compress, or taken in tincture form. Just don't smoke it.

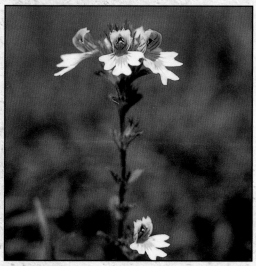

Eyebright could be called an eye, ear, nose, and throat doctor's dream, for in folk medicine, it's been used for conjunctivitis, hay fever, hoarseness, sore throats, coughs, and runny noses.

and clogged, no amount of relaxation, vasodilation, or antispasm strategy is going to relieve your pain. Different problem, different herbs.

"Sinus headaches are a whole other kettle of fish," says Winston. "Obviously, to cure sinus headaches permanently, you have to clear up the problems that cause the headaches in the first place." To treat the underlying infection, see page 356. To ease the pain of a sinus headache *now*, try one of these remedies.

Give eyebright the eye. "Although its name makes you think it's an eye herb, eyebright is specific medicine for the sinuses, and it's also used for earaches," says Winston. "Use eyebright when your sinus condition is accompanied by red, itchy, scratchy eyes. Be sure to use tincture made only from fresh, not dried, plants—it should say so on the bottle. If not, assume it is dried."

Dr. Low Dog recommends taking five milliliters every four to six hours until the pain and infection are gone.

Choose echinacea or thyme. When your sinus infection produces profuse green or yellow mucus or mucus streaked with blood, you should take a cooling, drying herb like echinacea, which will act as a decongestant, recommends Winston. He suggests taking 40 to 60 drops of echinacea tincture every three to four hours until the pain and infection are gone.

If your sinuses are infected (that is, if you have fever, sinus pain, or green nasal discharge), you should also take three milliliters of Oregon grape root, goldenseal root, or barberry root, says Dr. Low Dog.

If your sinus secretions are clear or white, you need a warming, drying herb like thyme, Winston says. Thyme is strongly antiseptic and is a specific and traditional remedy for respiratory infections. Drink a cup of thyme tea—made by steeping 2 teaspoons of dried thyme in 1 cup of boiling water for 10 minutes—three times a day. Alternately, take two to four milliliters of tincture of thyme three times a day.

Try an aromatic head massage. "I've found that people find their sinus pain eases if they gently massage a drop or two of essential oil of lavender into their temples a few times a day," says Winston. Tiger Balm, an oriental salve sold in health food stores, can also help ease sinus pain when it is gently rubbed into your temples, he adds. Just be careful not to get it in your eyes, he advises.

Heart Health

SMART SUPPORT FROM NATURE

There are no poignant pink ribbons, no 5-K races, no candlelight vigils, and no celebrity spokeswomen to trumpet the fact that for women, heart disease is the number one health enemy. In fact, it would have been truer to life if a couple of seasons ago, TV character Murphy Brown had been dealt a heart attack instead of breast cancer, because heart disease fells women *five*

times more frequently than breast cancer does.

If that statistic comes as news to you, you're not alone. In fact, surveys reveal that 65 percent of women don't know that heart disease is the number one killer of women, and only 33 percent know that women die from heart attacks far more frequently than they do from breast cancer.

Women aren't the only ones who need to speed-read up on their heart disease risks, either. Their own doctors may not realize that heart disease is such a formidable female foe. As a result, studies show that doctors order fewer tests, follow up less, and recommend lifesaving surgery less frequently for women than they do for men. That may partly explain why women with heart disease are more than one-and-a-half times more likely to die within a year of a first heart attack than men are.

And here's yet another heads-up: Heart disease isn't just an older woman's problem. True, before menopause, it's unusual for women to develop coronary heart disease. But right after menopause, your chances of developing high cholesterol, high blood pressure, and heart disease rise steadily. Believe it or not, more than 30 percent of the women who die of heart attacks are under the age of 55, according to the American Heart Association.

Why does menopause make women so much more susceptible to heart disease? In a word, estrogen. During your childbearing years, egg-rich ovaries produce estrogen. But just before, during, and after menopause, there are fewer and fewer eggs left, and your body produces estrogen in ever-dwindling amounts.

Estrogen helps your heart by raising the level of high-density lipoprotein (HDL) cholesterol, the "good" type that sweeps the "bad," gummy cholesterol, low-density lipoprotein (LDL), from your arteries. That helps keep your arteries open—and helps prevent heart disease.

What Herbs Have to Offer

In the absence of estrogen, your heart disease risk factors rise. You're at higher-than-normal risk if you smoke, are inactive, or have high cholesterol or blood pressure. Diabetes seriously increases your risk, as do obesity and even stress.

But if you take the advice of herbalists, you'll learn how to keep your cholesterol and blood pressure within safe limits. Adopt the right herbs, in combination with regular activity and healthy eating habits, and your years past menopause can be long, healthy, and vibrantly productive, comments Tieraona Low Dog, M.D., a family practice physician at the University of New Mexico Hospital, professional member of the American Herbalists Guild (AHG), and member of the Alternative Medicine Research Group at the University of New Mexico School of Medicine in Albuquerque.

Heed this caution, however: The recommendations in this chapter are for healthy women who want to help prevent high cholesterol and high blood pressure, not for women who are already under a physician's care for a heart condition. If you do have a heart condition or high blood pressure, it is also important to consult your doctor, since some herbs may have serious side effects or interactions with prescription medication.

One category of herbs called cardiac glycosides specifically affects the function and rhythm of the heart muscle, so self-prescribing could be dangerous. Foxglove, for example, can have a toxifying effect when taken beyond the recommended dosage, and it must be taken in smaller amounts when combined with other "heart-y" herbs such as English hawthorn. Since several prescription drugs for cardiovascular disease, such as digitoxin (Coramedan), are derived from foxglove and have the same action, taking both could result in a fatal overdose. So if you're being treated for heart disease, be sure you are working with a qualified health-care practitioner who knows the interactions and effects of these types of herbs.

"Well-trained phytotherapists (otherwise known as clinical herbalists, or health-care professionals clinically trained in the use of herbal medicine) may have striking results when using herbs to treat people with heart conditions," says David Winston, a professional member of the AHG and founder of Herbalist and Alchemist, an herbal medicine company in Washington, New Jersey. "But unless you're under professional care, use herbs to help *prevent* heart disease, not as a substitute for medication prescribed by your doctor," he says. "Like a low-fat, vegetarian diet and a regular exercise program, herbs that benefit the circulatory system are best used as one aspect of a healthy lifestyle," concludes Winston.

High Cholesterol

Your cholesterol is more than just a number. When cholesterol levels are high, the threat of atherosclerosis—the disease that Grandma called hardening of the arteries—looms large. Here's why: LDL carries cholesterol to the tissues, where it's deposited as fat. HDL, on the other hand, transports cholesterol to the liver for processing and excretion. In the arteries, cholesterol-based fat deposits become hardened adhesions called plaque. As plaque accumulates, the arteries narrow and harden, and blood flow can become blocked. If the arteries narrow enough to cut off the heart's blood supply, well, you're in trouble. One problem is that atherosclerosis is a silent disease. In fact, your first symptom—a heart attack—could potentially be your last.

But don't panic. For the most part, the deadly effects of this silent killer are easy to prevent. Where do you start? By maintaining healthy cholesterol levels.

Herbalists and the American Heart Association (AHA) agree on three ways to do just that. The first is a low-fat diet, with no more than 30 percent of your daily calories from fat and 10 percent or less coming from saturated fat.

"I like the Food Guide Pyramid from the U.S. Department of Agriculture and the Department of Health," says Winston. "It emphasizes foods based on whole grains, like pasta, bread, rice, and cereal, with more servings of vegetables and fruits than of dairy or protein foods."

Strategy number two you've heard before: Exercise is essential. Take three or four brisk 30-minute walks every week and up your activity in general, the AHA recommends.

Consider exercise your heart's best friend. In addition to a cornucopia of other body-friendly benefits, regular exercise strengthens the heart muscle, lowers blood pressure, and lessens the chances that your blood vessels will narrow.

Number three: Deal with stress. "We need to make the connection between what happens when we're stressed and what's happening in our bodies," says Dr. Low Dog. "Stress contributes to atherosclerosis because when we're stressed, we mobilize fat into fuel. That was really helpful when we needed energy to run from warring neighbors or fierce animals. But today, most of our day-to-day stress comes from non-life-threatening stuff, like running late or dealing with bad-mannered people. When we don't get enough aerobic activity to burn off the fat as fuel, those mobilized lipids have no place to go," she says. "As a result, the fat ends up floating around in your blood vessels and can end up as fatty deposits in your arteries."

Exercise, she notes, is an excellent antidote to stress. "The more stressful your life is, the more you need your exercise," she concludes.

Beyond diet and exercise, herbalists and heart doctors diverge dramatically on how to treat high cholesterol. Conventional medicine recommends drug treatment to lower your cholesterol if diet and exercise alone don't do the job. But each and every drug that lowers cholesterol may also offer some not-so-welcome side effects, such as liver or kidney problems, for example.

Instead of drugs, herbalists use several herbs that are mild yet show promise in lowering cholesterol. One or two of them might even be in your pantry right now.

All about Allium

Ask any herbalist which herb has the greatest potential for lowering cholesterol—and blood pressure, for that matter—and the answer will invariably be garlic, an herb in the Allium family.

"More than 30 years of research shows that garlic lowers cholesterol and triglyceride levels," says David Hoffman, a founding and professional member of the AHG, a fellow of Britain's National Institute of Medical Herbalists, assistant professor of integral health studies at the California Institute of Integral Studies in Santa Rosa, and author of *The New Holistic Herbal*. Since 1960, some 1,000 research papers have been published on this herb, and a considerable amount of research supports garlic's role as an aid to lowering the risk of heart disease.

In a study conducted at the University of Guelph in Canada, people with cholesterol levels higher than 200 milligrams per deciliter who took commercial garlic preparations lowered total cholesterol levels by nearly 12 percent. What's more, those taking garlic had significantly lower ratios of LDL to HDL compared with those who didn't take garlic. (A person is considered at greater risk for coronary heart disease if her level of LDL cholesterol is high when compared to that of HDL cholesterol.) For study participants who took garlic, LDL levels dropped about 15 percent, and blood pressure dropped slightly.

In addition to potentially lowering blood cholesterol levels, some research suggests that garlic further protects against heart disease by preventing the formation of blood clots that can block arteries.

"We know that garlic lowers the bad cholesterol and raises the good cholesterol," agrees Dr. Low Dog. "There's some question about how best to use it—cooked or uncooked—because garlic has so many active constituents, including over 60 sulfur compounds."

Nothing beats raw garlic for potency, so most herbal experts recommend that you eat garlic raw to get its medicinal benefits.

"Most of the garlic products on the market today—capsules, for example—are nowhere near as potent as raw garlic or other members of the Allium family such as onions, scallions, leeks, shallots, chives, and ramps (a relative of chives that grows in the wild). All members of the garlic family are good for you and your heart," Winston says. "For antibacterial purposes, I think garlic is best eaten raw. But for lowering cholesterol, it is also effective when used in cooking or when taken as one of the garlic products on the market," he adds.

Dr. Low Dog theorizes that since "people have a lower incidence of heart disease in the Mediterranean countries, where red wine,

Heart-Healthy Pesto

Many experts recommend raw garlic for its ability to lower cholesterol. Pesto, a hearty paste of raw garlic and basil used on pasta or bread, is a tasty way to take your medicine. Purists make it with a mortar and pestle, but you can also use a blender or a food processor. And although most recipes call for fresh basil, for convenience, you can freeze fresh basil in a little olive oil in ice cube trays for later use. You can also substitute flatleaf Italian parsley for basil.

Pesto is also a delicious snack spread on toasted slices of Italian bread or stuffed into large mushroom caps with bread crumbs and broiled until the crumbs are brown.

2½ **cups fresh basil**
4 **cloves garlic**

¼ **cup pine nuts or walnuts**
1 **tablespoon grated Parmesan cheese**
½ **cup extra-virgin olive oil**
Freshly ground black pepper

Chop the basil, garlic, and pine nuts or walnuts, then combine them in a large mortar. Pound the mixture until a thick paste forms. Add the Parmesan, then add the oil a tablespoon at a time until it is absorbed. Add pepper to taste.

To serve, toss with cooked pasta and vegetables. Add water if the pesto is too thick to toss evenly.

Makes 4 servings

---

olive oil, and cooked garlic are essential components of the cuisine," cooked garlic may have some cholesterol-lowering benefit.

And scientific evidence does suggest that cooked garlic helps lower cholesterol, says David Christopher, a founding member of the AHG and director of the School of Natural Healing in Springville, Utah, which was founded by his late father, the renowned herbalist John R. Christopher, N.D., in 1953. In a review of 16 studies involving 952 people, British researchers found that eating garlic—whether fresh or in powdered form—lowered total cholesterol by an average of 12 to 13 percent.

Raw or cooked, fresh garlic is a heart-healthy herb. Don't expect garlic to be a quick fix for high cholesterol, however. "Your arteries don't get clogged up overnight," says Douglas Schar, a practicing medical herbalist in London, editor of the *British Journal of Phytotherapy*, and author of *Backyard Medicine Chest*. "Similarly, garlic won't clear them out overnight. It takes 40 years to develop plaque in the cardiovascular system, so you should consider using garlic as part of your long-term prevention program." Here are some of the best, most effective ways to use it.

Toss it around. "Garlic becomes effective against cholesterol at around 3,000 micrograms of raw garlic, which is about three cloves a day," says Dr. Low Dog. Mince garlic and add it to salads or toss it in the pot just before serving time when you cook soups, sauces, or stews, she suggests.

Suck on a spoonful of honey. Raw

garlic—or even lots of cooked garlic—can give some people indigestion. "If raw garlic doesn't agree with you, try this three times a day, after meals," suggests Winston. "Chop up a clove of garlic, put it in a spoon, and mix it with a little honey, applesauce, or yogurt. Swallow it quickly and drink some water to help wash the garlic down."

Pop a garlic pill. "Since garlic doesn't agree with everyone, you may have to try one of the different brands of processed garlic," says Dr. Low Dog. "Several brands, like Kyolic, have studies backing them up, but I always say that the proof is in the pudding, so take the pills or capsules and have your cholesterol checked again in eight weeks. If it hasn't budged, switch products," she advises. She recommends taking capsules containing 3,000 to 4,000 micrograms of allicin (one of the active components of garlic) per day.

Beef up your diet with onions. "Since all the members of the onion and garlic family help lower cholesterol, it makes sense to include as many of them as possible in your diet regularly," says Winston. And don't think of onion and its cousins merely as a seasoning vegetable for other foods. Think heart-warming onion soups, stuffed onions, and sautéed onions.

Beyond Garlic

Garlic's not the only cholesterol-lowering herbal arrow in Mother Nature's bountiful quiver. Ginger and guggul, an herb used for centuries in Ayurvedic medicine (a healing system that originated in India), have promise, according to herbalists. So do other herbs that help support liver function.

Good-for-you guggul. Guggul is a gum resin closely related to myrrh. The herb has come into the spotlight for its ability to lower cholesterol. "I've had good experience using guggul to lower cholesterol," says Dr. Low Dog. "In my patients, it raises HDL by 20 percent, lowers LDL by 20 percent, and has a similar effect on triglycerides. It acts like some of the prescription drugs commonly prescribed for high cholesterol do, but without the side effects," she notes.

Guggul helps the liver create more receptors for LDL, which enables the liver to "catch" more LDL from the blood and excrete it from the body through the feces rather than having it floating around and creating fat deposits in your arteries, Dr. Low Dog says.

"I've used guggul to treat 16 or 17 men and women who refused to take other medication for high cholesterol," reports Dr. Low Dog. "They've had dramatic results taking guggul, with no side effects other than a little diarrhea, which is normal when you're getting rid of cholesterol."

If you can't find guggul in health food stores, it's available by mail order (see "Where to Buy Herbs and Herbal Products" on page 462). Look for products that offer it in standardized form, advises Dr. Low Dog. The recommended standardized dose is 25 milligrams three times a day. "If you take a non-standardized form, you have to take so much that it could irritate the stomach," she says. A person should take guggul until lipid levels have normalized and then reduce the dose to 25 milligrams once a day, she says.

Gravitate toward ginger. Ginger gives you a double bonus of protection because it temporarily lowers elevated blood pressure and reduces LDL while raising HDL levels, says Dr. Low Dog. "In addition, ginger can help ward off strokes and heart attacks because it keeps platelets from aggregating, or getting sticky, and blocking the arteries," she says.

Take one capsule of ginger, equivalent to

Guggul: A Brave New Medicinal from Bark

If you were hiking through the wilds in guggul's native habitat—Arabia or India—you might not even notice the thorny little tree that produces this herb, a resin believed to have medicinal properties. Naked of foliage for much of the year, the tree has bark that is unassumingly ash-colored and belies the healing power contained within.

If you peel back two layers of bark, however, and give the tree a little nick, it will exude an aromatic yellowish resin that smells of balsam. And that gummy resin is what all the excitement is about, because herbalists claim that it can lower cholesterol and ease arthritis pain with few side effects.

Guggul has traditionally been used in Ayurvedic medicine, which is practiced widely in India, for treating arthritis. But at one point, a researcher stumbled across an ancient Sanskrit text that suggested guggul as a treatment for obesity, high cholesterol, and related problems. Scientific studies ensued, and the results are promising.

In studies with animals that were fed a diet high in cholesterol, taking guggul prevented high cholesterol and stopped plaques from forming in arteries. A study with humans showed that 100 milligrams of guggul taken daily can decrease total cholesterol by almost 12 percent, and LDL and triglycerides also declined by about the same percentage.

Herbalists recommend guggul to lower high cholesterol and triglyceride levels, relieve arthritis, treat heart disease caused by inadequate blood supply to the heart, and diminish acne.

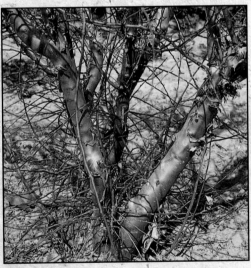

Guggul is recommended by herbalists for a variety of conditions, from high cholesterol to skin problems.

500 milligrams, three times a day, advises Dr. Low Dog. Then take more or less, depending on what your lipid profile looks like after eight weeks. Ginger remains medicinally potent when you cook with it, and crystallized ginger and pickled ginger (the kind you get in Japanese restaurants) are also effective—and delicious—she says.

Dig some dandelion. "When you're dealing with cholesterol, you want to do things that support liver function," says Betzy Bancroft, a professional member of the AHG and manager of Herbalist and Alchemist in Washington, New Jersey. "That's because cholesterol, which is a building block for hormones, is produced in the liver. Dandelion is a bitter, and bitters help normalize liver and pancreatic function, which affects the way your body metabolizes fat, including cholesterol," she says.

You can take a cup or two of dandelion root tea or 20 drops of dandelion tincture (also called an extract) in water before meals. Dandelion is considered a tonic herb that can be taken indefinitely, notes Bancroft.

High Blood Pressure

It's one of the leading causes of stroke, heart attack, congestive heart failure, kidney failure, and premature death. Yet one out of three people with high blood pressure (also called hypertension) doesn't even know that she has it. This is remarkable, since a blood pressure reading is one of the simplest and most available medical tests around.

Blood pressure is, simply put, the force exerted on your artery walls by the blood as it's pumped throughout your body. The pressure of the blood flow is determined by how vigorously your heart pumps as well as by your body's blood volume. Arteries that are clogged by thickened walls and those that have lost their elasticity cause problems, too, by increasing the resistance against which the blood circulates, in turn increasing the pressure at which the blood is pumped.

When the circulating blood exerts too much pressure on artery walls, it can cause scarring, thickening, and hardening. That makes matters worse, because your heart has to work even harder to pump blood through your body.

What Those Numbers Tell You

Blood pressure is expressed in two numbers: Systolic is the measurement of the pressure of blood flow when your heart is pumping; diastolic is the pressure measured between beats. A normal blood pressure is considered 120/80 (systolic over diastolic). Your blood pressure is said to be high when it consistently measures either a systolic pressure of 140 or higher or a diastolic pressure of 90 or higher.

Only a blood pressure test can tell you whether your blood pressure is too high. According to medical experts, you should have your blood pressure checked every two years if a first test shows that it's 130/85 or lower. If it's in the 130 to 139 over 85 to 89 range, check it annually. But if it's higher than that, follow the advice of your health-care practitioner.

"Under stress, most people experience elevated blood pressure, and that's normal. If someone has persistently high blood pressure, though, they have hypertension," explains Dr. Low Dog. "The most common type is essential (also known as idiopathic or primary) hypertension, which means that a person's blood pressure is high, but we don't know why.

"Many mainstream doctors simply prescribe blood pressure medication regardless of the cause. I like to take three blood pressure readings, spaced at least six hours apart, to see if it remains elevated or is reduced once the person relaxes," she continues. "If I'm able to rule out all secondary causes (such as kidney disease or stress), then I treat it as hypertension. My approach is to prescribe such herbs as hawthorn and lemon balm combined with relaxation and stress-management techniques. I also recommend a low-fat, low-salt diet."

Herbal Control Measures

Herbalists and medical doctors generally agree that if your blood pressure's too high, you should eat more healthfully, reduce your intake of sodium (which seems to raise blood pressure in some people), maintain a healthy weight, and get regular exercise. You'll also be told in no uncertain terms to quit smoking and perhaps to lighten up on the liquor, limiting yourself to a glass or two of wine (5 ounces each) or beer (12 ounces) or one cocktail (1½ ounces of liquor) a day.

"If you have high blood pressure, your diet becomes extremely important," says Dr. Low Dog. "Decrease your intake of alcohol while adding omega-3 fatty acids (fish oils)." Lowering the amount of sugar in your diet is a good idea, too, because diets high in sugar have been linked to heart disease.

When it comes to the role of medication for high blood pressure, herbalists differ from medical doctors. "High blood pressure isn't a disease, it's a *symptom* of a disease," emphasizes Christopher. "You can medicate high blood pressure away, but then you risk the side effects of the medication. In a sense, high blood pressure is like constipation of the arterial system, and as an herbalist, my job is to find out what's clogging things up in the first place," he says.

Herbalists like Christopher believe that the trick to reducing high cholesterol and lowering high blood pressure is to stimulate the liver, because it helps rid the body of cholesterol.

"Just be careful about what you use to stimulate the liver. Coffee enhances the flow of bile (which is partially composed of cholesterol), for example, but it does nothing to lower your blood pressure," Dr. Low Dog remarks.

Consider these herbal therapies for reducing your high blood pressure. If you're currently taking medicine for high blood pressure, don't stop taking it without the advice of your doctor. If you use herbal remedies, your medication may need to be adjusted. If your blood pressure is borderline high and you're not on medication, herbal remedies, along with dietary changes, may help you avoid the need for medication, says Dr. Low Dog.

Do be bitter. "Any herb that tastes bitter will stimulate the production of bile," says Christopher. "Herbs that are especially good for this purpose include dandelion, milk thistle, and blessed thistle," he says. "It doesn't matter what form you take these herbs in—teas, tinctures, or raw dandelion leaves. But to trigger bile production, you have to really taste them and get the bitter flavor."

Destress with melissa. "Lemon balm (also known as melissa) is an herb that's underutilized," says Dr. Low Dog. "This herb affects the limbic system—that is, the part of your brain responsible for thoughts and feelings—helping to reduce the daily toll that stress places on our hearts and spirits. 'Melissa makes the heart glad,' was its age-old reputation, and now we know it's true," she notes.

Lemon balm lowers blood pressure when its aromatic oils are inhaled. "The aroma of lemon balm concentrates itself within the limbic system," says Dr. Low Dog.

When you encounter fear or stress, the limbic system processes your feelings and produces a physical response, which can include increased blood pressure, dilated pupils, a rapid heartbeat, and other physical reactions, notes Dr. Low Dog.

German scientists have finally demonstrated what herbalist have known for centuries: When people are given lemon balm, it blunts their autonomic responses to fear and anger so that blood pressure doesn't take a steep climb when they're under a lot of pressure, says Dr. Low Dog. "Lemon balm is especially good for Type A people, who are impatient and easily angered," she comments.

To use lemon balm, just brew and drink two cups of tea a day or take five milliliters of lemon balm tincture twice a day for 12 weeks. Then recheck your pressure and continue taking as needed. In addition, you can inhale the aroma of the pure essential oil as often as needed, whenever you're stressed out or in especially tense situations, recommends Dr. Low Dog (see "Aromatherapy" on page 134 for tips on using essential oils).

According to Dr. Low Dog, if you use lemon balm tea or tincture religiously, you'll find that your blood pressure will fall nicely within six to eight weeks. "We don't know exactly how lemon balm works, but it's a perfectly safe remedy, and I love the way it makes me feel," she says. "The only time I'd exercise caution is if you're being treated for low-thyroid conditions, because lemon balm may compromise thyroid hormones."

Treat your heart to some hawthorn. "I like hawthorn because it strengthens the heart," says Dr. Low Dog. "As we age, the heart doesn't work as well as it did when we were in our twenties," she adds.

Hawthorn dilates the coronary arteries and helps relax other, peripheral arteries, providing more blood to the heart itself. In part, it works by blocking or slowing ACE (angiotension converting enzyme), which indirectly raises blood pressure. "There is a whole class of prescription drugs called ACE inhibitors that are designed to block this enzyme's actions," says Dr. Low Dog. "ACE is found in the lining of the blood vessels, and when you take hawthorn, you gently keep the enzyme from becoming active and help prevent constriction of the blood vessels."

The prescription ACE inhibitors have a few downsides. They are costly. Plus, they can produce a chronic dry, hacking cough—a side effect more frequently reported in women than in men—as well as produce dizziness and weakness and disturb your sense of taste.

In contrast, says Dr. Low Dog, "Hawthorn is a tonic for the heart, and it has lots of positive effects. It's important for the mildly aging heart, and it's a particularly important herb for postmenopausal women to consider, especially if they opt not to take hormone replacement therapy (commonly prescribed to ward off heart disease in women over the age of 50 or so)."

You can make hawthorn tea from the dried flower, leaf, and berry and drink it two or three times a day or take five milliliters of hawthorn tincture twice a day. Look for a 1:5 tincture (meaning one part herb to five parts alcohol/water mixture), recommends Dr. Low Dog. Hawthorn can be taken indefinitely, she says, but have your doctor monitor your heart if you are using it for more than a few weeks.

Hawthorn's beneficial effects may require that you take lower doses of other medicines, such as blood pressure drugs. If you have low blood pressure caused by problems with heart valves, don't use hawthorn without a physician's guidance.

Hemorrhoids

A COMBINED APPROACH TO RELIEF

Few human conditions are as humbling as hemorrhoids. They're painful, they can bleed enough to be downright scary, and they aren't easy to discuss, even among close friends.

Like varicose veins in your legs, hemorrhoids are simply swollen veins, but in the rectum. They may occur inside the anal canal (internal hemorrhoids) or protrude outside the anal opening itself (external hemorrhoids). Anything that puts pressure on the rectal veins can precipitate the problem, including constipation, pregnancy, extreme overweight, physical exertion (such as lifting a heavy suitcase), a low-fiber diet, and standing or sitting for long periods.

If you have hemorrhoids, you'll know it—they hurt, sometimes exquisitely, and they can itch, burn, and bleed.

Hemorrhoids aren't exactly rare: By some estimates, more than half of people over the age of 50 have them in some form or other. And pregnant women are especially susceptible because during pregnancy, hormones that slow the movement of food through the digestive tract are released. They cause constipation, which in turn causes hemorrhoids.

Fiber, Fluids, and Flora

Herbalists and conventional physicians agree on at least one phase of hemorrhoid treatment: Eat plenty of high-fiber foods (especially those rich in soluble fiber like that found in oatmeal and psyllium) and drink lots of fluids. The fiber-fluid combo helps bulk up the stool so it becomes softer and passes more easily through the rectum and anus. Beyond that sound advice, try these soothing herbal remedies.

Apply witch hazel. "One of my favorite remedies for hemorrhoids is good old-fashioned witch hazel," says Betzy Bancroft, a professional member of the American Herbalists Guild and manager of Herbalist and Alchemist, an herbal medicine company in Washington, New Jersey. Witch hazel is an astringent, which helps shrink swollen tissues, and it's very soothing when applied to painfully inflamed hemorrhoids, Bancroft notes. You can make a witch hazel decoction if you have access to fresh or dried witch hazel bark or leaves (to do so, follow the directions in "Decoctions" on page 90). You can also apply the decoction in a compress by soaking a washcloth and placing it on your battered bottom. Either way, apply freely as often as needed.

Park yourself in a sitz. Pour about a pint of witch hazel into a tub filled with a couple of inches of comfortably warm water. Sit in the sitz bath for at least 15 minutes, advises Bancroft.

Help yourself to tincture of butternut. "The root bark of the butternut tree is an excellent stool softener," says Bancroft. "Try taking 20 to 30 drops of butternut tincture three times a day for as long as the hemorrhoids are painful," she recommends. You can find the tincture (also called an extract) in health food stores with well-stocked herbal medicine sections or in mail-order catalogs (see "Where to Buy Herbs and Herbal Products" on page 462). If you are pregnant, check with your doctor before taking butternut.

De-itch with figwort. Figwort has been used as a hemorrhoid remedy at least since the seventeenth century, when British herbalist Nicholas Culpeper wrote, "The decoction of the herb . . . dissolves clotted and congealed blood within the body . . . (including) the hemorrhoids, or piles."

"'Fig' was an old slang term for hemorrhoids, which is how the plant got its name," Bancroft says. "Take 20 to 30 drops of figwort tincture—available in health food stores—three times a day. It works slowly, so you may not see any improvement for several weeks, especially if your hemorrhoids are chronic."

Herpes

UNLEASH THE ANTIVIRAL POWER OF HERBS

You might call herpes the unromantic side of intimacy. Sometimes, what starts as a kiss or a session of lovely, languid lovemaking ends up as a nasty little cluster of blisters erupting from reddened, sensitive skin on your lips, around your mouth, or on your genitals. Then, long after the afterglow of the encounter subsides, the blisters burst and tiny, painful ulcers emerge, taking a week to 10 days to heal.

There are two main forms of herpes, a viral infection of the skin or mucous membranes. Herpes simplex type 1 primarily causes cold sores around the mouth and lips, but it can also affect the genitals. Herpes simplex type 2 is the predominant cause of genital herpes.

If you've been diagnosed with herpes, don't feel like a pariah. Fifty to 80 percent of adults have some form of herpes. Nationwide, 20 percent of teens and adults—some of them your best friends—are infected with herpes simplex 2. Herpes is easily transmitted via sex: You are very likely to get the virus if you have sex with someone whose herpes is causing active eruptions, but you can also get it even if their herpes isn't active.

Herpes is a lot like Godzilla: Even after it disappears, it lurks below the surface and threatens to return. After a herpes outbreak heals, the virus becomes dormant and dwells symptom-free within nerve cells. Stimulate the sleeping virus with a known trigger—stress, sunburn, sex, or even your period—and the virus wakes to attack again, erupting in yet another outbreak near the primary site of infection. Fifty to 75 percent of people who contract herpes simplex 2 will have a recurrent infection within three months.

Subdue the Surly Virus

Medical books state that there's no cure for herpes. And it's a big issue for pregnant women, who can pass the infection to their babies during delivery. But according to herbalists, botanical remedies can ease outbreaks significantly and lengthen the time between episodes.

"I have worked with men and women infected with the virus who've been able to go for years without an outbreak," says Aviva Romm, a certified professional midwife, herbalist, and professional member of the American Herbalists Guild who practices in Bloomfield Hills, Michigan, and is author of *The Natural Pregnancy Book* and *Natural Remedies for Babies and Children*.

"Over the years, I have seen many cases of herpes respond remarkably well to natural treatment," agrees herbalist Rosemary Gladstar, director of the Sage Mountain herbal education center in East Barre, Vermont, and author of *Herbal Healing for Women*.

Here are some of the best ways to treat herpes, according to herbalists, as well as current wisdom on how to keep it dormant for as long as possible between outbreaks.

Start with a tonic. "The primary medicinal herbs that I use against herpes are burdock root and echinacea," says Romm. Echinacea stimulates the immune system, which helps prevent infection. Burdock also acts as a mild antiviral agent and is a gentle cleansing tonic.

"I suggest that women with herpes prepare a very strong infusion using 1 ounce by weight of each herb to 1 quart of water," says Romm. "Toss the dried herbs into a quart jar and fill it to the top with boiling water. Steep for 4 to

8 hours, then strain. To prevent recurrent outbreaks, drink ½ cup two to four times a day." The amount and frequency depend on the severity of the outbreaks you were having. If you do have an outbreak, increase the amount to four cups a day until the blisters disappear, then go back on the maintenance amount, Romm suggests. You can use this infusion for up to three months, then take a 3-day break after each 27-day stretch.

If you go three months with no outbreaks, you can stop taking the infusion, Romm says. If you're still having outbreaks after trying this treatment, see your health-care practitioner, she suggests.

Make yourself a stress formula. "Think of herpes outbreaks as stress barometers," says Romm. "When your stress level spikes, you're most at risk. Making your own herbal antistress formula is a powerful healer because it affirms your intent to keep stress at bay."

She suggests concocting either a tea or tincture (also called an extract) blend using equal parts of vervain (to relax tension and stress),

"Herbal healing is what Native American elders call 'good medicine.' Using herbs connects women to the healing power of nature and reminds us that we, too, are healers. For women, there is tremendous power in reclaiming our health care. Using herbs allows us to do this. In connecting with and using our inner wisdom and intellectual abilities, we gain in confidence. And in connecting with the healing forces of nature, we grow wiser about the ways of women's bodies—so closely attuned with the cycles of the Earth, the moon, and the seasons."

—*Aviva Romm, herbalist, midwife, and teacher*

Siberian ginseng (to help the body adapt to stress), St.-John's-wort (which calms tension and anxiety, helps reduce pain, and has antiviral properties), and passionflower (to ease pain from viral infections and help insomnia).

If you prefer a tea, blend the dried herbs together and then follow the instructions for making an infusion in "Teas and Infusions" on page 89. During times of above-normal stress, sip a cup of tea three times a day.

If you use tinctures, blend equal parts in a bottle large enough to hold them all. Take ½ teaspoon three times a day.

Make an antiviral lotion. Blend equal parts of lavender essential oil, an antiseptic that's effective for dry and weepy skin problems, and oil infused with lemon balm, which has been shown in studies to act against the herpes virus (see "Infused Oils" on page 101 for directions). Then apply a few dabs of this antiviral lotion on the affected area three times a day during herpes outbreaks for up to a week, recommends Romm. You can also add a dash or two of this formula to your bathwater, she suggests.

Don't do the wild thing. If you have a cold sore around your mouth—or even the tingling sensation that signals its onset—forget about performing oral sex until the blister is gone. Otherwise, you could transfer genital herpes to your lover, even though your herpes was not of the genital variety. Likewise, if your partner has a cold sore, refrain from being on the receiving end of oral sex. It goes without saying that you should also nix kissing while either of you has active oral herpes, experts say.

Abstinence makes the heart grow fonder. Obviously, if you or your partner has active genital herpes, don't even think about having genital contact of any kind, even with a condom, until well after the outbreak has healed. Even then, experts recommend that you always use a latex male condom or a female condom with spermicide to guard against transmission. Using a condom *during* an outbreak is a bad idea because sores may occur in an area unprotected by the condom. (If you and your partner both have inactive herpes and want to have a baby, talk to your health-care practitioner about options for safe conception and delivery.)

Infertility

Hormone-Balancing Botanicals Offer Hope

his is my son, John."
"Say hello to Christopher."
"My baby's name is Ray."
Women often approach herbalist David Christopher and introduce their children to him. "They tell me that they believe herbs were the reason they were finally able to conceive a child," says Christopher, a professional member of the American Herbalists Guild (AHG) and director of the School of Natural Healing in Springville, Utah. "Some have even named their children for my late father,

John Raymond Christopher, N.D., who created a simple herbal fertility formula using lobelia and false unicorn root."

Whether they realized it or not, these women followed a healing tradition that is thousands of years old. Long before fertility drugs, ovulation tests, sperm analysis, infertility specialists, or clinics specializing in high-tech "assisted reproduction" techniques, women relied on plant remedies in hopes of reversing infertility—or simply to better their baby-making odds.

"The women's herbs we use most often, including fertility herbs, often come from old Chinese and Native American practices," says Cascade Anderson Geller, an herbal educator and consulting herbal practitioner in Portland, Oregon. "When settlers arrived in the New World, they were amazed at the health of Native American women and their children. Their remedies became our remedies."

Today, herbalists recommend botanicals that may boost reproductive health by improving overall health, restoring vitality, and balancing hormone levels. As part of a program that emphasizes good nutrition, exercise, and stress reduction, herbs may assist a woman's body in creating the conditions necessary for fertility: Well-timed ovulation, the secretion of slippery, sperm-friendly cervical mucus, and a womb that's ready to receive—and hold onto—a tiny embryo, says Margi Flint, a professional member of the AHG from Marblehead, Massachusetts, who teaches herbal approaches to health at Tufts University School of Medicine in Boston.

Nourish and Strengthen Natural Fertility

At best, a woman should begin "feeding" her reproductive system and boosting well-being with nutritive herbs months—or even years—before she starts trying to become pregnant, Flint says. "You want to be in wonderful health before becoming pregnant. But even if you're already trying to conceive, the place to start is with nourishing herbs and foods." Herbalists suggest beginning your quest for heightened fertility with these nurturing botanical strategies.

Sip a gently nourishing cuppa. Mix your own blend of nourishing, fertility-enhancing herbs as tea, then enjoy one to three cups a day, suggests Flint. "These herbs contain vitamins and minerals and have an affinity for the reproductive system," she says. "They are also safe, tonic herbs that enhance well-being—more like food than medicine. So you can drink them every day for months or even years." Flint suggests rotating the herbs in your formula.

Combine equal amounts of herbs of your choice from the list that follows and store them in a glass jar. Make your tea using at least 1 teaspoon of the herb blend per cup of boiling water; "you'll need more if the herbs are fresh and chunky," Flint says.

Red clover. "This is the single most useful herb for establishing fertility," notes Susun S. Weed, an herbalist and herbal educator from Woodstock, New York, and author of the *Wise Woman* series of herbal health books, including the *Wise Woman Herbal for the Childbearing Year.* "It contains just what you need: protein, lots of minerals, and even plant hormones." Research has found that red clover tops contain genistein, a weak estrogen, as well as a wide range of trace minerals.

Nettle. One of the best plant sources of iron, nettle leaves also contain calcium and vitamin A, notes herbalist Rosemary Gladstar, director of the Sage Mountain herbal education center in East Barre, Vermont, and author of *Herbal Healing for Women*. Scientific research confirms that this plant, which herbalists regard as a food and tonic for the hormonal system, is indeed mineral-rich.

Raspberry leaf. Revered for centuries as *the* uterine tonic, raspberry leaf provides the extra calcium, iron, and vitamins that you will need during pregnancy as well as a compound that firms and relaxes uterine and pelvic muscles.

Alfalfa. Herbalists say that the dried cloverlike leaves of this common farm-animal food plant offer superior nutrition as well as phytoestrogens that can help your body make the best use of its own natural estrogen. High in protein, alfalfa also contains vitamins A, C, E, and K (a vitamin essential for blood clotting) and several B vitamins, along with calcium, potassium, iron, and zinc.

Rose hips. "Rose hips contribute vitamin C," notes Flint. "They also impart a lovely, garnet red color and a tart taste to your tea." According to Cherokee lore, red is the color for success, she explains.

Add a vitamin-rich herbal supplement. Herbalists suggest that women planning to become pregnant should start taking plant-based vitamin and mineral supplements even before trying to conceive—and continue throughout pregnancy. (To find plant-based supplements conducive to fertility, look for companies offering a wide range of health food products in "Where to Buy Herbs and Herbal Products" on page 462.)

Gladstar recommends taking a fertility-boosting supplement, that is, one that's rich in vitamins and minerals, daily. Take according to package directions.

If you're 40-something, consider a digestive aid. An "older" prospective mom may need to boost her body's ability to absorb nutrients, Flint says. "The body slows down the production of enzymes as we age," she notes.

"Herbs, taken as bitters before meals, can help encourage digestion and the uptake of important nutrients." Try 5 to 10 drops of dandelion root tincture right before you eat, she suggests. You can also add bitter "gourmet" greens, such as dandelion leaves and arugula, to your salads, she says.

Used traditionally to stimulate appetite and digestion, dandelion has been shown by research to contain bitter compounds that stimulate the secretion of bile, which aids digestion.

Strengthen your uterus with lady's-mantle. "Look at the leaves of this herb, and you see outstretched hands, like the beauty of the pelvic floor that holds the seed of life," says Flint. "In the morning, you will see it holding the first pearly dew as if it were in an outstretched palm. Lady's-mantle has been used throughout time for women's issues. It gets its Latin name, *Alchemilla*, from the alchemists who gathered the dew from its leaves and put it in nearly every compound they made."

Although not heavily studied, lady's-mantle has a long tradition as a uterine helper for easing menstrual pain, curbing heavy menstrual flow, and strengthening uterine muscles. Take nine drops of lady's-mantle tincture a day for at least three months, Flint suggests. "Put the drops in a full water bottle, label it so no one else drinks it, and sip all day," she says.

A Menu of Hormone Balancers

If you haven't conceived after three to six months of using nutritive herbs, you may want to add herbs that balance hormones, Geller says. "Add a fertility herb to your daily nutritive formula or use a fertility formula consistently for six months," she suggests. "If you haven't gotten pregnant by then, switch to a different formula. When considering

A Fertility-Boosting Salad Dressing

Turn your next vinaigrette into a mineral-rich salad splash with medicinal herbal vinegars featuring fertility-enhancing botanicals such as red clover or partridgeberry, suggests Susun S. Weed, an herbalist and herbal educator from Woodstock, New York, and author of the Wise Woman series of herbal health books, including the Wise Woman Herbal for the Childbearing Year.

"Think of minerals as the building blocks you need for a well-functioning reproductive system and for a healthy baby. The minerals and other healing compounds from these fresh herbs can be transferred into the vinegar. I use one or more tablespoons every day," says Weed, who serves a variety of medicinal herbal vinegars at lunch during herbal education workshops at her Wise Woman Center. "Every tablespoon is as nourishing as a glass of milk."

Fresh red cover, nettle, alfalfa, partridgeberry, raspberry leaf, or any kind of mint
Apple-cider vinegar

Cut the herbs finely and place in a clean glass jar. Fill the jar, but do not pack the herbs. Add room-temperature vinegar (Weed recommends using an organic variety). You'll need 6 ounces of vinegar to fill an 8-ounce jar filled with herbs. Seal with a clean, tight-fitting lid. Let stand for a few weeks, then enjoy. You don't have to remove the herbs unless you want to.

which formula to choose, it's a good idea to consult an herbalist. She can help tailor one to meet your particular needs."

If your biological clock is ticking loudly, and you feel you only have a limited amount of time left in which to conceive, you may want to switch formulas after just three months, Geller says. "In any case, the most important thing is to use the formula every day, as directed," she says. "That way, you get the full benefit of the herbs."

Turbocharge your tea with hormone balancers. Give your nourishing fertility tea a boost by adding a traditional hormone balancer, herbalists suggest. Here are their top choices.

Chasteberry. Also called vitex, this herb is good for fertility because it can help make your menstrual cycle more regular and stabilize the lining of the uterus during the second half of the menstrual cycle—the time when a fertilized egg would implant in the uterine wall, notes Amanda McQuade Crawford, a practicing herbalist in Ojai, California, professional member of the American Herbalists Guild (AHG), member of Britain's National Institute of Medical Herbalists, president of the American College of Integrative Medicine in Albuquerque, and author of *Herbal Remedies for Women.*

"Chasteberry seems to work by stimulating part of the pituitary gland to secrete more luteinizing hormone, which in turn stimulates the corpus luteum—the ovarian follicle that releases the egg—to produce more progesterone," says McQuade Crawford. "Progesterone helps keep the blood-rich lining of the uterus in place."

McQuade Crawford advises women who want to improve fertility to take a teaspoon of chasteberry tincture twice a day. You can add a dose to 2 cups of your fertility blend or make chasteberry tea by adding 1 ounce of crushed, dried chasteberries to a pint of boiling water, mixing in at least 2 teaspoons of your fertility blend, and steeping for 15 minutes. She recommends two to four cups a day. Use chasteberry for a minimum of three months, McQuade Crawford suggests.

False unicorn root. Considered *the* herbal antidote for infertility by many herbalists, this herb has yet to be researched scientifically. False unicorn root, which was included in many traditional fertility formulas, is believed to contain compounds called steroidal saponins that herbalists suspect may be responsible for its normalizing effect on female hormones. Use 5 to 15 drops of the tincture or take up to ½ cup of an infusion daily, sipped slowly throughout the day. Herbalists suggest using false unicorn root in fertility formulas for at least three to six months.

Herbalists say that wild false unicorn root is becoming rare and endangered in nature. Help protect this wild plant by buying products that use the cultivated herb. You can find these products in health food stores.

Sample a simple formula. Christopher's top choice among fertility formulas is his father's creation, a mix of three parts false unicorn root and one part lobelia. "You can make this up as a tea or as a tincture or grind the herbs finely and pack them into capsules," he suggests. "Women *and* men should take this three times a day. Take it as long as you need it—that could be six months or six years." For each of your three daily doses, have a cup of tea made with 1 teaspoon of the herb mix per cup of boiling water, 10 to 15 drops of tincture, or two capsules.

While lobelia is not a fertility herb, Christopher says that the small amount in this formula seems to act as a catalyst, enhancing the hormonal action of the false unicorn root. Do not increase the lobelia portion of the recipe; Christopher says larger amounts of lobelia can cause vomiting. You can also purchase the formula by mail.

Make a traditional mother's cordial. A formula popularized by the Eclectics, physicians of the nineteenth and early twentieth centuries who combined herbs with conventional medical treatments, mother's cordial actually has its roots in Native American herbal healing, Geller says. "The white folks who settled in North America were pretty astounded by the good-quality babies and good-quality mommies here on this land when they arrived," she notes. "If you go back and read old medical books, there was very big interest in what Native American women were taking to do so well. This formula contains some of those herbs."

Make this cordial as a tea by combining 1 ounce each of dried partridgeberry, false unicorn root, cramp bark, and blue cohosh. Add 1 tablespoon to 1 cup of water and simmer over low heat for about 15 minutes. Drink one cup a day, Geller suggests.

Yet to be heavily studied by researchers, partridgeberry is reported to contain saponins that herbalists believe are responsible for the herb's hormone-balancing effects. It has a long history of use among women preparing for pregnancy. Research has shown that cramp bark contains antispasmodic substances that herbalists believe make it effective in preventing miscarriage.

Try Cascade's fertility formula. Research shows that dang gui increases blood

False Unicorn Root: America's Native Fertility Reviver

*T*hanks to its gnawed-looking roots and its well-regarded use as a reproductive-system tonic, false unicorn root stars in a dramatic folk tale: Legend has it that this herb's beneficial powers so enraged the Devil that he tried to kill off the entire species by biting the roots of every single plant. He failed—false unicorn comes to life each spring with beautiful, star-shaped flowers—but one of this herb's folk names is Devil's bite.

For centuries, this botanical has found its way into fertility formulas for women and men, and it has been a women's remedy for everything from miscarriage to morning sickness to uterine prolapse. Barely studied by science, it contains a compound called chamaelirin, a steroidal saponin that may be responsible for its action in the body, according to herbalist Rosemary Gladstar, director of the Sage Mountain herbal education center in East Barre, Vermont, and author of *Herbal Healing for Women*.

"False unicorn root can help correct infertility," notes Susun S. Weed, an herbalist and herbal educator from Woodstock, New York, and author of the *Wise Woman* series of herbal health books, including the *Wise Woman Herbal for the Childbearing Year*.

While herbalists say that this plant can be taken safely for long periods of time, they also suggest that daily doses should be small: 5 to 15 drops of tincture or ½ cup of an infusion, sipped slowly. If mixed with other herbs in a tea blend, limit yourself to no more than three to four cups of false unicorn root tea per day. Larger doses may cause nausea and vomiting.

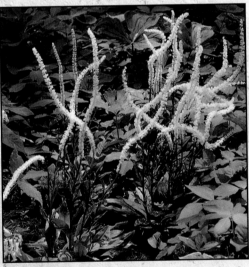

This well-regarded herb is becoming rare in the wild. Herbalists suggest protecting remaining wild false unicorn communities by purchasing products that use the cultivated herb.

flow to the uterus. It is used in Traditional Chinese Medicine to normalize painful, difficult, or abnormal menstrual flow. Both ginseng and he-shou-wu (also known as fo-ti) have long histories of traditional use as promoters of vitality and fertility. Dandelion leaf and root are shown to be digestive aids. Wild yam may have a mild hormonal action in the body, and it also helps improve digestion. Combined, these herbs are good for building the vitality and functioning of the reproductive system and the whole body, especially if a woman feels depleted, says Geller.

"I used it while I was trying to conceive," she says. "At the time, I had been traveling back and forth between the West and East coasts about a dozen times in six months. I was tired. I got pregnant two weeks after I started using it."

Combine one part each of tinctures of dang gui, ginseng, he-shou-wu, and a combined extract of dandelion leaf and root with two parts each of partridgeberry and wild yam tinctures. Mix well. Take 30 drops twice daily, before meals. Discontinue during your menstrual period. Repeat for up to four months, and discontinue if pregnancy occurs. If you are experiencing diarrhea, be aware that he-shou-wu may occasionally cause gastric distress.

Herbs, or the Fertility Clinic?

Herbalists are quick to note that if you're having a difficult time getting pregnant and are concerned, both you and your partner may want to consult a doctor who can help discover the reasons why.

Among the most common causes of infertility are stress, endometriosis, and uterine fibroids; scarring of the fallopian tubes, ovaries, or uterus by sexually transmitted infections like chlamydia or gonorrhea; cigarette smoking; caffeine; extremely low body fat; use of marijuana and other illicit drugs; and advancing age. Among four in ten couples experiencing infertility, the woman's reproductive system is not functioning optimally. For another four in ten couples, the problem is

low sperm production or poor sperm function in the man. For the remaining two couples in ten, the reasons are never known.

When are herbs the right choice for overcoming infertility? "Botanical remedies seem to work best for unexplained infertility," Geller says. "Over time, herbal treatments can help balance hormones and build up depleted body systems. They can also help with endometriosis, fibroids, and irregular menstrual cycles. But herbal remedies seem to be less helpful where there are adhesions (when tissues join or adhere abnormally) or scarring in the reproductive organs."

Women find many ways to use herbal fertility enhancers, according to top female herbalists. For some, botanical therapies are a last resort. For others, they are a first stop. Still others practice a kind of complementary medicine, sipping gentle, nourishing teas daily while undergoing high-tech infertility treatments. Herbalists caution, however, that you should not combine treatments on your own. Tell your doctor and herbalist what you are using.

Women often go to herbalists when they've tried everything else. "They've been through the emotional and physical ordeal of medical infertility treatment, and they're frustrated. They feel invaded. Herbs can help build and cleanse in a way that invasive surgeries and pharmaceutical drugs cannot," says Geller.

There are few studies measuring the effectiveness of herbal infertility treatments. German research has found that pregnancy seemed to be among the beneficial effects for women who took chasteberry. In fact, chasteberry is used by German gynecologists to resolve some forms of infertility. "But there are no studies on the success rate of herbal fertility formulas using several herbs, which is what we use most in America," Geller says, "so it's very difficult to know how many preg-

Herbal Contraceptives: Not Yet Ready for Prime Time?

Women looking for a means of natural birth control may be tempted to try wild carrot seeds. The small, oblong, tan seeds, culled from that common and lovely weed called Queen Anne's lace, are sometimes sold as herbal contraceptives.

But do they work? And how well?

"It's clear from research and tradition that women have used many herbs as anti-fertility drugs for thousands of years," says Adriane Fugh-Berman, M.D., medical officer for the contraception and reproductive health branch of the National Institute of Child Health and Human Development at the National Institutes of Health. "With wild carrot seeds, there's reason to think that they have some mild hormonal activity that might prevent conception. And there are plenty of stories of women who have used it after intercourse and haven't gotten pregnant. But without decent studies with human beings of how much to use, how to use it, and how well it works, I wouldn't trust it, or any other herb, if I really wanted to avoid pregnancy."

From ancient Egypt to the modern-day Appalachian Mountains of North Carolina come intriguing stories of herbal birth control involving plants as diverse as pomegranate, juniper, and cypress, among many others, says medical historian John M. Riddle, Ph.D., chairman of the history department at North Carolina State University in Raleigh, author of *Eve's Herbs* and *Contraception and Abortion from the Ancient World to the Renaissance*, and an expert on the historical use of anti-fertility herbs. "It's clear that women knew how to use these plants, and in some places, they still do. But the knowledge was discredited and lost to the Western world. We don't know enough about how women used these herbs to suggest that people use them today. We need good studies."

Even with word-of-mouth instructions for their use, herbal contraceptives are most likely not completely reliable, Dr. Fugh-Berman notes, because the levels of active chemical constituents in plants can vary significantly depending on growing and harvesting conditions. "They're risky. Even in the past, women could not completely control their fertility," she notes.

nancies can be attributed to herbs. Personally, I know a dozen couples who used one of my formulas regularly and conceived, and another 4 or 5 who gave it a good try and did not succeed. In those cases, there were serious problems like adhesions. Another 30 or 40 couples used the formula for a while and then quit. They got pregnant later on, but the role of the herbs is questionable."

Before You Build a Baby . . .

If you have a history of erratic menstrual cycles, painful periods (both possible signs of hormone imbalance), or a potential conception stopper like endometriosis, early herbal intervention may enhance your chances for pregnancy success later, Geller says. (For more information about herbal remedies for these specific conditions, see "Endometriosis" on page 225 and "Menstrual Problems" on page 296.)

Otherwise, herbalists suggest a gradual approach to enhancing fertility or reversing infertility. Begin with nourishing, vitamin- and mineral-rich herbs to boost vitality and help your reproductive system work optimally. Add hormone-balancing herbs and fertility formulas later, if there's evidence that your body needs more assistance.

"If you are in good health and have regular periods that seem normal, don't use fertility herbs right away," Geller notes. "Eat a healthy diet. Drink plenty of water. Get rest and moderate exercise. Relax and have fun. Trust your body. You may be pleasantly surprised to find that you can get pregnant fairly easily."

Top women herbalists suggest following these ground rules when using herbs to enhance fertility or overcome infertility.

Share with your man. Remember, it takes two to make a baby. "It's a misnomer to say that fertility herbs are female herbs. They're reproductive tonics for both sexes," notes Geller. "If a couple has unexplained infertility and the man's sperm count is fine, then herbal formulas can build vitality for both partners and may help lead to conception."

Finally pregnant? It's time to stop herbal treatments. Once you know, or even suspect, that you're pregnant, its best to stop using all herbs except those considered safe during the first trimester of pregnancy, says Aviva Romm, a certified professional midwife, herbalist, and professional member of the AHG who practices in Bloomfield Hills, Michigan, and is the author of *The Natural Pregnancy Book* and *Natural Healing for Babies and Children*. "I recommend using herbs very cautiously in the first three months of pregnancy," she notes. "The fetus is very delicate then." (For more information about safe herbs in pregnancy, see "Pregnancy" on page 325.)

Insect Bites and Stings

RELIEVE THE ITCH WITH PEPPERMINT AND MORE

Mosquitoes gotta munch. Wasps gotta sting. To a bug, biting and stinging are just basic survival skills. But when six- and eight-legged denizens of the creepy-crawly world descend on human prey, the results are unpleasant. Fiery pain. An unrelenting itch. Swelling. And sometimes infection.

Some bugs—including mosquitoes, fleas, and biting flies such as black flies, deer flies, and tiny biting midges known as no-see-ums—want to suck your blood. You may or may not feel the bite, but you can't ignore the itching later on. Other insects—most commonly yellowjackets and other types of wasps, velvet ants, and sometimes honey bees—jab you with stingers in self-defense. Only the females sting, prompting immediate, piercing pain followed by swelling and redness.

Fast Action with Herbs

First, some ground rules: Always remove a honey bee's stinger immediately so more venom won't be pumped into your skin. Scrape or pull out the stinger as fast as possible. If you have trouble breathing after a sting or develop hives along your arms, legs, or body, call your local emergency medical number or go to the nearest hospital immediately. And if, after a day or two, a bite or sting appears to be infected, with oozing, yellow crusting on top, a rapid increase in swelling, or onset of pain or fever, go to your doctor immediately. Otherwise, try these simple herbal soothers—as near as your kitchen or even your backyard.

Cool the itch and squelch swelling with mint. A tiny droplet of peppermint essential oil rubbed into the bull's-eye center of a bite or sting can bring quick, long-lasting relief, says Sharol Tilgner, N.D., a naturopathic physician, professional member of the American Herbalists Guild (AHG), and president of Wise Woman Herbals in Eugene, Oregon.

"Peppermint makes the area feel cool, so you don't feel itching," Dr. Tilgner says. "At the same time, it increases blood flow to the area, which helps to quickly carry off the little bit of venom the insect has deposited under the skin surface as well as the chemicals your body has produced in reaction to the venom. That means less swelling and less itching."

Peppermint oil has been used traditionally as an antiseptic and local anesthetic. Remember to wash your hands after applying it, Dr. Tilgner says, and don't use essential oils near your eyes, as they can be irritating. Mosquito and flea bites as well as bee and wasp stings all benefit from a little mint oil, she says, but don't use this remedy on large, serious bites such as those from a venomous spider or a snake, Dr. Tilgner adds. "In that case, you don't want to increase blood flow or circulate large amounts of venom more quickly through your body," she notes. If you are bitten by a poisonous spider or snake, get medical attention immediately.

In a pinch, pick plantain or chickweed. Plantain, the first choice of many herbalists for easing bee stings, is a traditional remedy for pain and swelling of the skin, and chickweed has a traditional reputation for easing itching and healing skin troubles (see "Backyard Medicine: A Field Guide" on page 193 for more on these herbs). So if you're bitten or stung when puttering in your backyard or hiking a backwoods trail, take advantage of "field medicine" by making an instant poultice of plantain or chickweed leaves, Dr. Tilgner suggests. "Just chew the leaves well or rub them together in your hands until they're juicy, then stick the wet leaves on the bite or sting," she says. Keep the leaves on for a minimum of 15 to 30 minutes or until they are dry, she adds. "These remedies have been used for hundreds of years, and I find that they work well."

Silence the sting with garlic. Around the globe, a popular medicinal use for "stinking rose" is treating bites and stings, says Paul Bergner, clinic director of the Rocky Mountain Center for Botanical Studies in Boulder, Colorado, editor of *Med-*

Herbal Bug Repellents

Deep in the Amazon rain forest, on a riverbank teeming with insects, herbalist Steven Foster once tried a field test that illustrates the power—and limits—of herbal bug repellents. "Someone had hung a sweat-soaked hat on a tree, and it was covered with big brown flies," he says. "We put a mixture of citronella and pennyroyal oil, among other oils, on a portion of the hat, and the flies stayed away from that section but still covered the rest."

Pungent essential oils *can* deter biting, stinging bugs, says Foster, a medicinal plant specialist from Fayetteville, Arkansas, and author of *Herbs for Your Health* and *Forest Pharmacy*.

Citronella oil, a top bug deterrent, has demonstrated anti-mosquito powers when applied to the skin and, in a study in an Ontario forest by researchers from the University of Guelph in Canada, when burned in bug-repellent candles. An often-used bug stopper, pennyroyal oil repels ants and has the power to kill some insects due to its main chemical compound, pulegone, says Foster.

Herbal repellents aren't perfect, notes Foster. Essential oils dissipate quickly in the air and must be reapplied as often as every half-hour, he says. And like most chemical anti-insect formulas, botanical bug stoppers may not be effective in extremely bug-infested places, herbalists say.

The best way to use them? As a tick repellent, try rubbing a few drops of pennyroyal essential oil (available at health food stores) on your shoe tops, socks, and the cuffs of your pants, Foster suggests. Ward off mosquitoes and ticks by dabbing citronella essential oil (also available at health food stores) on your clothing. You may want to reapply it after about a half-hour. "These will not leave oily marks on your clothes—they should dissipate," he says. You may want to test them on an inconspicuous place to make sure. "But do not use these pure essential oils directly on your skin. They can be irritating," adds Foster.

Or mix up this woodsy-smelling insect repellent spray formula, suggests Sharol Tilgner, N.D., a naturopathic physician, professional member of the American Herbalists Guild, and president of Wise Woman Herbals in Eugene, Oregon. Combine ½ cup of 70 percent isopropyl alcohol (available at drugstores) and ½ cup of water. To this mixture, add ¼ to ¾ teaspoon each of cit-

ical Herbalism, and author of *The Healing Power of Garlic* and *The Healing Power of Echinacea, Goldenseal, and Other Immune System Herbs*.

Try this traditional, quick kitchen cure for insect bites and stings, widely used in India and Arabic countries: Chew or crush a clove of garlic and dab it on the affected spot. Cover with a bandage or tape for up to 20 minutes, then wash, says Bergner. Remove it sooner if you see signs of irritation. You could dilute the garlic's strength by putting a little saliva on the bite just before applying the garlic, suggests Bergner.

ronella, pennyroyal, lavender, and rose geranium essential oils and pour it into a spray bottle. To use, shake well, then spray lightly on your clothing. Keep the spray away from your eyes, other mucous membranes, and open cuts. You may want to test the spray on an inconspicuous place on your clothing to make sure it doesn't stain. "The alcohol keeps the essential oils diluted," explains Dr. Tilgner. "This formula not only keeps bugs away, but it smells good, too." Reapply the spray when the oil evaporates or about once every hour, she adds. You can store the mixture for about two years if it's tightly capped.

Dr. Tilgner cautions that this formula should not be used on skin on a daily basis. "If you apply too much, too often, essential oils can have an effect on the skin and the nervous system," she says. "This is fine for a hike or a day out working in the yard, but don't use it more than once a week."

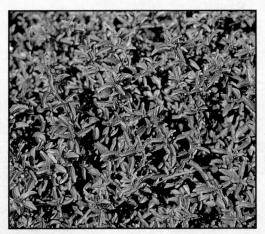 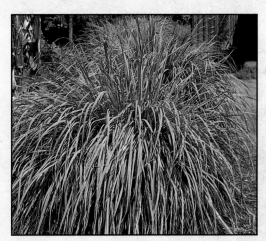

Before the invention of chemical insect repellents, outdoor enthusiasts relied on oils of pennyroyal (left) and citronella to keep bugs at bay.

Herbalists theorize that garlic's sting-easing action may come from enzymes that break down prostaglandins, the natural chemicals that your body releases in response to pain.

Rub out chiggers with menthol and camphor. Intensely itchy red welts can be a sign that tiny chiggers, the larvae of harvest mites, have attached themselves to your skin and are sipping fluid nourishment from your body. Nix them by showering, then rubbing on a salve containing essential oils of camphor and menthol such as Tiger Balm, suggests Steven Foster, a medicinal plant specialist from Fayetteville, Arkansas, and author of *Herbs for*

Your Health and Forest Pharmacy. "I know from personal experience that this works. Camphor and menthol are so strong that insects can't deal with them," Foster says. "It kills them."

For inflammation, add echinacea. When a bite won't heal or remains swollen and inflamed, an echinacea poultice can ease the inflammation, Dr. Tilgner says. If the bite appears infected or the inflammation increases, see your doctor.

For a small bite, combine a teaspoon each of echinacea tincture (also called an extract) and water, then mix in enough bentonite clay to make a thick paste. For a larger bite, try doubling the recipe. Dab the mixture on the bite and cover it with an adhesive strip bandage or gauze taped down with adhesive tape. Change it twice a day. You can use green facial clay instead of bentonite; look for these clays at health food stores.

At the same time, Dr. Tilgner suggests taking echinacea tincture internally. Try 60 drops of tincture in $\frac{1}{4}$ cup of warm water three times a day for up to two weeks.

In one large-scale German study, echinacea healed a variety of skin problems when used topically; it seems to work by regenerating tissue, reducing inflammation, and promoting more immune system activity at the site of the problem.

Use osha tincture. Osha tincture helps reduce inflammation, too, says 7Song, a professional member of the AHG and director of the Northeast School of Botanical Medicine in Ithaca, New York. Valued by Native Americans living in the Rocky Mountains as a potent antibacterial herb, osha is used extensively as an internal and external treatment by herbalists in that region today. "I use one to five dropperfuls of osha tincture (taken internally) an hour if infection is setting in," says 7Song. "I've found it to be very effective when insect bites are becoming swollen and reactive. I always start with one drop (not a dropperful) on the tongue to see how the person reacts to a tincture. I also use osha on bee stings and spider bites in a poultice made with a little clay and moistened with chaparral and osha tincture." If the infection does not show signs of improvement within a week, see your doctor.

Insomnia

REST EASY WITH HERBS

Nothing is worse than lying awake all night—except, of course, trying to get out of bed the next morning. Either way, most of us can relate. At some point, at least half of all Americans suffer from insomnia, a catch-all term for the inability to fall or stay asleep.

One night of poor sleep can be triggered by drinking alcohol or caffeinated beverages at night, exercising close to bedtime, or doing mentally challenging work before going to bed. Stretches of insomnia lasting up to three weeks or so are usually caused by stress. Insomnia that lasts a month or more may signal an underlying physical or emotional problem and may not clear up without advice from a doctor.

In women, drops in production of the female hormone estrogen that occur premenstrually or during menopause can contribute to insomnia. The National Sleep Foundation estimates that 40 percent or more of women have trouble sleeping, compared to 30 percent of men.

Prescription sleeping pills and over-the-counter sleep aids can do more harm than good. While they put you to sleep, they can also cause a "hangover" effect the next morning, say experts. If these products are used for long-term insomnia—that is, more than three weeks or so—there's also the risk of becoming dependent on or addicted to them.

The Herbal Alternative

Herbs used for their sedative effects do not have these drawbacks, says Aviva Romm, a certified professional midwife, herbalist, and professional member of the American Herbalists Guild (AHG) who practices in Bloomfield Hills, Michigan, and is author of *The Natural Pregnancy Book* and *Natural Healing for Babies and Children*. Most have been used for thousands of years to induce sleep, and they can help treat occasional sleeplessness gently, safely, and effectively.

Many of the herbs used as sleep aids, such as chamomile and lemon balm, have traditionally been consumed in the form of teas. That can be a good thing, as many women find the pre-bedtime ritual of measuring out the right amount of fragrant herbs, allowing the tea to steep, and inhaling the steam rising from a pretty cup a much-needed respite from the demands of the day, says Romm.

Along with herbal treatments for insomnia, herbalists recommend reworking your lifestyle in ways that promote sound, healthy sleep. Get out and exercise a few days a week—or every day, if possible. (If you don't exercise regularly, check with a physician before starting any new fitness regimen.) And learn some type of stress-management technique, such as meditation or progressive relaxation. Taking herbs that promote relaxation during the day can also help, says Romm. (For more information on relaxing herbs, see "Stress" on page 451.)

Good-Night Herbs

The following herbs can help remedy the occasional night of sleeplessness, according to herbalists. If you find yourself tossing and turning for more than a week, no matter what you've tried, consult your doctor.

Turn to valerian. One of the most widely used natural sleep aids in the world, "valerian is a safe and effective natural alternative to the harsh and potentially toxic synthetic sedatives that people take," says Christopher Hobbs, a professional member of the AHG from Santa Cruz, California, and author of *Valerian: The Relaxing and Sleep Herb*.

The herb's active ingredients include a group of compounds called valepotriates. Research indicates that components in valerian attach to the same brain receptors as tranquilizers like diazepam (Valium), but without causing dependency.

Health food stores sell valerian in several

Ten Tickets to Dreamland

Sometimes, it takes more than herbs to prime your brain for sleep. To increase the likelihood of getting a good night's rest, follow these tips from the National Sleep Foundation.

1. Go to bed and get up at the same time every day, regardless of when you went to sleep.
2. Steer clear of caffeine—in coffee, tea, and soft drinks—for at least six hours before bedtime.
3. Shun alcoholic beverages for at least two hours before bed.
4. If you smoke, don't light up two hours or less before going to bed.
5. Exercise every day, but not too close to bedtime.
6. Don't nap during the day.
7. Develop a nightly routine that enables you to wind down from the day's activity.
8. Keep your bedroom as dark and quiet as possible.
9. Don't use your bedroom for anything other than sleeping and making love. No working, reading, or watching television.
10. If you're not asleep 30 minutes after going to bed, get up and do something relaxing (or boring).

forms, including teas, tablets, and tinctures (also called extracts). Alas, however, valerian is not one of the better-tasting herbs, and it has the aroma of smelly feet. Most people prefer taking the tincture or tablets instead of tea. Hobbs recommends taking one to two dropperfuls (½ to 1 teaspoon) of the tincture in a little water or one or two capsules 30 minutes before bed.

Lighten up with lavender. Research shows that the volatile oil of this fragrant flower has a mild sedative effect. In a small preliminary study conducted in England, researchers found that lavender oil introduced into the air with a diffuser worked as well as prescription medication for people with insomnia. The study participants also appeared to sleep more restfully. Try rubbing lavender oil into your temples, suggests Penelope Ody,

a member of Britain's National Institute of Medical Herbalists and author of *The Complete Medicinal Herbal*, but be careful to avoid contact with your eyes.

Lick insomnia with lemon balm. Commission E, the expert panel that judges the safety and effectiveness of herbal medicines for the German government, has endorsed this fragrant herb as a treatment for sleep disturbances. To make lemon balm tea, place 1 to 3 teaspoons of the dried herb in boiling water. Cover, steep for 10 minutes, and strain. Drink one cup 30 minutes before bedtime, says Ellen Hopman, a professional member of the AHG who practices in Amherst, Massachusetts.

Nod off with chamomile. Chamomile, which Germans call *alles zutraut*, or "capable of anything," has been used to treat insomnia

Sweet-Dream Pillows

People have used dream pillows—small pillows stuffed with various fragrant herbs—to promote sound sleep and peaceful dreams for more than a century, says Susun S. Weed, an herbalist and herbal educator from Woodstock, New York, and author of the *Wise Woman* series of herbal health books.

What herbs should you use? Anything with a strong scent. Here are some of Weed's dream pillow suggestions that use various dried herbs. From each group, pick only one or two; do not use them all.

For insomnia: Flowers of hops, goldenrod, wild oregano, dill, catnip, or hawthorn.

For more vivid dreams: Flowers and leaves of mugwort (which Weed and some other herbalists call cronewort), mint, lavender, or lemon balm.

For peaceful dreams: Leaves of sassafras, sage, mullein, or potentilla (also called common cinquefoil); balsam needles (Weed recommends collecting needles of

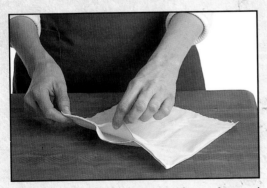

1. Cut and stitch. Cut two pieces of natural fabric, such as cotton, into the shape you want. Sew up three sides, leaving the last side open to receive the herbs.

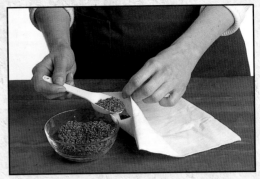

2. Add stuffing. Turn the fabric right side out so the stitching is inside. Then spoon in or stuff in the herb of your choice and stitch the opening closed. Place the dream pillow in a pillowcase on top of or under your regular pillow.

balsam or any other kind of evergreen outdoors if you are certain the tree has not been sprayed with chemicals); or chamomile flowers.

To remember your dreams: Flowers of lavender, rosemary, mugwort, catnip, bay, or heliotrope (which can be purchased from garden supply stores, grown, and dried.)

To banish nightmares: Leaves of rosemary, valerian, lemon balm, or anise.

To relieve headaches: Leaves of marjoram, mint, betony, or bay; flowers of bee balm (which can be purchased in garden supply stores, grown, and dried), roses, lavender; or nutmeg or cloves.

To dream of love: Flowers of yarrow or roses; leaves of dill, myrtle, coriander, or basil.

To ease heartache: Any evergreen needles, especially balsam or pine (the needles must be gathered); lavender flowers; or lemon balm leaves.

since antiquity. Most folks use chamomile as a tea. Pour 1 cup of boiling water over 1 tablespoon of dried chamomile, steep for 10 minutes, and strain. Drink one cup before bed, says Hopman.

Do as the Italians do. "When I was a student in Italy, I learned a remedy for insomnia from the peasants," says Hopman. "Simmer equal parts of fresh mint leaves, fresh lemon rind, and fresh chamomile flowers in some water for five minutes." Be sure to use organic lemons, she adds, because you are boiling the rinds. Add a bit of honey if you wish. Strain, cool, and drink one cup 30 minutes before bedtime.

Sip "insomniac tea." This sleep-inducing tea is brewed from chamomile, skullcap, oatstraw, and catnip—all herbs traditionally used for insomnia, says Hopman. Skullcap is a relaxing herb that's also used to relieve premenstrual tension. Oatstraw "is a fabulous remedy for insomnia," says Romm. And catnip contains nepetalactone, a mild sedative.

To make the tea, blend equal parts of all four herbs, fresh or dried. Boil 1 cup of water in a nonaluminum pot and pour over 2 teaspoons of the herb mixture. Cover tightly with a lid and steep for 20 minutes. Strain the herbs from the tea, then drink one cup 30 minutes before bed.

Mix up a bedtime tincture. Blend 1 ounce (or equal portions) each of tinctures of passionflower, hops, skullcap, wood betony, and catnip, suggests Hopman. Take 20 drops in a small amount of water two hours before bedtime and again right before you retire.

Passionflower, which has been used to capture sleep since the days of the Inca and Aztec Indians, contains harman, an alkaloid reported in laboratory studies to have tranquilizing effects. Hops is a folk remedy for insomnia; in fact, people in some European countries stuff their bed pillows with it to induce sleep. Wood betony is considered by herbalists to be a relaxant and nervous system tonic.

Jet Lag

RELIEF FOR TIME-ZONE JUMPERS

*I*magine flying to a meeting across the country, only to show up too fuzzy and foggy to conduct business. Or how about arriving in Paris too sleepy to stroll along the Seine.

Whether you are traveling for business or pleasure, jet lag can leave you feeling out of sorts both physically and mentally. When you fly across several time zones, it takes a while for your internal body clock to reset itself to the day/night cycle in your new locale. As a result, you can feel exhausted and irritable, your head may ache, and your digestion may be distressed.

Remedies from Those Who Know

Since herbalists are a pretty intrepid group, jetting off to conferences and botanical adventures all over the world, it stands to reason that they'd come up with some pretty effective jet-lag remedies. Here are some of their best.

Concoct Cascade's jet-lag elixir. Cascade Anderson Geller, an herbal educator and consulting herbal practitioner from Portland, Oregon, recommends a formula using Siberian ginseng, Korean ginseng, hawthorn flower, and gotu kola. These herbs are adaptogens, she explains, which means that they help your body cope with changing conditions. Specifically, Siberian ginseng protects the body and nervous system from stress, Korean ginseng eases depression caused by exhaustion, hawthorn flower is good for jet lag and times of poor circulation, and gotu kola is a tonic for the nervous system.

"This formula is great for jet lag because it helps the body adapt to changes in time, sleep patterns, and even elevation," says Geller. "It's also helpful for people on swing shifts and new moms who are sleep-deprived."

To make this formula, buy one-ounce bottles of Siberian ginseng, Korean ginseng, hawthorn flower, and gotu kola tinctures (also called extracts). Using a small funnel, pour the tinctures into a four-ounce bottle and shake well. Two or three days before you

fly, says Geller, use a clean dropper to add one dropperful of the blended tincture to $\frac{1}{4}$ cup of water. Take two to three dropperfuls of the diluted tincture a day. For your flight, fill a water bottle with a pint of water combined with one to two tablespoons of blended tincture and take it with you on the plane to sip throughout the flight. After you land, take two to three dropperfuls of tincture (each diluted in $\frac{1}{4}$ cup of water) a day for two or three days.

Sleep well with aromatherapy. Jane Buckle, R.N., an aromatherapist in Hunter, New York, and author of *Clinical Aromatherapy in Nursing*, jets back and forth between her homes in England and America. She uses this formula to sleep peacefully upon arrival.

On a tissue, dab a drop each of the essential oils of ylang ylang (used for depression and nervous tension), lavender (which eases insomnia), and frankincense (believed to soothe the spirit). "Pop the tissue under your pillow and get your Zzzs," advises Buckle. "If traveling disrupts your menstrual cycle or makes PMS worse, add a drop of rose geranium to the formula," she suggests. This herb helps to normalize hormones, and aromatherapists use it to treat PMS and menopause problems.

Inhale yourself awake. If you need to be at your best upon arrival in a new time zone, Buckle suggests an energizing blend of essential oils of rosemary (a nervous system stimulant), basil (which overcomes mental fatigue), eucalyptus (an energy enhancer), and peppermint (which counters mental fogginess).

Dab a drop each of the oils on a handkerchief, advises Buckle, and "breathe in every time your eyelids start to close."

Low Immunity

Sure, we all *get* sick. But who has time to *be* sick? If you're like a lot of women, there's a good chance that the last time you took to bed for more than a day was when you gave birth. Come hell or high fevers, more often than not, we try to tough it out. We throw off our covers to tackle another "to do" list, whittle away at another deadline, or troubleshoot another problem.

The reality is that while we're busy taking care of the world, our diets suffer. We don't get enough sleep. We worry, weep, and pick at our cuticles. Like it or not, we stress out. This kind of chronic stress can ravage the immune system.

Normally, the immune system functions as a sort of home security system. It silently patrols your body, ever alert to intruders such as viruses, bacteria, and other microorganisms that threaten your health. When the immune system detects these invaders, it sounds the alarm and, figuratively speaking, calls the cops—infection-fighting white blood cells that identify and liquidate microbial marauders. But like a high-tech burglar, stress deactivates the immune system, allowing these microbes to breach its defenses. The end result is a weakened immune system.

Adapting to Chaos

Enter the adaptogens, herbs that are thought to guard the immune system from the effects of chronic stress. The stress might be physical, such as a poor diet or fatigue, or emotional, such as workplace worries, relationship tension, or a family problem.

"Adaptogen herbs balance and nourish the immune system," says Betzy Bancroft, a professional member of the American Herbalists Guild (AHG) and manager of Herbalist and Alchemist, an herbal medicine company in Washington, New Jersey.

Adaptogens have a long history of use in world medicine. The Chinese and Japanese, for example, have recognized the medicinal value of garlic, astragalus, and certain mushrooms for thousands of years. Siberian ginseng has been used in the Far East for millennia and has been studied extensively for 50 years.

According to herbalists, adaptogens also strengthen the body's endocrine and nervous systems, both of which exert a powerful influence on the immune system. To take one example, adaptogens fuel the adrenal glands, two small glands that sit on the top of the kidneys and release the stress hormones epinephrine, norepinephrine, and cortisol into the bloodstream. These hormones rise and plummet during times of chronic stress, revving up the heart, brain, and other organs in the process, and may reduce immune function.

Adaptogens help keep these hormone fluctuations on a more even keel, explains Bancroft. Of course, these herbs work best in a well-rested, well-nourished body. "You can't hang out in smoky bars, sleep three hours a night, and live on cupcakes and expect herbs to keep you healthy," says Chanchal Cabrera,

Super Soup for Super Immunity

Brimming with garlic, astragalus, and shiitake mushrooms, this tonic soup can help keep your immune system in peak condition, says Sharleen Andrews-Miller, faculty member at the National College of Naturopathic Medicine in Portland, Oregon, and associate medicinary director at the college's public clinic. If possible, buy organically grown vegetables. Otherwise, scrub the veggies well to remove chemicals and pesticides, she advises.

- **1–2** tablespoons toasted sesame oil or organically grown olive oil
- **1** large onion, chopped
- **1½** cups chopped celery (include inner stalks and leaves)
- **6–7** large cloves garlic, chopped
- **1** piece gingerroot, 1" long, peeled and chopped
- **5–7½** quarts filtered water or broth
- **6** carrots, chopped
- **1** parsnip, chopped
- **1** turnip, chopped
- **1** medium burdock root, sliced
- **3** medium red potatoes, cubed
- **2** sticks dried astragalus root
- **1** cup fresh shiitake mushrooms, sliced
- **¾** cup fresh parsley, chopped, or ¼ cup dried parsley
- **½** cup fresh herbs, chopped, such as basil, sage, thyme, marjoram, oregano, and rosemary, or 3–4 tablespoons dried herbs
- **3** tablespoons low-sodium soy sauce
- **½** cup barley
- **½** cup lentils or dried peas (optional)
- **½** teaspoon turmeric
- **½** teaspoon paprika
- **1** tablespoon balsamic vinegar
- Finely chopped hot peppers or cayenne pepper
- Salt and pepper
- **½** cup chopped sweet red peppers
- **1** medium zucchini, chopped
- **1** cup spinach, cabbage, kale, or collard greens, chopped
- Freshly ground black pepper or crushed red pepper

In a large stockpot, sauté the onion, celery, garlic, and ginger in the oil until the onion turns translucent. Add the water or broth, carrots, parsnip, turnip, burdock, potatoes, astragalus, mushrooms, parsley, herbs, soy sauce, barley, and lentils or peas (if using). Simmer on low to medium heat for 1 to 2 hours, or until the root vegetables start to become tender. Stir in the turmeric, paprika, and vinegar. Add hot peppers or cayenne and salt and pepper to taste. Add the red peppers, zucchini, and greens. Simmer for another 30 to 60 minutes. Remove the astragalus root and garnish with black pepper or crushed red pepper.

Makes 25 one-cup servings

a member of Britain's National Institute of Medical Herbalists and a professional member of the AHG who practices in Vancouver.

Stay Strong for the Long Haul

Following are the adaptogen herbs most commonly recommended by herbalists. Since these herbs can take six weeks to three months to begin working, take them well in advance of cold and flu season or (if possible) a major life change such as a move, advises Bancroft.

Take a Chinese tonic. Native to northeast China, astragalus is one of that country's most valued medicinal herbs. The dried root, which resembles a leathery tongue depressor, is readily available in health food stores and is usually used to make tea. To make astragalus tea, place 2 teaspoons of the dried root in 2 cups of boiling water. Gently simmer for about 45 minutes, or until reduced by half. Drink one cup three times a day.

Research shows that astragalus root pushes infection-fighting white blood cells from their resting state into heightened activity and stimulates the production of interferon, a protein that slows the multiplication of viruses and boosts the activity of the body's killer cells. Polysaccharides, long, branched chains of carbohydrates that are believed to have powerful antiviral and immune-boosting properties, and saponins, another group of compounds believed to stimulate immunity, are thought to be its active constituents.

Buy only astragalus root that's of a uniform yellow hue, advises David Winston, a professional member of the AHG and founder of Herbalist and Alchemist, an herbal medicine company in Washington, New Jersey. (The Chinese name for astragalus, *huang-qi*, means "yellow leader.") If you see streaks of white, the root is of low quality.

Opt for extract. Health food stores also sell astragalus as a tincture (also called an extract). Take 40 to 60 drops in water two to three times a day, says Winston.

Say "da" to Siberian ginseng. Taken by about six million people in the former Soviet Union every day, Siberian ginseng is the root, root bark, or stem of a shrub in the ginseng family. This herb (actually a distant relative of Korean ginseng) has undergone extensive research. One study found that it reduced the number of sick days that Russian factory workers took during cold and flu season. Others found that the herb improved people's ability to cope with increased physical labor, high temperatures, and other physical stressors.

Siberian ginseng contains eleutherosides, substances that fuel the adrenal glands and help them to withstand emotional and physical stresses. It also contains polysaccharides.

You'll find Siberian ginseng in various formulations, all of which are available at health food stores. Most herbalists suggest taking the liquid extract or the tincture. Take 20 to 30 drops of the extract or 40 to 60 drops of the tincture, straight or in water, two or three times a day, recommends Winston.

Power up with Asian ginseng. In the winter, the Chinese serve their children soup laced with Korean ginseng (also known as Asian ginseng) root to keep them healthy. Asian ginseng root contains polysaccharides and saponins.

Health food stores and pharmacies are stocked with dozens of Asian ginseng products. Winston suggests cutting the dried root into two or three pieces and cooking it with rice. Or brew the root into tea: Place 3 small ginseng roots in a pan, add 3 cups of water, and simmer for 1 hour. Allow it to cool and then strain (the roots will become soft enough to eat, if you like). Drink one cup three times a day.

Drink up some drops. The next best thing to Asian ginseng root is a tincture of the herb, says Winston. He recommends taking 20 to 40 drops in water two or three times a day.

Brew up a tonic tea. If you enjoy herbal teas, you might consider making a pot of this immune-boosting tea suggested by Deb Soule, a practicing herbalist in Rockland, Maine, in her book *The Roots of Healing: A Woman's Book of Herbs*. Mix 2 parts astragalus root, 2 parts codonopsis root, 1 part Siberian ginseng root, 1 part schisandra berry, 1 part prickly ash bark, and ½ part licorice root. Soak 12 tablespoons of the mixed herbs overnight in 2 quarts of water. The next morning, transfer the mixture to a pot, cover, and simmer for 30 to 60 minutes. Strain and drink one to three cups every day. (If you have high blood pressure, skip the licorice, as large amounts can raise blood pressure.)

Codonopsis root, called *dang shen* in China, and schisandra berry "nourish and strengthen the immune system," says Bancroft. Licorice, another popular Chinese medicinal herb, has antiviral properties. All of these herbs are available in health food stores, Asian herb shops, or by mail order (see "Where to Buy Herbs and Herbal Products" on page 462).

Reach for the reishi. In Japan, street vendors sell medicinal mushrooms from pushcarts, like hot dogs. That's because the Japanese and Chinese—along with most Western herbalists—consider them the mother of all immune boosters. Pharmacological studies have shown that these fungi contain substances that build the body's resistance to viruses, bacteria, and stress.

Reishi (pronounced "ree-shee") mushrooms are one of more than 200 varieties of mushrooms used in traditional Asian medicine. The Japanese call the reishi mushroom the "10,000-year mushroom," and the Chinese named it "the mushroom of immortality." Whatever the label, this fungus is considered a classic prescription for longevity. Reishi contains hundreds of as-yet-unidentified compounds, but its healing powers are commonly attributed to polysaccharides.

The only catch is that the reishi is one evil-tasting mushroom, so most folks opt to take it in supplement form. Mushroom tablets formulated with a dried extract are more potent than capsules containing the chopped-up herb, notes Bancroft. Reishi supplements are available in health food stores and by mail order. Preparations vary, so follow the dosage directions on the label, she advises.

Stay strong with shiitake. In Japan, the shiitake mushroom was once reserved for the emperor and his family. Now it's that country's largest agricultural export. Traditionally used to increase vitality and fight the common cold, the shiitake contains lentinan, a substance that's been shown in clinical studies to stimulate the immune system.

Fresh or dried shiitake mushrooms are sold in most Asian markets or the bigger grocery stores. You can grill, sauté, or stir-fry the fresh mushroom and toss the dried variety into soups and stews. The traditional dose is one or two fresh mushrooms or 6 to 16 grams (about one to three teaspoons) of the dried variety.

Shiitake extracts, powders, and capsules are available at health food stores. Follow the dosage directions on the label.

Thrive on maitake. Pronounced "may-tak-ee," this monster mushroom (some weigh as much as 100 pounds) is believed to have antimicrobial and antiviral properties and to

Anti-Germ Warfare in an Instant

Adaptogenic herbs such as Siberian ginseng and shiitake mushrooms "tune up" the immune system and keep it running smoothly. But when your immune system needs a jump start, you turn to the AAA of herbs: garlic, thyme, and echinacea.

The herbs recommended below can boost immunity almost immediately, say herbalists, so they're valuable when you know that you're vulnerable. "If you're going to a nephew's birthday party and there will be 20 sniffling kids there, these are the herbs to take," says Betzy Bancroft, a professional member of the American Herbalists Guild (AHG) and manager of Herbalist and Alchemist, an herbal medicine company in Washington, New Jersey.

Help yourself to garlic. "Garlic is one of the most powerful medicinal plants there is," says David Winston, a professional member of the AHG and founder of Herbalist and Alchemist. Used as medicine for millennia, garlic has repeatedly shown an ability to kill viruses and bacteria. Researchers attribute its healing powers to allicin, a compound released when the bulb is cut or crushed.

Consume at least one teaspoon of crushed garlic a day, recommends Winston. If you'd rather take a garlic supplement, choose a gel-cap variety that contains pure garlic oil rather than an odorless tablet, he advises. "It's the oil that possesses the antibacterial activity," he explains.

Brew a cup of thyme tea. This common kitchen spice contains thymol, which has been shown to kill viruses and bacteria, according to Winston. "I use thyme for head colds and bronchitis," he says. To make a tea, pour 1 cup of boiling water over 2 heaping teaspoons of the herb. Let stand, covered, for 10 minutes, then strain. Drink one cup several times a day.

Get set with echinacea. This herb increases the levels of a chemical called properdin, which activates the part of the immune system that increases the body's defense mechanisms against viruses and bacteria. "When I feel a cold coming on, I take 15 to 25 drops of the tincture three times a day," says Rob McCaleb, president and founder of the Herb Research Foundation in Boulder, Colorado. The dose should equal at least 900 milligrams of echinacea per day, whether taken as liquid extract, capsules, tablets, or lozenges.

---

stimulate the immune systems of animals. Researchers attribute its therapeutic actions to the polysaccharides trehalose, chitin, and beta-glucan.

Some gourmet grocery stores sell fresh maitake mushrooms, but this variety can be difficult to find. You can find maitake supplements in health food stores, however. Douglas Schar, a practicing medical herbalist in London, editor of the *British Journal of Phytotherapy*, and author of *Backyard Medicine Chest*, suggests taking six 300-milligram tablets of maitake a day for a daily total of 1,800 milligrams.

Menopause

NURTURE THE CHANGE WITH GREEN MEDICINE

ook up *menopause* in a medical dictionary, and you'll find a simple definition: "Cessation of menstruation in the human female, occurring usually around the age of 50." That's it. No mention of hot flashes, depression, mood swings, or any of the other complaints that women associate with the changes in hormone production that prompt a permanent recess for menstruation and fertility.

Somewhere along the line, menopause evolved from a natural transitional phase to a trauma to be feared—or a medical condition in search of a cure.

Among herbalists—and many women—the old-fashioned view of menopause has given way in recent years to yet another perspective—a modern attitude of acceptance and sometimes even anticipation. Women herbalists describe this life cycle as a passage graced with knowledge and wisdom, echoing a philosophical legacy that goes back centuries and makes more sense than treating this transition as a disease.

"Menopause is not a disorder; it's a powerful and exciting transition," says herbalist Rosemary Gladstar, director of the Sage Mountain herbal education center in East Barre, Vermont, and author of *Herbal Healing for Women*. "As long as a woman takes really good care of herself and uses natural support, menopause doesn't have to be the trauma that so many of us fear," she adds.

"Hot flashes can awaken a woman to her greatest possible potential," says Susun S. Weed, an herbalist and herbal educator from Woodstock, New York, and author of the *Wise Woman* series of herbal health books, including *Menopausal Years: The Wise Woman's Way*. "Think of hot flashes as kundalini moving up your spine," she says. In yoga philosophy, kundalini is the life force that lies coiled at the base of the spine. Hot flashes occur when your kundalini energy awakens and rushes to your head. These surges can trigger true enlightenment.

"Think of hormones as specialized kinds of fat and kundalini as a kind of fire," encourages Weed. If you can envision what happens when you throw fat on a fire, you'll see how it is that kundalini plus extra hormones make flashes hot. To cool down, avoid extra hormones, whether synthetic, natural, herbal, or otherwise, advises Weed.

"I see menopause as a rite of passage," says Silena Heron, N.D., a naturopathic physician in Sedona, Arizona, who lectures widely on botanical medicine. "It's an opportunity for a woman to expend energy on her spiritual growth, or on the bigger community that surrounds us all."

"Theories about what menopause should be like are irrelevant," says Amanda Mc-Quade Crawford, a practicing herbalist in Ojai, California, professional member of the American Herbalists Guild (AHG), member of Britain's National Institute of Medical Herbalists, president of the American College of Integrative Medicine in Albuquerque, and author of *The Herbal Menopause Book*.

According to McQuade Crawford, menopause is a time to contemplate your relationship with others and with your world.

Puberty in Reverse

That said, it may take quite a leap of faith to make that spiritual connection to menopause when you're gripped by a face-reddening, brow-wetting hot flash in the middle of a meeting.

Suddenly, it seems, the body you've known so well for four or five decades just isn't behaving as it once did. Your periods change in ways subtle or dramatic, perhaps with more pain and bleeding and less regularity. Sensations of heat, which can range from brilliant red blushes to night sweats that bounce you out of bed, may overwhelm you occasionally or even regularly. Your vagina may not lubricate as lushly as it once did, and as a result, your interest in sex may dwindle. Your moods may become turbulent and roiling, with unaccustomed flashes of anger that meld into uncontrollable urges to cry over anything—or nothing at all.

Strictly speaking, menopause means that you've stopped menstruating for a period of 6 to 12 months. But well before that vague point in time, your body begins to change in many ways as it eases out of its reproductive responsibilities. This stretch before your periods actually cease is called perimenopause, and it can last for several years.

A basic knowledge about hormones is key to understanding your menopausal changes. And the first thing to learn is that, contrary to popular opinion, some hormonal activity actually *surges* during menopause. So if you think that menopause is all about the decline and fall of your estrogen levels, think again.

"Because taking estrogen supplements can sometimes relieve hot flashes, many women assume that hot flashes are caused by too few hormones," says Weed. But just the opposite is true, she claims. During menopause, the production of some kinds of estrogen does drop, she says, but production of other hormones, especially luteinizing hormone (LH) and follicle-stimulating hormone (FSH), increase by a factor of 30 to 60 percent.

Here's why: A woman is born with something like a million eggs in her ovary egg banks. That number declines by more than half at puberty, but only 400 or so of the eggs actually mature during your reproductive years. By the time you edge toward the age of 50, few eggs are left. The absence of active egg follicles (the egg and the surrounding fluid and cells that nourish it) causes estrogen and progesterone levels to drop.

But somehow, your pituitary gland (up there in your brain) misses the signal to slow down the reproduction plant. In a vain attempt to jump-start production, growth, and release of eggs, it boosts the production of two hormones, LH and FSH. During menopause, these two hormones are continuously secreted in copious quantities. With no egg follicles left to stimulate, LH and FSH have to find something else to do. So they prompt the ovaries and the adrenal glands to secrete increased amounts of androgen. Androgen is the hormone that promotes guylike characteristics like beard growth and a deep voice. Although the fat cells on your hips and thighs convert androgen to estrogen, your total estrogen levels are still far below what they were during your peak reproductive years.

This is all perfectly normal. The trouble is, when combined with other risk factors, decreased estrogen in your system puts you at increased risk for heart disease, which kills more American women than any other disease, including all cancers combined. As long as estrogen circulates through your system, your heart is well-protected because estrogen reduces your total cholesterol level, raises your "good" high-density lipoprotein (HDL) cholesterol, and lowers your "bad" low-density lipoprotein (LDL) cholesterol. LDL is the gummy cholesterol that can build up in your arteries, causing them to narrow and increasing your chances of a heart attack. HDL is like a street sweeper that helps keep your arteries clear and LDL-free.

With menopause comes another health risk: osteoporosis, the gradual loss of bone density that can lead to disabling, even life-threatening, fractures of the spine and hip. Until menopause, estrogen helps keeps bones strong, a benefit that's lost when estrogen supplies wane.

The Whys of Hormone Replacement

"Conventional medicine treats menopause as a deficiency disease of estrogen in much the same way that diabetes is considered a deficiency disease of insulin," says naturopathic physician Tori Hudson, N.D., professor at the National College of Naturopathic Medicine and director of A Woman's Time, a women's health clinic, both in Portland, Oregon. So just as physicians are quick to prescribe insulin for diabetes treatment, many are equally quick to prescribe estrogen and other hormones, called hormone replacement therapy (HRT), for heart and bone protection. HRT can also relieve hot flashes and other menopausal symptoms, notes Dr. Hudson.

"But menopause, unlike diabetes, isn't a disease process, and it's not something to be halted or reversed," says Dr. Hudson. "It's a perfectly normal part of life. All women stop menstruating—it's a part of normal aging. True, some women have problems associated with menopause, but we have to be realistic about treating those problems in a way that best suits the individual woman."

HRT uses either synthetic or natural female hormones, like estrogen (collected from the urine of pregnant mares or plant sources), to compensate for the normal decline in production experienced by women at midlife. Some herbalists and many M.D.'s agree that HRT may be an appropriate choice for certain women with severe menopausal symptoms or for those at high risk for heart disease and osteoporosis.

Using HRT does not necessarily guarantee a problem-free passage, however. Among women who choose HRT, roughly one out of three will stop using it before a year is up because of uncomfortable side effects. Fully 50 percent of all women who take HRT will experience one or more problems, including menstrual bleeding, bloating, premenstrual irritability, cramps, and breast tenderness. There can be other problems, too, like headaches, weight gain, depression, abnormal uterine bleeding, and changes in hair and skin. Using estrogen can double your chances of developing gallbladder disease. And many doctors tell women to shun HRT if they've had breast cancer or have a family history of the disease.

In other words, some women feel better, and may be better off, with the side effects of menopause than with the side effects of menopause medicine, says Dr. Hudson.

Phytoestrogens: Mother Nature's Hormones

Some herbs and other plants, notably soybeans, contain estrogen-like substances called phytoestrogens that have been used traditionally for menopause and other conditions now treated with HRT. Compared to the estrogen in HRT, phytoestrogens are quite weak—only about $1/400$ to $1/1,000$ as strong, in fact. So you'd think that phytoestrogens would be no match for forceful menopausal symptoms.

But even though phytoestrogens are weaker, they still work, because they have properties that make them more effective, even at low doses, says Dr. Hudson. When estrogen levels are low, phytoestrogens crank up their estrogen-like activity, increasing their estrogenic effects. And when estrogen levels are too high, the phytoestrogens bind to estrogen receptor sites, effectively competing with estrogen and decreasing its effects, Dr. Hudson explains.

More good news about phytoestrogens: Because they're chemically weaker than estrogen, using them poses fewer health risks than using HRT can—health risks that include increased risk of cancer, gallbladder disease, and blood clots, says Dr. Hudson. What's more, there's some data that suggests that phytoestrogens may even be effective in preventing breast cancer, she says.

Interestingly, because phytoestrogens do such a creative balancing act, it's common to find that the herbs recommended for excess estrogen problems (like PMS) are the same ones used for estrogen deficiency problems (like menopause).

In addition to foods like soybeans, legumes, and sprouts, there are a number of specific herbs that experts say can help relieve many of the symptoms of menopause. These herbs include licorice, chasteberry, and black cohosh, to name just a few. You'll often find them combined in menopause formulas because, although they can be individually effective, their benefits are even more powerful when they are combined, say herbalists.

Your Herbal Protection Plan

Heart disease and osteoporosis are associated with menopause, but they're often preventable problems caused by unhealthy aging, not menopause, points out Gladstar. "If we support our bodies all through our lives with healthy habits, including a good diet and adequate exercise, we'll be at much lower risk for the diseases associated with menopause," she says. "There are plenty of steps you can take while you're in your thirties and forties that will serve you well later on." Here are some to consider.

Use tonic herbs at 30-plus. "When you're flush with youthful vitality in your twenties and thirties, whether you're working outside the home or in it, raising small children, you don't pay too much attention to your body," says Gladstar. "My suggestion—my plea—to women in their thirties is to plan for a healthy menopause *now*. It will make a vital difference later and will enable them to enter menopause brimming with strength and vitality." Two herbs that are especially good for long-term use leading up to menopause are dang gui and lady's-mantle, says Gladstar.

Dang gui acts on the liver and endocrine system, helping to regulate and normalize hormone production, says Gladstar. The best way to take this herb is in the form of sliced and pressed root, which you can chop and make into an infusion or tincture (see "Teas and Infusions" on page 89 and "Tinctures" on page 92 for directions). If you'd rather not fuss, you can buy it as a tea, as an extract in the form of capsules, or in a tincture (also called an extract). Drink two cups of the tea daily or take two capsules three times a day, she explains. For a tincture, take ½ teaspoon mixed in a little water three times a day, says Gladstar. When taking dang gui for extended periods of time, stop taking it the week before your period starts and resume using it when your period is over.

Lady's-mantle has been used traditionally to treat menstrual irregularities. It contains salicylic acid, similar to aspirin, and has sedative properties, both of which help to ease cramps. According to Gladstar, "the magic and gentle power of lady's-mantle can be quite helpful" before and during menopause. Sip a cup or two of tea every day as menopause commences, she suggests. It has no known side effects.

Help your heart with hawthorn. Hawthorn helps keep your heart strong, which is vital as your supplies of heart-protective estrogen dwindle, says Lisa Alschuler, N.D., a naturopathic physician and chair of the department of botanical medicine at Bastyr University in Bothell, Washington. "I add a handful of hawthorn berries to an infusion of mineral-rich herbs like nettle, oatstraw, and red clover," she says. Alternately, you can make a tincture of hawthorn berries and add some to your tea for menopausal re-

lief, Dr. Alschuler suggests. Add ½ to 1 teaspoon of tincture to each cup of the herbal tea of your choice. Drink one to three cups of tea with the tincture added every day. Begin when you notice initial symptoms of menopause and continue indefinitely, making sure to take a week off every eight weeks, she advises.

Mineralize deeply and lavishly. Nettle leaves, oatstraw, and red clover blossoms are also excellent for helping keep bones strong. "Make mineral-rich herbal infusions part of your life," says Weed. You can enjoy these drinks every day with no adverse effects, she says. It is important to make a good, strong infusion, not a tea. "I let my infusions brew overnight and drink them throughout the next day or two," says Weed.

In some people, allergy symptomss worsen with nettle, so medical experts recommend taking only one dose a day for the first few days.

"I like raspberry leaf and horsetail infusion because they have lots of calcium, too," says Gladstar. "In addition, horsetail is high in silica, a trace mineral that helps build strong bones, healthy hair, and strong nails and helps the body better utilize calcium," she adds.

Help yourself to calcium-rich greens. "It's a good idea to concentrate on building and maintaining healthy bones early on," says Gladstar. "That means including plenty of dark, leafy green vegetables like watercress, nettle, and dandelion greens in your diet every day," she adds.

Add a dandelion tincture. "As I was going through menopause, I found that anything I did to strengthen my liver made me happier and healthier," says Weed. "Remember that menopause floods us with hormones, and the liver is responsible for clearing hormones from the blood and balancing hormone production." According to Weed, one of the best herbs for long-term liver support is dandelion. Try making a medicinal vinegar tincture with dandelion leaves and/or root (it's delicious, Weed says) and using it liberally on your salads and vegetables. (To make a medicinal dandelion vinegar, see "Tinctures.") Alternately, you can use 30 drops of dandelion tincture in $\frac{1}{2}$ cup of water before meals or 10 drops in $\frac{1}{2}$ cup of water when you have a hot flash.

Enlist flax. Flaxseed can do a menopausal woman a world of good, says Dr. Alschuler. "Not only do the seeds contain lignans, which help reduce your chances of getting some forms of cancer, but they also act as a potent phytoestrogen. On top of that, flax is a good source of fiber to keep your bowels moving. That's essential, because good bowel function improves the circulation of estrogen in your body. Finally, flax decreases inflammation and eases cramps and other menopausal aches," she says.

To use flaxseed, grind $\frac{1}{4}$ cup of raw seeds in a coffee grinder and add to cereal, yogurt, salads, or other foods. Store unground flaxseed in an airtight container, preferably dark glass, in the refrigerator. Flaxseed can quickly become rancid, so keep unground flaxseed for only three to six months, and throw out ground seed after one to three months. Make sure you take your flaxseed with at least six ounces of water, and avoid it altogether if you're chronically constipated.

Use caffeine-rich foods with respect. "This is one of the first things I say to women in their thirties," says Gladstar. "Caffeine can stress the adrenal glands, which are called upon to help manufacture estrogen during menopause." But it's never to late to wean yourself off the bean.

Stop smoking. Any medical expert will tell you that the single most important thing you can do for your health is to stop smoking. Unless you've been living in a yurt in outer Mongolia for the last 30 years, you know that smoking cigarettes is a major risk factor for heart disease. But did you know that smoking significantly increases your risk of having an early menopause? Smoking is also associated with infertility and miscarriage. Consider it another incentive to quit.

For individual menopausal problems, herbalists offer these remedies.

Hot Flashes

We don't really know what causes hot flashes (sometimes called hot flushes), but we do know that as many as 65 to 80 percent of women will experience them at some point during their transition to menopause. One theory implicates an instability in the way the body regulates heat when your hormone balance is in flux. Another suggests that hormonal changes irritate blood vessels and nerves, causing the blood vessels to overdilate and produce a hot feeling. Whatever the cause, they're unpredictable and uncomfortable. Here's how to chill out with herbs.

Turn down the heat with motherwort and black cohosh. "I like to start with the simplest things first," says Patricia Howell, a professional member of the AHG who practices in Atlanta. "I mix 2 parts of motherwort tincture with 1 part black cohosh tincture." (Black cohosh isn't a hormone per se, but it normalizes hormone fluctuations prior to menopause, she says.)

Start with ¼ teaspoon of the formula, mixed into a small amount of water or a cup of tea, three times a day. Herbalists sometimes recommend increasing the dosage to ½ teaspoon three times a day. But Howell cautions that at high doses, black cohosh makes some women nauseated. If that happens, take it less often.

Science supports motherwort's traditional use as a heart strengthener due to its ability to lower blood pressure, which may be why it's considered a hot-flash helper. Motherwort also has sedative qualities to ease the insomnia that troubles many menopausal women, notes Gladstar.

Consider an herbal combination. In a pilot study, Dr. Hudson used a formula that she calls Women's Phase II, consisting of dang gui, licorice, burdock, wild yam, and motherwort, which she gave to women who experienced hot flashes. The botanical formula reduced the frequency of hot flashes in 7 out of 10 women who participated and helped with other menopausal symptoms as well.

Try an herbal trio. "My own standard recommendation for hot flashes and other symptoms of menopause is a trio of traditional herbs," says Andrew Weil, M.D., director of the program in integrative medicine at the University of Arizona College of Medicine in Tucson and author of *Spontaneous Healing*.

Dr. Weil recommends taking one dropperful each of tinctures of dang gui, chasteberry, and damiana once a day at midday. Continue taking the herbs until your hot flashes cease, then taper off gradually.

Damiana is a nervous-system tonic, said to ease depression and anxiety. Chasteberry may counteract the effectiveness of birth control pills. Don't use dang gui while menstruating, spotting, or bleeding heavily, because it can increase blood loss.

Taming the volcanic hot flash. For some women, menopause follows surgical removal of the ovaries or chemotherapy or radiation treatments that can destroy the ovaries, says Weed. For them, hot flashes may be especially frequent and intense, she adds. "Volcanic hot flashes are to a normal hot flash as a tidal wave is to a normal wave," she says. Twenty-five to 30 drops of motherwort tincture can stem the tide, she suggests. And for the long term, she recommends 30 to 90 drops of chasteberry tincture three times a day for at least 13 months.

Night Sweats

Hot flashes that strike while you're asleep are called night sweats, and sometimes feelings of terror or anxiety will precede them. Here's how to help yourself through them.

Go with *au naturel* bedding. Shell out a little extra dough for all-cotton sheets, down or feather pillows, and a mattress of natural fibers such as a futon, suggests Weed. And

Sage: Herbal Relief for Night Sweats

Salvia officinalis may not need much introduction, especially if you're a cook or a gardener. With its long, leathery leaves, its earthy color of greenish purple, and its aroma—its unforgettable aroma—sage has been with us for as long as anyone can remember.

Like many ancient herbs, this one has been used to treat all kinds of problems. It was said to be good for preventing the plague, strengthening the liver, and blackening the hair. But perhaps its best-known modern-day use is as a stuffing seasoning for the big holiday bird.

Sage is useful for menopause because of its estrogenic action and because it dries up perspiration, which may explain why it's so effective for dampening night sweats, says Susun S. Weed, an herbalist and herbal educator from Woodstock, New York, and author of the *Wise Woman* series of herbal health books, including *Menopausal Years: The Wise Woman's Way.*

Pay strict attention to dosages recommended for sage, and don't take more than advised. In large quantities, sage's active ingredient, thujone, can provoke irritability, advises Weed. And don't use sage as a medicine when you're pregnant or breastfeeding, she adds, because it can stimulate the uterus, and it dries up breast milk. (Sage used in small amounts in cooking is fine, however.)

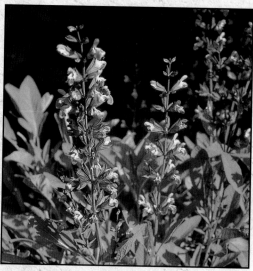

Sage was consumed in tea by the Chinese and has made its way into ales, perfumes, deodorants, and even insecticides.

sleep in all-cotton—or silk—nightwear, she adds. This is helpful because the usual polyester blend used in sheets, foam rubber bedding, and nylon nighties encourages flashes and leaves you feeling damp and clammy afterward, Weed adds.

Get some help from a sage. Garden sage is famed for the way it reduces or even eliminates night sweats. It acts fast, within a few hours, and a single cup of infusion can stave off the sweats for up to two days, says Weed. What's more, you probably have a bottle of sage sitting on your spice rack. Just make sure it's still nice and aromatic before you use it medicinally.

To make a sage infusion, put 4 heaping tablespoons of dried sage in a cup of hot water. Cover tightly and steep for 4 hours or more.

Irregular Periods and Flooding

Your cycles used to be regular, but now they're not. You used to know roughly how many tampons or napkins you'd use during each period, but now you haven't got a clue. Nothing about your period is as it used to be.

If you're like a lot of women, you wonder whether this new irregularity is a normal part of menopause or if it's a sign that something sinister is going on. More than likely, bleeding irregularities that begin in your forties or fifties—or even as early as your thirties—can be traced to the beginnings of menopause, says Weed. To distinguish normal from abnormal changes, keep records. You may find that there's a certain regularity to your irregularity. If your periods are indeed erratic or profuse, consult your doctor or other expert in women's health.

Sometimes herbs can even out irregular menses; sometimes they can't. Weed suggests trying these herbal remedies.

Turn to chasteberry. Although it's slow to act, chasteberry tincture is highly recommended for women who are bothered by menopausal irregularities. Weed recommends a dropperful in a small glass of water or juice two or three times a day for six to eight weeks after every irregular period.

Sip some cinnamon. Cinnamon bark invigorates the blood, helps regulate the menstrual cycle, and checks flooding, says Weed. For heavy bleeding, sip a cup of cinnamon infusion or use 5 to 10 drops of tincture once or twice a day, or chew on a cinnamon stick. You can also simply sprinkle cinnamon powder freely on food, advises Weed.

Visit a lady. In a clinical study, 5 to 10 drops of lady's-mantle tincture controlled menstrual hemorrhage in virtually all of the 300 women who participated, says Weed. When taken after flooding began, lady's-mantle took three to five days to become effective. When taken for one to two weeks before menstruation, it prevented flooding. Weed suggests using 5 to 10 drops of the fresh plant tincture three times a day for up to two weeks out of every month.

Keep your iron up. Try to consume more iron from herbs and food sources on the days that you bleed heavily, says Weed. You'll feel more energetic and alive within two weeks, and your flooding will diminish noticeably by your next period, she adds. Herbal sources of iron include dandelion leaves, milk thistle seed, dang gui, black cohosh, echinacea, and peppermint, according to Weed. Food sources include leafy greens, tofu, raisins, carrots, beets, pumpkin, tomatoes, cauliflower, mushrooms, soybeans, and salmon. Of course, lean red meat is the best source of iron, because it contains heme iron, which is readily absorbed by the body.

Reach for yellow dock root. Another iron source, yellow dock root contributes one milligram of iron per 20-drop dose of alcohol tincture or three-teaspoon dose of vinegar tincture, says Weed. Yellow dock also contains thiamin and vitamin C, which assists absorption of iron, as well as compounds called anthraquinone glycosides that stimulate bile production, thereby aiding digestion and nudging a sluggish liver. Either an alcohol or vinegar tincture is fine, taken daily in tea or water, advises Weed. Iron is absorbed a little at a time, so she suggests taking it throughout the day. Acids and proteins increase iron absorption, says Weed, so take your iron with some orange juice or milk.

Limit iron-eating foods. Coffee, black tea, soy protein (such as tofu or soy milk), egg yolks, bran, and calcium supplements over 250 milligrams impair iron absorption, Weed notes. Limit consumption of coffee and tea, and take your calcium at night or with meals that don't include iron-rich foods.

Vaginal Dryness

After menopause, your vaginal lining may begin to thin and dry out due to the lack of estrogen. As a result, having sex may hurt, and you may find yourself with a vexing vaginal infection. Here are some juicy herbal—and other—remedies to help keep your love life flowing.

Become a love goddess. There's no doubt about it—regular lovemaking increases blood flow to the vaginal tissues, and that improves their tone and lubrication, say herbal experts. To add lubrication, you can apply K-Y Jelly or a similar water-based lubricant before you have sex. Or take herbs that increase lubrication.

Lather up with Rosemary's liquid lube. Gladstar suggests a blend of equal parts of distilled witch hazel and pure aloe vera gel, used as needed before and during sex. "A friend of mine who goes camping a lot in Vermont mixed this up as a water-free cleanser," says Gladstar. "I tried it and realized it was the perfect vaginal lubricant for menopausal dryness. It's so soothing and lubricating and easy to make, I recommend it to everyone. This is also very nice if you mix it with some slippery elm powder, which makes the liquid even more, well, slippery," she says.

Massage yourself. Choose evening primrose oil or combine vitamin E oil and clary sage essential oil (5 drops per ounce) and massage your vaginal area daily or whenever you need extra lubrication, suggests McQuade Crawford. You'll find that with regular use of either oil, your vaginal tissues will become moister and more supple, she adds. She also explains that coconut oil can be used as often as needed, including during intercourse.

Call on comfrey. "Comfrey ointment is the ally of choice when skin needs flexible strength," says Weed. Use the ointment to keep vaginal tissues moist, strong, and supple by rubbing it in morning and evening and using it during love play. Your vulva will be noticeably plumper and moister within three weeks, Weed promises. You can also do what French courtesans used to do: Brew up 2 quarts of comfrey leaf infusion, then strain it, rewarm to a comfortable temperature, pour it into a small tub, and "sitz" yourself in it until it cools, says Weed.

Mood Swings

In menopause, you can be merry one moment and maniacal the next, without any rhyme or reason, it seems. According to one theory, the hormonal downdrafts and upsurges of menopause trigger mood swings in an interesting, indirect way. Unusual fluctuations in estrogen cause your body's sodium level to rise, and that means that the cells retain more water, says Gladstar. "Even a few ounces of excess water can cause breast tenderness, swelling, depression, and anxiety," she believes. Here's how to remedy the situation.

Drink, drink, drink. Contrary to what you might think, the solution to fluid reten-

Rosemary's Mood-Swing Tea

The herbs in this tea—oatstraw, chickweed, nettle, uva-ursi, and corn silk—work together to help the body shed excess water and the irritability and mood swings it can trigger, says herbalist Rosemary Gladstar, director of the Sage Mountain herbal education center in East Barre, Vermont, and author of Herbal Healing for Women. Oatstraw is a natural diuretic, and chickweed is a traditional remedy for the kidneys. Uva-ursi and nettle are well-known diuretics, and corn silk is a soothing diuretic. Use high-quality dried herbs for this tea. Drink three to four cups daily, says Gladstar. (Don't use uva-ursi during pregnancy, as it can stimulate the uterus.)

1	part chickweed
2	parts nettle
1	part oatstraw
1	part uva-ursi
2	parts corn silk

Use 4 to 6 tablespoons of herb mixture per quart of water. Place cold water in a saucepan, then add the herbs and slowly bring to a simmer over low heat. Remove immediately from the heat and keep the pot tightly covered. Let infuse for 20 minutes, then strain.

tion is to drink more fluid, not less, says Gladstar, because water is an absolute necessity for correcting fluid balance. Drink at least two quarts of water or mild diuretic herbal tea, like dandelion or nettle, daily. Unsweetened cranberry juice is a refreshing tonic for the kidneys, and if it is just too tart for you, dilute it with water and add a bit of honey, says Gladstar. If you can't find unsweetened cranberry juice, regular cranberry juice, like Ocean Spray, is just fine, she adds.

Soothe with oatstraw. Drinking oatstraw infusion freely can banish irritability and strengthen the nerves, says Weed.

Strengthen with skullcap. Skullcap tincture strengthens the nerves, eases oversensitivity, and helps promote deep, sound sleep, says Weed. She uses four to eight drops of the tincture mornings and evenings when she's feeling "fried, stressed out, wired, or just wound up." (Do not confuse it with Chinese skullcap, though, which has entirely different properties.)

Cold Hands and Feet

Menopausal women aren't the only ones troubled by icy extremities; lots of women complain of this chilly problem. According to botanical experts, there are three causes: thyroid problems, low levels of iron, and poor circulation. Some serious collagen and vascular diseases, like lupus, can also cause cold hands and feet. To find out what's putting the chill on yours, see your doctor for a complete physical. In the meantime, try this instant warm-up.

(continued on page 294)

A Naturopathic Approach to Menopause

As more and more women consult naturopathic doctors (N.D.'s) for everyday health problems, they're also consulting naturopaths for menopause-related issues. If you go this route, your experience may resemble a visit to an M.D. in some ways but differ in others.

Naturopaths are medically trained practitioners who use a variety of natural healing techniques to enhance wellness and prevent and treat disease. It's likely that, at least initially, you'll spend quite a bit more time during your appointment with a naturopath than you do with your medical doctor.

"I spend nearly an hour with a woman, and I take a thorough medical and family history," says Tori Hudson, N.D., professor at the National College of Naturopathic Medicine and director of A Woman's Time, a women's health center, both in Portland, Oregon. "I might also recommend some hormone testing, cholesterol testing, and a test to determine bone density. Only then can I determine her personal risk factors for heart disease, osteoporosis, breast cancer, and other diseases—and only then can I determine what she needs in the way of menopausal support," says Dr. Hudson.

After your naturopath has assessed your needs, she'll discuss your options. They range from the simplest and most side-effect-free lifestyle changes to hormone replacement therapy (HRT), an option that Dr. Hudson uses only when other choices are inappropriate.

Here's a rundown of the natural approaches to menopause (including herbs) that are taken by naturopaths.

Start with a diet high in phytoestrogens. The right diet is the starting point for all women approaching menopause. "Along with a good exercise plan, the correct diet may be all that some women, who have minor menopausal symptoms and low risk factors for heart disease and osteoporosis, need to take," says Dr. Hudson.

Your diet should be very low in animal fat and high in good sources of phytoestrogens, says Dr. Hudson. Foods high in phytoestrogens include soy products (look for soy foods that are made from soy flour and whole soy rather than those made from isolated soy proteins), nuts, whole grains, apples, alfalfa, flaxseed, and rye. In addition, foods from the Umbelliferous family, such as celery, parsley, and especially fennel, contain active phytoestrogens, says Dr. Hudson. A diet high in phytoestrogens is thought to be the reason that hot flashes and other menopausal symptoms rarely occur among women who eat mostly vegetarian diets, especially when they eat a lot of soy products, she explains.

Get your daily quota of real exercise. "I recommend that a woman approaching menopause and beyond take up a good, weight-bearing, aerobic exercise that she really enjoys," says Dr. Hudson. Walking, jogging, aerobics classes, or tennis will all do the trick. Your goal here is to exercise for 30 to 60 minutes at least every other day, she says. If you're new to exercise or it's been years since you exercised regularly, get medical clearance before you work out, especially if you're over the age of 40.

Results of a Swedish study showed that regular physical exercise definitely lowers the frequency and severity of hot flashes. What's more, the women who exercised regularly passed through a natural menopause without HRT. The women in the study who had no hot flashes were those who spent an average of 3½ hours per week exercising. In contrast, women who exercised less were more likely to have hot flashes.

Consider nutritional supplements. "I recommend routine mineral supplements to women approaching menopause," says Dr. Hudson. "Look for a mineral supplement complex that includes calcium, magnesium, vitamin D, zinc, and trace minerals like copper, boron, silica, and manganese. This combination helps guard against osteoporosis," she notes. A good brand to try is Osteocomplex, she suggests. (People with heart or kidney problems should not take supplemental magnesium; it may also cause diarrhea in some people.)

If a woman is beginning to have hot flashes, Dr. Hudson recommends 400 to 800 international units (IU) of vitamin E daily. (If you are considering taking more than 600 IU, discuss it with your doctor first.)

Add the right herbs. "If vaginal dryness, mood swings, and hot flashes become troublesome, I recommend black cohosh extract," says Dr. Hudson. "I use Remifemin, and I find that it works so well that I rarely need to add other herbs." Another combination of black cohosh extract and other herbal products is Women's Phase II. Always follow the label instructions exactly, she cautions.

"I usually steer women to take 20 to 40 milligrams twice daily of a standardized black cohosh extract," Dr. Hudson adds. If black cohosh isn't appropriate for a particular woman, or it doesn't work, a naturopath would be likely to blend a botanical formula based on a woman's specific needs.

Look to natural hormones. "Many women do well with diet, lifestyle changes, and herbs," says Silena Heron, N.D., a naturopathic physician from Sedona, Arizona, who lectures widely on botanical medicine. "When I see a woman who really needs hormone therapy because she's at high risk for heart disease or osteoporosis or one whose symptoms are severe, I may prescribe sublingual (under the tongue) natural progesterone alone or in combination with one or two of the three forms of natural estrogen," she says.

Spice up your gloves and socks.
"Simply sprinkle equal parts of ground cinnamon and cayenne pepper in your socks or
even in your gloves," recommends Ellen
Kamhi, R.N., Ph.D., of Oyster Bay, New
York, an herbalist, professional member of
the AHG, and host of the nationally syndicated radio show *Natural Alternatives*. "This
will increase circulation—and warmth—to
your hands and feet quite quickly." Be sure
to wash your hands after you take your
gloves off, so you don't accidentally get the
mixture in your eyes or nose, Dr. Kamhi
warns.

Herbal Formulas Cover All the Bases

Many herbalists have their own special
herbal tonics that they've used over the years
to treat not just isolated problems but a spectrum of menopausal symptoms. Say hot
flashes bedevil you. Your sleep isn't very deep
or very restful. Your moods are a touch volcanic. And the periods you're still having
could be less, well, bloodily intense. Nothing
you can't live with, mind you, but life could be
a whole lot more comfortable without this
cluster of annoyances. Here's what highly respected herbalists have to offer in the way of
help. These formulas help normalize out-of-
kilter hormones and should quell most of
your menopausal woes.

Keep in mind, though, that when it comes
to menopause, each woman is different. One
of these formulas may work better for you
than another, so you may have to experiment
to find the best blend. Remember, too, that
herbs work slowly, so you may not feel any results at all for three weeks or so. Weed urges
women to begin with one herb if they are
novices. If you take a lot of herbs at once and
one of them doesn't agree with you, you won't
know which one it is.

Try the menopause formula. Created
by herbalists Cascade Anderson Geller and
Valerie Perrine for the National College of
Naturopathic Medicine in Portland, Oregon,
"this formula has helped women who are experiencing menopausal changes," says Geller,
who is a consulting herbal practitioner and
herbal educator in Portland.

"If menopausal changes become increasingly intolerable, first consider improving
your diet and lifestyle. Stick to a low-fat,
high-fiber diet, drink lots of water, and exercise for at least 30 minutes every other day,"
advises Geller. "If these changes don't bring
relief, try my herbal formula. It has helped
countless women ease the effects of menopause. Have your doctor monitor your
progress," she says. "Tell your doctor precisely
what you're taking. Suggest that you may be
able to take less estrogen as a result. Ask her
to monitor you closely as you ease off your estrogen," suggests Geller. "Most M.D.'s are
more and more open-minded about herbs
these days, and it's very important that you let
your doctor know that you're taking herbs in
hopes of taking less estrogen."

To make this formula, use the following
herbal tinctures.

- 2 **parts licorice**
- 2 **parts dandelion root**
- 1 **part motherwort**
- 1 **part true unicorn root or false unicorn root**
- 1 **part wild yam**

Using a funnel, pour the tinctures into a
bottle large enough to hold seven ounces
(nearly a cup). To take, add one to three dropperfuls of the tincture mixture to a little water
and drink two or three times a day three to

five days a week. Always take the lowest dose possible and taper off as quickly as possible when symptoms diminish, advises Geller.

Into the change? Try this. According to Dr. Heron, chasteberry helps balance hormones, motherwort has anti-anxiety and antispasmodic effects, and false unicorn has hormonal and digestive benefits. Dang gui, licorice, black cohosh, and alfalfa help enhance estrogen activity. Black haw reduces spasticity that can promote hot flashes, and black cohosh relieves cramps. Sage decreases secretions, including sweat, which makes it useful for reducing both the frequency and severity of hot flashes. As a bonus, sage helps improve digestion, it's a source of zinc, and it kills germs, too. Dr. Heron includes St.-John's-wort in her menopause formula because of its ability to ease pelvic complaints and depression.

"A woman benefits most from herbal therapy when the formula is adjusted to her specific needs," says Dr. Heron. "But this basic formula has been so successful in relieving menopausal discomforts that many women return to my clinic just to have the prescription refilled."

Her formula is made by mixing the following herbal tinctures.

2	parts chasteberry
1	part motherwort
1	part false unicorn root
1	part dang gui
1–2	parts sage
1	part St.-John's-wort
1–2	parts black cohosh
½–1	part licorice
½–1	part black haw
½–1	part alfalfa

Blend the herbal tinctures together in a jar. Take ½ to 1 teaspoon three times a day on an empty stomach, straight up or mixed with a little water, advises Dr. Heron.

Opt for a hormone helper. This tonic will strengthen and tone the endocrine system, which is responsible for manufacturing your body's hormones. During menopause, the adrenal glands take on the role of producing estrogen after the ovaries cease doing so, and they often need a boost during the transition, says Gladstar. Each of the herbs in this formula helps revitalize the adrenal glands, she says. In addition, wild yam is known for its powerful effect on regulating hormone production, sarsaparilla is said to aid body functioning as a whole, and black cohosh has traditionally been recommended for menopausal pains and discomfort.

Gladstar recommends using high-quality dried herbs which you tincture yourself in good brandy or vodka. You can also make this formula from store-bought tinctures. The formula will last you a very long time. Use the tonic consistently over an extended period of time to assure steady, long-lasting results, she adds.

2	parts wild yam
1	part sarsaparilla
1	part black cohosh
2	parts Siberian ginseng
1	part dang gui
3	parts sage
3	parts licorice
3	parts dandelion root

Mix the herbs together. Put 4 tablespoons of the mixture into a wide-mouth bottle and cover with 1 pint of good-quality brandy or vodka. Cover with a tight-fitting lid, place in a warm, shaded area, and let stand for four to six weeks. Shake daily to mix the herbs with the alcohol. After four to six weeks, strain into a clean bottle through a strainer lined with cheesecloth. The recommended dose is ¼ teaspoon three times a day for three months or longer. Dilute the tincture in water, juice, or tea before drinking, Gladstar suggests.

To avoid irritability, you should avoid consuming caffeine and other stimulants while using ginseng.

Sip Amanda's menopause tea. If you prefer drinking tea rather than taking an alcohol-based tincture, try this blend. Use high-quality dried herbs. All quantities are dry weight, not liquid.

3 ounces chasteberry
2 ounces dang gui
1 organic orange or lemon rind (for flavor)
1 ounce Siberian ginseng or licorice
2 ounces St.-John's-wort
2 ounces horsetail
3 ounces motherwort

Mix the herbs together well. Infuse 1 ounce of herb blend in 2 pints of boiling water, cover and steep for 20 minutes, then strain. Drink one large glass three times a day, recommends McQuade Crawford.

Menstrual Problems

ANCIENT HERBS FOR MONTHLY WELL-BEING

Nearly 2,500 years ago, women in Greece plucked the pinwheel-shaped leaves of the chaste tree, soaked them in wine, and sipped this drink to relieve menstrual problems. Today, chasteberry preparations are widely prescribed by gynecologists in Europe for everything from premenstrual tension to heavy or irregular periods.

Meanwhile, on the other side of the world, the author of one of China's oldest herbal medicine texts recommended the slightly sweet, ivory-hued root called dang gui for menstrual difficulties nearly 2,000 years ago. Today, research suggests that this ancient herb eases menstrual pain and has a beneficial influence on the uterine muscle.

Herbal healers, it seems, have long known that the leaves, flowers, seeds, and roots from nature's pharmacy can have a profound, positive effect on common menstrual cycle problems. Fortunately, that knowledge is still with us today.

"Herbs can improve women's conditions in unique and important ways," says herbalist Rosemary Gladstar, director of the Sage Mountain herbal education center in East Barre, Vermont, and author of *Herbal Healing for Women*. "Plant remedies can help rebalance hormones and improve the functioning of the reproductive system by helping the body remember a state of wellness and return to it. If you use herbal remedies for premenstrual syndrome, cramps, or other problems for a few months or even a year, you get to the point where your body is well again. You won't need those herbs anymore. That's something drugs cannot do."

Today, science is beginning to identify the combinations of chemical compounds responsible for this unique brand of natural healing. At the same time that modern researchers are glimpsing these natural secrets, Gladstar says that modern-day women are using herbs to tune in to a natural experience that's often missing from our modern lives of computers, cars, microwaveable pizza, and 100-channel televisions. "I see herbs bringing women back into an earthy, intuitive relationship with the natural world," she notes. "Something in women responds to herbs on a very deep level. It's a kind of spiritual healing."

Think about it the next time you brew a mug of chamomile tea to ward off premenstrual insomnia. In the meantime, the world of herbal healing has many remedies in store for women's menstrual discomforts.

Premenstrual Syndrome

Natural rhythms aren't always nice. From weepiness and bloating to anger, acne breakouts, and headaches, the monthly drama of PMS may be as predictable as sunrise, snow in winter, or songbirds in spring. But for the 60 to 80 percent of women who experience it month after month, this premenstrual condition is hardly a welcome event.

Women's health experts say that the enormous hormonal changes associated with the menstrual cycle are bound to influence our bodies, our moods, and our behavior in some way. What they don't yet understand is why shifting reproductive hormones, especially levels of the female hormone progesterone, affect some women more profoundly than others, sometimes to the point where normal life is disrupted during the 5 to 15 hellish days before menstruation. They also don't know exactly why PMS, which can begin in your teenage years, may grow worse as you near menopause.

Herbalists and conventional health practitioners alike suggest that women who want to minimize PMS symptoms start with healthy eating (emphasizing low-fat protein and complex carbohydrates such as fruits, vegetables, and whole grains) and regular aerobic exercise (20 to 45 minutes a day three times a week is a good amount). Adding vitamin and mineral supplements can help, too. Experts generally suggest getting 1,000 milligrams of calcium, 50 to 100 milligrams of vitamin B_6, and 150 to 400 international units of vitamin E daily. (Note: Unstable gait and numb feet may occur with doses of B_6 that exceed 50 milligrams daily over a prolonged time.)

With more than 150 recognized symptoms, however, PMS isn't a simple condition to relieve. While conventional doctors may suggest drug therapy to brighten mood, lessen fatigue, and even adjust hormone levels, herbalists recommend plant-based remedies that a woman can blend to create a PMS formula that matches her specific needs. "Herbal remedies offer women benefits for PMS relief that drugs cannot," notes Gladstar. "Over a period of months, herbal teas, tinctures, or even capsules can correct imbalances so that your body functions in a healthier way on its own. You bring your body back to a state of well-being, based on your individual needs."

Start with Roots and Berries

Top women herbalists suggest that to improve PMS symptoms, begin with herbs that will help you relax, balance your hormones, and improve liver function. "These basic herbs alone can be very helpful," notes Amanda McQuade Crawford, a practicing herbalist in Ojai, California, professional member of the American Herbalists Guild (AHG), member of Britain's National Institute of Medical Herbalists, president of the American College of Integrative Medicine in Albuquerque, and author of *Herbal Remedies for Women*. "A woman may see improvement in just a month, as her muscles and nerves

relax, as her liver processes circulating hormones better, and as hormone levels themselves become normalized. But continue taking the formula every day for at least three menstrual cycles. It takes that long for a woman to begin seeing a permanent improvement in her health—an improvement that will last after she stops taking the herbs," she says.

You can mix the top three PMS herbs—skullcap leaf, dandelion root, and chasteberry seed—and take as a tea or as a tincture blend. For tea, use 1 to 2 teaspoons of the dried herb mix per cup of boiling water, steep for 20 minutes, and strain. Have three cups a day. If you prefer tinctures (also called extracts), mix the herbal tinctures together, then have one teaspoon of the mixture three times a day, McQuade Crawford suggests. (For more details about which herb or herbs to use and why, see the tips that follow.)

If you do not see any improvement after a month or two, change brands or check the quality of the herbs with a local herbalist. Once you're satisfied with the quality of the herbs, consider adding an extra dose per day, McQuade Crawford suggests. "These herbs are like strong foods," she says. "They are not like drugs. Women can relax and experiment with the dosage within these guidelines." If you still see no improvement after a month or more, herbalists suggest consulting a health-care practitioner for a diagnosis.

Unwind taut nerves with skullcap. "The simplest place to start for PMS relief is with skullcap," McQuade Crawford says. "Nearly 80 percent of women with PMS have anxiety and irritability, and this is the herb for those conditions. Skullcap is a mild but powerful muscle and nerve relaxer," she says. This native North American herb is a traditional nerve tonic and anxiety easer. While it is not well-studied, researchers know that it contains scutellarin, a mild sedative with antispasmodic actions. When making the PMS blend described above, start with 1 part dried skullcap.

Taken for one to two weeks prior to the first day of your period, skullcap can help prevent the teeth-on-edge tension that can build during the days before your period begins, says McQuade Crawford. You may continue throughout menses if needed, she adds. As a result, you will be able to nurture yourself better and cope more serenely with the extra stresses—at home or at work—that always seem to demand attention during that time of the month.

Support your liver with a dandy root. Add 1 part dried dandelion root and 1 part dried dandelion leaf to your tea or tincture mix. Bitter dandelion root and leaves are co-stars in the PMS formulas created by many top women herbalists, not because this common backyard weed can balance hormones but because it helps your liver and digestive system function more effectively, notes Chanchal Cabrera, a member of Britain's National Institute of Medical Herbalists and a professional member of the AHG, who practices in Vancouver.

"Dandelion is very bitter. It stimulates bile production and helps the liver decommission hormones, clearing them from your bloodstream so they don't build up in your body," she notes. "The leaf is also a potent diuretic, so it helps relieve water retention. The root is a gentle but effective laxative, which helps women who become constipated in the days before menstruation begins. When you're constipated, hormones that should be eliminated from your body can end up recirculating, which makes PMS symptoms worse."

Research has found that dandelion's jagged leaves and long taproot contain bitter compounds that boost bile secretion from the liver by as much as 40 percent. "When a woman with PMS improves the way the liver works, that helps balance hormones, eliminates excess water, helps diminish blood sugar shifts, and reduces cravings for starches and sweets," McQuade Crawford notes.

Balance raging hormones with chasteberry. Crunchy, gray-brown, peppercorn-size chasteberry seeds are *the* top herbal remedy for PMS, Cabrera says. "Everything else in a PMS formula revolves around it," she notes. So add 2 parts chasteberry to your tea or tincture mix. One caution: Some herbal experts say that chasteberry may counteract the effectiveness of birth control pills, while others believe it has no effect.

In one German study of 175 women with PMS, a chasteberry extract relieved end-of-cycle symptoms more effectively than vitamin B_6, a time-honored remedy for PMS. One-fourth of the women who took chasteberry for three menstrual cycles rated the treatment as excellent, and one-third stopped experiencing the discomforts of PMS entirely.

German herbal experts say that chasteberry seems to work by raising levels of progesterone, the female hormone that governs the second half of the menstrual cycle. Substances in chasteberry (researchers haven't yet identified which ones) apparently prompt the pituitary gland to release more luteinizing hormone, which in turn prompts the corpus luteum (the follicle that releases an egg from the ovary at ovulation) to produce more progesterone. The exact cause of PMS is unknown, but herbalists believe that an imbalance between levels of progesterone and estrogen may be one cause.

"Chasteberry helps with PMS by stabilizing and regulating the hormones," Cabrera notes. "It is safe to take throughout the entire menstrual cycle." The herb can improve PMS in as few as three menstrual cycles, but you may need up to 18 months to see lasting relief.

A Chinese Menu of Choices

You can further customize your basic PMS relief formula by adding herbs that can ease the specific symptoms that bother you most at this time of the month, Cabrera says. "If you go to an herbalist for help with PMS, you will get a customized formula," she notes. "I usually suggest herbs for hormone balancing and liver function and then two or three herbs for specific symptoms."

How can you tailor a formula at home? Begin with basic PMS herbs, then add two or three of the following herbs—depending on your symptoms—during the second half of your menstrual cycle (which is from about day 14 until you begin to menstruate), Cabrera suggests. "It's better to take these as premenstrual tension approaches," she notes. Take the same dosage—one teaspoon of a tincture mix or one teaspoon of tea blend per cup of boiling water.

Say hello to herbal hormone adjusters. If you'd like to add a second hormone-balancing herb to your personal PMS relief blend or you want to substitute something else for chasteberry, herbalists suggest these choices.

Dang gui. If your main PMS symptoms include depression, crying, forgetfulness, confusion, and insomnia, you may want to add 1½ parts dang gui root to your PMS formula or even substitute it for chasteberry, Cabrera notes. One of the best-selling traditional Chinese herbal remedies outside China, dang gui root can regulate the menstrual cycle, easing premenstrual cramping and pain. Research suggests that the herb improves blood flow to the uterus.

"Dang gui doesn't act like estrogen," says Gladstar, "yet it balances and regulates hormone production."

Don't use dang gui *during* menstruation, as it can stimulate bleeding, warns Cabrera. Stop taking it a week before menstrual bleeding begins and resume once menstruation ends. Women with heavy menstrual flow should not use dang gui at all.

Black cohosh. This native North American herb is also recommended when PMS leaves a woman "feeling gloomy—like a black cloud has descended on her life," notes Betzy Bancroft, a professional member of the AHG and manager of Herbalist and Alchemist, an herbal medicine company in Washington, New Jersey.

In lab studies, constituents found in black cohosh, including an isoflavone called formononetin, seemed to have an effect on levels of luteinizing hormone, mimicking estrogen by binding to estrogen receptor sites on cells. This smooths out estrogen's effect on the body and helps maintain estrogen balance, says Bancroft. As an herbal remedy for menstrual distress, it was used by Native Americans and later appeared in nineteenth-century patent medicines such as Lydia Pinkham's Vegetable Compound.

So if you're depressed, adding 1 part black cohosh to your PMS formula might help, suggests Bancroft. Do not use black cohosh if you suspect that you may be pregnant, because it stimulates the uterus and can cause premature contractions. And don't use it while nursing.

Smooth away stress and tension botanically. If your PMS experience includes tangling with tension, stress, and wakefulness, herbalists suggest adding one of these stress-taming, anxiety-easing, irritability-lifting herbs to your formula.

Valerian. If you have trouble falling asleep, McQuade Crawford suggests taking valerian root at bedtime. Avoid valerian if you're taking other sleep-enhancing or mood-regulating medications such as diazepam (Valium) or amitriptyline (Elavil), however.

"Despite its strong smell and taste, valerian is the best mild sedative for anxiety and insomnia," McQuade Crawford notes. Taken in ancient times for menstrual difficulties, valerian is widely used today in Europe to counteract insomnia and exhaustion. Research shows that it can slow down an agitated central nervous system, ease muscle spasms, and shorten the time it takes to fall asleep.

Passionflower. If you find that you cannot use valerian—either because it tastes and smells like dirty socks or because, as happens to a few women, it actually heightens insomnia—turn to passionflower for tension relief, McQuade Crawford suggests. Research shows that this beautiful North American and tropical vine can help ease anxiety, lower blood pressure, calm nervous tension, and induce sleep, probably due to the action of several compounds collectively called flavonoids. Use the aerial parts of this herb—the vine, stem, or leaf—in either dried form or as a tincture, says McQuade Crawford.

Bloated? Try a natural diuretic. If water retention is a major issue, address the problem with this botanical.

Yarrow. A mild diuretic, yarrow makes a useful addition to a PMS-easing formula because it also stimulates the liver, thereby helping to balance hormones, notes McQuade Crawford. Add ½ part yarrow leaf and flower to your PMS formula, but avoid it if you suspect that you might be pregnant, she cautions.

Sidestep bowel problems botanically. If you become constipated, experience diarrhea, or must cope with more intestinal gas than usual during the days before menstruation, these herbs can help.

Yellow dock. The root of this common weed has been used by traditional and modern herbalists alike to treat constipation and skin problems brought on by PMS, say McQuade Crawford and Bancroft. Herbal experts say that yellow dock contains compounds that nudge sluggish bowels and promote the flow of bile, helping the liver to better process hormones. Adding 1 part dried yellow dock root to your PMS formula may help. Do not use this herb if you suspect that you may be pregnant, however.

Blackberry root. If diarrhea is your premenstrual problem, then adding 1 part dried blackberry root to your PMS formula can help, McQuade Crawford says. A traditional diarrhea remedy, the bark of the blackberry root is high in tannins that have a gentle, astringent action in the intestines to reduce watery stools.

Chamomile. This is another traditional diarrhea remedy, and adding 1 part chamomile flowers can also ease intestinal gas before menstruation, McQuade Crawford says.

Find mental clarity with herbs. Forgetful? Confused? If PMS leaves your brain feeling foggy, these herbs can help restore you to clear-headedness.

Ginger. A small amount (½ part or less) of the warming herb ginger added to your PMS formula can help boost circulation and

Hearty Time-of-the-Month Soup

"In Traditional Chinese Medicine, there's not a big difference between food and medicine—people incorporate healing herbs into their meals," notes Cathy McNease, a professional member of the AHG from Ojai, California, and an instructor at the Santa Barbara College of Oriental Medicine and at Yo San University in Santa Monica.

If you have PMS or menstrual cramps or experience irregular periods, McNease suggests adding traditional hormone-balancing medicinal herbs like white peony root and bupleurum (available by mail) to a hearty chicken soup.

A handful each of white peony root and bupleurum, chopped

1 whole chicken, about 1½ pounds

3–4 cups chopped, mixed vegetables (such as carrots, shiitake mushrooms, spinach, broccoli, onions, garlic, and grated gingerroot)

6–7 cups cold water

Place the medicinal herbs in a cheese-cloth bag so that you can remove them when the soup is ready to eat.

Place the chicken, vegetables, and bag of herbs in a large saucepan, cover with water, and bring to a boil. Simmer for 1½ hours.

Remove the chicken from the pan and remove the meat from the bones. Dice the meat and return it to the pan. Remove the bag of herbs, season the soup to taste, and serve.

Makes 3 to 4 servings

---

improve mental alertness, notes Cabrera. In laboratory studies, ginger extracts have been shown to stimulate the heart and blood vessels.

Ginkgo. To help clear the mental fog that sometimes descends in the days before menstruation begins, add 1 part ginkgo in dried or tincture form to your PMS formula, Cabrera says. Don't take high amounts of ginkgo, as it can cause skin and digestive discomforts in higher doses. Also, you should only use ginkgo under the supervision of a qualified health-care practitioner if you also take pharmaceutical MAO inhibiters such as phenelzine sulfate (Nardil).

Add a finishing touch. To round out a PMS formula, herbalists also suggest the following options, depending on what's bothering you.

Sarsaparilla root. If you feel sluggish or experience skin problems or changes in digestion with PMS, adding 1 part dried sarsaparilla may help because it enhances the function of the body's lymphatic system, McQuade Crawford says. Science has yet to take a close look at this herb, but it has a reputation in folk medicine as a reproductive tonic.

Wild yam. The root of the wild yam vine helps with uterine cramping for many women. It's a specific remedy for hollow organ cramping, easing not only menstrual cramps but also pain from gallstones and kidney stones, says Geller. She suggests adding 1½ parts to your PMS formula.

Cinnamon. The spicy bark of the cinnamon shrub has been used traditionally for "female disorders," including cramping, as well as for diarrhea and abdominal pain. Geller suggests adding 1 part cinnamon to your PMS formula. (Use cinnamon for only a few months at a time.)

Other Herbs That Spell Relief

If PMS isn't a big deal for you, and you're just looking for a simple approach to anxiety, premenstrual headaches, or breast tenderness, experienced herbalists suggest focusing on the following herbal strategies.

Sip a calming blossom. Gentle, with a flowery, citrusy flavor, chamomile tea is used around the world to relax nervous tension, says Cathy McNease, a professional member of the AHG from Ojai, California, and an instructor at the Santa Barbara College of Oriental Medicine and at Yo San University in Santa Monica. Chamomile contains chamazulene and other antispasmodic compounds. It has been used traditionally to overcome insomnia and pain.

"Make a strong decoction by gently simmering ½ ounce (a small handful) of dried chamomile blossoms in a pint of water for 5 to 10 minutes. Strain, and drink two to three cups a day," McNease suggests. "Start a few days before PMS symptoms start making you uncomfortable and continue until your period begins." If you also get menstrual cramps, continue drinking the tea until cramps have subsided.

Enlist calcium-rich botanicals. High-calcium herbs, taken starting 10 days before your period begins and ending at the completion of your cycle, can ease and even eliminate premenstrual and menstrual headaches, Gladstar says. She recommends that women include high-calcium foods such as yogurt in their diets, add an herbal vitamin-and-mineral supplement such as Floradix, Iron and Herbs (available at health food stores), and drink three to four daily cups of what Gladstar calls her high-calcium tea blend.

Mix the blend using 1 part horsetail leaf, 2 parts each oatstraw and nettle leaf, and 4 parts each red raspberry leaf and peppermint leaf (for flavor). Add 6 to 8 tablespoons of the blend to a quart of warm water in a pot, bring to a slow simmer, then remove from the heat and steep for 20 minutes. Strain and enjoy.

Research shows that all of these herbs contain calcium, and conventional medical doctors note that some studies show that extra calcium eases PMS symptoms. (This approach may not work for all women, however.)

Recruit evening primrose oil. Some studies show that evening primrose oil significantly eases PMS symptoms, including breast pain and tenderness, as well as mood swings and irritability, notes Steven Foster, a medicinal plant specialist from Fayetteville, Arkansas, and author of *Herbs for Your Health* and *Forest Pharmacy*.

This oil provides essential fatty acids, including gamma-linolenic acid, which is found in significant quantities in only a few plants. Evening primrose oil may help correct fatty acid deficiencies that occur in the days prior to menstruation and can prompt PMS symptoms. Taking three to six capsules a day, for a total of three to four grams, with meals may help, says Foster.

Pau d'Arco: A Natural Hormone Balancer

In bloom, the South American tree known as lapacho or taheebo is crowned with a cloud of brilliant, magenta-and-pink flowers. As a healing herb, this plant's inner bark and heartwood—known as the herbal remedy pau d'arco—enjoy a reputation that stretches back to the days of the Mayan and Inca civilizations.

Today, pau d'arco is a controversial botanical. Used by doctors in Argentina and Brazil to help treat leukemia and other cancers, its anticancer activity was tested by the National Cancer Institute, with disappointing results.

American herbalists like Rosemary Gladstar, director of the Sage Mountain herbal education center in East Barre, Vermont, and author of *Herbal Healing for Women*, regard this herb as a liver-function booster and include it in some formulas for balancing women's hormones.

One buying tip: Look for organic, woods-grown pau d'arco to avoid pesticide-laden products and those that have been gathered from diminishing wild plant communities, Gladstar suggests. It's available at health food stores.

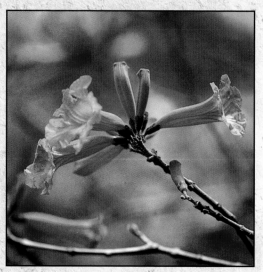

When mixed with other herbs, pau d'arco makes a pleasant tea.

Menstrual Cramps

Once dismissed as "all in your head, dear," the searing, grasping pain that 5 to 10 percent of women feel for the first hour or few days of menstruation is now recognized by medical experts as an especially vexing kind of muscle cramp.

But where do these cramps come from, anyway?

When hormones called prostaglandins are released during your menstrual period, they prompt uterine blood vessels to tighten, decreasing blood flow. This makes the uterine muscle clench, which you feel as a painful cramp.

While conventional medications for cramps include painkillers, nonsteroidal anti-inflammatory drugs such as ibuprofen that act as anti-prostaglandins, and stronger prescription drugs, herbalists suggest remedies that minimize cramping discomfort and that work over several months to regulate hormones so that cramping becomes less severe. Here are women herbalists' favorite remedies for this painful problem.

Vanquish pain fast with valerian and viburnum. Many women herbalists include two herbs in their quick-relief formulas for menstrual cramps: valerian and either cramp bark or black haw, which are both members of the Viburnum family. "These herbs help you moderate your cramps or eliminate them completely," Gladstar notes. Valerian contains several compounds that, working together, relieve muscle spasms and ease anxiety. Cramp bark and black haw are muscle relaxers that soothe painful spasms.

"You may still feel twinges, but the cramps won't incapacitate you. Chemical constituents in these botanicals work on the smooth muscle of the uterus to relax it. If you also put a warm heating pad over your lower abdomen, your uterus will relax even more," says Gladstar.

Gladstar recommends making a cramp-easing tea by slowly simmering 4 tablespoons of cramp bark or black haw with a tablespoon of grated fresh gingerroot in a quart of water for 20 minutes. (Ginger improves the flavor of this formula, helps boost circulation, and is a mild antispasmodic, according to Gladstar.) Turn off the heat and add 2 tablespoons each of dried valerian root and dried pennyroyal leaf, then let the mixture steep for another 15 to 20 minutes. Strain and sip ¼ cup every 15 minutes until your cramps abate. "Never use pennyroyal when you are pregnant," cautions Gladstar.

One note about pennyroyal: While the essential oil of this herb, like most essential oils, is extremely potent and can be fatal if taken internally, pennyroyal leaves and flowers are nontoxic and safe to use as herbs, Gladstar says. "Pennyroyal herb is one of the best for stimulating blood flow to the pelvis and for alleviating menstrual cramps," she says. And other herbal experts say that it relaxes spasmodic pain.

If your cramps are already building in intensity, and you need relief right now, Geller suggests mixing 3 teaspoons of cramp bark or black haw tincture with 5 teaspoons of valerian tincture. Then take 30 to 220 drops in a small amount of warm water as needed. "Every woman's cramps are different, so the amount of these herbs that will help to dispel cramps will also be different," Geller notes.

"After a month or two, as you improve your diet and use long-term herbal formulas to support your liver and boost calcium levels, cramp bark and valerian will probably be all you need when menstruation begins," says Gladstar.

Boost calcium and give cramps the boot. The same calcium-rich supplements and tea that can ease menstrual headaches can also help, over time, to reduce menstrual cramping, Gladstar says. Follow the directions on page 303 for relieving menstrual headaches, drinking three to four cups of high-calcium tea starting 10 days before menstruation begins.

Sip Rosemary's hormone-regulating tea for long-term help. Women who experience menstrual pain can lessen cramps, or even stop them before they start, by drinking a gentle, hormone-balancing blend that features dandelion, licorice, and yellow dock, among other herbs, Gladstar says.

"This tea helps improve liver function," she says. "It may sound like a funny place to start for menstrual cramps, but the health of the liver is dynamically related to the health of a woman's reproductive system. If the liver isn't functioning right, herbs like dandelion and burdock help stimulate it so that it processes hormones and nutrients optimally. In this formula, chasteberry helps balance hormone levels. And yellow dock and dandelion, among others, promote good digestion."

Combine ¼ part dried chasteberry with 1 part each of the dried roots of wild yam, ginger, and yellow dock, then add 2 parts each dandelion root, burdock root, licorice root, and sassafras bark. Brew the tea by adding 6 tablespoons of the blend to a quart of cold water in a medium pot. Simmer very slowly for 20 minutes, then strain. Have three to four cups daily for three weeks during each menstrual cycle. Stop drinking the tea while you are menstruating. If the tea is too bitter, try powdering the herbs in a blender and encapsulating them. (You can buy empty capsules at drugstores.) Take two capsules three times a day, says Gladstar.

Research has found that bitter compounds in dandelion root boost bile secretion from the liver. Yellow dock also contains compounds that research suggests can nudge sluggish bowels and promote the flow of bile, thus helping the liver to better process hor-

mones. Wild yam has been used traditionally for uterine pain and cramping. Ginger adds flavor and improves circulation, and Gladstar says that it brings better blood flow to the pelvis. Burdock, a traditional "blood purifier," has a diuretic action, research suggests. Licorice lends a sweet taste to this tea and has a place in traditional herbal medicine as a hormone regulator. Chasteberry is widely prescribed in Germany for menstrual problems. And sassafras is a traditional herb for improving liver function, Gladstar says.

Irregular Menstrual Cycles

Call it the myth of the "normal" 28-day menstrual cycle. While four weeks is often touted as the average or typical length of a woman's cycle, medical experts say that normal cycles for *real* women can actually range in length from 21 to 38 days. Younger women tend to have longer cycles—about 32 days for someone in her twenties—while women over 35 may have shorter cycles because of the natural aging of reproductive organs and the resulting hormonal changes.

In a perfect world, a menstrual cycle begins when the pituitary gland's hormones stimulate an egg to develop within a follicle in one of the ovaries. On the 14th day of the cycle, when you ovulate, the follicle bursts and the egg leaves the ovary, headed for the fallopian tubes and ultimately, the uterus. If the egg is fertilized, pregnancy begins. If not, the cycle ends with menstruation on day 28.

Then there are those month-to-month fluctuations. Your cycle can also vary in length due to illness, travel, or stress. And it's normal for cycles to become somewhat irregular as you approach menopause and hormone levels diminish.

So how do you know if your cycle is truly irregular and in need of "fixing"? If your periods are more than six weeks apart or less than three weeks apart, a hormone imbalance may be the problem.

"Herbs can help correct hormone imbalances, so a woman should not have to take hormone medications," Gladstar notes. "But first I look for situations that may not require herbal treatment. If a woman tells me she's just changed jobs, moved across the country, started a new relationship, or experienced some other life-changing event, I suggest that she wait a couple of months to see if her period will normalize itself. Often, it does. And if a woman has an unusual menstrual rhythm—she may have a three-week menstrual cycle and then a five-week cycle, for example—but has no other signs of hormone imbalance such as PMS, cramping, or ovulation problems, then my view is that this is simply her individual rhythm."

If your cycle is truly irregular, wildly fluctuating from month to month—short/long and without a pattern—these herbal strategies can help.

Start with chasteberry. "The single best herb for regulating menstrual periods is chasteberry," notes McNease. "Taken regularly as a tea or tincture, it will help balance

hormonal irregularities that lead to irregularities in the menstrual cycle."

McNease suggests taking one dropperful of chasteberry tincture three times a day in a small amount of warm water or having a cup of tea three times a day. Prepare the tea by lightly simmering 1 rounded teaspoon of crushed chasteberry seeds per cup of water for about 15 minutes. "Take a break during menstruation, and resume when bleeding has stopped," she suggests. "I think it's good to give the body a rest. Use chasteberry for two to four cycles to restore balance."

Chasteberry is widely used in Europe for menstrual and reproductive problems and is recommended to women there who have stopped using birth control pills to help reestablish normal menstruation and ovulation.

Add a sweet hormone balancer. Combine chasteberry with licorice root for sweet flavor and a more well-rounded hormone-balancing effect, McNease suggests. "Licorice contains phytoestrogens, which work on a different aspect of the menstrual cycle than chasteberry does, so the two can work well together. The body takes from both what it needs," she says.

Other herbalists also say that licorice root seems to regulate and normalize hormone production. And research suggests that when the body metabolizes licorice, some compounds become molecules with a structure like the body's own adrenal cortex hormones.

Combine the two herbs in equal parts: Take $\frac{1}{2}$ teaspoon each of chasteberry and licorice in tea three times a day, prepared as directed above, or a half-dropperful of each tincture three times a day for two to four menstrual cycles. Again, stop taking the herbs during menstrual bleeding.

Improve liver function with Chinese herbs. "In Traditional Chinese Medicine, the liver also regulates uterine function," McNease says. "You can't look at reproductive problems without considering the liver. My first choice for liver support that helps the uterus is the herb bupleurum (*chai hu*) in a Chinese herbal formula called *Xiao-Yao-Wan* or Bupleurum Sedative Pills. The meaning of the word *sedative* here is to relax the liver." You can buy this formula by mail from American companies that produce Traditional Chinese Medicine formulas (see "Where to Buy Herbs and Herbal Products" on page 462).

Among the herbs in this formula are bupleurum, which studies show can improve liver health, and white peony root, which has been shown to improve menstrual regularity and fertility.

"These are mild pills that can be taken for many months," McNease says. "Take 8 to 10 pills three or four times a day, for a total of 24 to 30 pills a day. These are dense, hard pills. If your digestion is weak, crush the pills, add them to hot water, and take as a tea. After a few cycles, you should notice that the timing is becoming regular. Then you can stop. But if you feel you need extra support after that, take the pills for the two weeks between ovulation and the start of menstruation."

Try Western liver-friendly plants. "I always treat the liver when I see a hormone imbalance," Gladstar says. "My women's 'root' tea combines liver-cleansing herbs like dandelion root with hormone balancers, including chasteberry and dang gui. And it tastes good. Any tea that you're going to drink for weeks at a time should taste really nice so you can look forward to your next cupful."

Blend Gladstar's tea by combining 1 part each of the dried root of licorice, pau d'arco, chasteberry, wild yam, and ginger with 3 parts sassafras bark, 2 parts dandelion root, $\frac{1}{2}$ part cinnamon bark, and $\frac{1}{4}$ part each of dang gui and orange rind (for flavor). For added sweetness, add a pinch of stevia (a naturally sweet herb), if desired. Add 4 to 6 tablespoons of this mixture to a quart of cold water in a medium pot, simmer slowly for 20 minutes, then strain. Drink three to four cups daily for three weeks of your menstrual cycle, pausing during menstruation, she suggests.

Use this tea for at least three menstrual cycles, Gladstar suggests. "You may see improvement sooner, but for a lasting change, I've seen good results with three months of treatment."

The actions of most of the herbs in this recipe were described earlier in this chapter. The pau d'arco is a liver-boosting botanical, says Gladstar.

Add a women's tonic. During menstruation, take a break from hormone-balancing blends and "feed" your reproductive system with a refreshing, vitamin- and mineral-rich tea, Gladstar suggests. The ingredients—red raspberry leaf, nettle, and peppermint—all contain calcium and other important nutrients.

Concoct this female tonic tea by mixing 2 parts each dried red raspberry leaf, dried nettle leaf, dried peppermint leaf, and dried lemongrass (for flavor) with 1 part each strawberry leaf and lady's-mantle. Add a pinch of stevia for extra sweetness if desired. Brew the tea by adding 6 tablespoons of this mix to a quart of cold water in a pan. Bring to a low boil, then remove from the heat and steep for 20 minutes. Strain, and enjoy three to four cups a day.

White Peony Root: Relief for Painful Menstruation—And More

As early as 900 B.C., the Chinese cultivated graceful, full-flowered peonies as both beautiful ornamental garden decorations and as widely used medicinal plants. White peony root, called *bai-shao* in Chinese, is a bitter, sour-flavored herbal remedy used for everything from abdominal pain to a charley horse in the calf and from abnormal or heavy menstruation to night sweats.

"White peony root has actions similar to dang gui in regulating menses," notes Cathy McNease, a professional member of the American Herbalists Guild from Ojai, California, and an instructor at the Santa Barbara College of Oriental Medicine and at Yo San University in Santa Monica. "While bai-shao nourishes the blood, dang gui both nourishes and moves it. In Traditional Chinese Medicine, we say bai-shao has a cooling effect, while dang gui has a warming effect. So if a person had feelings of heat, I would choose white peony root for helping with hormonal balance." It is available by mail order (see "Where to Buy Herbs and Herbal Products" on page 462).

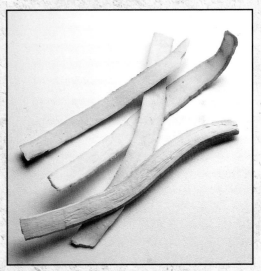

White peony can be found in Chinese botanical formulas, or you can add it to soups.

Heavy Menstrual Bleeding

If your menstrual flow soaks a tampon or sanitary pad every hour, or if your menstrual period lasts for more than seven days, you have what doctors call menorrhagia, an excessively heavy or long menstrual period.

Is copious flow a problem? It depends. For some women, heavy periods are simply an inconvenience. For others, they are debilitating and make life difficult for several days each month. And if your monthly flow is heavy, extra blood loss may lead to anemia, doctors say.

It also depends on what's behind the steady soaking. "If heavy bleeding comes on suddenly, a woman should first make sure that she is not having a miscarriage," notes Mary Bove, N.D., a naturopathic doctor, midwife,

Sarsaparilla: From Soft Drink to Digestive Aid

Once an ingredient in root beer, sarsaparilla's reputed healing powers have long been extravagantly touted—sometimes too extravagantly. An extract of this root was an ingredient in many nineteenth-century patent medicines promoted as blood purifiers and tonics, among other questionable uses.

More recently, sarsaparilla products have been advertised as performance-boosting, body-building stand-ins for anabolic steroids and marketed to athletes. Some products even claimed that sarsaparilla contained the male hormone testosterone. The trouble was, those claims could not be substantiated: Compounds in sarsaparilla called plant sterols haven't been shown to enhance athletic prowess and are not the same as human hormones.

But that doesn't mean that this native Latin American herb is useless. Research suggests that it has inflammation-fighting, liver-protecting actions. Herbalists today include sarsaparilla in women's health formulas to help heal skin problems and clear up digestive problems that can be associated with menstrual disorders.

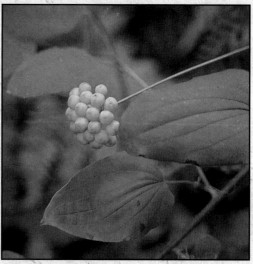

Traditionally, Mexican herbalists have recommended sarsaparilla for skin diseases and digestive problems.

and member of Britain's National Institute of Medical Herbalists who practices at the Brattleboro Naturopathic Clinic in Vermont. "Beyond that, the most common causes are fibroids, uterine polyps, dysfunctional uterine bleeding of unknown cause, and endometriosis."

If serious underlying causes have been ruled out or addressed and you still bleed heavily, herbalists suggest two strategies.

Press some astringent herbs into service. Astringent herbs such as yarrow, geranium root, and shepherd's purse can help stanch an episode of excessive menstrual bleeding, Dr. Bove says. Both shepherd's purse and yarrow have been used traditionally to slow profuse uterine bleeding, as have geranium root and lady's-mantle. Dr. Bove recommends using a formula that combines 2 parts shepherd's purse tincture with 1 part each of the tinctures of yarrow flowers, geranium root, and lady's-mantle. Take ½ to 1 teaspoon three or four times a day when menstrual flow is heavy.

Come to the aid of your liver. Correct hormone imbalances behind heavy bleeding by supporting liver function, Dr. Bove suggests. Burdock, dandelion, fennel, and milk thistle are traditional liver-support herbs. Milk thistle, the subject of more than 300 studies, contains silymarin, a substance that helps protect liver cells from toxic chemicals and at the same time stimulates the growth of new liver cells.

Create your own liver formula by using one or two of the herbs mentioned above. To take, make a tea using 1 teaspoon of herb or herb mix per cup of boiling water, steep 15 to 20 minutes, and strain. Have two to three cups a day. You can also take two milk thistle capsules three times a day or combine equal parts of the tinctures of your chosen liver herbs and have one teaspoon of the mix three times a day. You can take liver herbs for several months, says Dr. Bove.

Motion Sickness

PUT TRANQUILLITY BACK INTO TRAVEL

Conflicting information can make you sick, especially if you're in a car, plane, or boat.

If you're riding in the backseat of a car, in a boat, or on a plane, your brain is getting mixed signals. Your eyes scan the interior of the vehicle and tell your brain that you're sitting still, but your inner ear (which plays a role in balance) feels movement and tells your brain that you're going forward—fast. In some people, the confusion results in nausea, vomiting, cold sweats, and headache, especially if the ride is rocky.

Say you're on an airplane buffeted by head winds or rolling turbulence, for example. Your ears sense massive movement. But to your eyes, everything looks steady. In contrast, when you're at the wheel of a car or piloting a plane, your eyes tell you that you're moving, and so do your ears. So you don't get motion sickness when you're at the wheel or in the front seat, watching the scenery.

Herbs for Travelers

Some people are more prone to motion sickness than others. If it's a problem for you, you don't need to stay put. With the right herbs, herbalists say that you can enjoy travel on any conveyance short of an alien spacecraft.

Give ginger a thumbs-up. The clear winner in the race against motion sickness, gingerroot works better than dimenhydrinate,

Herbal Wisdom
Ginger Saves the Day

"I get motion sickness very easily. So on a recent trip, I took three ginger capsules before I left the hotel and three more just before getting on the boat. The trip lasted four hours. All around me, everyone was vomiting, but I was fine. I was really impressed with how well ginger worked."

—*Lois Johnson, M.D.*

the active ingredient in over-the-counter motion sickness medications such as Dramamine, says Daniel Gagnon, executive director of the Botanical Research and Education Institute, professional member of the American Herbalists Guild (AHG), and owner of Herbs, Etc., in Santa Fe, New Mexico.

In a one-of-a-kind study conducted in the 1980s, researchers blindfolded 36 students who claimed they were especially susceptible to motion sickness and asked them to sit in a tilted rotating chair. About 25 minutes before getting in the spinning chair, some of the students took a medication with dimenhydrinate, some took ginger, and some took a placebo. Of the students who took either dimenhydrinate or the placebo, none was able to last six minutes in the chair. But of those who took ginger, half endured the ride without getting sick.

Ginger may work by decreasing stomach movements caused by motion sickness or by dampening impulses to the brain that deliver messages about equilibrium. You need to give ginger time to kick in, says Lois Johnson, M.D., a physician in private prac-

tice in Sebastopol, California, and a professional member of the AHG. To be on the safe side, take either two ginger capsules, about a teaspoon of grated fresh ginger, or 60 drops of ginger extract (also called a tincture) an hour before your trip.

Use peppermint as a runner-up. Although not as effective as ginger, peppermint can also soothe your nausea. Like ginger, peppermint works most effectively when taken an hour before a trip, according to Gagnon. Pour hot water into a cup with a tablespoon of fresh peppermint. Cover it to keep the oils from escaping and let stand for five minutes. Then strain, says Gagnon. For times when you must travel at the last minute—say, your rich new friends invited you to drop everything and sail to Martha's Vineyard for lunch—keep a permanent stash of premade peppermint tea on hand. Then you can easily take a travel mug of tea along as you head out the door.

In a pinch, ask for chamomile. Although it's not as good as ginger or peppermint, chamomile can also help soothe away motion-induced nausea by calming the nerves in the stomach, says Gagnon. Because of its popularity, you may be able to find a chamomile tea bag during a flight or cruise (or take one along). Since fresh flowers are most effective, he says, keep a permanent stash of tea on hand so you can take a travel mug's worth with you to sip during trips. To make the tea, mix a tablespoon of the flowers with hot water and cover with a saucer. Let stand for 5 minutes, then strain.

Press Here for Relief

If you end up on a boat or plane or in a car with not an herb in sight, look to your wrist for relief.

Acupressure is the Chinese practice of pressing specific points to treat disease or relieve pain. Pressing the Neiguan point, located just below the crease between your palm and your wrist, can help ease nausea and symptoms of motion sickness, experts say.

Special elastic bands, available in drugstores, exert constant pressure on the Neiguan point throughout your trip. Or you can provide the pressure yourself when needed. Use the thumb of one hand to massage the underside of the opposite wrist just below the palm, says Dr. Johnson. If you exert enough pressure, you can suppress a wave of nausea.

Muscle Strains and Sprains

HERBAL SMARTS FOR ACHING PARTS

Sprains and strains can be so, well, stupid. It's one thing to twist an ankle on the tennis court. It's quite another to sprain it while doing something that you do every day, like stepping off a curb. Likewise, you feel less like a klutz if you hurt your back moving the couch than if you do it while lifting a basket of laundry.

But the fact of the matter is, strains (which affect muscles) and sprains (which affect joints) are embarrassingly common. With a strain, muscle tissue overstretches or tears outright, causing sharp pain followed by stiffness and tenderness. Strains usually affect the lower back and are often caused by lifting heavy objects incorrectly, such as by using your back instead of your legs, for example. A sprain, which forces a joint beyond its normal range of motion, is more serious. In a sprain, the ligaments—the tough bands of tissue that connect bones and hold joints in place—stretch or tear. The result: swelling, pain, and bruising. Sprains commonly affect the ankle, knee, finger, wrist, and shoulder.

Salves and Tinctures
à la Carte

Herbs can work as well as over-the-counter painkillers to ease the discomfort of a strain or sprain, says Douglas Schar, a practicing medical herbalist in London, editor of the *British Journal of Phytotherapy*, and author of *Backyard Medicine Chest*. And they won't upset your stomach, as aspirin and other nonsteroidal anti-inflammatory drugs sometimes can. What's more, "herbs contain agents that stimulate the healing process itself," says

Try RICE with Your Herbs

*T*he best way to reduce your risk of a sprain or strain is to keep in shape so that your muscles and joints are strong and flexible enough to withstand a sudden wrench or twist. But if, despite your best efforts, you sprain a joint or strain a muscle, use RICE—the standard treatment for joint or muscle injuries—along with herbal treatments.

The recipe for RICE (short for rest, ice, compression, and elevation) is simple. Keep the injured part immobile and don't put weight on it. Apply ice three times a day for 15 to 20 minutes at a time. Loosely wrap the injury in an elastic bandage to reduce pain and swelling. And elevate the injured part above the level of your heart, which will help reduce swelling.

If the pain is very severe, see a doctor immediately—it could be a sign of a fracture. If you have difficulty walking after hurting your back, seek medical help immediately.

Schar. Substances in some herbs, for example, increase the circulation of blood to the injured area, which encourages healing.

Any one of the following treatments suggested by herbalists may help ease the pain, swelling, and bruising of a strain or sprain.

Soak away the ache. A soothing aromatherapy soak can help ease the pain of a sprained ankle, and it smells heavenly, too. Add 5 drops of sandalwood oil, 5 drops of lemon oil, and 2 tablespoons of witch hazel to a basin of warm water. Soak the sprained area until the water cools. "Citron, a substance in the lemon oil, helps relieve pain, and the sandalwood promotes circulation to the area, which speeds healing," says Schar.

Sip some "herbal aspirin." "White willow bark is herbal aspirin," says Schar. It contains salicin, which is the natural version of salicylic acid, the active ingredient in aspirin. It also contains tannins, which help reduce swelling. So if bottled painkillers make you queasy, brew up some white willow bark tea. To make it, steep 1 teaspoon of white willow bark in a cup of boiling water for 15 minutes, then strain. Drink one cup three times a day until the pain and swelling subside.

Heal with a special kind of ginseng. Drinking tea made with a certain type of ginseng, *Panax notoginseng*, "is a fabulous treatment for strains," says Schar. In fact, Asian practitioners have long used this herb, also known as san qi ginseng, to treat sprains, strains, and bruises. To make a tea, steep 1 teaspoon of the herb in a cup of boiling water for 30 minutes. Drink one cup three times a day.

It's thought that substances called ginsenosides give san qi its healing power, but exactly how or why they work isn't known. Different ginsenosides are found in different varieties of ginseng. This type of ginseng (which should not be confused with more common ginseng species in the *Panax* genus) is hard to find, but it is available through some mail-order catalogs (see "Where to Buy Herbs and Herbal Products" on page 462).

Sip "sore muscle" tea. A tea made from poplar bark and cramp bark "can work wonders for sore muscles," says Schar. To brew up relief, add $1/2$ teaspoon of poplar bark and 1 teaspoon of cramp bark to a cup of boiling water. Simmer for 10 minutes, then strain. Drink one cup of this mixture four times a day.

This isn't the tastiest tea around, but it is good medicine, says Schar. Cramp bark contains scopoletin, which is thought to help fight pain, reduce swelling, and relax muscles, while poplar bark contains salicin, a natural painkiller. Cramp bark is sold through mail order. Poplar bark is difficult to find; try mail-order sources or Internet herb sites.

Comfort with comfrey. Comfrey, also known as bruisewort, is a traditional herbal remedy for joint pain and bruises. This comfrey poultice is an effective treatment for sprains, says 7Song, a professional member of the American Herbalists Guild (AHG) and director of the Northeast School of Botanical Medicine in Ithaca, New York. Chop a few handfuls of fresh comfrey and place it in a pot. Cover the herb with water and cook until tender. Let the mixture cool. When it's comfortably warm, strain off the water, place the herb directly on the sprain, and wrap the injury with an elastic bandage. When the comfrey cools, unwrap the bandage, rewarm the comfrey, and repeat. Apply this poultice two or three times a day until the pain and swelling improve.

Herbalists and scientists attribute comfrey's anti-inflammatory powers to a substance called allantoin. Tests in animals have shown that another substance in comfrey, rosmarinic acid, also reduces swelling.

Rub in relief. Substances in arnica called helenalins are believed to relieve pain and inflammation, while tannins in witch hazel bark relieve swelling and bruising. St.-John's-wort muffles or lessens pain signals to the brain and soothes the nerves irritated by inflamed muscles. A massage with oil containing all three combines the pain-relieving power of St.-John's-wort with the anti-inflammatory qualities of arnica and witch hazel bark, Schar says.

To make the oil, mix 4 ounces of tincture (also called an extract) of St.-John's-wort, 4 ounces of tincture of arnica flowers, and 1 ounce of tincture of witch hazel bark. Store the mixture in a glass jar. When you're ready to use it, blend 1 teaspoon of the mixture with 1 teaspoon of extra-virgin olive oil and massage into the affected area. Use the rub three times a day until the swelling and pain subside. (Don't use arnica on broken skin, however.)

Mix up some "dancing oil." Gently applied to the injured area, this blend of oils "is very effective for sprains and strains," says 7Song. First, combine equal amounts of infused oils of arnica, St.-John's-wort, and valerian root (see "Infused Oils" on page 101 for directions). Then add several drops of wintergreen and tea tree oil essential oils. To this, add vitamin E oil, which will help preserve the mixture, says 7Song. Lightly apply to the affected area as needed.

Rub on an ancient remedy. Consider seeking out an even stronger herb-based remedy called *Shang Shi Zhi Tong Gao* (translation: "attack and stop pain plaster"). This remedy includes clove oil, which contains the painkiller eugenol, and menthol, which eases pain and reduces swelling. The ingredients also promote the flow of blood and chi (qi) to the injury, says Eugene Zampieron, N.D., a naturopathic doctor, professional member of the AHG from Woodbury, Connecticut, and co-author of *The Definitive Guide to Arthritis*.

"It's a very effective remedy for sprains and strains," says Dr. Zampieron. Simply place the self-adhesive plaster directly over the injured area and leave it on for a day or so. (It's waterproof, so it won't come off in the shower.) Shang Shi Zhi Tong Gao is available in Chinese herb shops.

Try Tiger Balm. If you don't have any Shang Shi Zhi on hand or can't find it easily, try Tiger Balm, another old Chinese remedy that contains menthol and clove oils. It's not as strong, say Dr. Zampieron, but it's easier to find at health food stores.

Turn to a tincture. Sprains and strains add insult to injury when they confine you to your chair or bed. This remedy can help ease your discomfort, says 7Song. Combine the following tinctures (sometimes called ex-tracts): 3 parts passionflower, 2 parts mead-owsweet, 1 part valerian, 1 part motherwort, and ½ part St.-John's-wort. Take ½ to 3 dropperfuls at a time, as needed. "But always try one drop first of any internal remedy and watch for adverse reactions," says 7Song. "This is especially true for valerian."

Like white willow bark, meadowsweet contains the natural painkiller salicin, while motherwort helps relieve pain and muscle spasms. Passionflower and valerian are mild sedatives. And here's a surprise: While St.-John's-wort is most often used to treat mild depression, it also has a reputation among herbalists as a wound-healing herb.

Nicotine Withdrawal

QUIT SMOKING AND STAY CALM

Sara Spear, a 44-year-old writer from New York City, decided it was finally time to quit her pack-a-day habit. "I was reading about nutritional steps that women smokers could take to ease the health havoc smoking caused," says Spear, "and the further I got into the research, the more I realized that I had to quit—especially when I read that smoking could even make menopause more difficult. From that moment on, cigarettes began to taste terrible. But quitting terrified me. I worried that I would be tense and gain weight. And most of all, I dreaded giving up a ritual that had been a part of my life for so long."

But Spear did quit—cold turkey. And the first few days were absolutely hellish.

"I'd read that nibbling on cinnamon sticks or cloves was helpful for quitters, and it did help—a little," she recalls. "Whenever I wanted a smoke, I'd pop a clove into my mouth or I'd suck on the end of a cinnamon stick till the urge went away. But still I felt edgy and awful, and it was weeks before I felt remotely close to normal."

Herbal Liberation

If Spear had visited an herbalist, she might have had an easier, more peaceful transition. Here's one herbalist's take on tackling this tough challenge.

"When an herbalist advises someone who's

thinking about quitting, several questions should be addressed," says Douglas Schar, a practicing medical herbalist in London, editor of the *British Journal of Phytotherapy*, and author of *Backyard Medicine Chest*. "First, ask yourself whether you are really ready to stop smoking," he says. "Have you thought through how you're going to cope once you stop? Are you ready to make a commitment? Once a woman has considered all the angles and believes she's up to the challenge, she nearly has it made."

But commitment is only half the battle. Supportive herbal therapies can go a long way toward easing the cravings and calming your nerves.

Brew a calming infusion. "A blend of chamomile, skullcap, and catnip will help clear excess phlegm out of your lungs and will also calm you down," says Ellen Hopman, a professional member of the American Herbalists Guild (AHG) who practices in Amherst, Massachusetts. Chamomile is a gentle relaxant, as is skullcap, which has also been used to treat drug and alcohol addiction. Catnip is also a relaxant and has been used traditionally for respiratory ailments.

You can use either tinctures (also called extracts) or dried herbs, adding a total of 2 teaspoons of the three herbs per cup of boiling water. Brew as for an infusion for about ½ hour, says Hopman. (see "Teas and Infusions" on page 89). Drink ¼ cup four times a day.

Strengthen the nerves with herbs.

Herbal Wisdom
A Joyful Skill That Makes Sense

"In previous decades, older women taught herbalism as naturally as they taught their daughters and granddaughters how to sew and cook. But without the teachings of the grandmothers, we must find new ways to learn this ancient tradition. Thankfully, it's a remarkably easy and joyful skill to learn. Rooted in common sense and natural laws, much of what there is to learn about herbalism comes simply and naturally."

—*Rosemary Gladstar, herbalist, author, and teacher*

People smoke because it soothes their nerves, notes Schar, so the solution is to build up the nervous system with herbal medicines. He recommends a combination of St.-John's-wort and oatstraw in either tincture or tea form. "As a tea, I would suggest a tablespoon of oatstraw and a teaspoon of St.-John's-wort in a cup of boiling water three times a day. If using tinctures, I would suggest 3 milliliters of 1:5 St.-John's-wort and 3 milliliters of 1:1 oatstraw three times a day. Either, in combination with the patch or the nicotine replacement gum really works." (Do not use St.-John's-wort with antidepressants without medical approval.)

Try aversion therapy, at home. If, despite these herbal strategies, quitting is still tough, Hopman offers a way to turn off your cigarette urge permanently. Collect a few days' worth of your old cigarette butts and put them in a jar. Fill the jar with water and put it under your kitchen sink. Every morning, first thing, open the lid and smell the concoction. Eventually—probably sooner rather than later—you will develop an aversion to smoking, Hopman promises.

Overweight

MAKE HERBS YOUR ALLIES

*L*et's face it, ladies. If there really were a magic bullet for weight loss, we'd all have taken up target practice by now—and we'd be mighty good shots, too. But even herbalists say that the strongest natural remedies for unwanted pounds are still diet and exercise.

But wait: Don't discount herbs just yet. Chosen and used with care, they can give a sensible weight-loss program an extra edge, according to herbalists. "And under certain circumstances, herbs may make all the difference between success and failure," says Dana Myatt, N.D., a naturopathic physician in Phoenix.

The stakes are high. Obesity, caused by consuming more calories than your body can use, is often linked to your genetic heritage. Being overweight increases your risk of a host of chronic illnesses, including osteoarthritis, diabetes, high blood pressure, heart disease, and cancers of the breast, uterus, and colon. And it's not just the body that suffers. Overweight folks are also more likely to struggle with depression and anxiety.

Herbs can promote weight loss in a variety of ways, says Dr. Myatt. Some seem to trick your belly and brain into believing that you just aren't hungry. Others are thermogenic—that is, they rev up the body's metabolism so that it burns more calories more quickly. Still other herbs, classified as stimulants, contain substances such as caffeine that speed up certain body functions, such as circulation, heart rate, digestion, and respiration. Stimulant herbs are often also thermogenic. According

to herbalists, some of these herbs, like dandelion leaf, green tea, and nettle (described in more detail later) are as safe as, or safer than, prescription and over-the-counter weight-loss drugs. Herbal laxatives and preparations containing the herb ephedra (also known as ma huang), however, have been shown to have serious side effects, says Ara DerMarderosian, Ph.D., professor of pharmacognosy and medicinal chemistry at the Philadelphia College of Pharmacy and Science (for more information on these preparations, see "Weight-Loss Aids to Avoid"). And before you start any weight-loss program, check with your health-care practitioner.

As helpful as herbs can be, however, it's smart to remember the big picture.

First, woman does not lose weight by herbs alone. "Many people believe that there's one magic herb formula that will make the pounds just fall off their bodies," says Dr. Myatt. "No product can do that." So swallowing herbs along with a diet high in cheeseburgers and pastries or other high-fat, high-calorie foods isn't going to work.

Second, not all herbs have a lasting effect. Diuretics like buchu or uva-ursi, for example, simply rid your body of excess fluid. Water weight returns as quickly as it's lost—overnight.

An Herbal Arsenal

What this all boils down to is that when it comes to using herbs for weight loss, there

Weight-Loss Aids to Avoid

"Lose Weight Naturally." It's a powerful and seductive promise. But the truth is, "natural" doesn't always mean "safe."

Some natural weight-loss products contain herbs that are potentially dangerous or extremely toxic. Also, because the Food and Drug Administration (FDA) classifies weight-loss products as dietary supplements, not drugs, manufacturers don't need FDA approval to market them. This means that many of these products haven't been proven effective—or safe. In one case, the FDA strictly limits their use.

The FDA has linked the natural weight-loss products listed below to serious side effects and even death, so avoid them. Period.

Herbal laxatives. Commonly sold as "dieter's teas," laxative herbs include cascara, senna, buckthorn, aloe, and rhubarb root. These products can cause stomach cramps and diarrhea. If they're overused, your bowels may no longer function without them. Most serious, these products deplete the blood of the mineral potassium, which can lead to paralysis and irregular heartbeat. At least four women with a history of eating disorders have died after misusing these products.

Ephedra. Research on the effects of ephedra, also known as ma huang, on weight loss has been modestly favorable. But in high doses, it can raise blood pressure, increase heart rate, and overstimulate the central nervous system, which controls the brain. Since 1996, the FDA has received more than 800 reports of side effects linked with the use of ephedra, including heart palpitations, seizures, stroke, chest pain, and heart attack. This herb has also caused at least two deaths.

Herbal fen-phen. Ephedra is the active ingredient in this "natural" version of the dangerous diet-drug combination, fenfluramine and phentermine, which was pulled from the market when it was discovered that it caused heart-valve problems. Herbal fen-phen has not been shown to work in clinical trials. Also, its misuse is associated with severe side effects, from nervousness and heartbeat irregularities to death from heart attack and stroke.

are no easy answers, and no miracles, either. Still, when teamed with a sensible program of diet and exercise, you may find that herbs work for you, say herbalists. Here's the strategy that's most likely to aid your weight-loss efforts, starting with what you eat and drink.

Crunch, crunch, crunch. Most weight-loss experts agree: If you want to lose weight, eat more foods high in fiber, such as fruits, vegetables, beans, potatoes, and whole grains. High-fiber foods take up more space in your stomach than fat-laden fare, and they tend to be low in fat and calories.

But fiber-rich foods do more than shush a growling tummy. Fiber may slightly reduce the number of calories your body absorbs from food each day.

Fiber also stabilizes levels of glucose, or blood sugar, your body's main source of fuel, says Dr. Myatt. Some people produce higher-than-normal amounts of insulin, the hormone that controls the rate at which blood sugar is absorbed by cells. In response to this abnormally high insulin level, the body manufactures more fat cells than normal. The more fat cells you have, the slower your metabolism is likely to become, and the more likely you are to gain weight. Fiber-rich foods don't appear to stimulate the production of insulin as much as foods made with white flour, such as white bread and baked goods, do.

Consume from 25 to 30 grams of fiber a day, recommends Dr. Myatt. A sample high-fiber menu might include a bowl of all-bran cereal for breakfast (some brands contain as much as 20 grams of fiber per cup), a large fruit salad accompanied by a couple of slices of whole-grain toast for lunch, and a can of water-packed tuna over a mountain of crisp greens and veggies for dinner.

Consider a fiber supplement. Despite their best intentions, "many folks just can't eat 25 grams of fiber a day," says Dr. Myatt. If this sounds like you, consider taking two dietary fiber supplements three times a day, she suggests. Several studies have shown that taking five grams of supplemental fiber a day can help women shed pounds. Dietary fiber supplements are available in drugstores and health food stores. And don't skimp on water: Too much fiber plus not enough liquid can equal severe constipation. So swallow the capsules with a full eight-ounce glass of water at the beginning of every meal, she says.

Pepper your food with cayenne. Add a dash of cayenne pepper (also known as red pepper) or hot-pepper sauce (like Tabasco) to your food several times a day, suggests Dr. Myatt. The active ingredient in cayenne pepper, capsaicin, is a stimulant of saliva, salivary amylase (an enzyme involved in the digestion of starch), and hydrochloric acid, which improve the digestive process, she says. "People with sluggish digestion tend to gain weight. Those with efficient digestion tend to maintain a normal weight."

Capsaicin may also accelerate metabolism. In research conducted at Oxford Polytechnic Institute in England, dieters who added one teaspoon of red-pepper sauce and one teaspoon of mustard to every meal raised their metabolic rates by as much as 25 percent.

Go green. Drink one cup of green tea with a meal two or three times a day, suggests Dr. Myatt. Green tea contains caffeine, a stimulant that revs up metabolism, as well as theobromine, a compound similar to caffeine. Depending on how long it's steeped, one cup of green tea contains from 40 to 100 milligrams of caffeine—up to the amount in one cup of coffee. So if you're cutting back on caffeine for other reasons, don't drink more than two or three cups.

Green tea has something that coffee doesn't, however: It's rich in vitamin C and flavonoids, compounds that are potent antioxidants. These protective nutrients help reduce the risk of illnesses such as heart disease and cancer, especially of the colon. And it promotes weight loss due to its thermogenic effect, which improves metabolism, Dr. Myatt says.

Green tea is sold in health food stores and some supermarkets. It is sold as loose, dried tea leaves and in tea bags, which is an easier form to use for some people, she says. It also comes in capsule form. The recommended dosage is usually two capsules three times a day, says Dr. Myatt, but she prefers the tea because "you get a lot more of the antioxidants in a cup than you will in a pill."

Try a five-herb tincture. Schisandra berry (which means "five-flavor seed" in Chinese) grows in the most remote parts of the world. Gum guggul is extracted from a plant related to myrrh, and bladderwrack is a type of brown seaweed. Team these exotic ingredients with some basic herbs, and the result is a remedy that "very gently helps weight loss along by improving metabolism," says David Winston, a professional member of the American Herbalists Guild (AHG) and founder of Herbalist and Alchemist, an herbal medicine company in Washington, New Jersey. Blend the following tinctures (also called extracts) in an eight-ounce or larger bottle (all available at health food stores): 1 ounce of nettle, 1 ounce of dandelion leaf, 1 ounce of bladderwrack, 2 ounces of guggul, and 2 ounces of Chinese schisandra berry. Take ½ to 1 teaspoon three times a day. (Hold your nose, though: This concoction isn't the most pleasant-tasting around, says Winston.)

Bladderwrack is a folk remedy for overweight. Schizandrin, the active ingredient in schisandra berry, gently stimulates metabolism. Dandelion is used by herbalists to boost the liver's secretion of bile, which helps break down the fats in food. Nettle is rich in minerals, which help maintain overall health during weight loss, Winston says. And

Herbal Wisdom
Your Connection to the Green World

"Plants teach us about the magic and beauty of life, the life force inherent in the green world. Working with herbs, digging in the earth, making herbal preparations, and using them for health and healing is the best way possible to re-establish our connection to our wise woman tradition of healing."

—*Rosemary Gladstar, herbalist, author, and teacher*

guggul helps normalize thyroid function, which is sometimes disturbed in overweight people.

See about seaweed. In rare cases, a sluggish thyroid gland can cause weight gain. Seaweed is rich in iodine, a natural thyroid stimulant, says Ellen Hopman, a professional member of the AHG who practices in Amherst, Massachusetts. "It's also a good source of essential trace minerals, such as chromium," she says. Hopman recommends taking seaweed supplements (usually kelp, because of its especially high iodine content) with cayenne supplements. Take one capsule of each once in the morning and once at night, always right after meals. "Never take cayenne on an empty stomach. It won't hurt you, but it will cause a burning sensation," says Hopman.

You'll find kelp and cayenne supplements in most drugstores and health food stores. If you suspect that your weight problems are due to a sluggish thyroid, or if you're taking thyroid medication of any kind, you should check with your doctor before considering this remedy.

Poison Ivy, Poison Oak, and Poison Sumac

STOP SUMMER'S MOST ANNOYING RASHES

At work in the lush herb gardens of the California School of Herbal Studies in Forestville or at home on her family's organic farm in Sebastopol, herbalist Leslie Gardner has learned to keep a sharp eye out for the telltale look of a poison oak plant: Three leaflets with scalloped edges.

"Poison oak is even more common out here than poison ivy is on the East Coast," says Gardner, a professional member of the American Herbalists Guild (AHG) and a staff member at the school. "Even if you know what it looks like and know where it grows, sometimes you just can't avoid it, particularly in the winter in our mild climate. When poison oak loses its leaves, it looks dead, but it still retains its potency." Poison ivy and poison oak both cause rashes. So does poison sumac, a shrub or small tree with white berries. Even experienced, well-trained herbalists like Gardner occasionally find themselves coping with an itchy, blistery rash, courtesy of a run-in with a poison plant.

No matter where you live, if you brush against the leaves of poison ivy, oak, or sumac, you'll come in contact with urushiol—a thick, oily substance in the plant's resin that provokes that annoying rash. A few lucky people aren't allergic to urushiol and can hike through poison plants or rip them out of the garden without fear. But for most of us, it's a different story. Even indirect contact with urushiol—handling clothing or shoes that have brushed against a poison plant, for example, or petting a dog or cat that has just romped in the poison ivy patch—can raise those itchy blisters.

A severe case can cause unbearable itching, a possible infection may develop, or it may spread to your face or eyes. If that happens, a cortisone shot may help.

Fight Fire with Herbs

Herbal remedies can help minimize the results of a poison-plant attack. But the first order of business is to get urushiol off your skin.

"Pay scrupulous attention to cleaning your skin," says 7Song, a professional member of the AHG and director of the Northeast School of Botanical Medicine in Ithaca, New York, "Wash yourself as soon as possible with soap. Fels Naphtha soap is the classic, but any strong detergent soap will do. Take off all clothing and wash it. And be careful around animals that have had contact with poison plants." Then try these herbal anti-itch tactics recommended by top herbalists.

Scrub with jewelweed or mugwort. Out in the woods? Can't wash? Don't wait until you're back home to get rid of urushiol.

Herbalists say that the leaves and juicy stalks of jewelweed, a tall plant with succulent stems that grows in damp soil along roadsides and woodland edges, make an effective, poison-plant-stopping scrub. Research suggests that a compound in jewelweed called lawsone seems to block urushiol from latching onto skin cells by binding to the same spots. Lawsone may be most abundant in the knobby, red prop-roots that grow at the bottom of the stalk. After exposure to a rash-making plant, crush the leaves and stem and use this wad of greenery to rub down any exposed skin, suggests 7Song.

If jewelweed isn't common in your area, look for mugwort, which grows in the West, suggests Gardner. Crush the leaves and stems and rub on exposed skin the same as you would with jewelweed.

Soothe yourself with grindelia. A traditional remedy among Europeans and Native Americans alike, grindelia (also known as gumweed) is endorsed enthusiastically by herbalists from coast to coast for taming the itch of poison oak, poison ivy, and poison sumac.

As soon as possible after you've brushed up against one of these poison plants, wipe exposed skin with crushed grindelia leaves or grindelia tincture (also called an extract), or use alcohol wipes to help remove the oil, suggests Sharleen Andrews-Miller, faculty member at the National College of Naturopathic Medicine in Portland, Oregon, and associate medicinary director at the college's public clinic.

Stem the irritation with tincture or tea. If you're already itching, wash the rash with an itch-fighting grindelia tincture, Andrews-Miller suggests. Or add some grindelia tincture to an ointment and apply it to the rash. (For information on how to make an ointment, see "Salves and Ointments" on page 110.)

You can sip grindelia for relief, too. "When itching is intense, take 10 to 20 drops of grindelia tincture in ½ cup of hot water, as often as every four hours," Gardner adds.

Conquer itching with a clay and herb poultice. A simple "mud pack" made with bentonite clay (available at health food stores) and enough water to create a thick goo can help control the itch and dry up blisters, herbalists say. Spread the clay over the affected area and let air-dry. Keep it on until the clay wears off or gets itchy, says Andrews-Miller. Wash off the residue.

You can customize the pack by adding ¼ to ½ teaspoon of powdered Oregon grape root to fight off infection, suggests Gardner. A traditional antimicrobial, Oregon grape is widely used by modern herbalists to battle external infections. If the rash feels hot, add a droplet of lavender essential oil to the clay poultice, she suggests. "That will produce a cooling feeling," she says.

Or simply dab on some dry facial clay—the kind used for facial masks—to help dry up the rash, suggests 7Song. If you see pus or other signs of infection, visit your doctor.

Soothe inflammation with echinacea. An echinacea wash, made with 1 part echinacea tincture diluted in 3 parts water, helps fight inflammation of blistered, irritated skin, says Paul Bergner, clinical director of the Rocky Mountain Center for Botanical Studies in Boulder, Colorado, editor of *Medical Herbalism*, and author of *The Healing Power of Garlic* and *The Healing Power of Echinacea, Goldenseal, and Other Immune System Herbs*. Use the wash on affected skin several times a day. A review study in Germany showed that echinacea helps reduce inflammation when applied externally, says Bergner.

Leafy Relief for Poison-Plant Attacks

"Jewelweed and grindelia are the top herbs for poison ivy and poison oak," notes Leslie Gardner, an herbalist in Sebastopol, California, professional member of the American Herbalists Guild and a staff member at the California School of Herbal Studies in Forestville.

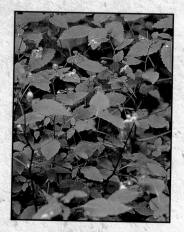

Found in shady wetlands from Canada to Georgia and west to Oklahoma and Missouri, jewelweed has a long history as an anti-rash botanical. The Potawatomi Indians used the juice of jewelweed leaves to relieve poison ivy's itch. The Omaha crushed the leaves and stems and applied them to rashes. Look for its tall, translucent stems and hanging, trumpet-shaped, yellow or orange flowers.

Grindelia, common in the West and Southwest, was used by Native Americans, including the Costanoan and Mahuna, to ease skin eruptions like poison oak. Look for its yellow, daisylike flowers with tiny, sticky leaves below the petals. Mugwort, which is also common in the West, can be used in the same way as jewelweed or grindelia. It has hairy stems, often red in color, and leaves that are dark green on top and whitish and woolly underneath.

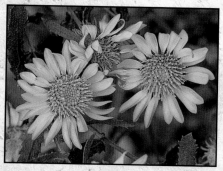

Outdoors, rub crushed grindelia leaves, jewelweed leaves and stalks, or mugwort leaves and stalks on bare skin that's been exposed to a poison-plant attack. (Contrary to what you may have heard, rescue plants like jewelweed don't always thrive conveniently close to troublemakers like poison ivy. Sometimes they do, sometimes they don't.) Grindelia is also available commercially as a tincture.

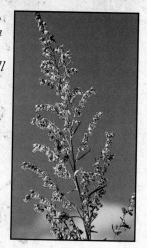

To stop a poison ivy, poison oak, or poison sumac rash before it even gets started, call on the itch stoppers: jewelweed, also known as touch-me-not (top); grindelia, also known as gumweed (center); and mugwort (right).

Sip a calming herb. Oatstraw, skullcap, valerian root, and passionflower—all traditional nerve-calming teas—can quiet the irritability that sometimes takes over when you've got a bad case of poison oak, ivy, or sumac, says Gardner.

"I've seen and experienced how these herbs called nervines can really help get you out of that intensely irritable state that seems to occur, especially with a poison oak rash," she says. Make a quick calmer by adding 2 to 3 dropperfuls of a tincture of one of these herbs to $\frac{1}{2}$ cup of hot water. Drink up to three half-cups a day, Gardner suggests.

Pregnancy

SAFE HERBS FOR MOTHER—AND CHILD

Pregnancy is a time of powerful new experiences: Hormones shift and surge, often taking your emotions along for the ride. New life stirs within. You watch as your body undergoes enormous changes. And you look ahead, with joy and a little trepidation, to a future changed forever by the arrival of a tiny new daughter or son.

Of course, you want the best for yourself and your growing child. So you eat well, take the recommended nutritional supplements, cut back on coffee (or stop the java jive entirely), give alcoholic drinks the cold shoulder, and don't even consider smoking. But on the nine-month journey toward motherhood, sometimes you need more: A morning-sickness soother or something to help you sleep better. A lotion that can help prevent stretch marks. Or a tea to quench heartburn.

That's where gentle, "pregnancy-approved" herbs, recommended by herbalists experienced at advising women during preg-

nancy, come in. Chosen wisely and used prudently, herbs can reduce or eliminate many discomforts commonly experienced during this special time, without harmful side effects for you or your baby, says Mary Bove, N.D., a naturopathic doctor, midwife, and member of Britain's National Institute of Medical Herbalists who practices at the Brattleboro Naturopathic Clinic in Vermont. That's good news for pregnant women, who usually must avoid many prescription drugs and over-the-counter medications.

But that's not all. Botanicals can also help a pregnant woman in two unique ways—by providing an extra source of nutrition that helps keep a mom-to-be healthy and by helping to prepare her body for the work of labor, birth, and breastfeeding.

And by taking time out for a cup of nettle-raspberry tea, rubbing your belly with lavender-almond oil, or even crushing a mint sprig under your nose to ward off morning sickness, you also give yourself much-needed moments of peace and calm. In those nurturing moments, you may feel closer to the natural world—a satisfying experience while your body builds a new human being.

Trustworthy Botanicals for Mothers-to-Be

Yes, you *can* use herbs with confidence during pregnancy—by following guidelines that top herbalists say will safeguard your baby's well-being and enhance a healthy pregnancy. The first rule of thumb: If you are pregnant, always check with your health-care practitioner before taking any herbs.

"Pregnancy is a special time," Dr. Bove notes. "You're carrying a delicate, developing baby. You have to remember that any constituent in any herb you choose to take might reach the fetus through the placenta and could affect the baby, especially during the first three months, when all organ systems are developing."

Your pregnant body is special, too. "New and changing hormone levels help to maintain your pregnancy," Dr. Bove says. "You don't want to take anything—including an herb—that might affect that delicate hormonal balance or stimulate the uterus, particularly in the first few months."

Few, if any, medical studies have examined the ways in which herbs can affect pregnant women and their babies, Dr. Bove says. "It would be unethical to expose a pregnant woman to something that might harm her," she explains. "So there hasn't been much research in this area, and we don't have a lot of information. As a result, caution is the best approach." Reputable herbal healers who work with pregnant women, therefore, offer these guidelines for using herbs safely and wisely during pregnancy.

Avoid herbs during the first trimester. Once you know that you are pregnant, stop taking fertility herbs, medicinal herbs, and even nutritional and tonic herbs, Dr. Bove suggests. "As much as I believe that herbs enhance health, the first three months of pregnancy can be a tenuous time. The fetus is delicate, your hormones are delicate, and the connection between you and the baby is delicate," she says. "Be healthy with good food, lots of water, gentle exercise, time spent in sunlight, love, laughter, and spiritual medicine. As much as possible, don't use herbs."

The exception to the rule is that if you have morning sickness, there are gentle herbal remedies you can try at home. But always consult an herbalist who's familiar with pregnancy and a health-care practitioner who's familiar with herbs about safe remedies.

Later, choose mild, nutrient-rich botanicals. Herbs such as alfalfa, dandelion root and leaf, lemon balm, nettle, oatstraw, and red raspberry are so gentle yet so packed with vitamins and minerals that herbalists regard them as "food herbs," not as medicinal plants. These herbs can be used daily during pregnancy with no residual buildup in your body, notes herbalist Rosemary Gladstar, director of the Sage Mountain herbal education center in East Barre, Vermont, and author of *Herbal Healing for Women*.

"Many of these herbs also complement the body's work during pregnancy," says Dr. Bove. When sipped as a tea, for example, red raspberry leaf adds vitamins and minerals and also contains a compound that helps the uterine muscle function effectively during labor and birth. Nettle, another nutrient-rich herb, also helps prompt milk production after birth. And fennel seed, a gentle morning-sickness soother, also has enjoyed a centuries-long reputation as a galactagogue—an herb that promotes lactation.

Steer clear of herbs that work against pregnancy. So many herbs are considered off-limits during pregnancy that herbalists often find it simpler to suggest a few safe herbs for home use and leave it at that. But it is helpful to know *why* many herbs that are normally considered beneficial are unsafe for a woman who is carrying a child.

According to Gladstar, pregnant women should avoid hormone-influencing herbs that can stimulate the menstrual cycle, such as dang gui, pennyroyal, yarrow, and motherwort. They could cause premature contractions and even miscarriage. Herbs that contain strong alkaloids, such as goldenseal, poke root, and blue cohosh, could be potentially damaging due to their marked physiological action on the body. Herbs with a strong action on the bowels, such as senna, may cause uterine contractions. Herbs rich in volatile oils, such as peppermint, may irritate the fetus's central nervous system and should not be taken internally. And any herb with a powerful medicinal effect, such as goldenseal, could irritate your system or your baby's in unknown ways if taken internally. Topical use of goldenseal—in a salve, for example—is fine, however, says Gladstar.

Less is more. A woman's metabolism slows down during pregnancy, thanks to hormonal changes. "Digestion slows down. The bowels slow down. So any herb you eat, drink, or take in capsule form will stay in your body longer," notes Aviva Romm, a certified professional midwife, herbalist, and professional member of the American Herbalists Guild who practices in Bloomfield Hills, Michigan, and is the author of *The Natural Pregnancy Book* and *Natural Healing for Babies and Children*. "The longer it stays, the more gets absorbed," she explains.

Therefore, herbalists recommend pregnant women use smaller quantities of herbs. "When I suggest a tincture (also called an extract), such as a ginger tincture for nausea, the dosages are much lower for a pregnant woman," says Romm. "This can be advantageous because its economical. You can use much less and still get good results."

The amount in a daily dose of tincture is perfectly safe, says Lisa Murray-Doran, N.D., a naturopathic doctor and instructor at the Canadian College of Naturopathic Medicine in Toronto.

In doubt? Consult an expert. If you have an ongoing illness or develop a health problem that doesn't respond to the gentle home remedies suggested here, consult an herbalist who is familiar with pregnancy and a health-care practitioner who is familiar

Aviva's Pregnancy Tea

This citrus-and-mint-flavored beverage supplies a pregnant woman with fluid as well as small amounts of nutrients and herbal constituents that can help with birth and breastfeeding, according to Aviva Romm, a certified professional midwife, herbalist, and professional member of the American Herbalists Guild who practices in Bloomfield Hills, Michigan, and is the author of The Natural Pregnancy Book and Natural Healing for Babies and Children.

According to Romm, the raspberry leaves contain calcium and magnesium and help prepare the uterus for labor. Nettle, which contains vitamins and minerals, can help prevent hemorrhaging during delivery, and lemon balm, which adds a pleasant, citrus-mint flavor, has a calming influence. Oatstraw is also a nerve soother. Rose hips contain vitamin C and add a tart flavor and cranberry red color to the tea. Alfalfa contains vitamins A, D, E, B_6, and K as well as calcium, magnesium, and iron. Spearmint adds another minty note.

"Start drinking this tea in the second trimester, at about the 12th week of pregnancy," Romm says. "You can continue enjoying it throughout pregnancy, during labor, and after delivery, too. It helps with milk production." Drink one to four cups a day, she suggests.

"We keep a jar in the refrigerator, and everyone in my house drinks it," notes Romm, who has four children. "It tastes great hot or cold."

This tea is also good frozen. You can suck on ice pops made with it (just freeze it in small paper cups or ice-pop molds) during labor. Or drink it as a nutritive iced tea after labor, suggests Lisa Murray-Doran, N.D., a naturopathic doctor and instructor at the Canadian College of Naturopathic Medicine in Toronto.

Here's the recipe.

8 tablespoons raspberry leaf
8 tablespoons nettle
4 tablespoons oatstraw
2 tablespoons lemon balm
2 tablespoons rose hips
2 tablespoons spearmint leaf

Combine the herbs and store in a jar or airtight container. To prepare the tea, add 4 tablespoons of the herb blend to a quart jar, then fill the jar with boiling water. Cover and steep for at least 30 minutes. Strain and sweeten with honey, if desired.

Makes 4 cups

with herbs, suggests Romm. "Because you can't see what's happening with the baby, extreme caution is required when choosing and using herbs," she notes. "Pregnancy is not a good time to experiment with herbs. It's a time to be safe."

For general well-being, try Aviva's Pregnancy Tea. For gentle herbal remedies that soothe pregnancy- and birth-related discomforts, try these suggestions from herbal-healing experts. And remember to talk with your health-care practitioner about any pregnancy-related discomfort you may experience, no matter how small.

Morning Sickness

Herbal remedies for the nausea and vomiting of morning sickness work best if taken as soon as you begin feeling mild queasiness, notes Dr. Murray-Doran. There is no single cure-all for morning sickness. The fact is, one remedy may help you for a while, then suddenly have little effect. If that happens, try another, Romm suggests.

Carry "relief seeds." Tote a small handful of aniseed in a plastic bag in your pocket or purse and nibble two or three at the first sign of queasiness, Romm suggests. "This is a gentle, traditional anti-nausea remedy," she notes. Research shows that volatile oils in aniseed have stomach-settling properties. And expectant moms may get an herbal bonus from anise: This herb has also been used traditionally to prompt milk production, perhaps thanks to estrogenic compounds that include dianethole and photoanethole.

Sweeten a roiling tummy with meadowsweet. Herbal experts say that meadowsweet contains pain-relieving, digestion-settling constituents that reduce excess acidity and ease nausea. Use 1 tablespoon of meadowsweet per cup of boiling water, steep 20 minutes, and strain. Have up to two cups of this gentle tummy soother a day, Romm suggests.

Nix nausea with minty scents. Sniffing peppermint oil or inhaling the scent of crushed fresh peppermint leaves can quell queasiness, Romm notes. Aromatherapists often recommend smelling peppermint for nausea. While research shows that volatile oils in peppermint relax smooth muscles in the digestive system, experts aren't sure why the aroma of peppermint also seems to quell nausea.

"Put a few drops of peppermint essential oil on a little cotton ball or small piece of cloth and carry it in a little glass jar with a tight-fitting lid or a plastic bag with a zipper closure. Open it and sniff when you feel the first waves of nausea," she suggests. "Or pick a sprig of fresh mint and keep it in your pocket. That's what I did when I was pregnant and had to ride in the car. The smell of peppermint oil relaxes that spasmy, sick feeling."

One caution: Never take peppermint essential oil, or any essential oil, internally. Even small quantities can be toxic. And pregnant women should not drink peppermint tea: The volatile oils may overstimulate an unborn child's nervous system, according to Romm.

Discover dandelion. Research shows that bitter compounds in dandelion stimulate digestion. Taken as tea or a tincture, dandelion can very effectively neutralize that vexing, sour taste in the back of your throat that comes with morning sickness, Romm notes. Use 20 to 40 drops in a small amount of warm water (about $1/4$ cup) as often as every two hours. "Do not exceed six doses a day," she says.

Go for ginger-aid. In small quantities, ginger is a safe anti-nausea herb for most pregnant women, Dr. Bove says. "Ginger works effectively in small amounts. It helps digestion and warms up the digestive tract. Try adding a teaspoon of tincture to 2 tablespoons of water, then take 10 to 15 drops of that diluted mixture every 15 minutes or so." Or make a tea by adding 1 teaspoon of grated gingerroot or a one-inch-long chunk of peeled gingerroot to a cup of boiling water and steep for 10 to 20 minutes, suggest Romm and Dr. Murray-Doran. Strain and sip throughout the day. Have two to three cups a day, they suggest.

Are Tinctures Okay for Moms-to-Be?

Herbalists agree that gentle teas are the best way to take herbs during pregnancy. Sometimes, however, if an herb is extremely bitter-tasting or you don't have time to make tea, you may want to reach for a ready-made tincture (also called an extract). But most tinctures are alcohol-based. Are they safe to use during pregnancy?

"In small quantities, alcohol-based extracts pose no problems for most women and babies," notes Aviva Romm, a certified professional midwife, herbalist, and professional member of the American Herbalists Guild (AHG) who practices in Bloomfield Hills, Michigan, and is the author of *The Natural Pregnancy Book* and *Natural Healing for Babies and Children.* "You can evaporate some of the alcohol by slowly adding your drops of tincture to ¼ cup of boiling water."

Some alcohol will remain, however, prompting some herbalists to recommend glycerin-based tinctures as an alternative during pregnancy. "They are another option," Romm notes, "but glycerin does not extract all the compounds in an herb that alcohol can, so glycerin tinctures are not always as effective as alcohol-based tinctures. And for a woman with morning sickness, glycerin may be too sweet—it could make you feel nauseated all over again."

If you use glycerin-based tinctures, limit yourself to 2 teaspoons per day, suggests Amanda McQuade Crawford, a practicing herbalist in Ojai, California, professional member of the AHG, member of Britain's National Institute of Medical Herbalists, president of the American College of Integrative Medicine in Albuquerque, and author of *Herbal Remedies for Women.* Glycerin can be slightly laxative.

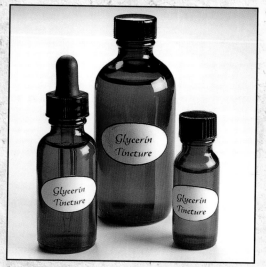

Glycerin-based tinctures are an option for women who want to avoid any trace of alcohol during pregnancy.

"If morning sickness is bad, try adding ½ teaspoon each of spearmint and meadowsweet to the ginger tea," Dr. Murray-Doran suggests. "The combination tastes wonderful."

You can also create your own ginger ale by mixing ¼ to 1 teaspoon of ginger syrup with 1 cup of seltzer water. Dr. Bove recommends Ginger Wonder Syrup, available in health food stores and by mail order (see "Where to Buy

Herbs and Herbal Products" on page 462). "It's really quick and tastes really good," she notes.

Researchers have found that ginger allays nausea associated with motion sickness more effectively than widely used motion sickness medications. One caution: Do not use ginger if you have a history of miscarriage, and do not exceed recommended doses. In larger amounts, ginger could cause miscarriage in early pregnancy, Dr. Bove says.

Heartburn and Indigestion

If fiery heartburn pain makes post-meal-times miserable, remember a few basic rules: Avoid spicy food, eat small meals, and don't lie down for two to three hours after eating, Dr. Murray-Doran suggests. Beyond that, these botanicals can quench heartburn discomfort that seems to come later in pregnancy and promote good digestion.

Soothe with slippery elm.   To quell that fiery feeling, stir 1 teaspoon of slippery elm powder into a cup of boiling water or warm milk. Add a dash of cinnamon and a teaspoon of honey, then sip. "Slippery elm can be taken during a bout of heartburn and can also be taken on a regular basis to help prevent it," Romm notes.

The soothing power of slippery elm comes from its rich supply of mucilage, slippery substances that coat and protect inflamed mucous membranes, including those burned by stomach acids when heartburn strikes, experts say.

Pour a citrus-mint digestion-helper. Perk up your digestive system and overcome indigestion with this delicious after-meal tea: In a teapot or heatproof quart jar, combine 1 teaspoon each of lemon balm, meadowsweet, chamomile, spearmint, crushed aniseed, and organic orange or tangerine rind (for flavor), Romm suggests. Add 2 cups of boiling water and steep for 15 minutes. Strain, sweeten with 1 teaspoon of honey if desired, and sip while warm.

Lemon balm, a traditional digestion calmer, is approved in Germany for easing digestive spasms. Research has found that volatile oils in chamomile relieve spasms and also calm digestion. Spearmint eases digestion and calms the stomach, says Romm.

Cool the burn with fennel.   Aromatic oils in fennel seed also ease heartburn pain, Gladstar notes. Make some tea by adding 1 cup of boiling water to 1 teaspoon of crushed fennel seeds. Steep for 15 minutes, then sip.

Constipation

Hormonal shifts are only the first of many possible reasons for constipation in pregnancy, Dr. Murray-Doran notes. "Later in pregnancy, when the uterus is huge, it can press on blood vessels that supply the intestines," she says. "This can slow things down even more. So can a lack of exercise—if you're feeling really big, you may not want to get up and walk around. But a half-hour walk every day can really help get your bowels moving."

So can eating fiber-rich fruits and vegetables and drinking eight eight-ounce glasses of water daily, she notes. Beyond constipation-easing lifestyle changes, these gentle herbal remedies can also help get your bowels moving normally again.

Move it with dandelion.   Dandelion root tincture can give sluggish bowels a

Relieve Heartburn with Slippery Elm Lozenges

For quick and convenient relief from heartburn during pregnancy, suck on slippery elm lozenges, suggests Aviva Romm, a certified professional midwife, herbalist, and professional member of the American Herbalists Guild who practices in Bloomfield Hills, Michigan, and is the author of *The Natural Pregnancy Book* and *Natural Healing for Babies and Children.* "Just make sure the lozenge does not contain other herbs," she notes.

The lozenges are available in health food stores or by mail order (see "Where to Buy Herbs and Herbal Products" on page 462).

Or you can make your own. Here's Romm's recipe: Combine ¼ cup of slippery elm powder with enough honey (about 2 to 3 tablespoons) to make a moist, nonsticky dough. Add 3 to 4 drops of vanilla flavoring, if desired. Roll the dough into a long, thin cylinder on a cutting board dusted with slippery elm powder. Cut the roll into pea-size pieces, roll them into small balls, and place them on a baking sheet. Bake at 250°F for 1 hour. Cool and store in an airtight container. The lozenges are best if used quickly, but if they're thoroughly dried, they can be stored for two weeks.

---

nudge, thanks to bitter compounds that improve bile flow and other constituents that have a slight laxative effect, experts note. Have 30 drops in warm water or tea three times a day, Dr. Murray-Doran suggests. "You could take dandelion root tincture for up to a month," she notes. "If you took a tincture with mixed dandelion root and leaf, it would help with minor water retention at the same time."

Just the flax, ma'am. Flaxseed also contains mucilage, which helps bowel movements slide easily from your body, Dr. Murray-Doran says. Grind flaxseed to a fine powder in a clean coffee grinder, then soak in water overnight. "The powder will absorb the water and become mucilaginous and gel-like," she explains. In the morning, add 3 tablespoons of flaxseed gel to your breakfast cereal, she suggests. Be sure to drink at least six ounces of liquid. "Do this until you're regular again," she notes. If the flax causes diarrhea, discontinue taking it. Diarrhea can cause uterine contractions, Dr. Murray-Doran adds.

Always buy whole flaxseed in airtight bags. If it smells like shellac, it's rancid, so don't buy it. Store whole flaxseed in the refrigerator or freezer and grind it fresh each time you want to use it.

Insomnia and Anxiety

Toward the end of pregnancy, a good night's sleep may be more elusive than the perfect wallpaper for the nursery. "It's hard finding a comfortable position. A woman may need lots of pillows, propping up her belly, between her knees, anyplace," Dr. Murray-Doran says. Anxiety about childbirth, caring for a new baby, working during late pregnancy, or your relationship with your spouse can also flare up. In these tense moments, try a calming herbal remedy that can soothe body and soul.

Ease into dreamland with chamomile. A cup of gentle, flowery-flavored chamomile tea can calm raw nerves, ease stress, and pave the way to a night of restful sleep, says Romm. Research shows that chamomile, used since ancient times to treat insomnia, contains volatile oils and other soothing compounds that promote sleep.

"But have respect for chamomile," Dr. Bove notes. "This herb contains a smooth-muscle relaxant that might relax the uterine muscle too much. One to two cups of chamomile tea a day is fine, but more could be a problem."

Also, chamomile can cause miscarriage, so take this tea in the second and third trimesters only, stresses Dr. Murray-Doran. If you have a history of miscarriage or spotting during early pregnancy, limit yourself to one cup of tea a day, Romm suggests. Make the tea by adding 1 teaspoon of the herb to a cup of boiling water, steep for 10 to 15 minutes, then sip.

Shop for a ready-made bedtime blend. Look for a ready-to-use herbal blend in the supermarket tea aisle that includes chamomile, such as Celestial Seasonings Sleepy-Time tea or Lipton Soothing Moments Quietly Chamomile, suggests Dr. Bove. "That's a very safe way to use chamomile because its already mixed with other gentle herbs and comes in small quanti-

ties in tea bags, so you can't overdo it," she says.

Sip Aviva's flowery balm. "For a lovely-tasting, lovely-smelling tea that's so relaxing, combine 1 tablespoon of lemon balm and 1 teaspoon of chamomile flowers with a pinch of lavender in a cup of boiling water. Steep for 15 minutes, then sip," Romm suggests. "The lavender is wonderful, calming aromatherapy," she adds.

Make this or any of these relaxing teas part of a nurturing ritual, Romm says. Each night before bed, set aside a half-hour or more to unwind quietly with a cup of tea, she advises. One practical suggestion: To avoid being awakened by the call of nature, Romm suggests having your tea an hour or so before bed and then urinating before you go to sleep.

Blend a bedtime relaxer. You can concoct your own nerve-calming evening tea by combining 2 cups each of oatstraw, lemon balm, and chamomile, suggests Dr. Murray-Doran. About an hour before lights-out, pour a cup of boiling water over 1 teaspoon of the blend in a cup and steep for 15 minutes, then sip the brew while you relax, she suggests. Or look for a tincture that contains some or all of these herbs and take 40 drops in a half-cup of hot water about one hour before dreamtime. Oatstraw, rich in calcium and magnesium, is a traditional relaxing herb. Herbalists say that it calms the nervous system.

Stubborn insomnia? Try a calming tincture. If tea doesn't send you into dreamland, try two doses of a relaxing herbal tincture in the evening, Romm suggests. "Have one dose around 7:00 P.M., the other around 9:00, and go to bed by 10:00," she says.

For each dose, sip one of these herbs as an alcohol tincture mixed with ¼ cup of warm water: 10 to 15 drops of lavender, 10 to 15 drops of passionflower, or 20 to 30 drops of lemon balm. Lavender, like the other herbs suggested here, is a well-studied nervous-system calmer.

This formula is for use only in the second and third trimesters when you are having difficulty sleeping, explains Dr. Murray-Doran.

Stretch Marks and Sore Muscles

Inside that bulging belly, a miracle is taking place. But outside, your skin and muscles may be paying the price in the form of stretch marks—those silvery patches where skin is pulled taut—and achy back muscles. Here's herbal relief.

Ahhh! A saintly rubdown for sore back muscles. As your pregnancy progresses and you (and the baby) gain weight, your lower back muscles may start complaining. Ease the soreness by rubbing in about a teaspoon of St.-John's-wort oil, Romm suggests.

St.-John's-wort has a traditional reputation for soothing sore muscles and nerve pain, Dr. Bove notes. The oil also relieves muscle pain in the lower back during labor, she says.

You'll find St.-John's-wort oil in health food stores or by mail order, or you can make your own (see "A Saintly Burn Soother" on page 185).

Sidestep stretch marks with an herbal "belly balm." Minimize or even avoid stretch marks by taking preventive action, suggests Dr. Bove. Create a belly balm by combining 4 ounces of almond oil or a combination of almond and olive oil with a few drops of lavender essential oil. You could also add an ounce or more of calendula infused oil, an ounce or more of cocoa butter or coconut oil, or a few teaspoons of vitamin E oil. All are available at health food stores or by mail.

"Starting early in your pregnancy, rub this all around your belly—from the top of your pubic bone to the bottom of your rib cage—every day," she suggests. "The oils and herbs will keep the skin supple and help it stretch without leaving stretch marks behind. This is especially good for second-time moms who already have stretch marks and know that they're likely to get more."

Lavender essential oil is soothing and antimicrobial, according to herbal experts, while calendula has properties that assist in healing the skin.

Labor, Birth, and Beyond

Herbs can play an important role in preparing a woman's body for the hard work of labor and delivery, says Dr. Bove. Afterward, botanical skin washes and a simple "recovery tea" can soothe stretched skin and help the uterus begin contracting. Here's how.

Ask about mother's herbal helper. "There are specific herbs that herbalists, naturopaths, and herbally trained midwives recommend for birth preparation," Dr. Bove notes. "But they should only be used in the last month of pregnancy and under the supervision of a health-care professional." Dr. Bove suggests asking your caregiver about the formula for birth preparation. "The herbs in this formula help the cervix soften and shorten so that it can dilate more easily," she notes. "They also help prime the uterine muscle so it's ready to contract smoothly during labor and clamp down after birth to prevent hemorrhaging." If you are interested in trying this, speak to an herbally trained health practitioner. Do not take this without medical supervision because taking too much or using it too soon can cause premature labor.

Drink raspberry tea daily. Herbal experts call raspberry leaf *the* top pregnancy herb. "Raspberry leaf is rich in vitamins and minerals and contains a substance that helps prepare the uterus for labor and birth," notes Romm. Drink a cup or two of tea daily during the second and third trimesters of pregnancy, Dr. Bove suggests.

"It helps the whole uterine muscle get coordinated so it can contract effectively during labor," Dr. Murray-Doran notes.

To make raspberry-leaf tea, pour a cup of boiling water over 2 tablespoons of the herb and steep for 20 minutes. Or try Aviva's Pregnancy Tea (see page 328).

Laboratory studies show that raspberry leaf extracts nudge uterine contractions into a more regular rhythm. The effect may be due to an alkaloid that is found in high concentrations in raspberry leaves. As a bonus, raspberry can increase the flow of milk after childbirth.

Prepare your perineum with lavender, calendula, and oils. Some herbalists say that massaging the perineum (the area around the outside of the birth canal) with oil can help minimize tearing at birth. The same oils and herbs that make a good belly balm can help make your perineum supple and more stretchable during delivery, Romm says.

Dr. Bove suggests rubbing your perineum daily during late pregnancy with a teaspoon of the balm.

Ease labor pain with aromatherapy. During labor, lavender essential oil can help ease tension, while peppermint essential oil can ease any feelings of nausea that you may experience, Dr. Bove notes. "Put a few drops on a tissue and sniff as you need it," she suggests.

Rest more comfortably with passionflower. Take the edge off early labor pains and help yourself rest between contractions with passionflower tincture, Dr. Bove says. Research shows that passionflower, called a "rest-provoking agent" by herbal healers in the late nineteenth century, has sedative, anxiety-relieving properties in animal studies.

"Passionflower is good during the early dilation stage," she notes. "It can help you stay calm so you don't waste energy that you'll need for the birth." Take 30 drops of tincture in a little warm water. "If needed, take up to three doses 15 to 20 minutes apart, then wait four or five hours," Dr. Bove suggests.

After the birth, rinse with healing herbs. Soothe a stretched, torn, or surgically stitched perineum with Dr. Bove's perineal wash: Mix 2 parts comfrey root and 1 part each of calendula, yarrow flowers, lavender, and rosemary leaves. Add a handful to a pint of boiling water, steep until cool, then strain. "Pour the cool liquid into a clean peri bottle (a squeeze bottle for washing the perineum, available at medical equipment or surgical supply stores) and rinse with it after urinating instead of using toilet paper," Dr. Bove suggests. "If you have stitches, use the rinse for five days, then you can also use the same formula in a sitz bath for 10 minutes a day. If you don't have stitches, you can use a sitz bath right away."

According to Dr. Bove, calendula works as an anti-inflammatory, reducing swelling; comfrey speeds tissue repair, thanks to a substance called allantoin; yarrow is an astringent

Alfalfa: The Mother's Herb

At first glance, alfalfa, with its dainty purple flowers and little leaf clusters, is just a modest food plant for farmyard animals. But this well-studied herb has a reputation in folk medicine for promoting the production of breast milk, whetting the appetite, and boosting vitality.

It's small wonder, then, that alfalfa shows up among women's herbs for fertility and pregnancy. The dried leaves contain a wealth of vitamins and minerals, including vitamins A, B_6, B_{12}, C, E, and K, as well as niacin and folate, an important nutrient that can prevent birth defects.

"Alfalfa is loaded with vitamins, plus eight digestive enzymes and numerous trace minerals," notes herbalist Rosemary Gladstar, director of the Sage Mountain herbal education center in East Barre, Vermont, and author of *Herbal Healing for Women*. It is among her top herbs for alleviating fatigue during pregnancy.

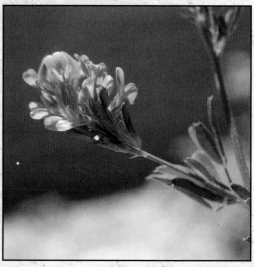

In 1915, one doctor praised alfalfa as "a superlative restorative tonic."

that draws torn skin together and also has antimicrobial actions; and rosemary is said to be an antiseptic and astringent that also stimulates circulation, which promotes healing.

Sip "recovery tea." To support milk production and help your uterus contract to prepregnancy size, begin sipping a tea blend made with 2 parts raspberry leaf and 1 part each of nettle, red clover, vervain, and lemon balm, Dr. Bove suggests. "I suggest that women start drinking this immediately after delivery," she says. "It helps heal the site where the placenta was attached to the uterus, calms the nerves, and helps balance hormones, thanks to the red clover. The nettle promotes milk production." Use at least 1 teaspoon of this blend per cup of boiling water, steep for 15 minutes, then sip. Have up to three cups a day.

Healing after Cesarean Section

If you have a baby by cesarean section, you'll face all of the typical challenges and joys of new motherhood (from breastfeeding to finding time for sleep), plus one: The added need to gain strength and heal after major surgery, Dr. Bove says.

"Remember, you've had a significant surgical procedure, and your body needs time to rest," she notes. "Take it easy for 7 to 10 days, or even longer. Don't lift anything heavier than your baby for about a month. Get help—have someone else do the laundry, wash the dishes, and prepare the meals."

Natural therapies after a C-section can help boost your body's ability to knit together layers of skin and muscle that were opened during the surgery, Dr. Bove says. "Topical herbal remedies can help the skin heal so that the scar isn't red or inflamed. And herbal tea can help the uterine muscle mend smoothly. When that muscle is well-mended, the endometrial lining inside the uterus will be very smooth, which will make things easier if you become pregnant again," she notes.

In addition to botanical treatments, Dr. Bove suggests that women who have had C-sections take zinc (15 to 20 milligrams), bioflavonoids (500 to 1,000 milligrams), vitamin C (1,000 to 3,000 milligrams), vitamin E (400 international units), and evening primrose oil as daily supplements for four to six weeks. "These help tissue mend and reduce inflammation," she says. (Doses of more than 1,200 milligrams of vitamin C may cause diarrhea in some people.)

Her post-C-section treatment plan also includes two homeopathic remedies. "I suggest that a woman take a single, 1-m dose of homeopathic arnica within the first day after her surgery and then take a 6-c or 12-c dose of arnica twice daily for a week after that. In addition, on the second day after surgery, take a 200-c dose of staphysagria. Both of these homeopathic remedies will prevent some swelling and tenderness." (Homeopathic remedies, which can be found in health food stores, come in doses marked "m," "c," or "x.")

Dr. Bove also suggests refraining from abdominal exercise and from any strenuous physical activity for the first six weeks. "Give the muscles time to mend. You can still do gentle stretching exercises for your arms, legs, hands, and feet to keep circulation moving and your muscles limber," she says.

After-Surgery Soothers

These herbal helpers can help you heal inside and out, Dr. Bove says.

Sip a healing tea. Pleasantly savory, Dr. Bove's special six-herb blend performs triple duty for new moms who are caring for a new baby and recovering from a C-section. "This tea can help heal tissue, normalize hormone levels, and support breastfeeding," she says.

Mix equal parts of raspberry leaf, partridgeberry, nettle, oatstraw, fennel seed, and lemon balm in a glass jar with a tight-fitting lid. To make the tea, steep 1 teaspoon of the blend in 1 cup of just-boiled water for 5 minutes, then sip. "Have one to two cups a day for at least a month," Dr. Bove suggests.

According to Dr. Bove, the herbs in this blend have many benefits. Raspberry leaf can help the uterus contract and return to its prepregnancy state, while partridgeberry can help regulate hormones and also helps the uterus contract. Nettle, rich in minerals, can help support milk production, and it is also a classic herb for convalescence, as it contains nutrients that help you regain strength after illness or surgery. Oatstraw is a calming herb that also builds stamina, fennel is a traditional breastfeeding herb that can increase milk production, and lemon balm helps soothe frayed nerves, she says.

"You can substitute lavender flowers for the lemon balm if you'd like," Dr. Bove notes.

"And if you don't like the taste of fennel, you can add spearmint to the blend for a minty taste or substitute milk thistle, which also supports milk production."

Wash with healing herbs. Once your incision starts to heal—when the skin is knitting back together, no longer weeps any fluid, and shows no signs of infection—you can help support the healing process with a skin wash made with yarrow, plantain, and calendula, Dr. Bove suggests. Calendula contains substances that reduce inflammation, combat infection, and even help the skin mend itself. Research shows that yarrow helps wound healing and is anti-inflammatory and antiseptic. Plantain also helps heal wounds.

Combine equal parts of the herbs, then steep 1 tablespoon of the mix in 2 cups of just-boiled water for 10 to 15 minutes. Cool to room temperature. Gently pour some of the mixture onto the incision and let it stay—don't rinse. Do this twice a day, Dr. Bove suggests. You can also use sterile gauze pads or a clean washcloth to apply the wash, she adds. The wash can be stored in the refrigerator for up to three days. Use it until the incision is healed.

Lubricate and massage gently with an herbal oil. Once the incision heals, you can help promote the regrowth of nerve tissue and reduce redness and swelling of the scar with St.-John's-wort oil, vitamin E oil, and lavender essential oil, Dr. Bove says.

"Add ½ ounce (1 tablespoon) of vitamin E oil and 3 to 5 drops of lavender essential oil to 1 ounce (2 tablespoons) of St.-John's-wort oil," she says. "Shake well, then put a little on your finger and apply it daily to the incision with tiny circular motions, gently rubbing it in." St.-John's-wort helps nerve cells regenerate and can reduce pain, while vitamin E can promote healing and lavender can reduce inflammation, Dr. Bove says. (Vitamin E oil and St.-John's-wort infused oil are available in drugstores and health food stores; lavender essential oil is also sold in health food stores.)

"Be patient," she says. "Healing the scar well could take four or five months. Keep using the oil. Remember that it will improve."

*P*soriasis

HALT A RUNAWAY RASH, HERBALLY

Too many new cells, too fast: The secret cause of the red rashes and silvery scales of a psoriasis outbreak lies hidden beneath the surface of the skin, says Sherry Briskey, N.D., chair of the botanical medicine department at the South-west College of Naturopathic Medicine and Health Sciences in Tempe, Arizona.

"In psoriasis, skin cells divide many times faster than normal. They pile up in clumps that look like scales on the surface of the skin," she says. This heartbreaking skin con-

Oregon Grape Root:
A Soother for Psoriasis

Coal tar, topical steroids, and prescription drugs are the conventional treatments for psoriasis. But some herbalists recommend a natural remedy for this itchy, scaly skin condition: Oregon grape root.

At least one scientific study has concluded that the root of this plant does indeed offer relief. Researchers in Germany tested Oregon grape root's effectiveness on 82 people with the condition. After four weeks, the symptoms of 78 of the people had improved.

The inner bark of the root is rich in berberine, which has been shown in clinical studies to be a strong antimicrobial. It also contains berbamine and oxycanthine, substances that are reported to reduce skin eruptions.

Oregon grape root extracts and capsules are available in health food stores or by mail order (see "Where to Buy Herbs and Herbal Products" on page 462). Follow the dosage directions on the label.

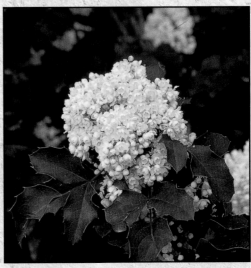

The root of this tall shrub with shiny, spiny leaves is a folk remedy for psoriasis, eczema, and other skin conditions.

dition may be inherited, but outbreaks come and go, often provoked by injuries, stress, infections, or a change of season.

Hope and Help for Outbreaks

Conventional medical treatment for psoriasis includes tar- and steroid-based creams, says Lisa Murray-Doran, N.D., a naturopathic doctor and instructor at the Canadian College of Naturopathic Medicine in Toronto. "Naturopathic doctors soothe the surface of the skin, too. But they also look deeper for the cause of the psoriasis," she notes. "We work on the connection between liver function and healthy skin.

"Naturopathic doctors believe that when the liver can't process the toxins, hormones, fats, and other substances in the bloodstream completely, some toxins are sent to the skin to be eliminated," Dr. Murray-Doran says. "If these things irritate the skin and you are prone to psoriasis, it will make matters much worse." Here's how herbal

Coleus Forskohlii: An Ancient Allergy Fighter–And More

A kind of mint native to the high, dry slopes of the Himalayas, coleus forskohlii has long been used in Ayurveda, India's ancient system of medicine. And judging by recent scientific research, this plant's active ingredient may be a natural treatment for a variety of ailments.

This substance, forskolin, appears to activate enzymes in the body that regulate cellular activity. In particular, it raises cell levels of a substance called cyclic adenosine monophosphate (cAMP). Theoretically, too little cAMP alters the workings of immune cells. A fall in cAMP is thought to contribute to the development of allergic conditions such as eczema, psoriasis, and asthma. Preliminary research also indicates that forskolin lowers blood pressure.

Coleus forskohlii root is available as an extract or capsules at health food stores or through mail order (see "Where to Buy Herbs and Herbal Products" on page 462). Sherry Briskey, N.D. a naturopathic physician and chair of the botanical medicine department at the Southwest College of Naturopathic Medicine and Health Sciences in Tempe, Arizona, suggests taking 60 drops of extract three times a day or following the package directions for capsules. She advises taking it for three to four months.

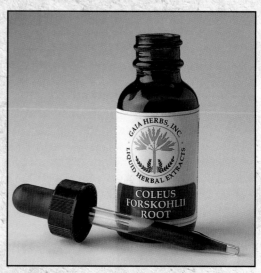

Because it's been shown to improve the heart's ability to contract, the active ingredient in coleus forskohlii root may be a future treatment for angina and congestive heart failure.

healers soothe psoriasis—inside and out.

Apply a soothing herbal cream. "Look for a heavy cream made with calendula and beeswax among the ingredients listed," suggests Dr. Murray-Doran. "You want to seal in moisture and help the skin heal as much as possible. Calendula is great for that."

Calendula can help ease swelling and red-ness, protect the skin from infection, and prompt healing, research shows. The beeswax in the cream heals the skin and seals the open psoriasis sores from the air, Dr. Murray-Doran says. Beeswax also has antimicrobial properties. (For more external herbal skin soothers appropriate for psoriasis care, see "Eczema" on page 222.)

Support your liver.   Herbs that support and boost liver function can benefit skin conditions such as psoriasis by helping the liver filter out toxins that irritate sensitive skin, Dr. Briskey says. "For psoriasis, my first choices would be milk thistle, Oregon grape root (don't use if you are pregnant), and sarsaparilla tinctures," she says.

Dr. Murray-Doran also suggests yellow dock, dandelion, and burdock, traditional skin healers that stimulate liver function. Take any combination of these herbs as tinctures (also called extracts), 30 to 60 drops straight or in up to 1/4 cup of warm water, two to three times a day for six to nine months, the doctors suggest.

Research shows that Oregon grape root contains a liver aid called berberine. Milk thistle's shiny black seeds contain silymarin, which research suggests changes the structure of cells along the liver's outer membrane, preventing toxic chemicals from entering. At the same time, this compound stimulates production of new liver cells.

In one study, sarsaparilla prevented bacterial bits called endotoxins from leaving the intestines. When endotoxins circulate in the bloodstream, they can aggravate skin conditions like psoriasis, Dr. Briskey says.

Slow cell growth with an Eastern herb. According to preliminary research, coleus forskohlii, which is native to India, Nepal, and Sri Lanka, contains compounds that seem to help balance enzymes that regulate cell production, Dr. Briskey says. "When you slow down production of skin cells, psoriasis gets better," she notes.

"One of the herb's active ingredients is forskolin," Dr. Briskey says. "I suggest taking 60 drops of coleus forskohlii extract three times a day for three to four months."

Think twice about red-pepper cream. While some herbal experts recommend creams containing tiny amounts of capsaicin, one of the active constituents of red pepper, Dr. Murray-Doran cautions women with psoriasis to handle this cream with care. "Red pepper is very irritating," she notes. "The cream could irritate skin that's already very sensitive and rash-prone."

Respiratory Problems

BREATHE BETTER WITH MEDICINAL HERBS

*T*he Grand Canyon. Monet's *Water Lilies.* Mel Gibson. All can steal your breath away. And that's a pretty sweet thing. Unfortunately, not everything that's breathtaking is necessarily enjoyable. In fact, lots of pretty unpleasant stuff can leave you breathless. And unlike landscapes, paintings, and handsome men, their effects aren't so fleeting.

Cold and flu season alone brings 200

viruses that descend upon your airways, causing infection and choking your upper respiratory tract with inflammation and congestion. In folks with allergies, dander and dust from dogs and cats and anything they drag in can make your nose run and your eyes itch and weep. Cigarette smoking can cause chronic bronchitis and the incessant coughing that goes with it. And stubborn inflammation in the lungs can set the stage for asthma attacks that close off the bronchial airways so that you feel as if you're sucking air through a swizzle stick when you try to inhale.

Physicians often recommend combating these breath thieves with synthetic drugs like decongestants, anti-inflammatories, antihistamines, and bronchodilators. In some circumstances, such as asthma attacks, such drugs can be lifesavers. But often, these over-the-counter remedies simply cover up the symptoms—suppressing a cough, for example, or eliminating congestion—without addressing what is making you sick. And stronger prescription medicines like those found in inhalers for asthma also may have unpleasant side effects, such as making you jittery or leaving you with a pounding headache.

Herbal remedies can offer a better alternative for respiratory conditions of all kinds, say herbalists, because they not only help provide relief from nagging symptoms, they also get right to the root of the problem by stimulating your immune system so that your body can heal itself. The other benefit of herbal treatments is that disease-causing bacteria are less likely to become resistant to them, says David Winston, a professional member of the American Herbalists Guild (AHG) and founder of Herbalist and Alchemist, an herbal medicine company in Washington, New Jersey. "Most drugs contain just one active ingredient. Herbs are chemically complex. They have not just one but many active ingredients, so it's harder for bacteria to develop resistance to their activity."

The herbal route takes patience, though.

"With some herbal treatments, especially ones that activate the immune system, it can take up to 24 hours before you feel the benefits," says Feather Jones, a professional member of the AHG and director of the Rocky Mountain Center for Botanical Studies in Boulder, Colorado. "That's because they aren't just masking symptoms, they are fighting the element that is making you sick."

What follows is a rundown of some common "breath-taking" respiratory disorders and the herbs that may help.

Asthma

Of all of the respiratory ills, asthma may be the most mysterious. What doctors know is that people with asthma have bronchial tubes that are easily aggravated by cold, dust mites, pollen, and a host of other triggers. When these sensitive airways are irritated, they clench down, making breathing a struggle. And to make matters worse, your body also produces excess mucus with asthma, further clogging up your airways. Chronic inflammation of the lungs seems to be the underlying problem, although no one knows why it occurs.

Because asthma varies from one person to the next, herbalists apply distinctly different approaches, "so if you have asthma and want to try herbs, it's a good idea to see a qualified herbalist first," says Jones.

If you are taking medicine for asthma, however, you should check with your doctor before taking herbs, says Thomas Platts-Mills, M.D., Ph.D., professor of medicine and head of the division of allergy and immunology at the University of Virginia Medical Center in Charlottesville.

Jones also recommends that people with asthma be checked for food allergies—a factor that she finds can aggravate asthma.

Janis Gruska, N.D., a naturopathic physician, professor of clinical medicine, and department chair of naturopathic medicine at the Southwest College of Naturopathic Medicine and Health Sciences in Tempe, Arizona, recommends that people also try acupuncture and homeopathy. "Both therapies complement herbal treatments, making them effective," she says.

Finally, don't ditch your inhaler just because you're starting an herbal plan, warns Jones. "Treating chronic or acute respiratory problems like asthma can be a long process," she says. While you should never stop taking your asthma medicine unless you have your doctor's approval, there are things you can do to help yourself breathe easier. Here's how experts recommend starting.

Favor flavonoid-rich fruits and vegetables. To fight the inflammation that accompanies asthma, Dr. Gruska emphasizes a diet loaded with flavonoids—tiny crystals in foods like onions, apples, blueberries, and prickly pears that give them their blue, yellow, or reddish hues. "Flavonoids not only strengthen the capillary walls, they're also antioxidants," she says. "So they help protect the membranes in the airways from being damaged by pollution. People with asthma should eat a couple of servings of flavonoid-rich foods every day."

Strengthen with horsetail. People with asthma need to strengthen their lungs and alveolar sacs—the sacs at the bottom of the bronchial tubes where your body exchanges carbon dioxide for oxygen—with respiratory tonics, says Jones. She suggests horsetail, an herb that comes from a fernlike weed. "It not only contains flavonoids, it also contains other compounds like silica and other absorbable minerals that can help your alveolar sacs maintain their elasticity," she says. "I recommend using 20 drops a day of horsetail tincture. But don't expect results overnight. It will take between six weeks and six months for the herb to really take effect. You can take it continuously, although I recommend taking a break during your menstrual period just to give your body a rest." This tincture (also called an extract), which can be found in health food stores, can be taken straight or diluted in soda or apple juice, says Jones.

Get some grindelia. You can help prevent asthma spasms with the dried buds of the grindelia plant, says Jones. "Grindelia is very good as an antispasmodic, which means that it helps relax smooth muscles like those found in the airways. So it works nicely to prevent the bronchial tubes from constricting. It's also a bronchodilator, so it opens bronchi that are already constricted." To prevent asthma or bronchitis, Jones suggests taking 20 to 30 drops of tincture (available at health food stores) two or three times a day.

Give ginkgo a go. Although more research needs to be done on its effectiveness against asthma, some herbalists recommend taking the ancient Chinese herb ginkgo. When you have asthma, histamine, along with several other substances, is released when you're exposed to an allergy trigger like pollen or animal dander. These substances, one of which is called platelet-activating factor (PAF), cause spasms of the bronchial muscles. Ginkgo contains compounds called ginkgolides that inhibit PAF, an action that some herbalists believe could help improve some types of allergies linked to asthma. If you want to try ginkgo, Daniel Gagnon, professional member of the AHG, executive director of the Botanical Research and Education Institute, and owner of Herbs, Etc., in Santa Fe, New Mexico, recommends taking 20 to 30 drops of alcohol-based ginkgo extract up to four times a day. Extracts can be diluted in water, juice, or herbal tea.

Ease asthma with ephedra. Also known as ma huang, ephedra has taken a public beating for its use and abuse as a diet aid, says Dr. Gruska. "But while its effectiveness is questionable and it can be potentially dangerous when used for weight loss, used wisely and with supervision, it can be a real help for serious respiratory illness."

The fact is, if you currently take prescription medication for your asthma, you're probably already taking a synthetic version of this natural airway opener. Used in Chinese medicine for the past 5,000 years, ephedra contains a compound called ephedrine that stimulates the sympathetic nervous system, which in turn relieves the bronchial spasms that trigger asthma attacks. Ephedrine from herbs is more effective than synthetic ephedrine, say herbalists, because the herb contains other compounds that reduce inflammation as well.

But ephedra "can make you jittery, along with causing other side effects, like insomnia, that are associated with stimulants," says Dr. Gruska. "So you don't want to take too much ephedra or take it for too long. I also recommend that you be monitored by a qualified health-care practitioner to see how much the herb is helping," she says.

It's also a good idea to take it in conjunction with Siberian or American ginseng (the peeled and dried root) or other herbs that strengthen and support the adrenal glands, which may be weakened by the constant stimulation from ephedrine, adds Gagnon. The recommended dose is one capsule or 20 drops of alcohol-based extract a day.

Don't take more than 20 drops of ephedra, divided into four doses a day, and then only when absolutely necessary, says Gagnon.

To make tea, add ½ pint of boiling water to 1 heaping teaspoonful of herb and let it steep for 10 minutes, says Varro E. Tyler, Ph.D., professor emeritus of pharmacognosy at the Purdue University School of Pharmacy and Pharmacal Sciences in West Lafayette, Indiana, in his book *Herbs of Choice*. It should not be taken habitually for more than seven days, cautions Dr. Tyler.

"You should not use it if you have high blood pressure, glaucoma, or heart problems," warns Gagnon. Anyone who has diabetes or thyroid disease should also avoid ephedra. And never use it along with asthma medications—the additive effects could be dangerous. It may increase the action of MAO inhibitors or any other prescription drugs. Individual doses should not exceed eight milligrams in dry form.

Bronchitis

When the bronchi—the air passages that carry oxygen to the lungs—are exposed to heavy doses of pollution or certain bacteria, they can become irritated and inflamed. Your body responds by secreting mucus to soothe them. At the same time, the mechanism that removes mucus slows down, leaving a surplus of gunk that causes the deep chest cough that you get with bronchitis.

Bronchitis may be acute or chronic. Acute bronchitis is caused by a viral infection and clears up in a week or two. Chronic bronchitis is caused by airborne pollution and is most common in people who smoke. Obviously, if you're among the latter, you should stop

Boneset: Nature's Aspirin

Although Native Americans did use boneset tea to bathe broken bones, that's probably not how this plant got its name. Known as a healing herb on both sides of the Atlantic, boneset was used to treat influenza, malaria, typhus, and dengue fever, diseases that made a sufferer's bones ache so badly that they felt broken.

Native Americans passed boneset along to the colonists, and it soon became so popular that one herbal historian calls boneset "the aspirin of the European settler."

Boneset contains sesquiterpene lactones and sterols, which have anti-inflammatory properties. That could be why herbalists use boneset to help reduce fevers and ease the aches and pains that accompany the flu. Boneset also contains quercetin, a flavonoid that has significant antiviral activity against cold, flu, and herpes viruses.

Boneset can be made into a tea, but it is very, very bitter, so herbalists recommend taking boneset tincture instead. In large doses, boneset can cause vomiting and may act as a bowel purgative. If you are prone to allergies/hypersensitivities, particularly to chamomile, feverfew, ragweed, or other members of the daisy family, you may also have an allergic reaction to boneset.

Do not confuse boneset with comfrey (see "Comfrey" on page 45). Although boneset is one of comfrey's common names, the two herbs are unrelated. True boneset is also known as feverwort, Indian sage, and ague weed. Boneset tincture and tea are available at health food stores. The dried herb can be purchased through mail-order sources (see "Where to Buy Herbs and Herbal Products" on page 462).

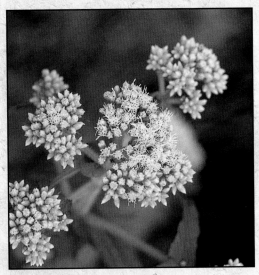

Herbalists say that boneset clears mucus congestion from the upper respiratory tract and acts as a mild laxative.

smoking. Otherwise, a number of herbs may help soothe your inflamed air passages and clear your congestion. Just remember that bronchitis is a potentially serious disease, so you should always see your doctor before trying any self-treatments.

Make it mullein. For a sudden episode of bronchitis, Andrew Weil, M.D., director of the program in integrative medicine at the University of Arizona College of Medicine in Tucson and author of *Spontaneous Healing*, recommends mullein as a good first line of herbal defense. Ironically, although it's traditionally been used to treat respiratory ailments, especially chest congestion and dry bronchial coughs, Native Americans actually used to smoke mullein instead of tobacco, he says. Although Dr. Weil certainly doesn't recommend smoking anything, he does recommend taking a dropperful of mullein tincture in a little warm water every four hours while you're ill.

Knock it out with grindelia. Grindelia has exceptional mucus-cutting ability, which makes it a prize-fighting herb against bronchitis, says Jones. "Grindelia traditionally has been used against the kind of thick, ropy, tenacious mucus found in chronic bronchitis. It's antimicrobial, so it fights the germs that cause infection. It is also known as anti-tussive, maning that it helps put an end to unproductive cough." Take 20 to 30 drops of tincture five times a day when you have a bronchial infection, advises Jones. It can be taken straight or diluted in fruit juice.

Crunch some cloves—of garlic, that is. Garlic makes a great addition to herbal treatment for acute and chronic bronchitis, says Gagnon. Herbal wisdom says that this odoriferous herb contains powerful antibiotic compounds that are actually excreted through the lungs, so they help treat bronchial conditions from the inside out. He recommends eating a clove of raw garlic during the day or taking an enteric-coated garlic capsule or tablet.

Ease bronchitis with elecampane. The root of this sunflower-like plant is a respiratory tonic, so it strengthens lungs that are weak from acute or chronic bronchitis, say herbalists. "It is also good at breaking up congestion, fighting infection, and acting as an expectorant," says Ed Smith, a professional member of the AHG and founder of the HerbPharm in Williams, Oregon. Pour 1 cup of cold water onto 1 teaspoon of shredded elecampane in a saucepan and gently simmer it for 15 minutes. Sip by the cupful three times a day.

"Just be prepared; elecampane is on my list of the 10 most unpleasant-tasting herbs," adds Winston. "But it *is* one of the primary herbs for respiratory tract infections like bronchitis and pleurisy." To ease elecampane's bitter edge, keep a honey jar close by and gulp a teaspoonful. The herb can be found in some health food stores and mail-order catalogs (see "Where to Buy Herbs and Herbal Products" on page 462). Don't chug this stuff, though: Large doses of elecampane can upset your system.

Rub on some thyme. This aromatic herb is good for breaking up and getting rid of thick, infected phlegm and congestion that accompany acute and chronic bronchitis, says Smith. You can even make your own chest rub, say herbalists, by mixing 10 drops of essential oil into 20 milliliters (approximately 1 teaspoon) of almond oil.

Relax your airways with soothing tea. Aniseed makes your bronchial cough more productive. Coltsfoot does the same while also reducing inflammation. Marshmallow contains mucilage, which helps soothe irritated airways. And mullein reduces inflammation while stepping up fluid production to clear the lungs. Mix them all together and you have a soothing concoction that is ideal for the irritating, unproductive cough that often accompanies acute bronchitis, according to David Hoffman, a founding and professional member of the AHG, fellow of Britain's National Institute of Medical Herbalists, assistant professor of integral studies at the California Institute of Integral Health Studies, and author of *The New Holistic Herbal*. He recommends combining equal parts of the four herbs and using 2 teaspoons of the blend per cup of boiling water. Infuse for 20 minutes and drink hot several times a day.

Chicken Soup à la Herbs

Nothing heals like hot chicken soup when you're down with a cold. Well, here's a simple yet super-healing recipe from Daniel Gagnon, a professional member of the American Herbalists Guild, executive director of the Botanical Research and Education Institute, and owner of Herbs, Etc., in Santa Fe, New Mexico. "It's delightful," says Gagnon.

1   **whole organically raised chicken**
2   **onions, finely chopped**
5   **carrots, sliced**
5   **cloves garlic, minced or crushed**
    Pinch of fresh or dried thyme
    Matzo balls

Place the chicken in a soup pot, cover with water, and bring to a boil. Add the onions, carrots, garlic, and thyme. Simmer for 2 hours. Strain the broth, add matzo balls for good measure, and eat hot.

Makes 3 quarts

Colds and Flu

If you're fighting to keep your nose from dripping on this page as you read, it won't make you feel better to hear that the best treatment for colds and flu is preventing them, says herbalist Roy Upton of Soquel, California, vice president of the AHG. There are 200 viruses that can infect your body and cause the inflammation and congestion of the common cold, "so it's a good idea to start taking herbs as soon as the weather turns cold to bolster your immune system," says Upton. That said, if you manage to avert only 199 of those viruses and come down with a cold anyway, there are some herbs that can help hasten your recovery as well, he says. Here's how to prevent and care for colds and flu.

Toast the season with astragalus. These days, you think cold and flu, you think echinacea, but top experts say that there's one straggling herb that you should put first in line—astragalus. "The difference between echinacea and astragalus is that echinacea is an immune-system stimulant. You take it when you need something to act quickly. Astragalus is an immune-system tonic, or strengthener—you take it so that you won't need the echinacea," says Gagnon. Studies have shown some immunity-stimulating benefits, and the herb has 2,000 years of history as an immunity strengthener in Chinese medicine.

"Astragalus helps boost interferon production in the body," says Gagnon. "I liken interferon to the Paul Revere of the body. When a cell is challenged by a virus or bacteria, it releases interferon, a substance that tells the adjacent cells what kind of bug is attacking and what it needs to do to protect itself. It also tells disease-fighting white blood cells where the virus is attacking. The idea is to build your resistance so you won't even know that a cold or flu bug has attacked."

Astragalus is a pleasant-tasting herb, says Upton. You can make it into a tea by using 1 teaspoon of the herb per cup of boiling water and letting it steep in a covered container for

10 or 15 minutes. Or you can add astragalus sticks to soups. "Use four to six sticks of astragalus per pot of soup," says Upton.

"I recommend taking astragalus in courses," adds Gagnon. "Take it for a month, then take two weeks off, and so on. If nothing else, take it a few months before and during the cold and flu season."

"My favorite form of astragalus is a classic Chinese preparation known as Jade Screen," says Upton. "It consists of three herbs, with astragalus being the primary component. It gets its name because people used to say it protected against the cold winds as if you were surrounded by a screen of jade." You can find it in stores or from mail-order companies that specialize in Chinese herbs.

Rush to reishi. Although reishi mushrooms are a fungus, not an herb, Upton also recommends taking reishi mushroom extract at the beginning of cold and flu season to fend off bacterial and viral illnesses. Seventy drops daily of a normal-strength (1:5) tincture is a good start, he suggests. "Reishi is rather bitter, though you can drink it in a tea if you don't mind the taste," says Upton. You can make reishi tea with 3 to 6 teaspoons of the dried herb per cup of boiling water. "Or you can take capsules or tablets as the label directs," he says. Reishi products are sold in health food stores. In rare cases, reishi can cause dry mouth and stomach upset when used for more than three months.

Drop echinacea. If, despite your best preventive efforts, you awaken with a scratchy throat, stuffed nose, and other telltale signs of an oncoming cold or flu, the first herb to reach for is echinacea, says Jones. "Whether you put it in your favorite beverage, drink it with water, or drop it under your tongue, be sure to get echinacea into your system," she says. "Echinacea is an antimicrobial, so it kills bac-

teria. More important, it contains polysaccharides and other compounds that are potent immune-system stimulants, meaning that it helps boost your immune system so it's better able to handle the assault from the virus or bacteria that are making you ill."

Jones recommends taking 20 to 30 drops of echinacea tincture every half-hour to hour while you're ill. "I like tinctures for colds and flu because they work more quickly than capsules, which have to be digested. Plus, echinacea has a fairly nice taste," she says.

Echinacea is one of the most studied medicinal herbs, with about 400 papers published on its effects. Most of the research has been done in petri dishes and with animals, primarily in Germany. Unfortunately, most also weren't the type of controlled trials that carry the most clinical weight. The good news is that the one human study done in recent years had positive results. In a study of 180 people with the flu, researchers discovered that 900 milligrams of echinacea significantly reduced their symptoms.

Although echinacea is largely safe for almost everyone, you should not take it if you have an autoimmune condition such as lupus, tuberculosis, or multiple sclerosis or if you are allergic to flowers in the daisy family, such as chamomile and marigold.

Find your elders. When you have that even-my-hair-hurts, overall achy and feverish feeling that signals that it's not just a cold but the flu that's coming on, try a shot of elderberry, says Gagnon. "If you take elderberry extract early enough, you may be able to head it off at the pass before it becomes a full-blown flu," he says. "Elderberry extract contains substances that break down an enzyme that the virus uses to penetrate your healthy cells and reproduce," he says. "It works within 24 to 48 hours after you take it."

Elder: Made to Order for Chills and Fever

It's said that the seventeenth-century British drank elderberry wine as a way to prolong their lives. Maybe it did, maybe it didn't. But they also credited the sweet berry extract with curing the common cold.

Commonly used for hedges in the British Isles, the elderberry shrub is a backyard medicine chest. Herbalists say that elder flowers are laced with essential oils that increase circulation and open pores, which may help reduce fever. Commission E, the expert panel that reports on the safety and effectiveness of herbal medicines for the German government, endorses using two to three teaspoons of elder flowers a day to treat feverish chills. Elder leaves are often used externally for bruises, sprains, and other minor injuries.

Elder's most potent plant part, however, could be its dark berries. In a clinical study in Israel, 27 people who had the flu were given an elderberry extract rich in flavonoids (called Sambucol) or a dummy fluid. After just two days, almost all the folks in the elderberry group were feeling much better, while those who drank no elderberry were sick for four more days.

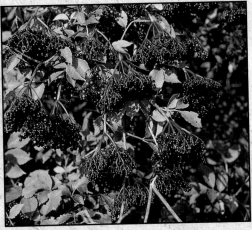

The leaves, flowers, and berries of the elder bush have been studied for their medicinal value.

The best way to take elderberry is as fresh berry juice, he says. But that's very hard to find. "Instead, you can buy the alcohol-based extract and take 40 drops every four hours the first day you feel sick." Continue to take it for three days, he says. You can dilute the extract in water, juice, or herbal tea.

Researchers in southern Israel put elderberry to the test against an outbreak of Panama flu. They gave 15 flu sufferers four tablespoons of the extract and gave 12 a dummy fluid. Within two days, 93 percent of those taking the elderberry had improved. Those stuck with the dummy fluid endured their symptoms for six days.

Take a soak. Another way to make the flu more bearable is with tea tree essential oil, according to Hoffman. At the very onset of your flu—when that first bit of achiness appears—put three or four drops of tea tree oil (more can be irritating for people with sensitive skin) in a moderately hot bath and

Botanical Dan's Failsafe Cold and Flu Formula

*I*f you take these four things at the very first signs of a cold or flu, you'll beat it 99 percent of the time, says Daniel Gagnon, a professional member of the American Herbalists Guild, executive director of the Botanical Research and Education Institute, and owner of Herbs, Etc., in Santa Fe, New Mexico.

1. Take one dropperful of echinacea extract every hour.
2. Take 500 milligrams of vitamin C every hour. (Excess vitamin C may cause diarrhea in some people. If you develop loose stools, cut back on the dosage.)
3. Take plenty of garlic—one clove, one capsule, or one tablet every four hours.
4. Top it off with chicken soup.

"If you're a vegetarian, use a vegetable broth instead of chicken soup," says Gagnon. "Take all four, and by the end of one day, your cold or flu will be gone," he adds.

---

soak for as long as you're comfortable. Repeating the bath for the next two or three days may ward off a full-blown attack, he notes. Plus, the warm bath will help induce restful sleep. (Tea tree oil is toxic if ingested or undiluted, so it should be kept out of reach of children.)

Breathe deep. Inhalants can be a wonderful way to get medicinal herbs to the place colds and flu often hit your breathing hardest—the lungs, says Jones. "I like to use antimicrobial oils, which kill bacteria, as inhalants," she says. "My favorites are eucalyptus, tea tree, and bergamot, which is a citrus essential oil." But Jones doesn't recommend pouring the oil directly into the inhaler, because it can gunk up your machine. Instead, put a shallow dish filled with the oil somewhere on or near the vaporizer's nozzle so the hot steam picks up the essential oil as it passes over.

Using inhalants has a dual effect. First, just the act of breathing in hot steam helps to loosen congestion, says Jones. Second, because they're antimicrobial, these essential oils will help kill the germs that are making you sick.

Pull some pungency. Upton believes that people can choose from an array of effective herbs to find the one that fights their cold the best. The most important thing is to try to catch it early, he says. "As soon as you feel a cold coming on, you should begin using herbal diaphoretics, which are spicy or pungent herbs that are most commonly taken in teas, immediately. This is the quickest means of turning a potentially persistent, lingering cold into nothing more than a few sniffles," he says. Try teas of any of the following: peppermint leaf, yarrow leaf and flower, elderflower, lemon balm leaf, chamomile flower, lemon verbena, lemongrass, gingerroot, sage leaf, thyme leaf, rosemary leaf, or basil leaf.

Generally, use 1 to 2 teaspoons of dried herb for every cup of water. Place the herb in a mason jar or teacup, pour boiling water over it, cover the container, and steep for 10 minutes. You can add honey to taste.

"These herbs have a stimulating effect on circulation," says Upton. The exact mechanism of how they work to prevent a cold from taking hold isn't clear, but history has shown them to be effective, he says. You can also use these in combination with the other remedies.

Try a garlic cocktail. Garlic is a favorite home remedy for killing the germs that cause colds and flu, says Smith. "It's great for fighting colds and breaking up congestion," he says. It is also an expectorant, which will help get all of that broken-up congestion out of your body.

Some herbalists suggest eating about six fresh cloves of garlic a day while you're sick. A painless way to do this is to blend three garlic cloves into ½ cup of carrot juice and drink it down, says Paul Bergner, clinical director of the Rocky Mountain Center for Botanical Studies in Boulder, Colorado, editor of *Medical Herbalism* and author of *The Healing Power of Garlic* and *The Healing Power of Echinacea and Goldenseal and Other Immune System Herbs*. If that much garlic irritates your stomach, experts recommend taking it with ginger or fennel seed tea. You can also eat parsley to help eliminate the garlic odor on your breath. Commission E, the expert panel that reports on the safety and effectiveness of herbal medicines for the German government, advises that fennel not be used for a prolonged time without direction from a qualified herbalist.

Warm up in the kitchen. To take the chills out of your cold, Hoffman suggests that you make a beeline to the kitchen and fix yourself a traditional herb-and-spice cold remedy. Combine 1 ounce (by weight) of sliced fresh ginger, one broken-up cinnamon stick, 1 teaspoon of coriander seeds, three cloves, one lemon slice, and 1 pint of water. He recommends simmering this combination for 15 minutes and straining. Then drink a hot cupful every two hours. Sweeten with organic honey to taste, he suggests.

To get well and stay well, use astragalus. "The biggest mistake that people make is not engaging in some type of preventive health program after they have been sick," says Upton. "Most people will treat the sickness with antibiotic substances, whether natural or synthetic, and get over the sickness, but then get sick again two or three weeks later." He recommends that people address the underlying deficiency in their immune systems that led to their getting ill in the first place. "Again, I suggest taking astragalus or reishi mushroom the same way you would to prevent a cold."

Congestion

Anything from tobacco smoke to cold and flu viruses can attack your delicate nasal membranes and leave you with stuffy congestion as the blood vessels in your nasal tissues become inflamed and swell so the mucus stagnates rather than flows. Here's what experts recommend to get the mucus moving.

Set a teatime. "I highly recommend fresh ginger tea to break up congestion," says Jones. "It's easy to make. Just use 1 tablespoon of grated fresh ginger for every cup of water. Simmer it for about 10 minutes, then let stand, covered, for 20 minutes. Strain it, add a squeeze of lemon, a dash of cayenne, and some honey, if you like. Then add more water, as needed, until you like the taste." Ginger tea will not only make you feel warmer, it will also loosen up sinus and chest congestion, says Jones. "Plus, it's a circulatory stimulant, so it will help move blood in and out of those congested areas, which will help clean the infection out of your system," she says. "Ginger is also antimicrobial and antibacterial, so it will help kill the germs that are making you sick to begin with. And it opens up your pores to help you sweat."

Apply an onion poultice. There's a great old-time onion recipe for breaking up congestion that has settled in your chest, says Jones. "Take one or two onions—enough so that when they're chopped, there's plenty to cover your chest area—and dice them up. Place the pieces in a pan and steam them with a little oil until they are transparent. Let them cool, and then lay them across your chest. Cover the onions with a piece of plastic wrap that is 1/2 to 1 inch larger than the area. Then lay a warm water bottle or a warm towel on top of them. Leave the onions in place for about a half-hour," she says. "The essential oils coming off the onions are antimicrobial, and they are slightly vasodilating, which opens the pores and helps these healing elements get through the skin. An onion poultice also stimulates circulation in your chest, so it'll help bring blood in to break up the congestion and carry out the waste," says Jones.

Get steamy. "The headaches and congestion from colds can be treated by inhaling the steam from steeping diaphoretic teas," says Upton. "My favorites for these symptoms are peppermint, rosemary, yarrow, ginger, thyme, and lemon verbena." He suggests taking a handful of your favorite of these herbs and tossing them into a pot of boiling water. Turn off the heat and place the pot on the kitchen table. Then cover your head with a large towel and bend over the pot with your head about 8 to 10 inches above it. Breathe in the vapors alternately through your nose and

mouth for 10 to 15 minutes. As the steam cools, you can put your face closer.

"The hot vapor helps to liquefy mucus, the essential oils help to combat certain pathogens, or germs that cause disease, and the fragrance helps to open up the sinuses and bronchioles," says Upton. You can do this whenever you need some stuffy-head relief.

Break it up with horseradish. Another timeless herbal remedy for respiratory ills is horseradish. And if you've ever inhaled its pungent vapors, it's easy to understand why, says Smith. "Horseradish is very high in polysaccharides, which stimulate the immune system. It's also rich in aromatic sulfur compounds, which are what you need to kill viruses and bacteria. And there's no doubt that it's good for breaking up congestion," he says. "The best way to get horseradish into your system is to just eat it. A teaspoonful on some crackers should help clear you right up."

Coughs

Like mosquitoes, car alarms, and so many other nuisances in life, coughs actually serve a purpose.

"Cough is the body's way to expel the mucus that is trapping pathogens and blocking the airways," says Upton. "So while it's okay to use treatments that soothe your throat and lessen dry, unproductive coughing, you don't want to completely eliminate your cough. You're best off using expectorants, which expel phlegm, not cough suppressants."

Herbs can help soothe your inflamed throat and eliminate phlegm and congestion. But the herbs you choose depend upon your cough. If you have a thick, congested cough, Upton recommends using a remedy that helps thin and liquefy mucus so it is expelled more easily. If your cough is dry and hacking, he suggests mucilaginous herbs that soothe and create a little healthy mucus so your cough will be more productive and you can expel whatever germs or irritants, like pollen, are making you cough. Finally, if your cough contains mucus that isn't clear, that could mean there's an active infection and you should take antimicrobial herbs, he says, because they kill the bacteria causing the cough. "Getting rid of whatever is causing the cough is more important than just getting rid of the cough itself," he explains.

Mull over mullein. "Mullein is excellent for a dry, hacking cough because it contains mucilage, which soothes throat irritation and cough," says Jones. Traditionally used to treat children with croup, mullein creates a thin layer of mucus in the lungs and airways, which soothes tickly throats and also helps heal throat irritation from all that coughing, she says. "It also makes a nice expectorant. Unfortunately, mullein doesn't taste very good, so you don't want to make it into a tea. If you have an acute cough, I recommend taking about 20 to 30 drops of mullein tincture five times a day."

Give it the slip with slippery elm. Native Americans used to make slippery elm into a throat-soothing beverage because it contains large amounts of mucilage, which also acts as an anti-tussive, or mild cough suppressant, says Dr. Tyler in *The Honest Herbal*. Although you can drink slippery elm as a tea, he recommends taking slippery elm in throat lozenges instead, because they provide a steady stream of mucilage to the throat. You can buy slippery elm "cough drops" at most health food stores, he says.

Have a little horehound. "Horehound is a good antispasmodic as well as a decongestant, which makes it a good cough remedy," says Patricia Howell, a professional member of the AHG in Atlanta. To make horehound into a tea, steep 2 heaping teaspoons of the dried herb in 1 cup of boiling water. If you don't like the taste, which Howell says can be "disgustingly bitter," you can buy horehound hard candy, which is frequently used as a cough lozenge, says Dr. Tyler in *Herbs of Choice*. Or you can steep horehound overnight, strain out the herb, and simmer the liquid until it's reduced by half. Then stir in an equal amount of honey and sip, says Howell.

Clear up with elecampane root. Elecampane root is also useful when you have a congested cough, says Howell, because it helps expel mucus while also drying out mucous membranes. Plus, it contains mucilage, so it also has a relaxing effect on a sore, irritated throat. To make a medicinal tea, Howell recommends pouring a cup of cold water onto 1 teaspoon of the cut root in a saucepan. Simmer for about 20 minutes, strain, and drink it warm. Drink the tea three times a day while you have a cough. Just remember that elecampane is quite bitter, so add some honey to sweeten it a bit.

Give it thyme. Thyme is a good herb to clear a congestive cough because it not only acts as an expectorant and an antiseptic, it also relieves bronchial spasms, says Smith. You can prepare thyme tea, which you can drink up to three times a day when you're sick, by steeping 1 teaspoonful of thyme leaves in 1 cup of boiling water, says Dr. Tyler in *Herbs of Choice*.

You can also put 1 teaspoon of thyme tincture in a bowl of steaming water and use it as an inhalant, says Smith. "That way, it goes directly into your lungs, where it stimulates blood flow and helps clear up the congestion."

Develop a liking for licorice. "Licorice is a key herb for cough," says Smith. "That's why they made those old-fashioned cough drops with it."

Kitchen Herbs That Soothe Sore Throats

One of the very first and decidedly least pleasant harbingers of a cold or the flu is a raw, scratchy sore throat. Fortunately, there are plenty of herbs that not only soothe your sore, inflamed throat but also fight the germs that are making you sick to begin with, says Roy Upton of Soquel, California, vice president of the American Herbalists Guild (AHG). Here's what Upton and other herbalists recommend.

Gargle away infection. "If your throat is infected and mucusy, I recommend gargling with teas made from infection-fighting, inflammation-soothing herbs such as sage, thyme, goldenseal, echinacea, or myrrh," says Upton. "The nice thing about using sage and thyme is that you can take them right out of your kitchen spice rack, make them into tea, and gargle. You don't have to run out to the drugstore." The other herbs can be found in health food stores.

To make these kitchen-cabinet teas, just take a teaspoonful of the herb, add boiling water, let it infuse in a covered container for 10 minutes, and strain, says Upton. You can use the liquid as gargle as often as necessary.

"I also recommend adding some echinacea to the mix whenever you have an inflammatory condition," says Ed Smith, a professional member of the AHG and founder of Herb Pharm in Williams, Oregon. "It stimulates your immune system so your body can get rid of the infection faster." For a sore throat, Smith recommends putting 30 to 40 drops of echinacea tincture into a glass of water and gargling with it several times a day.

Coat it with marshmallow. Mucilaginous herbs—herbs that reduce irritation and inflammation in the mucosal surfaces of the throat, bronchial tubes, and sinuses—are very soothing to a sore throat, says Feather Jones, a professional member of the AHG and director of the Rocky Mountain Center for Botanical Studies in Boulder, Colorado. "Marshmallow is one of my favorites," she says.

Marshmallow root is 35 percent mucilage when it's dried. To draw out the plant's mucilage properties, make a cool marshmallow tea, suggests Jones. Boil 8 ounces of water, then turn off the heat and add 1½ teaspoons of finely chopped marshmallow root. Put a lid on the pan and let stand for 30 minutes. Strain it and keep it in a covered glass container in the refrigerator. Sip it throughout the day, says Jones. Because bacteria like this rich mixture, experts advise that you make a fresh batch daily.

Chew on some licorice. If you're going to be out and about with your sore throat, Upton recommends chewing on an occasional stick of licorice root. The root comes in sticks the size of a pencil. The mucilage in licorice is especially good for soothing dry, scratchy sore throats, he says.

Suck some slippery elm. Another soothing treatment for a dry, scratchy sore throat is slippery elm in the form of a cough lozenge, says Upton. Slippery elm is also rich in soothing mucilage. It protects irritated mucous membranes, he says. Keep some lozenges in your pocket and take them as necessary.

"Licorice is anti-inflammatory," he explains. "And it's a mucilage, so it's soothing. Plus it is an antiviral herb, so it will help kill the organisms that are causing you to be sick to begin with." Licorice is effective as a tincture or as a tea. If you take it as a tincture, take $\frac{1}{2}$ to 1 teaspoon three times a day. To make a tea, use 1 teaspoonful per cup of boiling water. "Just be sure to let it simmer for about 20 minutes for full effectiveness," says Smith. You can drink it three times a day as you need to. But it's important to note that you can overdo licorice. In some cases, people who have consumed copious amounts of the herb—several ounces to a pound a day—have experienced headaches, water retention, high blood pressure, and, in very extreme cases, cardiac arrest.

Soothe with onions and honey. "My all-time favorite cough remedy is onions and honey," says Smith. "Simply dice a large onion and put it into a bowl. Then cover the diced pieces with honey and let stand overnight. The honey will draw the essential oils from the onions. In the morning, strain the mixture through a kitchen strainer into a bottle and take it by the tablespoon as you would a regular cough syrup," he says. The mixture will help kill your cold germs and act as an expectorant. "Plus, it tastes quite delicious," adds Smith.

Use a little eucalyptus. Eucalyptus is another aromatic herb with a long-standing history as a cough remedy. If you've used such over-the-counter medications as Vicks VapoRub, Mentholatum Chest Rub, or Halls cough drops, you've used this cool, aromatic herb to fight a cold. Eucalyptus leaves contain a chemical called eucalyptol that loosens phlegm in the chest and kills influenza and cold viruses and bacteria. Smith suggests putting 5 to 10 drops of eucalyptus oil in a teaspoon of honey and taking that as a quick cough syrup. "Or if you prefer, you can simply rub a few drops on your hand and breathe it in that way. The aromatic vapors are a powerful antiseptic, and they'll stimulate blood flow in your lungs to help clean them out," he says.

Hay Fever

Every year, it's the same thing. The magnolias flower, the tulips bloom, and while the world is awash in sights and scents, you can't see or smell any of it because your eyes are running and your nose is stuffed up.

Hay fever is essentially your immune system gone haywire. Instead of reserving its attacks for harmful bacteria and viruses, it also goes after harmless stuff like pollen and dust, flooding your body with chemicals such as histamine to fight the invaders. Unfortunately, that flood of chemicals also causes congestion, inflammation, and other irritating symptoms. If you're one of the 14 million Americans who have hay fever, these herbs might help.

Nose up to nettle. "Nettle is one of my favorite herbs for hay fever," says Jones. "It contains trace amounts of histamine, which is the substance that triggers allergies. So nettle has a homeopathic effect: When you take these trace amounts of histamine, your body builds up its immunity to the substance through its own natural antihistamine, and you are able to handle the attack of histamine during allergy season," she says.

You can drink nettle as a tea, or you can even eat it. For a tea, just pour 1 cup of boiling water onto 1 to 3 teaspoons of dried nettle and steep for 10 to 15 minutes. Drink three times a day (in some people, allergy symptoms get worse with nettle, so medical experts recommend taking no more than one dose a day for the first few days). Or you can just eat steamed nettle leaves, says Jones. "You don't want to eat them raw, because the plant is covered with fine hairlike needles that excrete a stinging acid when you rub up against them. But cooking takes away the sting. Nettle cooks up like spinach and is sweet and delicious. I would eat a cup two or three times a week." Jones recommends beginning to take nettle one month before allergy season begins and taking it continuously until one month after it ends.

De-stress with Siberian ginseng. If you can keep your mast cells (basic elements of your immune system) from becoming hypersensitive and spewing histamine at every slight assault, you can help ward off hay fever attacks, says Gagnon. "I recommend Siberian ginseng to cool down the adrenal glands, which are the glands responsible for causing stress in the body. Ginseng can help make the body more resistant to the wear and tear of stress." He recommends that you start taking one dropperful of alcohol-based extract twice a day beginning a month before you typically suffer from allergies and continuing throughout allergy season. To avoid irritability, avoid consuming caffeine and other stimulants while using ginseng.

Brighten your eyes with eyebright. As its name implies, eyebright can help clear up weepy, allergy-stricken eyes, says Jones. "It tones and strengthens the ocular membranes behind the eyes, so it helps clear up runny eyes and nose," she says. Herbalists suggest taking one to four milliliters of eyebright as a tincture three times a day, as you need to.

Hit it with goldenrod. If the mucous membranes in your nasal and bronchial passages are inflamed, you might want to hit them with a dose of goldenrod, says Jones. "Goldenrod is a good anti-catarrhal, which means that it relieves inflammation of the air passages. It also works as a demulcent, which means that it can help soothe mucous membranes that have been irritated by coughing,

hacking, and sneezing," says Jones. You can take goldenrod as a tea. Just pour a cup of boiling water over 2 to 3 teaspoons of the dried herb. Allow it to steep for about 10 to 15 minutes, then strain. Experts suggest drinking this three times a day when you need relief from sinus inflammation.

Use ephedra with care. If you are so congested from hay fever that you can't even see straight to take any other medicinal herb, a shot of ma huang, or ephedra, extract may be just what the herbalist ordered, adds Gagnon. "I use ma huang when there is so much blockage that the person simply cannot breathe through their nose and they need symptomatic relief," he says. "Ma huang, which is a powerful Chinese decongestant herb, will work within 45 minutes." All you need is a teaspoonful when you're seriously blocked up.

"As in the case of using ephedra for asthma, I only use small doses for hay fever, and I prefer that people be monitored by a qualified health-care practitioner," says Dr. Gruska.

"Because it's a powerful stimulant, you shouldn't take ephedra if you have high blood pressure, glaucoma, or heart problems," cautions Gagnon. "It can also cause insomnia. You should use it *only* under medical care." And don't use ephedra along with over-the-counter or prescription medicines—the additive effects can be dangerous.

Sinus Problems

Colds and allergies can cause the healthy, moistening mucus that naturally flows in and out of your sinuses to become trapped, leaving it to build up and cause uncomfortable congestion. Blocked sinuses generally can be cleared with the same teas and inhalants you would use for congestion, says Jones. But when a little blockage becomes major sinus stoppage, bacteria can set up camp in the stagnant mucus, causing an infection called sinusitis that leads to headaches and nasty postnasal drip. For sinus relief, the following herbs may help.

Strengthen with goldenseal. Sinus problems are where goldenseal can shine, says Gagnon. "Goldenseal works wonders on subacute (somewhat lingering and severe) and chronic bouts of inflammation of the mucous membranes, such as sinusitis," he says. "It'll kick the problem out so fast, you'll wonder what happened." He recommends taking 10 to 25 drops of alcohol-based goldenseal extract, depending upon the severity of your condition, up to five times a day. You should use it only until your sinus inflammation has cleared, he says. "It's not meant to be used daily, long-term, as you would a strengthening, tonic herb."

Unplug with pleurisy. "Pleurisy root is a very stimulating expectorant," says Jones. "It's especially good for loosening up thick, tenacious mucus, whether it's in the lungs or in the sinuses," she says. It works by allowing the body to produce healthy mucus, which helps to loosen the thick, unhealthy mucus that is stuck there.

"In the old days, they used to grind up the dried root and snort it to get it directly into the sinuses," says Jones. "These days, you can take about 20 drops as an extract. It doesn't work as instantly, but it's still relatively quick." It is available at some health food stores. Pleurisy root can cause nausea and vomiting, so if it disagrees with you, stop taking it.

Clear up with yerba santa. When your sinuses feel like they're filled with mud, herbalists often suggest yerba santa, a Southwestern herb that's available through mail order. "Yerba santa is very aromatic," says Smith. "You can take it as a tea or liquid extract, and it will help stimulate blood flow to the mucous membranes and slough off thick, stubborn congestion." Experts recommend taking up to two ounces (by weight) a day as a tea for symptom relief when the condition flares up. Make the tea as you do most herbal teas, says Smith. Add a cup of boiling water to a heaping teaspoonful of herb and infuse for 10 or 15 minutes, then drink it hot.

Herbal Wisdom
Linked to Cycles of the Moon, Sun, and Seasons

"For thousands of years, women collected plants from meadows and woodlands and used them to create healing medicines. They gathered herbs by the waning and waxing of the moon, artfully created preparations, and developed herbal formulas. The best of these remedies were added to the lore, and the wisdom was transferred from mother to daughter, from wise woman to apprentice, for countless generations. This is the legacy we have inherited. Healers, wise women—these women were the center and source of medicine and healing for their communities. They understood the cycles of the season, the ebb and flow of the universe, the sun, the moon, the stars, and the natural rhythms of their bodies."

—*Rosemary Gladstar, herbalist, author, and teacher*

Slow-Healing Wounds

HERBS THAT MEND BROKEN SKIN, FAST

In a perfect world, cuts, scrapes, nicks, and even surgical incisions would knit themselves back together swiftly and neatly. There would be no infection, no enduring red marks, and no need to sport a bandage for weeks on end. But this isn't a perfect world, and everything from dirt to microbes to poor circulation can slow the healing process to a crawl, leaving you with an unwanted souvenir from that time you tripped over the neighbor kid's tricycle two weeks ago or nicked your leg while shaving a month ago.

Fast-Forward Therapy

The herbal solution for slow-healing wounds begins with a good cleaning. Wash the injury well with mild soap and water. Then call on these tissue-mending herbs that can make hurt skin whole again. If you have poor circulation due to diabetes or hardening of the arteries, however, you should see a doctor rather than try to self-treat slow-healing wounds.

Soak out debris. "An herbal soak can help draw out small pieces of dirt and lingering infection that can prevent a wound from healing," notes Sharol Tilgner, N.D., a naturopathic physician, professional member of the American Herbalists Guild (AHG), and president of Wise Woman Herbals in Creswell, Oregon.

If the wound is on a part of the body that you can soak in a basin or large bowl, make a strong tea using a quart of water and ½ cup of wild geranium, oak bark, or witch hazel, she suggests. Simmer the tea for at least a half-hour, then strain. Soak the wound in the comfortably hot tea for at least 15 minutes, Dr. Tilgner says.

If the wounded area cannot be soaked easily, use the strong tea mixture as a compress, Dr. Tilgner suggests. Soak a clean cloth in the tea but don't wring it out. Lay the very wet cloth over the wound. "Every few minutes, rinse the cloth in the tea and reapply to the wound," she says. "Keep the tea very warm; gently heat it up if necessary."

Herbs like oak bark, geranium, and witch hazel are astringents that were used traditionally to clean and heal wounds, Dr. Tilgner says. "Astringent herbs make skin tissue contract," she says. "Bits of debris come loose and are pulled out of the wound. Combined with a warm liquid, an astringent herb acts like a vacuum cleaner, pulling out the debris." So if the wound is infected or bits of foreign matter remain in it, you may see the debris floating in the soaking liquid or clinging to the cloth, Dr. Tilgner says. "If a wound is very dirty, you may have to change the soaking liquid several times to keep it clean," she notes.

Fight inflammation with echinacea. A compress made by mixing 1 part echinacea tincture with 3 parts water and applied to the wound with clean cloths or gauze pads can fend off inflammation in a hard-to-heal wound, notes Paul Bergner, clinical director of the Rocky Mountain Center for Botanical Studies in Boulder, Colorado, editor of *Med-*

Calendula: The Blossom That Erases Scars

You can avoid unsightly scarring after a wound or surgical incision heals by rubbing calendula-infused olive oil into freshly healed skin, suggests Sharol Tilgner, N.D., a naturopathic physician, professional member of the American Herbalists Guild, and president of Wise Woman Herbals in Creswell, Oregon. "Start rubbing a little in every day, as soon as a wound heals," she notes. To protect your clothing, cover the area with a bandage or apply the oil at night. "If you're patient, you can also use calendula oil on any existing scars," says Dr. Tilgner. "It can take months or even a year to erase an older scar this way, but I've seen it work."

Calendula's traditional use as a wound healer has been substantiated by research that shows this herb promotes the skin-mending process. You can order calendula-infused olive oil by mail (see "Where to Buy Herbs and Herbal Products" on page 462). Or make your own by infusing 2 parts olive oil with 1 part dried calendula petals (for directions, see "Infused Oils" on page 101).

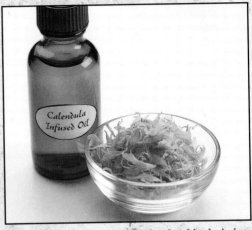

Substances in calendula help the skin knit itself together after a wound.

ical Herbalism, and author of *The Healing Power of Garlic* and *The Healing Power of Echinacea and Goldenseal and Other Immune System Herbs.* Apply the compress for 10 to 15 minutes, Bergner says, and reapply a compress four times a day until the wound is clearly healing.

If a wound hurts, heals slowly, and is swollen and red or discharges pus or liquid, most likely it's infected, says Dr. Tilgner. If, despite self-treatment, it shows no sign of healing within a week, see a doctor.

Close clean, shallow wounds with comfrey and calendula. Once the wound is clean and infection-free (there's no debris in the wound or pus around it), give the healing process a nudge by applying comfrey and calendula, Dr. Tilgner suggests.

Both herbs have traditional reputations as skin menders. Comfrey contains a substance called allantoin that prompts rapid tissue repair. Research shows that calendula prompts the body to produce healthy new skin cells at a wound site. In Europe, calendula creams are widely used for slow-healing wounds.

"Plain comfrey is the best healer," says Dr. Tilgner. "If you grow this herb, harvest the roots and make a slurry with a little water and the root in a food processor or blender. Soak the wound in it or dip a clean cloth in it and lay it over the wound, bound with another cloth on top to hold it in place. Do this twice a day until the wound heals. You can leave the comfrey on overnight and change the cloth in the morning."

You can also apply a comfrey and calendula cream that's available at health food stores and by mail order (see "Where to Buy Herbs and Herbal Products" on page 462). One buying tip: "Look for a cream or salve that's a rich, dark green. The color should tell you there's a lot of comfrey in it," suggests Jenny McFeely, a member of Britain's National Institute of Medical Herbalists and a professional member of the AHG who teaches courses on herbalism through her Herbal Healing and Research Center in Scottsdale, Arizona.

You can prepare your own comfrey-calendula salve, Dr. Tilgner suggests. First, infuse 2 cups of olive oil with ½ cup of comfrey and ½ cup of calendula petals. Then use the infused oil to concoct a simple herbal salve (see "Infused Oils" on page 101 and "Salves and Ointments" on page 110 for directions).

One caution: Don't use comfrey on wounds that are deep or show signs of infec-tion, Dr. Tilgner warns. Comfrey promotes such quick cell regeneration that the surface of a wound could heal, leaving infected or damaged skin underneath. If you're not sure whether a wound is clean or too deep for comfrey, don't use it, she says. Use a cream or salve that contains only calendula instead.

Increase circulation with prickly ash. If a wound is white rather than pink, that's a sign that it's healing slowly, notes McFeely. "If a wound is healing slowly because circula-tion in the area of the wound is poor, then one remedy I suggest is prickly ash bark, which improves blood flow to the periphery of the body, such as the hands and feet," she says. "Improving circulation brings more of the body's own healing substances to the wound site."

McFeely suggests using a tincture of American prickly ash bark, which has a tra-ditional reputation for stimulating periph-eral circulation, by taking 30 drops of the tincture two or three times a day for a month. You can find prickly ash at some health food stores.

Sunburn

COMFORT SCORCHED SKIN WITH NATURE'S SOOTHERS

Ultraviolet rays of the sun stalk un-defended skin—unprotected, vul-nerable spots such as the nose or the back of the neck where that smear of sun-block didn't quite cover. Bombarded on the ski slopes, at the beach, on the golf course, or in the garden, your skin first feels warm, then tender, then assaulted. Later comes proof that you've spent too long catching rays—your skin is red, swollen, painful, and perhaps even blistered, all signs that blood vessels near the skin's surface have dilated.

Fair-skinned women and those with blond, red, or brown hair are at highest risk for skin damage from the sun. But anyone, regardless of skin tone, can get a sunburn. Unfortunately, there's no such thing as an herbal sunblock, says Jenny McFeely, a member of Britain's National Institute of Medical Herbalists and a professional member of the American Herbalists Guild (AHG) who teaches courses on herbalism through her Herbal Healing and Research Center in Scottsdale, Arizona. Your best bet, as always, is to buy a sunscreen with an SPF (sun protection factor) of at least 15 and stay covered up or indoors when the sun is brightest in the middle of the day.

Look for a PABA-free sunscreen, recommends Gayle Eversole, R.N., Ph.D., a nurse practitioner, medical herbalist, and professional member of the AHG in Everett, Washington. And don't use sunscreen as an excuse to prolong sun exposure to the maximum.

Relief for Solar Accidents

If for some reason you neglect to adequately protect your skin, herbalists offer remedies to relieve the pain and swelling and promote healing. If you have blisters, a fever, chills, or severe pain, you could have what is commonly called sun poisoning. Get medical attention immediately. These symptoms could also indicate the presence of heat exhaustion or heatstroke.

Vanquish the pain with aloe. Aloe vera gel cools and soothes painful sunburn and also seals in the skin's natural moisture, which helps healing, says McFeely. "The aloe forms a coating on the surface of the skin, helping to prevent dehydration from the inside out. This is important, especially with a bad, blistering sunburn," she notes. "When the body becomes dehydrated, healing is more difficult."

The best aloe treatment? Gel from your own plant, McFeely says. "Just cut off an outside leaf, slit it open, and scrape out the gel. Pat it onto sunburned areas with your fingers." Or put the gel on gauze and gently lay it on the burn, but don't rub, she adds. Don't have an aloe plant on your windowsill? "Look for aloe in health food stores or mail-order catalogs," she suggests (see "Where to Buy Herbs and Herbal Products" on page 462). "Although the juice has a higher concentration of real aloe than skin lotions that contain aloe, some aloe preparations don't contain a lot of juice. Read the label and ask an expert."

Mix an aloe-lavender "smoothie." Aloe vera and lavender essential oil combine to cool sunburn, reduce swelling and redness, and prevent infection, says herbalist Mindy Green, a professional member of the AHG, faculty member at the Rocky Mountain Center for Botanical Studies and director of education at the Herb Research Foundation, both in Boulder, Colorado, and co-author of *Aromatherapy: A Complete Guide to the Healing Art.* To make an herbal soother, combine 4 ounces of aloe vera gel, $\frac{1}{2}$ teaspoon of lavender oil, 1 teaspoon of apple-cider vinegar, and 2 capsules (400 international units each) of vitamin E oil (to use the oil, just prick the capsule with a clean needle or knifepoint, then squeeze out the oil). Or you can buy a small jar of vitamin E oil, says Dr. Eversole. Shake the mixture before applying it.

Gently pat your aloe vera smoothie on painful, inflamed sunburn. Reapply as needed to keep skin cool and comfortable, Green says.

Cool down with tea. The tannic acid in tea soothes sunburn pain, says Dr. Eversole. "Just make regular tea with black or orange pekoe, and when it's cool, pat it on your sunburned skin," she suggests.

"The tannic acid actually helps restore the natural acid balance of your skin. Sunburn throws off that balance, contributing to the pain," Dr. Eversole notes. While some herbal teas also contain tannins, the high tannin content of regular black tea makes it the top choice when it comes to soothing sunburn.

The tannins also prompt proteins in the top layers of your skin to form a protective covering, "kind of like a natural bandage," notes Sharol Tilgner, N.D., a naturopathic physician, professional member of the AHG, and president of Wise Woman Herbals in Creswell, Oregon. You can pat the tea onto your skin with your fingertips or soak a cotton ball in the tea and apply it. Start using this remedy as soon as you notice sunburn pain. If pain returns, reapply as needed, says Eversole.

Pat on St.-John's-wort or calendula. For a cooling splash or compress, combine 1 part St.-John's-wort or calendula tincture (also called an extract) with 9 parts cool water, Dr. Tilgner suggests. Pat it on sunburned areas or soak a clean cloth in the mixture and lay it on scorched skin for at least 15 minutes. St.-John's-wort can relieve pain caused by nerve damage, Dr. Tilgner says, and, in one study, it also helped heal burns. Calendula is a traditional skin mender that has been shown in research studies to have anti-inflammatory activity. The cool water also helps ease sunburn pain and swelling.

Bathe in apple-cider vinegar. Another plant-based product, apple-cider vinegar, can also soothe sunburn pain, Dr. Tilgner says. For all-over sunburn relief, try adding a cup to a bathtub full of cool water, then soak. "Apple-cider vinegar is astringent. It soothes sunburn pain much the way black tea does," Dr. Tilgner notes.

Soak in your oats. If your sunburn is fading but your skin feels dry, tight, and itchy, relieve the discomfort with an oatmeal bath, Dr. Tilgner suggests. "It really soothes the skin," she notes. Try colloidal oatmeal, available in drugstores as Aveeno, which you can add directly to the bathwater. Or, in a pinch, you can use noninstant breakfast oats. To avoid a messy cleanup job, wrap the oats in a handkerchief or an old pair of panty hose and fasten it with a rubber band.

Urinary Tract Infections

HERBS THAT STOP THE BURN

Another bladder infection, another round of antibiotics. If you're on this frustrating merry-go-round, take heart. Herbalists say that it may be possible to stop the ride without filling yet another prescription.

That's good news, especially for women. Urinary tract infections (UTIs) account for over seven million doctor visits each year. And women get UTIs—sometimes called cystitis—25 percent more often than men. That's because a woman's urethra, the tube that empties urine from the bladder, is shorter than a man's. (Ours are 1½ inches long; theirs are 8 inches.) This quirk of feminine plumbing makes it easy for bacteria from the vagina or rectum to move up the urethra into the bladder.

Less-than-sanitary toilet habits contribute to the risk. So does using a diaphragm and its spermicides, as well as products such as douches and feminine deodorants.

The result is symptoms that include burning during urination, strong-smelling or cloudy urine, and an urgent need to urinate. Left unchecked, bacteria from the urethra or bladder may work their way into the kidneys, causing a potentially serious kidney infection.

A Revolutionary Alternative

Antibiotics are the standard treatment for UTIs—they wipe out the bacteria that cause bladder infections. Herbal treatments for UTIs go one step further, says Douglas Schar, a practicing medical herbalist in London, editor of the *British Journal of Phytotherapy*, and author of *Backyard Medicine Chest*. "Women who get chronic UTIs also need to protect the mucous membrane that lines the urinary tract so that bacteria have a hard time moving in," he explains. "Herbs can both kill bacteria and maintain the mucous membranes so they can resist infection. They do double duty."

Certain herbs also act as diuretics, substances that increase your output of urine. Urinating more often helps to flush out bacteria.

"We almost never recommend antibiotics for UTIs," says Ellen Kamhi, R.N., Ph.D., of Oyster Bay, New York, an herbalist, professional member of the American Herbalists Guild (AHG), and host of the nationally syndicated radio show *Natural Alternatives*, who works in tandem with Serafina Corsello, M.D. "We focus on herbs and lifestyle changes, and we use antibiotics only as a last resort."

Herbs work best when they're teamed with good hygiene and healthy habits, explains Dr. Kamhi. Wipe from front to back after you go to the toilet to keep bacteria away from the urethra. Drink up to eight glasses of filtered water a day to speed bacteria-infected urine on its way. And go when you feel the urge: Holding it in allows bacteria to flourish.

Herbal Soothers for Bothered Bladders

If you've had UTIs in the past and your doctor has ruled out kidney problems, you might want to try herbal remedies for a few days. So the next time you have to go . . . and go . . . and go . . . give these treatments a try.

Soak away discomfort. Sitting in an herbal sitz bath can help relieve the external burning of a UTI and hasten healing, says Feather Jones, a professional member of the AHG and director of the Rocky Mountain Center for Botanical Studies in Boulder, Colorado. She recommends using uva-ursi and marshmallow root powder. To make this soothing soak, boil 1 gallon of water and add a handful of powdered uva-ursi leaves (approximately 1 ounce by weight). Steep for 20 minutes, then strain. Add 1 ounce of marshmallow powder. Transfer the brew to a large pan, be sure the water is comfortably warm, and soak for 20 minutes. Jones suggests doing this once or twice a day for several days or as long as it's needed.

"Uva-ursi is an astringent, so it will help reduce swelling, and the marshmallow root soothes irritated tissues," says Jones. You can find powdered uva-ursi and marshmallow root in some health food stores or purchase them through the mail (see "Where to Buy Herbs and Herbal Products" on page 462).

Use a tincture trio. When combined, uva-ursi, corn silk, and echinacea tinctures are known as urinary tract antiseptics. Because uva-ursi tincture can be irritating by itself, it's usually mixed with other tinctures (also called extracts). Jones suggests 10 drops of uva-ursi tincture, 10 drops of corn silk tincture, and 10 drops of echinacea tincture.

Add this mixture to ½ cup of water or a noncitrus juice and drink to help as an antiseptic in the urinary tract, she says. You can buy one-ounce bottles of the tinctures already combined at health food stores.

Smooth on a salve. A salve made from chickweed and calendula can ease the external burning of a UTI, says Dr. Kamhi. To make the salve, put a handful of each herb in a nonaluminum pan and cover them with 2 to 3 cups of extra-virgin olive oil. Warm the mixture over low heat for 30 minutes. Discard the herbs, then mix in 1 tablespoon of melted beeswax per 2 cups of olive oil. Let it cool. Apply the salve to irritated tissue as needed. You can store the salve in the refrigerator for up to a year, says Dr. Kamhi.

Some herbalists say that chickweed soothes irritated tissue, while calendula contains glycosides and carotenoids that reduce swelling. Both of these herbs are sold in bulk in some health food stores and through mail order. Health food stores also carry ready-made salves made with these ingredients.

Go with parsley. Parsley is an excellent diuretic, says Varro E. Tyler, Ph.D., professor emeritus of pharmacognosy at the Purdue University School of Pharmacy and Pharmacal Sciences in West Lafayette, Indiana, and author of *Herbs of Choice*. This herb contains myristicin and apiol, compounds that are thought to help increase the output of urine by increasing the flow of blood to the kidneys. To make a tea, pour a cup of boiling water over a few sprigs of crushed fresh parsley or 1 teaspoon of dried parsley. Let the herb steep for 5 to 10 minutes, then strain and drink. Consume one cup two or three times a day until the infection clears up, says Dr. Kamhi. (Using

Custom Herbal Mixes
for Urinary Tract Infections

*U*va-ursi, juniper berry, and nettle have long been used to treat urinary tract problems, says herbalist Ellen Kamhi, R.N., Ph.D., of Oyster Bay, New York, a professional member of the American Herbalists Guild and host of the nationally syndicated radio show *Natural Alternatives*, who works in tandem with Serafina Corsello, M.D. The active ingredient in uva-ursi, arbutrin, cripples infection-causing bacteria, says Dr. Kamhi. Juniper berry is an antimicrobial that disinfects the urine, and it contains terpenes, which act as a diuretic. Nettle also has a diuretic effect, studies show.

Health food stores sell teas, tinctures, and capsules that contain herbs used specifically to treat UTIs. But because of labeling laws, they won't say so. Look for brands that contain the herbs that are recommended here. "They're excellent," says Dr. Kamhi. If you decide to try one of these products, follow the directions on the label, she says. The usual dosage is two capsules four to six times a day or 10 drops of tincture three or four times a day. You can drink the teas several times a day until the infection clears up. If you opt for a tea, make sure that what you buy is fresh, so that it still has active ingredients. Ask someone at the store how long it's been on the shelf—more than three months is too long.

parsley as a vegetable condiment during pregnancy is fine, but don't use it as a tea in high amounts, she cautions.)

Sip a berry good remedy. Virtually all of us have heard that cranberry juice helps clear up UTIs, and research shows that this old folk remedy really works. A substance in cranberry keeps infection-causing bacteria from sticking to the lining of the bladder and urethra. If bacteria can't stick, they're less likely to trigger infection.

Cranberry is available in different forms, all of which you can find at health food stores, says Dr. Kamhi. If you opt for juice, she suggests that you choose an unsweetened variety, available at health food stores. "The sugar in commercial brands weakens the ability of the immune system to fight off the bacteria," she says. "If the juice is too tart, sweeten it with the herb stevia. One to two drops per glass should suffice." She recommends drinking eight ounces of cranberry juice a day, the amount used in research studies, until the symptoms subside.

For convenience, consider capsules. Cranberry also comes in capsule form. And, like cranberries, the capsules are safe for pregnant women, says Eric Yarnell, N.D., a naturopathic doctor in Sedona, Arizona, who is on the board of the Botanical Medicine Academy. He suggests taking two or three capsules containing at least 400 milligrams each of cranberry extract every day until the infection clears up.

Make a berry tea. If at all possible, Dr. Kamhi prefers a tea made from whole cranberries. She recommends purchasing fresh, organically grown berries (available in health food stores or in the organic food section of supermarkets) in the fall, when they're harvested. "Stock up, put them in plastic bags, and pop them into the freezer," says Dr. Kamhi. "You'll have them all year long." To make fresh cranberry tea, place a handful of berries in a pot and cover them with water. Gently simmer the berries (don't boil) for 30 to 45 minutes. When the berries are white and the water is bright red, discard the berries, let the tea cool, and drink. If the flavor is too tart, add a drop or two of stevia as a sweetener. Drink three to four cups a day until the infection clears up.

If you can't find fresh cranberries, use the dried variety, says Dr. Kamhi. Fill a tea ball with dried cranberries, place the ball in a cup of boiling water, steep for 20 minutes, and drink. Consume three to four cups a day during an infection.

Make tea with a triple punch. Besides using cranberries, you might want to try drinking tea made with equal parts of buchu, corn silk, and couch grass (also known as triticum or dog grass), recommends Schar. To make the tea, add 1 teaspoon of each herb to 1 cup of boiling water and steep for 10 to 15 minutes. Drink three cups a day until the unpleasant sensations have subsided. "This tea is especially good for a sudden, painful bladder infection," says Schar. "You'll feel better in a matter of days."

Buchu contains pulegone, a volatile oil that kills some bacteria in the urine, while the corn silk acts as a diuretic, says Schar. The couch grass contains anti-inflammatory substances that help to soothe burning and inflammation. (Do not take buchu while pregnant.)

Whole-Body Herbal Helpers

In addition to recommending the problem-specific herbs mentioned above, herbalists advise women who are prone to UTIs to take steps to boost their overall immunity to infection. Here's what they advise.

Build resistance with echinacea. First used by the Native Americans, echinacea has been shown in clinical tests to stimulate the immune system. Researchers aren't sure why echinacea works, but they think it boosts the production of interferon and properdin, two protein substances that resist viruses and bacteria.

Some people take echinacea in tea or tincture form, but Schar doesn't recommend the tincture, as he says it tastes "real bad." Some people like the tea, and some people don't. Thus, you may prefer to take capsules. Schar suggests taking two 500-milligram capsules of pure echinacea root three times a day for three to six months to end the cycle of repeated UTIs.

Heal with goldenseal. "Goldenseal is an excellent mucous membrane tonic," says Schar. It's also a powerful antimicrobial agent, and herbalists have used it for the last century to treat infections. Schar recommends taking four 500-milligram capsules of goldenseal root a day. It can take up to three months for the herb's healing properties to take full effect, he notes, but during that time, you're likely to get fewer UTIs that pass more quickly. Do not take goldenseal if you are pregnant, however.

Vaginal Problems

HERBAL REMEDIES FOR IRRITATIONS AND INFECTIONS

For women, vaginal trouble ranks right up there with fatigue and headaches as a nearly universal complaint. Vaginitis—a catch-all term for irritation, redness, and swelling of the vulva and vagina—is responsible for nearly half of all the visits that women make to their doctors. One study reported that 72 percent of young, sexually active women had one or more forms of vaginitis, and another determined that vaginal infections are six times more common than urinary tract infections.

Why does this oh-so-common problem prompt millions of women to seek medical attention? Because quite frankly, vaginitis can disrupt a woman's life at its most intimate level. Besides itching, burning, irritation, and swelling, you may also experience an odd-looking or odoriferous discharge. Urination may be painful—and that goes double for sex.

Gyn-Ecology

Vaginitis can be caused by irritants, infections, hormonal disruptions following menopause, or the surgical removal of the ovaries. (Read more about vaginitis due to hormonal disruptions in "Menopause" on page 281).

Irritant vaginitis occurs when the vaginal area is chafed or otherwise injured. Causes include wearing tight pants or panty hose, overly vigorous sex, and allergies to feminine hygiene products or medications. Leaving a tampon or other foreign object in the vagina can also contribute to irritant vaginitis.

As for infectious vaginitis, the causes will likely remind you of sophomore biology class. That's because the vagina is an ecosystem that's home to billions of organisms—yes, tiny little living fungal or bacterial beings—that flourish democratically in its warm, moist environment. Maintaining the vagina's healthy balance means maintaining a certain, slightly acidic pH level, explains Kathleen Maier, a physician's assistant, professional member of the American Herbalists Guild (AHG), and former advisor on botanical medicine to the National Institutes of Health.

Disturb the "ecology" of the vagina—via a nutrient-poor diet, energetic sexual activity, a sexually transmitted disease (STD), pregnancy, frequent use of commercial feminine hygiene products, or some prescription drugs, notably antibiotics—and war breaks out, as the vaginal population of bacteria or fungi increases disproportionately and runs amok. An imbalance in the organism population leads to various uncomfortable symptoms.

A short list of organisms causes an overwhelming majority of vaginal infections. The most common cause is bacteria. Second to bacterial vaginitis are infections caused by the yeastlike fungi candida and monilia, which are referred to as yeast infections. Trichomoniasis (commonly called trich) is caused by a single-celled bug called a protozoan and is the third most prevalent type of vaginal infection. Less frequently, culprits include herpes simplex (a virus), chlamydia (a parasite), *Neisseria gonorrhoea* (a bacterium), streptococci, staphylococci, and human papillomavirus.

Each variety of vaginitis has signature symptoms, says Aviva Romm, a certified professional midwife, herbalist, and professional member of the AHG who practices in Bloomfield Hills, Michigan, and is author of *The Natural Pregnancy Book* and *Natural Healing for Babies and Children.*

"Vaginal infections caused by bacteria may have a strong-smelling yellow, grayish, white, or mucusy discharge, possibly streaked with blood, with a foul, fishy odor. Itching may be present. A yeast infection usually involves moderate to severe itching and burning, and the tip-off is a thick, cheesy discharge with a yeasty smell," says Romm. Trichomoniasis often reveals itself with a frothy green or yellowish discharge, may smell bad, and can cause burning when you urinate. The itching is severe.

"I think the three main factors in any case of vaginitis are diet, hygiene, and sexuality," says Maier, who is also the director of Dreamtime Center for Herbal Studies, an herbal school and free herbal clinic in Flint Hill, Virginia.

"Many vaginal infections are sexually transmitted to women by men—who, unfortunately, have no symptoms 95 percent of the time. What often happens is this: A woman gets a bacterial or yeast infection, has intercourse with her partner, and passes it on to him. She gets treatment and clears up her problem, but if her partner remains un-treated, she then becomes reinfected. To prevent this scenario, her partner needs to be treated, too, at the same time. He needs to make the same commitment to the treatment as she does," Maier says.

You need to know what kind of vaginal infection you have in order to determine the best course of treatment. Seek the help of a health-care professional to identify the type and to choose the proper course of action. Women can safely treat themselves for most yeast infections that last no longer than 10 days to two weeks. If your condition persists, consult your heath-care practitioner for advice and treatment, says Maier. After you've been diagnosed, consider the following courses of action.

A Nondrug Approach to Yeast Infections

Herbalists and other holistic practitioners treat vaginitis differently than conventional physicians do, says naturopathic physician Tori Hudson, N.D., professor at the National College of Naturopathic Medicine and director of A Woman's Time, a women's health clinic, both in Portland, Oregon.

"Instead of the 'raid and defoliate' approach that conventional doctors often use, we try to 'improve the soil,' so to speak," says Dr. Hudson. "That means that we work to balance the vaginal environment and correct the underlying deficiencies that caused it to get out of whack in the first place, rather than simply killing the offending flora."

"A few nutritional adjustments are the first line of defense for vaginal yeast infections," says Romm. "Good nutrition for you means bad nutrition for yeast, so you need to eliminate the kinds of food that yeast organisms crave—sugar, breads and other baked goods, and alcohol. These foods contain the medium that allows yeast to thrive.

"In fact, I have found that many women seem to be prone to yeast infections around the holidays, when they're getting married, or when they've done some extra-heavy partying," notes Romm. "That's because party foods like cocktails, wine, and sweet foods fuel yeast infections. And as a double whammy, social occasions, especially weddings, often coincide with stressful times. Stress weakens your immune system and can allow yeast infections to invade and flourish," she adds.

A diet that promotes vaginal health is high in low-fat proteins like fish and chicken and includes plenty of steamed vegetables—sans starchy, yeast-promoting foods like potatoes, Romm says. And for women who have recurrent yeast infections, Romm also suggests peeling fruits and vegetables before eating them raw, since the skins can attract yeast.

A Potpourri of Remedies

For irritations and yeast infections, herbalists recommend the following remedies.

Slather on some yogurt. "Live-cultured yogurt is full of friendly bacteria called *Lactobacillus acidophilus*. They gobble up the bad yeast and restore acid balance to the vaginal area," says Romm. To use yogurt as a remedy for vaginitis, choose plain yogurt with live cultures, such as Dannon. Yogurt labels often

Herbal Wisdom
Medicine That Nourishes and Heals

"What I like about herbs is that they span the spectrum between food and medicine. Herbs enhance our food when we are hungry, nourish our bodies when we are depleted, and provide pharmacological interventions when we are ill. Herbs are generally less specific and more supportive than drugs."

—*Adriane Fugh-Berman, M.D., medical officer at the National Institutes of Health*

tell you whether or not the product contains live cultures.

Scoop a few tablespoons of yogurt into a dish and let it to come to room temperature so you don't have the shocking experience of putting icy yogurt on sensitive tissues, recommends Romm. Stand with one foot resting on the edge of the bathtub and dip your fingers into the yogurt. Work some up inside your vagina and all around the outer vaginal area. Discard any unused yogurt in the dish. "You can do this several times a day, or you can put some yogurt on a sanitary pad and wear it, changing the pad and adding fresh yogurt several times a day," suggests Romm. Continue to use the yogurt treatments for five to seven days, she recommends.

You could also insert a capsule of acidophilus as a convenient alternative, suggests Dr. Hudson.

Squirt on an herbal rinse. "Herbal rinses are the best," says Romm. "They're cooling, soothing, and antimicrobial, which means that they attack the bad organisms and leave the good ones intact," she adds. You can use this in addition to the yogurt treatment suggested above.

To make Romm's herbal rinse, blend equal parts of dried calendula, yarrow flowers, lavender, and comfrey root. Put 2 ounces of the mixture in a 2-quart pot and cover with 2 quarts of boiling water. Cover and steep for 30 minutes. Allow the infusion to cool to lukewarm and strain. Add 4 ounces of the infusion to a peri bottle (a plastic squeeze bottle designed for washing the outer genital area—available at surgical or medical supply stores and some drugstores) and squirt the mixture over your vaginal area after you urinate, suggests Romm. Alternately, you can saturate a washcloth with the infusion and apply it as a compress to the vaginal area for several minutes. Repeat several times a day until the solution is used up, advises Romm. You can store the herbal rinse in the refrigerator for up to three days.

The calendula eases inflammation and, like lavender, is antimicrobial. Comfrey root is soothing and contains allantoin, which promotes cell growth and helps heal any little fissures or irritations. The yarrow, an astringent, eases inflammation and tones the tissue.

Douche with Aviva's rinse. If your vaginitis is very uncomfortable and there's no possibility that you're pregnant, Romm suggests using the herbal rinse described above as a douche, once a day for a week. If you want to try this remedy, check with your health-care practitioner about how often you should douche. If overused, douching can dry out the vagina and upset its natural balance. "If you try this, use a regular douche bag and fill it with about two cups of the herbal rinse. Keep the tip very low in the vaginal canal and let the rinse flow very slowly," advises Romm.

Alternately, you can purchase a premixed commercial douche, empty the contents completely into the sink, and fill the bottle with the herbal rinse. Then use as described, Romm suggests.

Take a powder. You should keep the area around your vulva dry, because a moist environment encourages the growth of yeast, fungi, and bacteria, suggests herbalist Rosemary Gladstar, director of the Sage Mountain herbal education center in East Barre, Vermont, and author of *Herbal Healing for Women*. She recommends using this fine herbal "yoni powder" whenever you feel the need.

1	cup fine white clay (available in many health food stores)
1/2	cup cornstarch
2	tablespoons black walnut hull powder
2	tablespoons myrrh powder
1	tablespoon goldenseal powder
1–2	drops tea tree essential oil

Using a wire whisk, mix the ingredients together. Put some in a clean spice jar with a shaker top for easy application. The remainder can be stored in a glass jar with a tight-fitting lid. Keep the mixture away from moisture and it will last indefinitely.

It's reported that the tannin in myrrh is an antiseptic that helps kill bacteria and viruses. Traditionally, the berberine in goldenseal has been used to counter fungi and bacteria, and tea tree oil is a potent antiseptic that specifically combats vaginal yeast infections and often works when other remedies have failed, says James A. Duke, Ph.D., a botanical consultant, former ethnobotanist with the U.S. Department of Agriculture, and author of *The Green Pharmacy*, who specializes in medicinal plants.

Tea Tree Oil: Nature's Antiseptic

When the early settlers arrived in Australia, they were given a gift: the pale yellow oil of the tea tree. The aborigines, Australia's native people, used the oil as a local antiseptic and passed its use along to their recently landed neighbors. Most likely, the new folks on the block welcomed the gift gratefully, for the oil came in mighty handy for treating the insect bites, cuts, abrasions, burns, athlete's foot, and other problems endured during the taming of their rugged new homeland.

Later, tea tree oil played a supporting role in abetting the Australian Allies during World War II. The oil was added to the machine "cutting oils" used in munitions factories, thereby reducing the number of infections suffered by the plant workers, who were bedeviled by nicks and cuts from the metal filings and turnings flying around in the course of making munitions.

In the laboratory, evidence shows that tea tree oil inhibits the growth of candida and other yeast and fungal infections.

Tea tree is available as an essential oil at health food stores. Like other essential oils, it is meant for external use only (don't drink it) and should be kept well out of children's reach. Even a few teaspoons can be fatal.

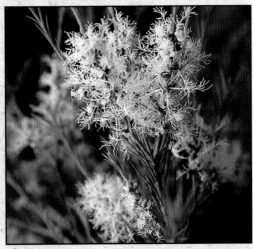

Researchers have found that, among other benefits, tea tree oil fights the kind of bacteria that may help cause acne.

Add aloe. "Aloe vera gel is very cooling, and it quells inflammation fast," says Romm. "You can use the gel fresh from an aloe plant or buy pure aloe vera gel from a health food store. Apply it to the vaginal area as often as needed."

Apply apple cider. An old folk remedy, douching with diluted apple-cider vinegar, really works, says Maier. It restores the vagina's pH balance, she says. To 2 cups of water, add ¼ cup of organic apple-cider vinegar and douche using a douche bag or a commercial douche bottle whose contents have been discarded. For the first three days, douche twice a day with this solution, says Maier. For the next four days, douche once a day. Many doctors discourage women from douching more than once a month, at most, so if you decide to follow this procedure, check with your health-care practitioner as to how often you should douche, based on your individual health history.

Blend a healing formula. This formula, a blend of tinctures (also called extracts), provides immune-system support and can be used along with any local or other treatment for bacterial vaginitis and trichomoniasis, says Dr. Hudson. (But don't use it if you are pregnant.)

Blend ¼ ounce of licorice tincture, ¼ ounce of echinacea tincture, ¼ ounce of usnea tincture, and ¼ ounce of goldenseal tincture. Using a standard measuring spoon, take ½ teaspoon of the tincture mix three times a day for 10 to 14 days, advises Dr. Hudson.

Licorice is considered a blood purifier and is used to quell internal inflammation. Echinacea stimulates the immune system, helping it increase the body's resistance to bacterial infection. Some herbalists report that usnea eliminates trichomonas, and goldenseal contains berberine, which fights bacterial infections, says Dr. Duke.

Varicose Veins

TOUGH HERBS FOR DELICATE VEINS

*I*t's small consolation, but varicose veins usually look a lot worse than they feel. The word *varicose* means swollen, and that's just how the affected veins appear: Tortuously dilated and easily visible, they seem to nearly pop from the skin. Since standing upright exerts tremendous pressure on blood vessels in the legs, veins lying under the skin of the legs are most commonly affected.

Four times as many women as men get varicose veins, perhaps because pregnancy increases the pressure in leg veins. In addition, extreme overweight, aging, and standing for hours on the job also encourage swelling. Although it's uncommon to have severe symptoms, varicose veins can make your legs feel heavy, tight, and tired. Less frequently but more seriously, varicose veins involve obstruction and valve defects of veins deeper in the leg, which can lead to dangerous circulatory complications. If you experience sudden, painful swelling of one leg with tenderness of the calf muscle, seek medical help right away. It could mean a blood clot in one of the deep veins of the leg.

"Treating varicose veins with herbs focuses on strengthening the blood vessels themselves as well as improving overall circulation," says Betzy Bancroft, a professional member of the American Herbalists Guild and manager of Herbalist and Alchemist, an herbal medicine company in Washington, New Jersey.

Butcher's Broom:
A Toner for Weak Veins

*I*t groweth in copses, and upon heaths . . . it shooteth forth its young buds in the spring . . . the branches of leaves abiding green all the winter." Thus did Nicholas Culpeper, the seventeenth-century herbalist, describe butcher's broom, a Mediterranean evergreen that is related to lilies and asparagus. In Culpeper's day, butcher's broom was considered a handy herb to "openeth obstructions, provoketh urine, and helpeth to expel . . . women's courses."

Today's herbalists describe this spiny, leathery bush somewhat less romantically as a specific remedy for varicose veins. In clinical trials, butcher's broom extracts have shown effectiveness in constricting bothersome veins. Largely, that's because butcher's broom is generously laced with natural yet steroidlike compounds called ruscogenin and neoruscogenin. Believed to be effective at inhibiting inflammation and constricting the blood vessels, these compounds may have the ability to shrink swollen varicose veins by strengthening and constricting the walls of the veins. Butcher's broom is used internally as well as externally and is available in various forms wherever herbs are sold.

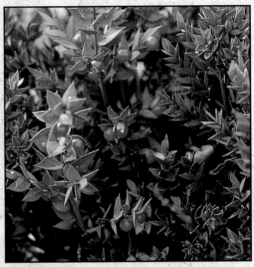

Compounds in butcher's broom strengthen weak veins and may also help shrink hemorrhoids.

To Bancroft and other like-minded herbalists, minimizing the possibility of varicose veins means keeping the walls of the blood vessels strong and elastic. "I do that by recommending herbs and other foods rich in flavonoids, because flavonoids are believed to increase the muscle tone of the vein's walls," says Bancroft. So be sure to maximize flavonoid-rich foods such as red peppers and dark fruits like cranberries in your diet, she suggests.

Other herbalists agree. Claudia Wingo, R.N., a member of the National Herbalists Association of Australia, says that she also treats varicose veins by improving circulation as well as the flexibility of the vein's walls.

Improve Your Circulation with Herbs

Several herbal remedies may help varicose veins. Here are some of the most effective, according to herbal practitioners.

Buy a premade vein-toning formula. A compound in horse chestnut called aescin helps to strengthen capillary cells and reduce fluid leakage. When capillaries swell and leak blood and fluid, varicose veins can develop. Strengthening capillary tone can improve the appearance of varicose veins.

Horse chestnut is best used as a minor ingredient in an overall formula that includes other herbs, Bancroft says. Look for such formulas that contain some horse chestnut; they are most often available through mail order (see "Where to Buy Herbs and Herbal Products" on page 462). Don't take horse chestnut during pregnancy or while breastfeeding, however.

Make your own "vein tonic." Although it's almost impossible to reverse varicose veins once they're established, this make-at-home formula can prevent them from getting any worse, Bancroft notes. Using herbal tinctures (also called extracts), combine 2 parts ginkgo, 1 part ginger, and 1 part cinnamon. Take 30 drops of the tincture, mixed with another liquid such as tea, juice, or water, three times a day, recommends Bancroft. Take this remedy for about four weeks, then re-evaluate your condition.

Ginkgo is highly effective in the treatment of various blood vessel disorders, Bancroft says. Ginger benefits the cardiovascular system, and as a bonus, it helps lower cholesterol.

Try butcher's broom. The herb butcher's broom is high in rutin, a component of vitamin C, and other compounds that actually help tone up vein walls, Wingo says. It is used extensively in Europe for varicose veins and hemorrhoids.

She adds this herb to a varicose vein formula that may also help improve the function of the circulatory system. Other herbs in the formula include cramp bark, which is high in flavonoids; buckwheat, which is also rich in rutin; ginkgo, which may improve peripheral circulation; hawthorn, believed to strengthen blood vessels and the heart muscle; and rosemary, a circulatory stimulant.

Make this varicose vein tonic by combining 1 part each of hawthorn, ginkgo, cramp bark, and buckwheat with $\frac{1}{2}$ part butcher's broom. Add 3 to 4 drops of food-grade rosemary essential oil per 8 ounces of tincture. Take two milliliters three times a day for two months, then gradually decrease the dosage, says Wingo. This tincture tastes bitter; try mixing it with 8 ounces of water or orange juice to dissipate the taste.

Make a massage lotion. When varicose veins make your legs feel tired and sore, give yourself a 10-minute rubdown while seated with your legs up on an ottoman. Then keep your legs elevated for at least a half-hour before you resume other activities, advises Wingo.

Use equal parts of distilled witch hazel and strong comfrey infusion (see "Teas and Infusions" on page 89). Add a few drops of essential oil of cypress, which is available in health food stores. Massage the lotion directly on the area that hurts or apply it to compresses held in place with an elastic bandage for up to an hour.

Comfrey is traditionally known as a skin-healing herb, and witch hazel is a soothing astringent. Oil of cypress is an astringent that's considered soothing and relaxing. Use dried comfrey only, and do not apply to broken skin.

Water Retention

BOTANICALS THAT DEFLATE PUFFINESS

*S*wollen feet? Sore breasts? Puffed-up cheeks? A bloated tummy? Premenstrual water retention is often the result of declining levels of progesterone. When levels of this female hormone drop a week or so before menstruation, salt levels in your body rise, and you retain water, a condition also known as edema.

Herbal experts and conventional medical practitioners alike say that women with water retention can help themselves by reducing salt intake and drinking more fluids. It sounds crazy, but adding extra fluid helps dilute sodium and aids your kidneys in excreting it. Beyond that, turn to the herbal pharmacy for more gentle diuretics that help your body flush away excess fluids.

"It's safe to treat minor water retention problems on your own, such as slightly swollen ankles or the tender breasts and swollen tummies women can get premenstrually," notes Ellen Kamhi, R.N., Ph.D., of Oyster Bay, New York, an herbalist, professional member of the American Herbalists Guild (AHG), and host of the nationally syndicated radio show *Natural Alternatives*. "But if you have a condition called pitting edema, in which you've retained so much water that pressing on a swollen spot leaves indentations on your skin, you should consult a health-care practitioner. You should also consult your doctor if you experience water retention during pregnancy," she says.

If you are considering using herbal remedies for edema, heed these cautions. First, don't mix herbal diuretics with prescription or over-the-counter pharmaceutical diuretics. "You could actually flush too much fluid from your body that way and become dehydrated," notes Cathy McNease, a professional member of the AHG from Ojai, California, and instructor at the Santa Barbara College of Oriental Medicine and Yo San University in Santa Monica. And if you tend to retain water, avoid using licorice as an herbal remedy. In larger doses, this herb can prompt your body to hold onto fluids or make an existing problem worse, she says. Otherwise, these herbal diuretic strategies may be worth a try.

Get corny. Corn silk—that smooth, yellow tassel that you find on a fresh, unshucked ear of corn—has a safe, effective diuretic action, according to research. "Make corn silk tea by steeping 1 tablespoon of the dried silk in a cup of just-boiled water for 5 minutes," Dr. Kamhi suggests. "Have up to three cups a day. But you might not want to drink this tea late in the evening if you want to sleep straight through the night, as this herb will have you waking up to visit the bathroom."

Dr. Kamhi suggests buying dried corn silk from a health food store or mail-order herb company (see "Where to Buy Herbs and Herbal Products" on page 462) or saving the silk from organically grown ears of corn. Dry it in a cool place for a few days, then store it in an airtight container. "Don't use silk from

Corn Silk: Nature's Diuretic

Corn silk—those fine, soft, threadlike strands jutfting from the top of an ear of corn like a mop of yellow hair—has long been used in folk medicine as a soothing diuretic that prompts the kidneys to flush out fluid. For the corn plant, this vegetal silk, which grows to eight inches in length, is a crucial part of its female flowers. The fresh yellow silks are better to use than the dark, dried ones, and they have a fresher taste, says Cathy McNease, a professional member of the American Herbalists Guild (AHG) from Ojai, California, and an instructor at the Santa Barbara College of Oriental Medicine and Yo San University in Santa Monica.

Researchers aren't certain which compounds account for the herb's fluid-flushing abilities, but they know it works. "And the tea tastes really good—just like corn," notes Ellen Kamhi, R.N., Ph.D., of Oyster Bay, New York, an herbalist, professional member of the AHG, and host of the nationally syndicated radio show *Natural Alternatives*.

You can also use this tea as basic stock in soup recipes, says McNease. "For a soup that helps ease water retention, start with a few cups of corn silk tea, then add celery and parsley, which also act as mild diuretics. I'd also put in carrots, onions, ginger, and garlic, or whatever vegetables and seasonings you like, to make a pleasant soup."

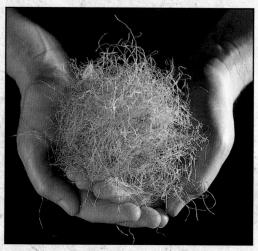

For women, corn silk makes a pleasant-tasting tea that fights water retention.

the regular corn you buy in the supermarket," she says. "If it isn't labeled organically grown, it probably has pesticides on it." You could also use corn silk tincture (also called an extract); take about 10 drops in a cup of warm water three times a day.

"You get an immediate effect from corn silk and will find that you need to urinate in an hour or two," Dr. Kamhi says. "Use corn silk for minor water retention for up to four days."

Pick some dandelions. Better known as an herb that supports healthy liver function, dandelion leaf and root also have scientifically documented diuretic properties, and they are mild enough to use for longer periods of time—for four to six weeks, Dr. Kamhi says.

"If you regularly retain water—say, right before your period—start taking dandelion at the first sign of bloating and breast tenderness," she says. Make a tea using 1 rounded teaspoon of the herb per cup of boiling water (use a tea ball or strain before drinking) and sip two to three mugfuls daily, she suggests. For long-term use, you can take dandelion six days a week for up to six weeks. It may be more convenient to use a dandelion tincture than tea; tinctures are available at health food stores.

Dandelion leaf may be one of nature's most clever diuretics. "It's very rich in potassium, which helps replace potassium you're excreting," McNease says. "In spring, you can also add fresh, clean dandelion greens to salads. Pick them from a place where you know no pesticides or other chemicals have been sprayed. Spring greens are best—by summer, they're very, very bitter."

Sip nettle. "Stinging nettle is the perfect mild diuretic," McNease says. "It nourishes you with vitamins and minerals, helps the lymphatic system, and can reverse water retention." And don't worry—once the leaves are dried, the stingers are not a problem.

Research shows that nettle has a proven diuretic effect, confirming its use in European and American folk-medicine traditions. This deep green, rich-tasting herb also contains calcium, magnesium, and iron.

To make nettle tea, use at least 1 teaspoon of the herb per cup of just-boiled water, steep for 15 minutes, then strain and sip. Have up to three cups a day for several weeks or months, says McNease. "You can also buy nettle as capsules or tinctures. Follow the directions on the label for those," she adds.

Quaff a parsley infusion. Fresh or dried, parsley contains two compounds, myristicin and apiole, that can help the body flush out excess water. Some herbal experts suggest consuming only small amounts of parsley (about as much as you'd use as a seasoning in food); the same compounds that make this herb a good diuretic can, in large quantities, cause giddiness, deafness, and kidney problems.

It is safe to consume a daily cup or two of parsley-leaf tea for up to one week, McNease notes. Brew the tea by adding a small handful of fresh parsley leaves or a teaspoon of dried parsley to a cup of just-boiled water. Steep for 15 minutes, strain, and enjoy.

Try uva-ursi. Also known as bearberry, rockberry, or hogberry, uva-ursi is an effective remedy for bladder infections, but it can also help relieve simple bloating caused by water retention, McNease notes. "Use 1 teaspoon per cup of boiling water, steep for 15 minutes, strain, and drink," she says. She recommends two to three cups a day for up to one week.

A traditional remedy, uva-ursi is used today in commercial diuretics and laxatives. Pregnant women and people with kidney disorders should avoid this herb.

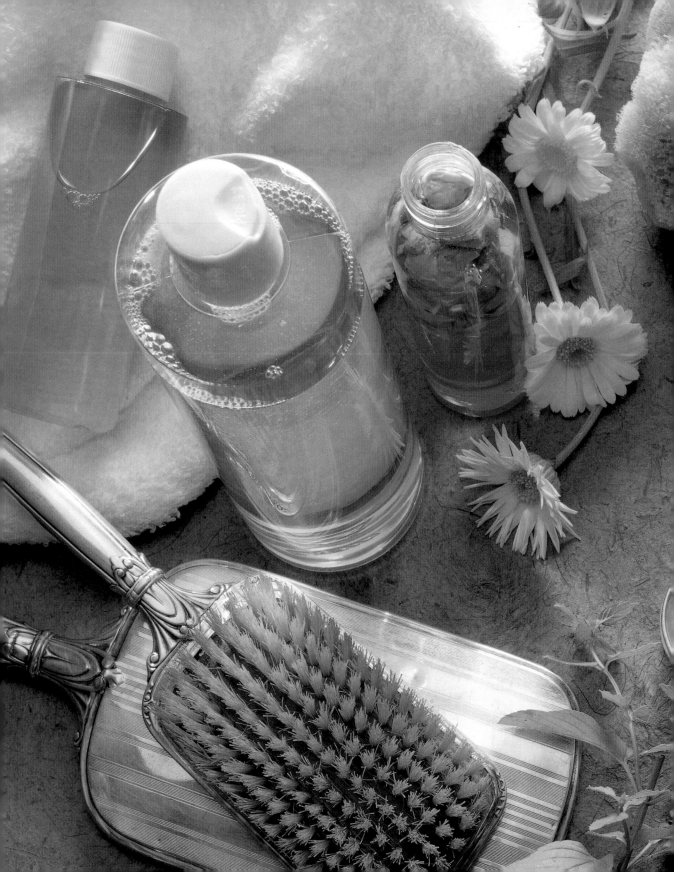

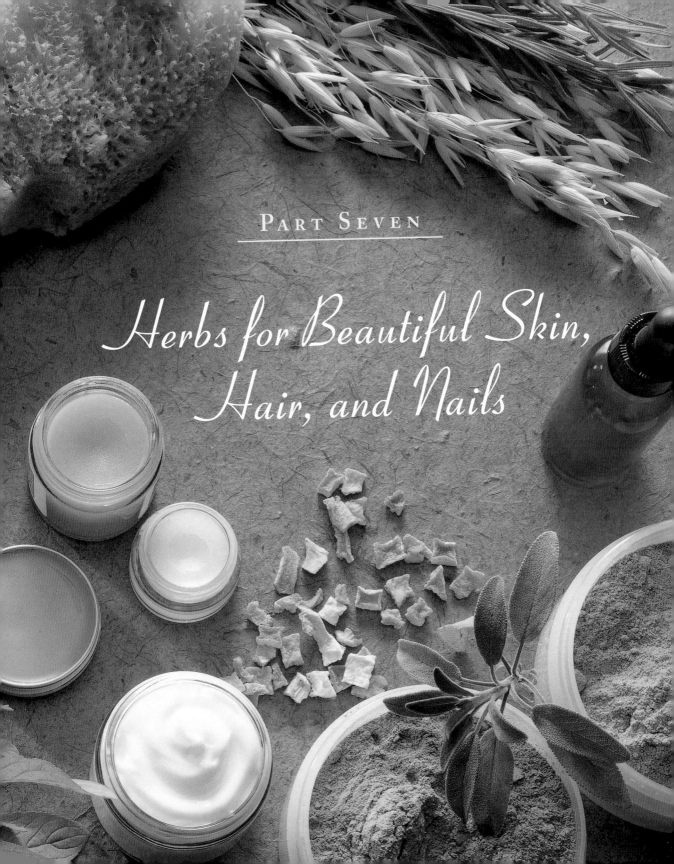

PART SEVEN

Herbs for Beautiful Skin, Hair, and Nails

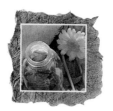

A Potpourri
of Botanical Blends

Visit the Dry Creek Herb Farm in Auburn, California, on "herbal beauty day," and you'll find women snipping fresh lavender and calendula in the garden, concocting aromatic facial steams, or napping on the lawn while herb-scented clay masks draw impurities from their pores.

You may not have the time to vacation at an herb farm. And you may not be ready to try napping on your lawn with an herb-scented mask. But herbalists say that you can easily blend your own herb-based shampoo, rinse, facial scrub, cleanser, mask, toner, lip balm, bleaching cream, or anti-wrinkle cream—without leaving your kitchen.

Natural Benefits

Why spend time mixing together herbal body-care products when the shelves of pharmacies, beauty-supply shops, health food stores—even supermarkets and convenience stores—are packed with dozens of different commercial products? Herbalists who champion natural cosmetics tout various benefits from trying at least a few homemade concoctions, even for the busiest women.

Protection for your skin's natural moisture barrier. Natural shampoos, rinses, skin scrubs, and toners can help your skin and scalp maintain their first lines of defense, says Mindy Green, a professional member of the American Herbalists Guild, faculty member at the Rocky Mountain Center for Botanical Studies and director of education at the Herb Research Foundation, both in Boulder, Colorado, and co-author of *Aromatherapy: A Complete Guide to the Healing Art.*

"The goal of good skin care is to maintain the natural barrier your skin provides," says Green. "The thin layer of moisture and oil (a natural moisturizing factor) that coats your skin is the best moisturizer of all. This layer also has a natural acid balance and is your skin's first immune barrier, protecting your body from infection and toxins in the environment."

Handmade herbal products help maintain your skin's natural moisture barrier, Green says. The result is that all skin types, from dry to normal to oily, from wrinkled to sun-damaged, may look and feel healthier. Oily hair becomes easier to control, and dry hair looks better-conditioned.

Ingredients that you can trust. Homemade body-care products contain no colorings, additives, or synthetic chemicals, notes Donna Bryant, an herbalist in Pembroke, New Hampshire, who teaches at the Sage Mountain herbal education center in East Barre, Vermont. "You know exactly what's in your shampoo or rinse or skin-care lotion," she says. "They don't contain the synthetic ingredients found in commercial products and even in some so-called organic and natural cleansing and conditioning products. That can be especially important if you know that you're sensitive to certain additives."

One caution: If you have acne or dermatitis, check with your doctor before applying herbs of any kind to your skin. "Some herbal remedies—such as tea tree oil or herbal toners—can aggravate dermatitis," says Mary Ruth Buchness, M.D., chief of dermatology at St. Vincent's Hospital and Medical Center in New York City and associate professor of dermatology and medicine at the New York Medical College in Valhalla. "And abrasive scrubs can make acne worse."

Customized beauty care. Cool mint. Relaxing lavender. Invigorating lemon. Sweet rose. When you create your own products, you choose the scent. Beyond fragrance, you can also choose ingredients that enhance your natural assets (such as chamomile to bring out the highlights in blond hair) or help you overcome problems with your hair, skin, or nails. A facial steam for a woman with dry skin, for example, might include comfrey and lavender, while a woman with oily skin might choose peppermint and yarrow. "The aroma is wonderful, and the herbs help heal your skin at the same time," Bryant notes.

Having fun. "When the women I teach start creating cosmetics, they become very enthused and excited. They love it," says Gail Ulrich, an herbalist and founder/director of the Blazing Star Herbal School in Shelburne Falls, Massachusetts. "It's true that herbs and herbal beauty treatments—like an oatmeal scrub or a clay mask—can be messy. But if you approach the experience in a childlike way and get your hands into the mixing bowl, you'll have fun."

Your Springboard to Inner Healing

Women herbalists say that for many, making natural cosmetic products serves as an excellent introduction to the world of healing herbs. "When you start out, you think you can't possibly make anything as good as you could buy in a store. But you quickly discover that your own products are even better," says Bryant "It's incredibly inspiring."

Many women who first experience the power and loveliness of herbs by concocting homemade beauty products go on to make and use herbal remedies for health conditions, says Shatoiya de la Tour, herbalist and founder of the Dry Creek Herb Farm and Learning Center, who presents workshops on herbal body care at the annual Women's Herb Conference in Peterborough, New Hampshire. Sometimes, she says, the most exciting moment is the simplest: Creating a balm for chapped lips. "Making a simple lip balm has turned so many women on to herbs," she notes. "They say, 'Oh, my gosh, I *made* this. And it works. And it smells great. What else can I try now?'"

Acne

Skin-Pleasing Herbs for Blemishes and Breakouts

Like the common cold, acne is a health condition in want of the ultimate cure. Dermatologists blame the clogged pores, blackheads, pimples, and angry red blotches that typify acne on two things: Hyperactive oil glands in the skin and a tendency for cells lining the pores to clog. The medical route relies on various over-the-counter and prescription drugs to control these two tendencies.

Herbalists take the explanation one step further. They say that clogged pores, pimples, and reddened skin are symptoms of internal imbalance, not simply a problem with overactive oil glands. As such, herbalists suggest remedies that control acne from the inside out. They offer gentle acne-fighting cleansers, masks, toners, and moisturizers. But first, top botanical healers recommend herbs that, when taken internally, reportedly help to normalize hormone levels, boost immunity, regulate bowel function, detoxify the body, and prompt the liver, skin, lymphatic system, and digestive system to work more effectively.

"If a woman with acne has flare-ups before her period or through menopause, I would strongly suspect that the skin changes are hormonally based," says Amanda McQuade Crawford, a practicing herbalist in Ojai, California, a professional member of the American Herbalists Guild (AHG), member of Britain's National Institute of Medical Herbalists, president of the American College of Integrative Medicine in Albuquerque, and author of *Herbal Remedies for Women*.

If you've had hepatitis or another liver disease, have difficulty digesting fats, or consume a diet high in salts, fats, meats, and dairy products, you may, in McQuade Crawford's view, have what herbalists call liver congestion. "An overworked liver cannot deal with wastes effectively," she says. "This can show up as skin problems."

McQuade Crawford says that still other acne-prone women may have sluggish lymph flow. In other words, the body's lymph system, designed to help fight infection, is working slowly.

Balance and Detoxify

How do you know for sure what's responsible for breakouts and which herbs to choose? "In reality, many women with problem skin have several of these conditions without any clear signs of obvious disease to go on. So it's helpful to work on hormonal health and liver health at the same time, starting with gentle herbs that can be taken safely over time," McQuade Crawford says. These are her recommendations.

Burdock. Burdock is a botanical remedy with a long history of traditional use for skin problems and as a laxative. McQuade Crawford says burdock helps the body eliminate waste through the liver and skin and is often combined with yellow dock for skin conditions like acne.

Calendula. Laboratory studies demonstrate that calendula's bright yellow and orange flowers can boost immunity and soothe inflammation.

Chasteberry. Research shows that the small, grayish fruits of the chaste tree improve hormonally caused problems, including PMS, menstrual cramps, infertility, and cyclical breast pain. McQuade Crawford says that in her experience, chasteberry helps balance female hormones, especially by regulating higher progesterone levels that herbalists believe may be a factor in acne. "Chasteberry is a specific remedy for problems with skin that occur with PMS and for women nearing menopause who find the same acne returning that they experienced in their teens," McQuade Crawford notes. You can buy chasteberry (often called vitex) in health food stores and by mail order (see "Where to Buy Herbs and Herbal Products" on page 462).

Dandelion. This herb was used traditionally to stimulate liver function, and research shows that bitter compounds in the root help the liver by increasing bile flow.

Sarsaparilla. Although sarsaparilla has been used through the centuries to alleviate skin problems, research is scarce. This New World plant is the root of several South and Central American and Caribbean species of *Smilax*, a genus in the Lily family. Based on what she has observed in her practice, McQuade Crawford says that it appears to balance hormones and improves functioning of the lymphatic system, two effects that can help clear the skin. Sarsaparilla is available by mail order.

Yellow dock. Used traditionally and by modern herbalists, yellow dock clears chronic skin problems, promotes good liver function, and encourages regular bowel movements. McQuade Crawford notes that herbalists believe that constipation can be a background factor in skin problems.

Teas and Tinctures for Acne

McQuade Crawford suggests taking the appropriate herb or herbs as a tea or tincture (also called an extract).

As a healing tea. Combine ¼ ounce of each of your herbs of choice. Then steep 1 teaspoon of the mixture in 1 cup of boiling water, McQuade Crawford says. Drink one to three cups a day for one to two weeks before your period if your acne is related to your menstrual cycle. Continue for a period of three months to one year, until your symptoms subside.

As a tincture. Take a total of 1 teaspoon of tincture diluted in 8 ounces of water three times a day. And be patient. "It takes a minimum of two weeks for the herbs to have any effect, and for long-standing problems, it may take three months to a year to make a permanent improvement so that you can stop taking the herbs without symptoms returning," says McQuade Crawford. "This is especially true if you're trying to balance hormone problems or improve liver function."

Pamper Your Skin with Anti-Acne Herbs

Herbalists also suggest botanical skin-care regimens that they find are gentle yet effective for women with acne. And as a bonus, they will leave your skin clear and glowing.

Wash gently with oatmeal. "It's important, even with problem skin, to leave natural oils in place to protect and moisturize," notes beauty expert Stephanie Tourles, a licensed aesthetician in Hyannis, Massachusetts, and author of *The Herbal Body Book*. "This is hard to understand when you have acne because you just want to get all that oil off your face to try and solve the problem. But that only

Blemish-Be-Gone Herbal Cream

Pimples show up in the most inconvenient places and at the most inconvenient times—at the tip of your nose as you stare down a pool cue at your rival, at midchin as family and friends snap photos of you blowing out the candles on your 40th-birthday cake, or on your cheekbone just before you're scheduled to pitch a radical new idea to the town council or PTA. Pimples are part inflammation, part infection. In time, they may heal on their own. But who can wait?

Never pop a pimple—you'll only make it worse. Instead, work with nature to ease the inflammation and fight the infection. Use this herbal pimple cream recommended by Gail Ulrich, an herbalist and founder/director of the Blazing Star Herbal School in Shelburne Falls, Massachusetts.

To prepare the cream, mix together ½ teaspoon of powdered goldenseal, ½ teaspoon of green clay or bentonite clay, 12 drops of tea tree essential oil, and 12 drops of grapefruit seed extract, a powerful, concentrated herbal extract. (All of these ingredients are available at health food stores and by mail; see "Where to Buy Herbs and Herbal Products" on page 462.) It should form a paste. If it's too runny, add a little more clay, and if it's too thick, add 1 to 2 drops of either liquid.

Apply the cream to blemishes at night or any other time you can leave the mixture in place for a few hours. Rinse it off with warm water.

"The goldenseal, tea tree, and grapefruit seed extract are all antibacterial. The clay holds the cream together, helps draw infection from the blemish, and helps soothe," Ulrich says. "You could also add 4 drops of Rescue Remedy flower essence to the paste for extra soothing."

Rescue Remedy is a brandy-and-water-based extract of blossoms that flower-essence practitioners say can evoke feelings of calm. It's available by mail and in health food stores. Or look for 5-Flower Formula, produced by Flower Essence Services, which is analogous to Rescue Remedy.

---

makes your skin produce more and more oil. The goal of cleansing is to remove dirt and oil without stripping. That's where oatmeal comes in."

To prepare a simple oatmeal scrub, grind old-fashioned or instant rolled oats in a food processor or clean coffee grinder, she says. Mix 2 teaspoons with about 1 tablespoon of water to make a paste. Gently wash your skin and rinse with warm or lukewarm water.

To scent the oatmeal scrub and fight bacteria, mix 1 teaspoon of ground dried lavender or rosemary leaves or cinnamon powder into each cup of ground oatmeal mixture, says Tourles.

Apply a calming mask. A clay mask draws excess oils and debris to the surface of your skin, boosts circulation to tighten the skin and stimulate blood flow, and whisks away dead skin cells that can clog pores, says

Mindy Green, a professional member of the AHG, faculty member at the Rocky Mountain Center for Botanical Studies and director of education at the Herb Research Foundation, both in Boulder, Colorado, and co-author of *Aromatherapy: A Complete Guide to the Healing Art.* You can add herbs and essential oils to soothe inflamed, painful skin and fight bacteria that inflame clogged pores into blemishes, she says.

To prepare a mask, make a tea with 2 tablespoons of comfrey in ½ cup of boiling water. Steep for about 15 minutes, let cool, and strain. Then combine small amounts of the tea with 1 tablespoon of bentonite clay or other plain facial clay (available at health food stores or by mail), 1 teaspoon each of ground dried American elder flowers and strawberry leaves, and 1 drop of lavender essential oil to form a paste. (Elder flowers and strawberry leaves are available through mail order.) Pat a thin layer of the mixture on your face (except around your eyes) and leave on for 5 to 10 minutes. Rinse with lukewarm water.

Tighten and soothe with benzoin. A toner featuring tincture of benzoin and calming yet astringent herbs can further help clear acne-plagued skin by soothing inflammation, fighting infection, and controlling oil, says Tourles. "You can find tincture of benzoin in drugstores or order it from herb companies," she notes. "It's a tightening, astringent fluid made from the resin of the benzoin tree."

To mix a benzoin-and-herb toner, first make a strong tea with 1 tablespoon each of yarrow and calendula or chamomile in 2 cups of boiling water. Steep for 30 minutes and strain. Add 15 drops of tincture of benzoin and 6 drops of peppermint essential oil. Pour the mixture into a plastic bottle with a tight-fitting lid and store it in the refrigerator.

Apply with a cotton ball. "Peppermint makes the toner very cooling," Tourles notes.

Tone with cabbage. "Of all things, cabbage is great for acne," notes Kathlyn Quatrochi, N.D., a naturopathic physician and herbalist in Oak Glen, California, and author of *The Skin Care Book: Simple Herbal Recipes.* "Cabbage contains sulfur, a mineral that helps dry blemishes and fight bacteria. At the same time, the toner restores the acid level of your skin to normal, re-establishing the 'acid mantle' that protects against infection."

To prepare your own cabbage toner, combine 4 ounces of witch hazel and one 1-inch-square piece of cabbage leaf in a wide-mouth plastic bottle. Cover with a tight-fitting lid. Let the mixture steep for 24 hours. "You can leave the leaf in the bottle after that," Dr. Quatrochi notes. The mixture can be stored at room temperature or in the refrigerator and will keep for up to a week. "Pat the mixture on your face with clean fingers, blot off with a water-dampened washcloth, and then apply a non-petroleum-based moisturizer." Petroleum smothers skin, causing it to heat up and enlarging the pores, Dr. Quatrochi says. Petroleum doesn't allow your natural oils to escape, but it does allow dirt and bacteria in, she explains. Non-petroleum-based moisturizers are available at health food stores.

Moisturize with confidence. *Add* moisture to skin with acne? "It sounds like heresy, but a light moisturizer helps the skin," Dr. Quatrochi says. "Pat on a small amount of a light oil, like jojoba (available by mail order) or sunflower at night. During the day, use a non-petroleum-based moisturizer. You could mix in a drop or two of lavender essential oil for each ounce of oil. Skin that's moisturized is not likely to overproduce oil. This can help reduce acne."

Age Spots and Sun-Damaged Skin

GARDEN-VARIETY HERBS THAT FADE BLOTCHES

Think of unsightly age spots—those brownish blotches that crop up on a woman's face, chest, hands, and any other expanse of skin that is repeatedly exposed to the sun—as little suntans that just won't quit.

Whether you sunbathe, bask at a tanning salon, drive around in your car, or work in your garden, your skin is flooded with ultraviolet light. In response to those rays, your skin produces melanin, a naturally dark pigment. An occasional suntan will fade. But if you catch enough rays, over time, this pigment stays dark in patches. These patches are what we call age spots. They are not directly related to how many birthdays you've had but are more closely linked to your history of days in the sun.

Age spots feed on sunlight like zucchinis in July. The more these spots are bombarded by sunlight, the greater the chance that they'll grow and multiply. To discourage the appearance of newer and more noticeable age spots, herbal beauty experts advise women prone to age spots to avoid the sun or wear sunscreen (or both).

"The main thing is to stay out of the sun so they don't get any darker," says beauty expert Stephanie Tourles, a licensed aesthetician in Hyannis, Massachusetts, and author of *The Herbal Body Book*.

Herbal Spot Removal

If, like many women, you already have a few age spots, you can fade the blotches with a two-step herbal spot-removal regimen recommended by Tourles and other herbal beauty practitioners. First, apply nature's own natural bleaching and peeling agents to fade and lift away the upper layer of overpigmented, spotty skin. Second, moisturize with rejuvenating skin conditioners that promote the growth of new, younger-looking skin cells. Here's how.

Use elderflowers to look younger. A paste of dried or fresh American elderflowers with lemon juice and water will help bleach age spots over time, says Kathlyn Quatrochi, N.D., a naturopathic physician and herbalist in Oak Glen, California, and author of *The Skin Care Book: Simple Herbal Recipes*. "The lemon is bleaching, and so is the elderflower," she says. Elderflowers and lemon juice contain alpha hydroxy acids, which promote peeling of the upper layer of the skin. Age spots get a one-two punch—they fade and, over time, are sloughed off as the natural acids loosen old, dead cells and surface discolorations, she says.

In a food processor or blender, combine 1 tablespoon of fresh or dried elderflowers and 1 teaspoon of lemon juice mixed with

Wipe Out Blotches with Oats

Uneven skin tone, blotchiness, and age spots all respond to this easy-to-make combination facial scrub and mask made with yogurt, oats, and salt, says beauty expert Stephanie Tourles, a licensed aesthetician in Hyannis, Massachusetts, and author of *The Herbal Body Book*. Acids in yogurt act as a mild skin peel, lifting old cells from the skin surface; oatmeal and sea salt whisk away dirt and debris.

Mix 1 tablespoon of plain yogurt, 2 teaspoons of ground old-fashioned or instant oats, and 1 teaspoon of sea salt, then massage it into your face and neck. Leave it in place for 20 minutes, Tourles says, then rinse with cool water. Use once a week.

---

enough water to form a paste. Apply with your fingers to clean skin, being sure to avoid the area around your eyes and lips, and leave in place for no more than 5 minutes—less if it stings. "A little sting is okay, but anything else means that you should take it off," Dr. Quatrochi says. Rinse it off with tepid water. "Over time, as your skin gets used to the mixture, you can add more lemon juice and less water," she says. Eventually, you should be using only lemon juice and no water. Use the treatment three times a week. Over three months, expect to see age spots diminish, she says.

Substitute parsley. Green, leafy parsley (the curly variety) can be used in place of elderflowers in the same quantity, Dr. Quatrochi says. "Parsley also has bleaching qualities," she says. Be sure to follow the application of all pastes with a non-petroleum-based moisturizer available at health food stores. Petroleum tends to smother skin and enlarge pores, allowing dirt and bacteria to clog them, Dr. Quatrochi says.

Think helichrysum. Essential oil extracted from helichrysum (common strawflower) helps skin look younger and fresher, says Mindy Green, a professional member of the American Herbalists Guild, faculty member at the Rocky Mountain Center for Botanical Studies and director of education at the Herb Research Foundation, both in Boulder, Colorado, and co-author of *Aromatherapy: A Complete Guide to the Healing Art*. Add 12 drops of helichrysum essential oil to an ounce of moisturizing oil—Green suggests chamomile-infused olive oil—and use regularly to help regenerate neglected skin, she suggests. Helichrysum oil is available by mail order (see "Where to Buy Herbs and Herbal Products" on page 462).

This herb protects young, growing skin cells, according to Kurt Schnaubelt, Ph.D., founder and scientific director of the Pacific Institute of Aromatherapy and director of Original Swiss Aromatics, both in San Rafael, California, and author of *Advanced Aromatherapy*.

Add carrot seed oil. The essential oil of carrot seed also ranks among Green's top choices for restoring youthfulness to overexposed skin. Extracted from the tiny seeds of the wild carrot, this oil (available by mail order) works well when combined with herbal products that lighten or peel the skin, Green says. While it won't fade age spots, Green says that in her experience, this oil helps accelerate the production of new skin cells, giving your complexion a younger, fresher look.

"It makes skin look healthier and regenerates new skin cells more quickly," she says. "Skin-cell production slows down as we age.

These essential oils can speed it up and plump up those cells a little. It gives skin some tools for repairing and rebuilding."

Green suggests mixing 6 drops each of carrot seed and helichrysum essential oils into a carrier oil, such as olive oil. You could also use 4 drops each and add 4 drops of lavender essential oil, which has antibacterial qualities.

Chapped Lips

HERBAL BALMS THAT SOOTHE AND SMOOTH

Dry winter heat. Summertime air conditioning. Burning sun. Biting winds. All sorts of indoor and outdoor conditions can conspire to leave you with dry, scaly, chapped lips. Once lips start to chap, they don't stop until they look like Mick Jagger's kisser. Worse, chapped lips can really hurt.

Balms for What Ails You

Conveniently tucked into your pocket, backpack, or purse, an herbal lip balm can go a long way toward maintaining moist, attractive lips. Once you master the basics of making your own formula (see "Herbal Lip Balm" for a basic recipe), you can customize your balm in various ways, depending on your needs or desires, says Shatoiya de la Tour, herbalist and founder of Dry Creek Herb

Farm and Learning Center in Auburn, California, who presents workshops on herbal body care at the annual Women's Herb Conference in Peterborough, New Hampshire. Here's how.

Infuse the oil. Before beginning the recipe, infuse your chosen base oil with an herb to add scent and healing power to your balm (see "Infused Oils" on page 101 for directions). Lavender, calendula, plantain, nettle, chamomile, and comfrey are all good choices that soothe and promote healing, she says.

Add a drop of an essential oil. Short on time? Adding 1 drop of essential oil to a cup of the plain base oil is a shortcut that lends aroma and healing qualities to your balm, de la Tour says. Try peppermint, lavender, chamomile, or rose.

Add blister relief. If you tend to get fever blisters or sun blisters on your lips, make

Herbal Lip Balm

LIP PROTECTION IN A POT

You can make a basic protective and moisturizing herbal lip balm in just a half-hour, says Shatoiya de la Tour, herbalist and founder of Dry Creek Herb Farm and Learning Center in Auburn, California. Here's her formula, which can be customized by adding essential oils or tints as needed.

De la Tour recommends using olive oil, almond oil, or a mixture of the two, but you can experiment with other oils to find one you like best. And for storage, "you can buy little jars and lip-balm tins from catalogs, or you can save jars," de la Tour says. "I love little pimiento jars—they're just the right size." If stored away from extreme heat, balms can last for years, but if you detect a rancid odor, the balm has gone bad.

What You'll Need

Before you start, assemble all of your materials so that you can work quickly.

- ✓ A teaspoon
- ✓ Oil
- ✓ A small saucepan
- ✓ Beeswax (available by mail)
- ✓ Measuring cups
- ✓ Small jars with tight-fitting lids

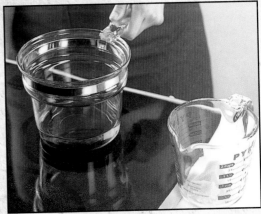

1. Warm the oil. First, put the teaspoon in the freezer to chill. Then gently warm 1 cup of oil in a saucepan over very low heat. While the oil warms, put 1¼ ounces of beeswax into a glass measuring cup and melt on low heat in the oven for about 20 minutes.

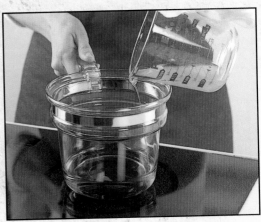

2. Add wax. Pour the melted beeswax into the warm oil.

(continued)

Herbal Lip Balm—Continued

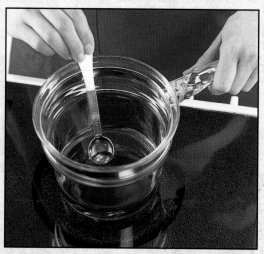

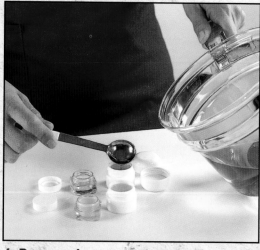

3. Test the consistency. Dip the frozen spoon into the warm mixture, then put it back in the freezer for about 30 seconds. When you remove the spoon from the freezer, rub your finger through the balm. It should be soft enough to apply to your lips but not runny. "If the balm is too soft, add more beeswax," says de la Tour. "If it's too hard, add more oil. You can customize the mixture by adding more beeswax or oil to create a softer balm for home use or a harder balm that won't melt so easily for travel." At this point, you can add essential oils or other custom ingredients to the basic lip balm, depending on your needs.

4. Pour and store. Finally, while the balm is still a warm liquid, spoon it into clean jars. Lay wax paper over the tops of the open jars while the balm cools to keep it clean. Cap the jars after the balm has completely hardened.

a protective balm. Start with a ready-made infused oil from a catalog or health food store, or make your own, says de la Tour. Replace ¼ to ½ cup of the base oil with oil infused with St.-John's-wort, which has antiviral properties. Then infuse the new oil with usnea, a bacteria-fighting lichen (available through mail order; see "Where to Buy Herbs and Herbal Products" on page 462).

Rushed? Reach for castor oil. If you have absolutely no time to whip up lip balm, go for castor oil, suggests Stephanie Tourles, a licensed aesthetician in Hyannis, Massachusetts, and author of *The Herbal Body Book*. "Get a little bottle at the drugstore," she says. "It's really thick and costs very little money. When I want a lip treatment with staying power, I use castor oil. It coats your lips with a thick lacquer of shine."

If your lips are really chapped and sore, add tea tree or eucalyptus essential oil. "Use 10 drops of essential oil in a 2-ounce bottle of castor oil," Tourles says. "Both are very soothing and healing."

All This, and Beauty, Too

Mauve Madness? Really Red? Pale Purple? Homemade lip balm doesn't have to be a prim, colorless gleam, say herbalists who create kitchen cosmetics. To add a rainbow of hues to your next pot of lip-shiner, use the techniques that follow. Perfectly Pink, anyone?

For a reddish tint: Steep a teaspoon of alkanet in the base oil for your lip balm for 10 minutes, strain the oil, then proceed with the recipe, suggests de la Tour. "This root adds a slight red color," she says. "It's a nice touch." Look for alkanet at health food stores or in mail-order catalogs.

For a custom color: Warm 2 ounces of castor oil in a small saucepan and stir in half a tube of your favorite color of moisturizing lipstick until it melts. Stir thoroughly and pour it into a small wide-mouth glass or plastic jar. Add the color as desired to the basic lip balm recipe. "That way, you get exactly the lip gloss color you're looking for," she says.

Crow's-Feet

SAY *ARRIVEDERCI* TO FINE LINES

Call them smile lines or wrinkles, laugh lines or squint lines. Crow's-feet, those fine lines that radiate from the outer corners of your eyes, are really nothing more than tiny wrinkles—and an often unwanted testament to aging skin and sun exposure.

You can't do anything about aging: Time passes, and birthdays come and go. But you can hold the line on crow's-feet.

"First, you should protect your skin against further wrinkling by wearing a sunscreen," notes beauty expert Stephanie Tourles, a licensed aesthetician in Hyannis, Massachusetts, and author of *The Herbal Body Book*. (You can buy moisturizers and foundation makeup that contains sunscreen.)

Some of the best natural remedies for minimizing crow's-feet come from the plant world, say herbalists. Acidic fruits like pineapple work like alpha hydroxy acids, substances in commercial creams that are derived from natural acids found in sugarcane, fruit, and milk. Like the wrinkle removers found in drugstores, fruit acids peel away scrunched-up skin cells to reveal younger-looking skin below. Some strong herb teas can also create mild peeling. "Over time, a peel will start erasing evidence of crow's-feet," Tourles notes.

Reach for a Botanical Peel

Before you attempt a face peel, check with your dermatologist. If you have lupus or broken capillaries, a face peel may aggravate your skin. Here's a peel that's tasty enough to eat.

Do the papaya peel. "If you're looking for an alternative to store-bought wrinkle creams or costly facial peels by a dermatologist, all you need is a papaya and maybe a little fresh pineapple juice," says Tourles. By loosening and removing old, wrinkled cells on the skin's surface, the peel will reveal fresher-looking skin underneath that is smooth and toned.

Find a papaya, an orangey green–skinned tropical fruit, in the supermarket produce aisle. It doesn't even have to be ripe. Take it home, mash ¼ cup of pulp, and apply it to the wrinkled skin around your eyes and even to

your entire face and neck. "You're tenderizing your face," Tourles says. "This is also good for those little wrinkles that form along the top of the lip line." Be careful not to get the pulp in your eyes. If you do, rinse immediately with copious amounts of cool water, Tourles recommends.

Leave the pulp on your skin for 10 to 15 minutes, then rinse with either warm or lukewarm water. Like alpha hydroxy cream, papaya pulp will probably sting slightly, which is a sign that it's working. "If it hurts, though, take it off," Tourles advises. Repeat twice a week. Tourles suggests adding 1 teaspoon of fresh pineapple juice, if available, to the pulp to enhance its skin-peeling properties.

Follow the papaya peel with a clay mask. To help remove loosened skin cells, Tourles recommends a simple mask. Combine 1 tablespoon of facial clay (available in health food stores or by mail order; see "Where to Buy Herbs and Herbal Products" on page 462) with enough liquid to make a smooth paste. Use water for oily skin, milk for normal skin, and dairy cream for dry skin. Apply the paste to dry skin and allow it to dry thoroughly, then rinse it off gently with warm or lukewarm water.

Exfoliate with tea. Strong rose hip tea also works as a mild facial peel, says Kathlyn Quatrochi, N.D., a naturopathic physician and herbalist in Oak Glen, California, and author of *The Skin Care Book: Simple Herbal Recipes*. Rose hips have antibacterial and antioxidant properties, and their ascorbic acid content aids in peeling away the upper layer of skin, she explains.

Prepare a rose hip peel with 1 tablespoon of dried rose hips (available at health food stores) in ½ cup of boiling water. Steep for 15 minutes, then cool. Use your fingers to pat the cooled tea on the skin over crow's-feet. Leave it in place for up to five minutes, then rinse with tepid water. To make a rose hip paste instead of a tea, mix 1 teaspoon of rose hips with enough water to make a paste, apply over your crow's-feet, leave on for three minutes, and then remove with a warm, wet cloth.

If you get some of either mixture in your eyes, rinse immediately with tepid water. Follow either treatment with a very light application of olive oil to moisturize the skin.

Dandruff

FIGHT THE FLAKES WITH HERBAL SCALP SOOTHERS

*B*lack sweaters cause dandruff.

Well, not really. But like an Elvis painting on velvet, a black sweater sure gets noticed when it's covered with dandruff.

Those embarrassing specks can be caused by several factors, including oily hair, yeast infections of the scalp, or the overzealous production of new scalp cells, which prompts your head to shed dead skin cells in large clumps. Seasonal changes that dry out your scalp, such as sunburn, only make matters worse. And if you happen to stand too close to an Elvis painting—well, you're just asking for trouble.

If dandruff is persistent and your scalp is red and very itchy, see your doctor. You may need treatment for a fungal infection or for seborrheic dermatitis, an inflammation of the oil glands. For milder dandruff, herbal beauty practitioners recommend gentle herbal remedies like rosemary, burdock, and calendula that control the inflammation, itching, and flaking.

Herbs That Work from the Inside—And Outside

To control dandruff effectively, herbalists often suggest botanical remedies that work on the scalp itself as well as remedies taken internally, says Gayle Eversole, R.N., Ph.D., a nurse practitioner, medical herbalist, and professional member of the American Herbalists Guild in Everett, Washington. While hair rinses control dandruff at the surface, herbalists also view skin problems like dandruff as a sign of impaired liver function, Dr. Eversole notes.

"If you have dandruff, perhaps this is a sign that it is time to evaluate your diet," she says. "If your liver can't effectively deal with the chemical by-products of the body's metabolism, that is reflected in the skin," she notes. "When the liver isn't working effectively, herbalists believe that the skin is called upon to eliminate more and more by-products. When it can't keep up, problems like oily scalp and dandruff appear." Here's what Dr.

Eversole and others suggest for fighting off flakes.

Sip your burdock. Burdock tea has a historical reputation as a gentle blood and liver cleanser, notes Dr. Eversole, and it is often suggested for skin problems. "Burdock is the herb of choice for skin disorders like dandruff because it cleanses the blood and improves liver function," she says.

Prepare burdock tea with 1 to 2 teaspoons of root per cup of boiling water. Fresh grated root is the best, but it is only available in season (generally late spring through late summer/early fall.) Dried, organic roots are most readily available and most convenient. Quality botanical extracts are also an option. You can put 2 to 3 drops in a cup of hot, distilled water, Dr. Eversole recommends.

When preparing a tea with the dried root, it is important to boil the roots in water for 15 to 20 minutes. "You do not extract the fullness of the root's medicinal qualities otherwise," Dr. Eversole explains. After boiling, strain the tea and drink up to three cups a day, she says. "In about a month, you should start seeing changes," she says. "Natural healing takes time, but it works."

Rinse with rosemary. Make a strong rosemary tea using at least 2 tablespoons of the dried leaf in a cup of boiling water. Steep for at least 20 minutes, then strain and cool. You can also add a few drops of rosemary essential oil to the tea. Use as a hair rinse after shampooing. If you choose to, you can rinse it out after a few minutes, but it is not necessary. This rinse will not leave a film on hair. "Rosemary, in my view, is the preeminent hair-strengthening and revitalizing herb. It helps control the overproduction of scalp oil, called seborrhea, that can lead to dandruff," Dr. Eversole says.

Rosemary is often used to darken hair, so blonds should avoid it. If you have blond hair, use chamomile for the rinse instead of rosemary.

Massage with jojoba. "Jojoba oil massaged into the scalp, covered with a plastic bag, and wrapped in a towel for 30 minutes is a good way to clear the scalp and hair follicles," Dr. Eversole recommends. She also suggests adding rosemary, sage, or lavender essential oils to the oil to help the process. "Add about 5 drops of therapeutic quality essential oil to 1 ounce of jojoba oil," she says.

Dr. Eversole also warns against using shampoos containing sodium lauryl/laureth sulfate (SLS). "These shampoos are toxic and very harmful to the head and scalp," she explains.

Splash with vinegar. Apple-cider vinegar with herbs and witch hazel helps to maintain the natural acid balance of your scalp, which boosts general scalp health, while the herbs also soothe inflammation, says Shatoiya de la Tour, herbalist and founder of Dry Creek Herb Farm and Learning Center in Auburn, California, who presents workshops on herbal body care at the annual Women's Herb Conference in Peterborough, New Hampshire.

Concoct an herbal splash by infusing any combination of calendula, plantain, and comfrey in the vinegar. Use a quart jar half-packed with dry herbs or fully packed with fresh herbs and covered with vinegar. Steep for three to six weeks, then strain. For every ³⁄₄ quart or 3 cups (both equal the same amount) of vinegar, add 1 cup of distilled water and 1 ounce of witch hazel. To use, mix "a splash"—about 2 tablespoons—in a pint of water and use it to rinse your hair after shampooing, says de la Tour.

Dry and Sun-Damaged Hair

NATURAL CONDITIONERS FOR MOISTURE AND LUSTER

Examine dull, brittle, fly-away hair under a microscope, and you'll discover hair shafts that look as bristly as bottle brushes. "That's the real problem with dry hair," herbalist Mindy Green, a professional member of the American Herbalists Guild, faculty member at the Rocky Mountain Center for Botanical Studies and director of education at the Herb Research Foundation, both in Boulder, Colorado, and co-author of *Aromatherapy: A Complete Guide to the Healing Art*. "If your scalp doesn't produce enough oil to keep the hair shaft moisturized and protected, the hair grows brittle, and the cuticles on the surface of the hair, which should lie flat, stick up," she says.

While healthy, smooth hair looks shiny because light reflects off the sleek cuticles, dry hair looks dull and lifeless. But don't blame Mother Nature alone. Hair-care regimens such as bleaching, coloring, straightening, perming, blow-drying, and primping with a hot curling iron can all fry your hair, as can exposure to sun, wind, and chlorinated swimming pools.

Give Your Hair an Herbal Shiner

As with most herbal beauty treatments, restoring your hair's natural luster calls for remedies that treat dryness from the inside out. To add much-needed moisture and help make dry hair shiny and manageable, herbalists recommend the following herbal solutions.

Supplement with evening primrose oil. The oil of this medicinal plant is rich in essential fatty acids, which are vital to healthy skin and hair. As such, a daily dose of evening primrose oil can help nourish dull, dry hair, notes Shatoiya de la Tour, herbalist and founder of Dry Creek Herb Farm and Learning Center in Auburn, California, who presents workshops on herbal body care at the annual Women's Herb Conference in Peterborough, New Hampshire. Herbalists recommend one to three 250-milligram capsules of evening primrose oil one to three times a day.

You could also substitute flaxseed oil for evening primrose oil, notes Green, since it contains some of the same essential fatty acids.

Sip oatstraw, the anti-dryness tea. Invite some oatstraw into your teacup. For many women, dry hair is part of an overall problem. As women approach or pass menopause, they may notice that every part of their body, from their heels to their heads and everywhere in between, tends to dry out. "For women who want to retain natural moisture throughout their bodies, oatstraw is incredible," de la Tour says. "And it tastes nice." Herbalists suggest using 1 teaspoon per cup of water and drinking one to three cups a day. Oatstraw combines well with other herbal teas, so if you already drink herbal tea regularly, you can simply add oatstraw to the blend, de la Tour notes.

Slather up with an essential oil. Add body and shine to dry or sun-damaged hair with an easy, deep-conditioning treatment using botanical oils, suggests Stephanie Tourles, a licensed aesthetician in Hyannis, Massachusetts, and author of *The Herbal Body Book*.

She suggests using about ¼ cup of olive, jojoba, or sweet almond oil, available at health food stores and by mail order (see "Where to Buy Herbs and Herbal Products" on page 462) with about 10 drops of lavender or rosemary essential oils added.

For thick, heavy hair, try coconut oil, says de la Tour. "For Polynesian and Latina women, coconut oil is wonderful for the hair," she notes. Dampen your hair, then rub the oil mix in until the hair is thoroughly coated.

Cover with a shower cap and a warm towel for a half-hour, then shampoo twice.

Rinse with marshmallow root. Made with 2 teaspoons of dried marshmallow root to a cup of boiling water, this tea has a natural moisturizing quality, says Kathlyn Quatrochi, N.D., a naturopathic physician in Oak Glen, California, and author of *The Skin Care Book: Simple Herbal Recipes*. "Strain the tea and cool it in the refrigerator, then use it as a rinse," she suggests.

Oil the ends. Condition brittle, fly-away ends with a few drops of sandalwood oil, Green suggests. Mix the sandalwood in a carrier oil such as olive or jojoba. Rub it on your palms, then across the ends of your hair.

Dry Skin

TONERS AND MASKS FOR A DEWY COMPLEXION

Itching. Flaking. Inflammation. Crinkly little "dry lines." Dry skin is prone to all sorts of uncomfortable and unsightly problems and is often made worse by the low humidity of heated and air-conditioned rooms as well as sun, wind, and winter cold.

Gentle botanical remedies can rescue desert-dry skin by adding moisture and relieving itching, redness and other problems, herbalists note. But they also say that herbal remedies for dry skin work best if you first moisturize from the inside

"Drink plenty of water, at least eight eight-ounce glasses a day," says Kathlyn Quatrochi, N.D., a naturopathic physician and herbalist in Oak Glen, California, and author of *The Skin Care Book: Simple Herbal Recipes*. "And make sure there's some fat in your diet; your skin needs it. (Oils high in monounsaturated fats—such as olive or canola oil—are preferred.) And I recommend taking at least 400 international units of vitamin E a day (look for a brand that specifies mixed tocopherols on the label). For some women, that's enough to clear up dryness. But it may take as long as three weeks to notice a difference in your skin."

Herbal Moisturizers That Ditch the Itch

If you're drinking plenty of water and supplementing with vitamin E and your skin is still dry, herbalists offer these suggestions.

Clean with oats. The gentle cleansing power of oats seems tailor-made for dry skin, says Stephanie Tourles, a licensed aesthetician in Hyannis, Massachusetts, and author of *The Herbal Body Book.*

To make an oatmeal scrub, grind enough rolled oats in a clean coffee grinder or food processor to make ½ cup of ground oatmeal. Combine with ⅓ cup of ground sunflower seeds, 4 tablespoons of almond meal, ½ teaspoon of peppermint leaves (both available at health food stores), and a dash of cinnamon powder. Store in a resealable plastic bag or a plastic container with a tight-fitting lid.

"Before you take your morning or evening shower, put 2 teaspoons of this mixture in a small plastic bowl, add 3 teaspoons of heavy dairy cream, and stir. Let it thicken for a few minutes, then lightly scrub it onto your face and neck. It leaves skin silky-smooth," Tourles says. "The heavy cream melts away grime and makeup without stripping away precious natural oils from your skin. I use this mix all winter long."

Make an oatmeal paste. For a quicker mix, simply use ground oats mixed with cream or whole milk, suggests Dr. Quatrochi. "For dry skin, combine a tablespoon or two of regular rolled oats—not instant oats—with enough whole milk or heavy cream to form a paste. Let it sit for a few minutes, until the oats start to plump a little, use it to gently scrub your face, then rinse," she says.

Take a whole-grain bath. If your whole body feels parched and dry, an oatmeal bath will relieve the itch, says Gayle Eversole, R.N., Ph.D., a nurse practitioner, medical herbalist, and professional member of the American Herbalists Guild (AHG), in Everett, Washington. "The same slightly gummy characteristic that you see in a bowl of oatmeal is very soothing in a bath," she says. "Oats are slippery—a quality that soothes and moisturizes. That's what heals your skin."

To prepare an oatmeal soak, place ½ to 1 cup of old-fashioned rolled oats in a muslin bag or a handkerchief closed securely with a rubber band. Place the bag in the tub and run warm water. "Don't just pour oats out of the box into the tub—they'll clog the drain and make a real mess," Dr. Eversole advises.

Tone with aloe and orange blossoms. Toners are usually suggested for oily skin, but even dry skin benefits from a toning splash to restore the skin's natural, protective acid balance, boost circulation, and help heal other skin problems such as blemishes and eczema, says herbalist Mindy Green, a professional member of the AHG, faculty member of the Rocky Mountain Center for Botanical Studies and director of educational services at the Herb Research Foundation, both in Boulder, Colorado, and co-author of *Aromatherapy: A Complete Guide to the Healing Art.*

To prepare a mild toner, mix 2 ounces of aloe vera gel, 2 ounces of orange-blossom water (available in health food stores and some supermarkets), 1 teaspoon of apple-cider vinegar infused with calendula petals (available at health food stores), 5 drops of helichrysum essential oil (available by mail order; see "Where to Buy Herbs and Herbal Products" on page 462), and 800 international units of vitamin E oil. (To make infused vinegar, follow the directions in "Infused Oils" on page 101.) You can buy vitamin E capsules in a supermarket or drugstore and squeeze out

(continued on page 400)

Herbal Masks

A Recipe for Fresher Skin

According to herbalists, herbal masks deep-clean pores, soften dry skin, peel away dead skin cells, and boost circulation, bringing a glow to a tired complexion. But herbalists also like herbal masks because they provide built-in relaxation time.

"While the luscious, liquid goo slowly dries on your face, you can relax on the sofa or take a warm bath," says Shatoiya de la Tour, herbalist and owner of Dry Creek Herb Farm and Learning Center in Auburn, California, who presents workshops on herbal body care at the annual Women's Herb Conference in Peterborough, New Hampshire.

During cosmetic workshops at her herb farm, de la Tour and the women she teaches nap on the lawn for 10 minutes to a half-hour after applying herbal masks.

What You'll Need

Masks may contain everything from egg whites to papaya, oatmeal to roses, whipped cream to clay. De la Tour recommends the following recipe, which is suitable for dry, oily, or combination skin. Test it on a small area on the inside of your arm and wait 24 hours before applying it to your face.

- ✓ A food processor or clean coffee grinder
- ✓ A large bowl
- ✓ A plastic storage container
- ✓ 1 cup oatmeal, ground to a very fine powder
- ✓ ½ cup almonds, ground to a very fine powder
- ✓ ½ cup dried lavender or roses, ground fine
- ✓ ¼ cup powdered kelp
- ✓ 1½ cups green clay or other facial clay
- ✓ A mixing spoon or small rubber spatula
- ✓ A small bowl
- ✓ A measuring cup
- ✓ Water
- ✓ 1 teaspoon honey

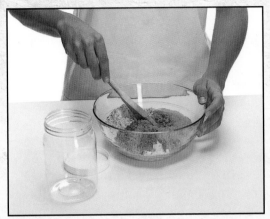

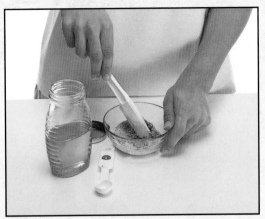

1. Make a basic mask mix. In a large bowl, combine the ground oatmeal, almonds, lavender or roses, kelp, and clay (powdered kelp and facial clay are available in health food stores). Work through the mixture with your hands to find and remove any large, unground almond pieces. Store the mixture in a plastic container with a tight-fitting lid.

2. Add water. For one mask, combine ⅛ cup of the dry mask mixture in a small bowl with enough water to make a paste with the consistency of loose mud or sour cream. Add the honey and blend completely, until the paste is smooth.

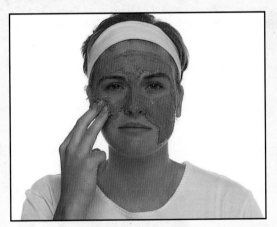

3. Apply. Spread the paste on your face with your fingers, avoiding the tender area around the eyes. Leave the mask in place for 10 to 30 minutes, then rinse thoroughly with warm water.

Herbal Face-Saving Strategies for Broken Capillaries

If your nose and cheeks are mottled with a fine network of broken-looking blood vessels, herbal medicine may offer some help, says herbalist Mindy Green, professional member of the American Herbalists Guild, faculty member at the Rocky Mountain Center for Botanical Studies and director of education at the Herb Research Foundation, both in Boulder, Colorado, and co-author of *Aromatherapy: A Complete Guide to the Healing Art.* "There's a lot of controversy about repairing broken or dilated blood vessels near the surface of the skin," Green says. "Herbalists disagree over whether the condition can be reversed and how to do it. But I believe that you can improve the look of your skin by working from the inside and the outside." Here's her herbal repair formula.

Start with supplements. Dermatologists and herbalists alike know that when blood vessels swell after drinking alcohol and eating spicy foods, capillaries can weaken, making them less elastic and more easily broken. The herbal route to stronger capillaries? Green recommends daily herbal supplements of ginkgo, hawthorn, and bilberry, plus vitamin C, taken according to package directions. These herbs are used traditionally to protect blood vessels and could help prevent more broken capillaries, according to Green.

Apply chamomile and friends. To improve skin tone, Green suggests applying moisturizers and toners containing essential oils of chamomile, helichrysum, rose, orange, neroli, and lavender, which ease inflammation and soothe the skin.

Opt for aloe, not vinegar. Choose toners that contain gentle-on-your-skin aloe vera instead of witch hazel or vinegar, which could irritate sensitive skin and capillaries.

Above all, be gentle with your skin. Wash your face with tepid water, not hot or cold; avoid facial steams; and don't scrub, says Green.

the oil. Combine, pour the mixture into a bottle with a tight-fitting lid, and shake.

In this formula, aloe vera acts as a moisturizer; apple-cider vinegar maintains proper acid balance, softens skin, and eases itchiness; helichrysum essential oil stimulates new growth of skin cells; and calendula soothes, Green notes.

Calm your skin with essential oils. A simple witch hazel and essential oil toner can calm irritated dry skin, "especially the type that gets red and inflamed across the cheeks and bridge of the nose," notes Tourles.

Combine ½ cup of witch hazel (the drugstore variety is fine) with 10 drops of one of the following oils: lavender (for regenerating skin cells and protecting against infection), sandalwood (for soothing chapped skin and skin rash), blue chamomile (a special form of chamomile oil that eases inflamed, sensitive skin), or rose geranium (for rejuvenating skin cells). Pour the mixture into a bottle with a tight-fitting lid and shake well. Apply morning and evening with cotton balls, avoiding the upper and lower eye area. Follow with a moisturizer.

Whip up a calendula mask. Rich with whipped cream, olive oil, and avocado, a lavish moisturizing mask made with calendula and lavender soothes dry skin and protects against infection, says Dr. Quatrochi.

To prepare the calendula mask, combine ¼ cup of whipping cream, ½ teaspoon of olive oil, 2 tablespoons of mashed ripe avocado, and 1 teaspoon each of calendula petals and lavender flowers. "Let it stand for 5 minutes so the liquid soaks up the herbs, then whip by hand or in the food processor," Dr. Quatrochi suggests. "Then slather it on clean skin and let soak in for at least 5 minutes. It's wonderful because it feeds your skin the water and fat needed to stay moist." (If a ripe avocado is hard to come by, you can omit it.)

Slather on an herbal salve. Red clover, plantain, and chickweed star in a kitchen-made salve that stops the scratching while giving dry skin a welcome drink of moisture, says Shatoiya de la Tour, herbalist and founder of Dry Creek Herb Farm and Learning Center in Auburn, California, who presents workshops on herbal body care at the annual Women's Herb Conference in Peterborough, New Hampshire.

To prepare your own anti-itch salve, first infuse any or all of those herbs in olive or almond oil. When the oil is ready, use it to make the salve (for directions, see "Salves and Ointments" on page 110). To help preserve the salve, add a few drops of lavender, rosemary, and thyme essential oils. Store it in the refrigerator or in a cool, dry place. Salves may last for years, but if it smells rancid, it's gone bad. Throw it out.

"If you have very dry skin, you'll probably want to apply a salve after you've showered or bathed, to seal in moisture," de la Tour says.

A word of advice: "Don't let anyone else stick their fingers in your salve. We all have our own personal bacteria. You don't want strange bugs growing in your skin cream," says de la Tour. (After all, you wouldn't share your toothbrush, right?)

Dull, Brittle Nails

GIVE YOURSELF AN HERBAL MANICURE

Rushing around from choir practice (hers) to soccer practice (the kids'), from golf lessons (hers) to tennis lessons (his), and from swim meets (the kids') to parent-teacher meetings (all), the average woman has little time to care for her nails. The result isn't pretty: Dried-out nails that break easily, ragged cuticles, or nails surrounded by skin cracked from overexposure to water, cold, heat, or wind.

Many a pair of brand-new panty hose has fallen victim to neglected (and unsightly) fingernails. Here's what herbalists have to offer.

Strengthen and Nourish

Herbal treatments may feed, condition, and protect dry, dull, or brittle nails, restoring shine and luster. Choose the option best suited for the problem at hand.

Soak in horsetail. This herb looks like the tassel on a mare's nether parts. High in silica, horsetail lends strength to weak, lackluster fingernails, says Shatoiya de la Tour, herbalist and founder of Dry Creek Herb Farm and Learning Center in Auburn, California, who presents workshops on herbal body care at the annual Women's Herb Conference in Peterborough, New Hampshire.

Combine ½ teaspoon of dried horsetail, available in health food stores and through mail order (see "Where to Buy Herbs and Herbal Products" on page 462), with 1 teaspoon of comfrey in a cup of boiling water. Comfrey has been used traditionally by herbal healers to soothe and heal wounded skin, so this herb can help soothe dry, cracked skin around your nails. Steep the herbs for 15 to 20 minutes and let cool to a comfortable temperature. Then soak your nails in the mixture for 5 to 10 minutes several times a week, de la Tour suggests. You can also make the soak using 1 teaspoon of horsetail and 1 teaspoon of dill, which contains calcium, she says.

Brush with comfrey. You can also soak your nails in a horsetail tea bath and then brush your cuticles with a comfrey paste, suggests Kathlyn Quatrochi, N.D., a naturopathic physician and herbalist in Oak Glen, California, and author of *The Skin Care Book: Simple Herbal Recipes.* Instead of adding the comfrey to the tea, mix it with enough water to make a paste and then brush it on your cuticles with an old nail polish brush. To soften cuticles, rub in a light application of olive oil after the horsetail and comfrey treatments, Dr. Quatrochi recommends.

Lubricate with chamomile and oil. If your nails are dry and split easily, rub them with chamomile-infused olive oil, de la Tour suggests. "This soothes and moisturizes," she says. (You can buy the oil through mail order or make your own, following the directions in "Infused Oils" on page 101.)

Try a soothing herbal salve. To ease dryness, cracked skin, and minor infections that can occur when the skin around your nails is damaged and vulnerable, herbalists suggest hand-and-nail relief salve, infused with horsetail, comfrey, and usnea, de la Tour says. Make your own by following the directions in "Salves and Ointments" on page 110. Begin by infusing your base oil with the three herbs.

"Rub it into your fingers at night, and you'll really start to feel the difference," de la Tour says. The comfrey soothes, the horsetail strengthens, and the usnea helps fight infection (all three herbs are available by mail). "A lot of nurses, who have their hands in water all day, love this formula," she notes.

Massage with herb-enriched castor oil. For dry, ripped cuticles, rub a drop of castor oil into the cuticle of each nail, suggests beauty expert Stephanie Tourles, a licensed aesthetician in Hyannis, Massachusetts, and author of *The Herbal Body Book.* "Castor oil is thick and has lots of vitamin E, so it's like food for the cuticle skin. And it makes the nails shiny," she says. You could also add a drop or two of carrot seed, lavender, or sandalwood essential oils to a two-ounce bottle of castor oil for an herbal nail treatment, she says.

Graying Hair

Natural Ways to Color and Highlight

Coffee. Walnuts. Rosemary. More than tasty foods and spices, these common kitchen items have the power to color graying hair, herbalists say. With natural dyes, which work like modern-day shampoo-in hair-coloring treatments, you get natural-looking color, complete with highlights.

"You can keep young-looking color in your hair without using a commercial dye or wash-in color," says Shatoiya de la Tour, herbalist and founder of Dry Creek Herb Farm and Learning Center in Auburn, California, who presents workshops on herbal body care at the annual Women's Herb Conference in Peterborough, New Hampshire. "In fact, women were using old-fashioned wash-in colorants made from herbs centuries before you could buy them in a box," she comments.

The Herbal Colorist

As with commercial coloring agents, the herbal approach you take will depend on your original hair color and the effects you want. If your hair is partially gray (less than 50 percent), all of the coloring techniques recommended here will add a dark tint over time and with repeated use. If your hair is more than 50 percent gray, the walnut-nettle rinse will impart more subtle tones, while the henna treatment will give you bolder color, de la Tour says. "The first time you color your hair, be cautious. Leave the mixture on for the shortest period of time to gauge how well your hair picks up the color." Here's what nature has to offer your graying hair.

Wash with sage or rosemary. To gently darken brown or black hair that's beginning to show signs of gray, rinse with a strong cup of sage or rosemary tea, suggests de la Tour. "Make the tea using 2 teaspoons or even 1 tablespoon of dried herb in a cup of water," she says. "Then let it cool, strain it, and use as a rinse after shampooing. Don't rinse it out. After using it several times, it should darken all of your hair."

Add walnuts and nettle. Make a strong tea with 8 cups of boiling water; $\frac{1}{4}$ cup each of dried sage, rosemary, and nettle; $\frac{1}{2}$ cup of black walnut hulls (available by mail order; see "Where to Buy Herbs and Herbal Products" on page 462); and 2 tea bags of regular black tea, suggests beauty expert Stephanie Tourles, a licensed aesthetician in Hyannis, Massachusetts, and author of *The Herbal Body Book*. Steep for 3 hours, strain, then add 2 teaspoons of sweet almond or olive oil and refrigerate.

To apply, wash and rinse your hair, then don rubber gloves and apply $\frac{1}{2}$ cup of this mixture. Don't rinse the mixture out. Just leave it on for a minute or so, then simply towel-dry your hair, using a dark towel so stains won't show. "This works well on hair that's brown, auburn, or medium to dark gray (as opposed to silver or white hair)," notes Tourles. "The dark color might look harsh on a woman with lighter gray hair."

Go for henna and coffee. When artfully applied, henna can impart beautiful dark tones and golden streaks to your hair, notes de la Tour. Available in health food stores in shades ranging from red to blond to jet black, henna is an herbal product made from powdered privet leaves (for blond and red henna) or from powdered indigo (for black henna).

De la Tour's henna regimen takes up to 2 hours and leaves hair conditioned and shiny. "But mix it up wrong, and it can be really brassy or yellow-looking," she says. "That's why I've added brewed coffee instead of water to my henna formulas. It's lovely." Her coffee-henna combination makes this coloring technique appropriate for women whose hair is more than half gray, she says, because it imparts natural-looking highlights.

How much henna you use and which color you choose depend on your hair. For the most satisfying results, de la Tour offers these guidelines.

🍃 Use 4 to 5 ounces (by weight) for short hair, 5 to 6 ounces for medium-length hair, and 7 to 8 ounces for long hair.

🍃 If you have dark hair, choose red henna. For jet-black hair, use black henna. If you have red hair, mix half red henna and half neutral henna. For blond hair, mix half blond henna and half neutral henna.

"Buy henna in bulk at the health food store. It's of better quality than packaged henna treatments because packaged hennas usually contain additives and bulk hennas are the pure herb," de la Tour says. Here's how to apply it.

🍃 Work some olive oil into your dry hair to moisturize it before applying the henna, which can be drying.

🍃 Rub unpetroleum jelly (available at health food stores) around your forehead, neck, and ears so the henna won't stain your skin.

🍃 Don rubber gloves and prepare the henna. Place it in a glass, ceramic, or stainless steel bowl (don't use plastic, as the henna will stain it) and add small amounts of regular-strength brewed coffee. Stir with a wooden or plastic spoon until the mixture is the consistency of mayonnaise.

🍃 Apply the henna to your hair, working down to the roots. Rinse the bowl with a little water and pour it slowly over your head to help the henna soak in. Press a washcloth to your forehead to keep water out of your eyes.

🍃 Cover your hair with a plastic grocery bag, leaving your ears exposed. Wipe any excess from your skin with an old towel or cloth.

🍃 Wait 45 minutes to 2 hours, then rinse your hair with water and let it air-dry. The first time you use henna, rinse after 45 minutes to see how well your hair takes up the color. If you want a darker shade, leave it on longer the next time you apply it. "When you rinse, you won't get all the henna out," de la Tour says. "When your hair is dry, you can brush the rest out. It brushes out like dirt, so you may want to do it outside." Clean your sink or tub right away to prevent staining.

🍃 After 24 hours, shampoo your hair.

Bear in mind that the color will be very bright for the first three days, but it will slowly fade for the next three months. "Your hair will look lush, soft, and shiny," says de la Tour. "This treatment coats the hair shaft, so your hair will be protected from sun and wind damage, too."

Oily Hair

WASH LIFE INTO YOUR HAIR WITH HERBS

Women with dry hair covet a little oil, figuring that you can always shampoo away the excess and still have enough to give hair life and luster. But oily hair presents a special challenge. Sure, you can lather up your scalp until you get repetitive strain injury from shampooing to excess. Yet frequent shampooing can dry out the ends, leaving them dull and brittle—especially if you use harsh commercial shampoos.

Easy-Does-It Oil Control

The herbal rescue regimen? Mild shampoos. Rinses that discourage overenthusiastic oil production. Teas that can help tame overactive oil glands. And a special mopper-upper for emergency oil slicks.

Wash gently. Oily hair may need frequent shampooing, but it doesn't need harsh shampoos, says Mindy Green, a professional member of the American Herbalists Guild, faculty member at the Rocky Mountain Center for Botanical Studies and director of educational services at the Herb Research Foundation, both in Boulder, Colorado, and co-author of *Aromatherapy: A Complete Guide to the Healing Art*. If you find that your hair is dull and dry after shampooing, you may be stripping too much oil from your hair and scalp, Green notes. This can happen if you wash your hair with harsh shampoos or use too much.

End the wash-grease-wash cycle by making a simple, mild shampoo that's gentle enough for everyday use (see "Herbal Shampoo and Rinse" on page 406). Use sage or lemongrass where the recipe calls for herbal tea, and add essential oil of clary sage or cypress to reduce oil gland secretions and for a refreshing scent, Green suggests.

Herbalize your favorite shampoo. Transform shampoo from the drugstore or health food store into a mild, herb-rich, and hair-friendly potion by diluting it and adding essential oils, suggests Donna Bryant, an herbalist in Pembroke, New Hampshire, who teaches at the Sage Mountain herbal education center in East Barre, Vermont.

Dilute an eight-ounce bottle of shampoo by half with water and add about 20 drops of essential oil of lavender, lemongrass, or patchouli. Observe the usual cautions for use of essential oils: Don't get the mixture in your eyes, and if you notice any skin irritation, stop using it.

Rinse with nettle and sage. Control runaway oil with an easy final rinse, suggests Bryant. "This rinse is simply a strong tea," she says. "The nettle and sage are astringent, so they help ease oil production."

Pour 1 quart of boiling water over $\frac{1}{2}$ cup each of nettle and sage. Steep for 10 to 30 minutes, then strain and let cool. Pour as much as you need over your hair as a final rinse. "An easy way to make this is in a one-quart canning jar," says Bryant. "It can be stored in the refrigerator for two to four days."

Finish with lemongrass and rose geranium. For an invigorating finale, combine

(continued on page 410)

Herbal Shampoo and Rinse

A Cleansing Routine for Perfect Hair

Wouldn't you love an orange-lavender shampoo that conditions dry hair or rosemary-and-sage-scented suds to gently cleanse oily tresses? You can concoct a mild, all-natural shampoo that's easy on your hair—and your wallet—with herbs that will help your 'do' look and feel healthy, says Mindy Green, a professional member of the American Herbalists Guild, faculty member at the Rocky Mountain Center for Botanical Studies and director of educational services at the Herb Research Foundation, both in Boulder, Colorado, and co-author of *Aromatherapy: A Complete Guide to the Healing Art.*

All you need is a shampoo base, some herb tea, essential oils of your choice, and perhaps a splash of vinegar. Shop for a gentle, unscented shampoo at a health food store. If you can't find an unscented version, look for a mild shampoo, such as baby shampoo, with as few ingredients as possible, suggests Green. Dilute it by half with strong herb tea before making an herbal shampoo.

Include vinegar in your homemade shampoo if you have dandruff or an itchy scalp or if your shampoo base is extremely alkaline. "Alkaline shampoos disturb the natural acid balance of the hair and scalp, which protects against dryness and skin irritation," notes Green. Check alkaline levels with nitrizine testing papers, available in drugstores, which measure pH. A balanced shampoo base will fall in the 4.5 to 5.5 pH range—midway between acidic and alkaline, Green says. "Vinegar's downside is that it cuts the suds. But the shampoo still cleans well," she adds. "And don't worry about the vinegar smell. It goes away in an hour or so."

What You'll Need

Before you get started, assemble your equipment. To make your shampoo, choose herbs from those listed in the table on page 408.

- ✓ A medium saucepan with a lid
- ✓ ¼ cup boiling water
- ✓ 6 tablespoons fresh or 3 tablespoons dried herbs
- ✓ A fine-mesh strainer
- ✓ A medium bowl
- ✓ ¼ cup unscented shampoo base
- ✓ ¼ teaspoon essential oil
- ✓ 1 tablespoon vinegar (optional)
- ✓ Measuring spoons
- ✓ A mixing spoon
- ✓ A 4-ounce plastic bottle with a tight-fitting lid

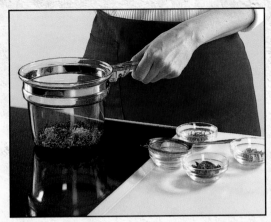

1. Mix it up. Make a strong infusion or decoction with the boiling water and herbs. (For more information on infusions and decoctions, see "Teas and Infusions" on page 89 and "Decoctions" on page 90.) Strain and cool.

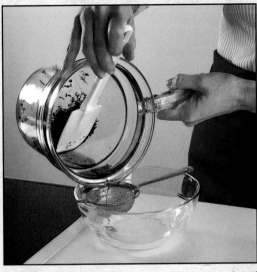

2. Add the tea. Place the shampoo in a bowl and pour in the tea.

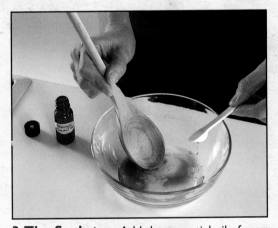

3. The final step. Add the essential oil of your choice and the vinegar, if desired. Store the shampoo in a plastic container with a tight-fitting lid for up to six months.

(continued)

Herbal Shampoo and Rinse—Continued

Customized Hair Care

You can create personalized shampoos and rinses by choosing from among these herbs and essential oils suggested by Green.

Hair Type or Condition	Herbs	Essential Oils
Dry	Orange peel, calendula, and comfrey root	Sandalwood, palmarosa, and rosewood
Oily	Sage, lemongrass, and burdock	Lemongrass, clary sage, and cedarwood
Dandruff	Burdock, sage, and willow bark	Sage, geranium, and tea tree
Thinning	Nettle and peppermint	Basil, cedarwood, and ylang-ylang
All types	Lavender, chamomile, rosemary, and rose	Lavender, Roman chamomile, carrot seed, and rosemary

FINISH WITH AN HERBAL RINSE

This simple, gentle rinse, used after you shampoo, adds shine and improves the health of your hair and scalp, says Green. The vinegar or lemon juice restores the natural acid-alkaline balance (or pH balance) that can be disrupted by some commercial shampoos, which have alkaline levels that leave hair looking stiff and dull, Green says.

To enhance the shine, start with an herb tea blended to enhance your natural hair color. If you're a natural blond, try chamomile or crushed rhubarb root. If you're a redhead, try calendula. If your hair is brown or black, choose from sage, rosemary, or crushed walnut hulls. To get the most out of your hair rinse, leave it on freshly washed hair for a few minutes, then rinse it out with water.

What You'll Need

You don't need a lot of equipment to make your own hair rinse.

- ✓ A plastic pint bottle with a tight-fitting lid
- ✓ Measuring spoons
- ✓ A funnel

- ✓ 3–5 drops essential oil
- ✓ 1 pint water or herb tea
- ✓ 1 tablespoon apple-cider vinegar or lemon juice

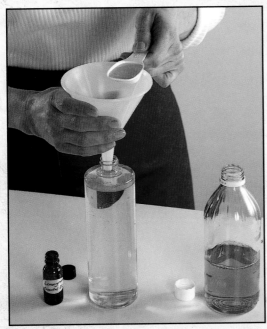

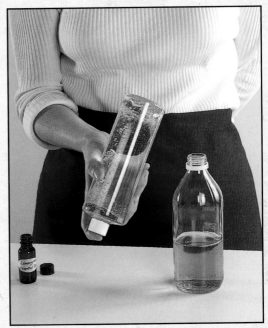

1. Fill the container. Using a funnel, pour oil, water or tea, and vinegar or lemon juice into a plastic bottle.

2. Shake to mix. Close the bottle tightly with the lid and shake thoroughly.

the fresh herbal scents of lemongrass and rose geranium in a rinse, suggests Jeanne Rose, an aroma herbalist from San Francisco and author of *The World of Aromatherapy* and *Herbs and Aromatherapy for the Reproductive System*.

To prepare a strong tea, use ¼ cup each of lemongrass, organic lemon peel, and rose geranium. Add the herbs to 2 cups of boiling water, steep for 10 to 30 minutes, strain, and let it cool. Add 8 drops each of rose geranium and lemon essential oils.

Pour about one cup through your hair several times. Put the remainder in a labeled glass jar and store it in the refrigerator. Make it in small quantities, Rose suggests, because the herbal-tea base won't keep for more than four days, even in the refrigerator.

Try burdock two ways. "Burdock root has a balancing effect on sebaceous glands, the oil glands in the scalp," says Gail Ulrich, an herbalist and founder/director of the Blazing Star Herbal School in Shelburne Falls, Massachusetts, and author of *Herbs to Boost Immunity*.

Rinse your hair with burdock root tea or make the tea to drink, using about 1 teaspoon of the herb per cup of boiling water. Have one cup a day. "To maintain healthy hair and skin, you can use burdock as an internal and an external treatment," Ulrich notes.

Refresh with herbs. If your part becomes an oil slick while the rest of your hair stays clean, swab down that grease puddle quickly with an herbal toner created by Stephanie Tourles, a licensed aesthetician in Hyannis, Massachusetts, and author of *The Herbal Body Book*.

To prepare the toner, mix ½ cup of vodka, ¼ cup of witch hazel (or ¾ cup of witch hazel and no vodka), and 1 teaspoon each of sage, yarrow, chamomile, rosemary, lemon balm, peppermint, spearmint, and strawberry leaves. Store in a tightly sealed bottle in a cool, dark place for two weeks, then strain and refrigerate. Use a cotton ball to dab the toner on the hair along your part, then let your hair dry naturally. Refrigerated toner will keep for up to six months.

Oily Skin

PLANT-BASED CONTROL TACTICS THAT WORK

Love that oil.

A shiny nose, glistening chin, or smudgy forehead can be signs of overeager sebaceous glands, tiny derricks that pump out a little more lubrication than most women want or need. The natural tendency is to attack oily skin aggressively with industrial-strength products, such as soaps and astringents that may be too harsh.

Herbalists and beauty experts who use herbal products say that by working *with* oily skin, you can help calm overproductive oil glands without sacrificing precious natural moisture that protects and softens your face.

"One of the hardest things for women with oily skin to realize is that when you strip all the oil off your skin with harsh soaps and astringent lotions, it sends a signal to your oil glands to produce more oil," says Mindy Green, a professional member of the American Herbalists Guild, faculty member at the Rocky Mountain Center for Botanical Studies and director of education at the Herb Research Foundation, both in Boulder, Colorado, and co-author of *Aromatherapy: A Complete Guide to the Healing Art.* "The film of sweat and oil that naturally coats the skin is one of the best moisturizers there is," she says. "It's also acid-balanced, so it protects against infection. Strip all that away, and your skin is vulnerable."

Degreasers from Nature

The best approach to taming oily skin is to remove excess oil while leaving some behind, says Green. The following herbal formulas, from cleansers to masks to face peels and moisturizers, do just that.

Wash with oats and herbs. Plain old-fashioned or instant rolled oats cleanse oily skin without robbing it of its protective oils, says Kathlyn Quatrochi, N.D., a naturopathic physician and herbalist in Oak Glen, California, and author of *The Skin Care Book: Simple Herbal Recipes.* "Make a paste with 1 tablespoon of oats, 1 tablespoon of warm water, 1/2 teaspoon of fresh or dried lavender, and 1 teaspoon of honey," Dr. Quatrochi suggests. "Let the paste soak for 1 hour and then wash gently as you would with soap. Lavender is antibacterial, yet soothing," she says.

Make a strawberry-lavender mask. Control oil with a clay mask that features strawberries and lavender, Green suggests. "This formula helps regulate overactive oil glands and sebaceous secretions," she says. "It leaves your skin feeling clean, not heavy with oils."

Make the mask by combining 1 tablespoon of facial clay (available at health food stores), 1 tablespoon of witch hazel, 1 mashed strawberry, and 1 drop of lavender essential oil. Apply to your face (except the area around your eyes), and leave in place for 10 to 15 minutes, then rinse with warm water.

Mop oil with rose water. Instead of washing with harsh soaps that strip too much oil off the surface of your skin, carry cotton pads and a bottle of hydrosol, an herb-scented water such as rose water or orange-blossom water that's available in health food stores and through mail order (see "Where to Buy Herbs and Herbal Products" on page 462). Use it to wipe away excess oil gently throughout the day, suggests Green. "This keeps down the oily shine but protects the moisture in your skin," she notes.

Tone with sage and peppermint. Sage helps to control oily skin, and peppermint adds a cool tingle. Combined with witch hazel, these herbs create an aromatic toner that restores the skin's protective acid mantle, says Dr. Quatrochi.

Add a teaspoon each of sage and peppermint to 4 ounces of witch hazel, then steep for one to three days. You can use this toner without straining it. Store it in an airtight container in or out of the refrigerator for up to two months.

Splash with vodka and herbs. Tone, tighten, and whisk away oil with an astringent featuring vodka, suggests beauty expert

A Fruit-Herb Refresher for Your Skin

Sunflower seeds and pineapple juice. It sounds more like an afternoon snack than a beauty treatment, but combined, these two gifts from the plant world create an effective skin wash that works like cleansing grains and a face peel all in one, says Stephanie Tourles, a licensed aesthetician in Hyannis, Massachusetts, and author of *The Herbal Body Book*.

How? Juice from a fresh pineapple contains natural fruit acids that slough off dead skin cells, much like the alpha hydroxy acids found in commercial face creams. Ground sunflower seeds exfoliate the skin, gently removing the dead cells to reveal newer, younger-looking cells. "The oils in the sunflower seeds also take off makeup and excess oils beautifully, without stripping moisture from the skin," she notes. "Used weekly, this will also even out the redness of blotchy skin."

To make your own facial wash, grind the seeds in a food processor or a clean coffee grinder. Then combine 1 tablespoon of sunflower seed meal with 1 tablespoon of fresh pineapple juice (canned won't work because the pineapple has been heated and the beneficial enzymes killed off). "If you don't have pineapple juice, substitute a half-and-half mixture of lemon juice and water," Tourles suggests.

Gently massage the fresh mixture onto your face. Let it dry for 10 minutes, then rinse in warm water. The mixture will sting a little when you apply it, which is a sign that it's working. If you experience severe stinging, rinse the mixture off right away and make a half pineapple juice/half water solution the next time you make the face wash. One note of caution: If you have a latex allergy or have acne, don't use pineapple on your skin.

Stephanie Tourles, a licensed aesthetician in Hyannis, Massachusetts, and author of *The Herbal Body Book*. "This is great after working out or as a quick, oil-removing cleanser in the middle of the day or when you're dashing out of the house," she says. "It won't overdry your skin."

To make an herbal astringent, mix ½ cup of water, ½ cup of vodka, ¼ cup of witch hazel, and 1 teaspoon each of dried sage, yarrow, chamomile, rosemary, lemon balm, peppermint, spearmint, and strawberry leaves. Store in a tightly sealed bottle in a cool, dark place for two weeks, then strain.

"The liquid will be pale green and have a floral, herbal fragrance," Tourles says. Apply with cotton balls and let your skin dry naturally. This astringent can be stored for up to six months at room temperature or up to one year in the refrigerator.

Slather with yarrow. Even women with oily skin need a moisturizer, says Shatoiya de la Tour, herbalist and founder of Dry Creek Herb Farm and Learning Center in Auburn, California, who presents workshops on herbal body care at the annual Women's Herb Conference in Peterborough, New Hampshire. "If you have combination skin, where part is oily and part is normal to dry, or if the surface of your skin dries out due to too much sun, wind, or washing, a yarrow moisturizer is nice," she says. "When the surface of your skin dries out, your oil glands produce more and more oil. A moisturizer prevents that from happening."

Adding yarrow to a homemade face cream can help reduce the appearance of large pores and tighten oily skin, she says. To prepare your own cream, first infuse yarrow in olive or almond oil (for directions, see "Infused Oils" on page 101). Then use the infused yarrow oil in the moisturizing cream recipe in "Creams" on page 104.

"Other herbs to infuse for oily skin are plantain, sage, or rosemary," de la Tour says. "Plantain is soothing. Sage and rosemary are more astringent, so they work like yarrow and are also antibacterial."

Puffy Eyes

BACKYARD REMEDIES FOR THAT SLEEPLESS LOOK

You're driving down a lonely road; suddenly, you're abducted by aliens. After several days, you're returned to your family. They notice that your eyes are puffy and ask what happened. You explain that you haven't slept for a week. Homesick, you've been crying for days. And while you were on the alien spaceship, you seem to have aged a couple of years. And they believe you.

Everyone knows that too little sleep, crying, and age can leave your eyes puffy. So can anything that interferes with your body's ability to transport and excrete fluids. You're more likely to wake up with puffy eyes if you're menstruating or pregnant and retaining fluid, for example, regardless of whether or not you've spent time on a UFO. The same is true if you eat salty foods.

Earthly Solutions

Whatever the cause, waking up with those little fluid-filled pouches beneath your eyes is no fun. Instead of hiding them with makeup, try these gentle herbal solutions that may deflate under-eye puffiness.

For instant relief, turn to chamomile. Need instant relief for puffy or tired eyes? Keep chamomile tea bags in your purse or your desk at work, suggests Shatoiya de la Tour, herbalist and founder of Dry Creek Herb Farm and Learning Center in Auburn, California, who presents workshops on herbal body care at the annual Women's Herb Conference in Peterborough, New Hampshire. "In a pinch, just wet two tea bags with warm water, let them stand for a minute or two, and apply them to your closed eyes for 3 to 10 minutes. Nothing could be quicker!"

Make a cold fennel compress. If puffy eyes are a recurring problem, make this cool-comfort remedy in advance, suggests Stephanie Tourles, a licensed aesthetician in Hyannis, Massachusetts, and author of *The Herbal Body Book.* "Pour a cup of boiling water over 2 teaspoons of fennel seeds and cover. Let steep, then put the whole pot in the refrigerator overnight, leaving the seeds in. In the morning, strain the cooled tea. The tea will have a nice licorice aroma and be kind of slippery—moisturizing and soothing," she says.

Cut patches from rolls of beautician's cotton (available at beauty supply stores), or use paper towels, and soak them in the cool fennel tea. "Lie down with your head elevated on a pillow and cover your closed eyes with the patches," Tourles says. "Rewet the patches whenever they warm up. After 10 to 15 minutes, your eyes will look and feel much better." This mixture will last for four days in the refrigerator, Tourles says.

Drink dandelion tea. Dandelion is a cleansing diuretic that flushes out excess fluid accumulation. Drinking one to three cups a day can help reduce water retention, including puffy eyes, says Amanda McQuade Crawford, a practicing herbalist in Ojai, California, a professional member of the American Herbalists Guild, member of Britain's National Institute of Medical Herbalists, president of the American College of Integrative Medicine in Albuquerque, and author of *Herbal Remedies for Women.* To make dandelion tea, use 1 teaspoon of dried dandelion leaf and 1 teaspoon of root per cup of boiling water. "Steep in a teapot or covered container for 10 minutes, then strain. Drink three cups a day until

symptoms improve," she says. You should see improvement in one to five days.

The root may also improve liver function, which helps the body break down and eliminate waste, among other jobs. Puffy eyes are a signal that the body needs improved liver and kidney function, according to McQuade Crawford, "so if your eyes are often puffy, try this remedy."

Slice up a cuke. Cucumber, a traditional external remedy for puffy eyes, also works well internally, says McQuade Crawford. "Externally, cucumber slices on closed eyes are cooling and astringent. They tighten up bags while soothing and reducing redness and irritation," she notes. "In addition, cucumber is a diuretic tonic that improves the elimination of excess fluids. So eat a few slices, and put some on your eyes. Cucumber has healing benefits inside and out."

Salve with violets. An eye-care salve made with fresh violets and dried chamomile and eyebright (available at health food stores and by mail order; see "Where to Buy Herbs and Herbal Products" on page 462) can perform double duty as a makeup remover and a soother for puffy eyes, notes de la Tour.

To concoct a salve, start by infusing a light oil, such as grapeseed oil (available at health food stores and through mail order), with the herbs. For instructions, see "Infused Oils" on page 101. Then use the infused oil to make a salve, following the directions in "Salves and Ointments" on page 110.

"Pat it gently under your eyes and leave it in place," de la Tour suggests. Apply whenever you are suffering from puffy eyes. The salve will keep for up to a year if stored in a cool, dark place such as a cupboard.

Brew an eye refresher. Don't have time

to make a salve? Then brew a cup of eye-bright-chamomile tea, using ½ teaspoon of each herb in 1 cup of boiling water. "Strain it well—chamomile has fine 'hairs' that you would not want to get in your eyes—and cool," de la Tour suggests. "Dip a clean, dry washcloth in the cool tea and lay it over your closed eyes. The coolness helps reduce swelling, and chamomile is very gentle on sensitive under-eye skin."

This mixture will keep for three days in the refrigerator, says de la Tour. "You can also put some in a misting bottle and spritz your closed eyes," she says.

Tired Skin

FRESHEN YOUR FACE WITH HERBAL SCRUBS AND TONERS

Riled or pasty, sallow or soiled, nothing beats nature for reviving a tired complexion. Herbalists swear by two time-honored techniques—scrubs and toners—to perk up skin that's lost its luster.

"I use a face and body scrub that's gentle enough to use every day," says Donna Bryant, an herbalist in Pembroke, New Hampshire, who teaches at Sage Mountain herbal education center in East Barre, Vermont. "It cleans. Softens. Exfoliates. Smells great. And my husband keeps remarking on how soft and smooth my skin is!"

Herbalists also suggest that after cleansing, scrubbing, or applying a mask to your face, you apply a toner. Versatile and fragrant, toners boost circulation, soften skin, and, perhaps most important of all, restore the skin's natural acid mantle. This slightly acidic surface, which is often washed away by harsh soaps, plays the vital role of protecting skin from bacterial invasion, says Mindy Green, a professional member of the American Herbalists Guild, faculty member at the Rocky Mountain Center for Botanical Studies and director of educational services at the Herb Research Foundation, both in Boulder, Colorado, and co-author of *Aromatherapy: A Complete Guide to the Healing Art*.

"A lot of women want to skip the toner because they think it's unnecessary. But it's very important, because keeping the acid mantle in place protects the skin from infection," notes Kathlyn Quatrochi, N.D., a naturopathic physician and herbalist in Oak Glen, California, and author of *The Skin Care Book: Simple Herbal Recipes*. "Pat on the toner after you cleanse your face and before you moisturize. The only time you don't really need one is after using a skin peel, because skin-peeling formulas are already acidic."

A Daily Regimen for Smoother, Fresher-Looking Skin

An Herbal Scrub for Face and Body

This basic cleansing formula, from Donna Bryant, an herbalist in Pembroke, New Hampshire, who teaches at the Sage Mountain herbal education center in East Barre, Vermont, combines the smoothing, soothing power of oats, the dirt-lifting oils and exfoliating properties of poppy seeds or almonds, and the pore-cleaning ability of facial clay.

What You'll Need

To make Bryant's herbal scrub, you'll need the following equipment and her suggested ingredients. "Look for kaolin clay at health food stores or by mail order," she says. "It works best. For this recipe, bentonite clay does not work well." (See "Where to Buy Herbs and Herbal Products" on page 462 for suppliers.)

For eye and nose appeal, Bryant suggests you add ground herbs, choosing from the options listed. Not only do herbs like calendula, comfrey, and chamomile look and smell pretty, but they're also soothing, and they can protect your skin from inflammation, Bryant notes. Lavender has infection-fighting properties. Roses are astringent and are also used for their scent in this formula.

When you make the scrub, pay attention to texture and consistency. "A coarse grind will tear up your skin," Bryant says. "A fine powder will exfoliate your skin beautifully and is gentle enough for everyday use."

- ✓ A food processor or clean coffee grinder
- ✓ A large bowl
- ✓ A wire whisk
- ✓ A quart jar with a tight-fitting lid
- ✓ 1 cup ground oatmeal (from rolled oats, not instant)
- ✓ 2 cups cosmetic clay
- ✓ ¼ cup ground almonds or poppy seeds
- ✓ ⅛ cup ground dried lavender, roses, calendula, comfrey, or chamomile, or any combination (optional)

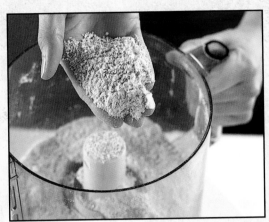

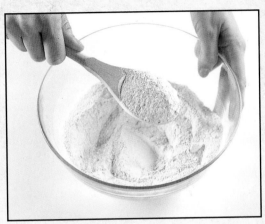

1. Grind the oatmeal. Place the oatmeal in a food processor or coffee grinder and grind it to a fine powder. Transfer to a bowl, then grind the almonds or poppy seeds to a fine powder.

2. Mix it up. Combine the ground oatmeal and seeds with the clay and herbs in a large bowl. To store, place the mixture in a glass jar with a tight-fitting lid; it can be stored for a year.

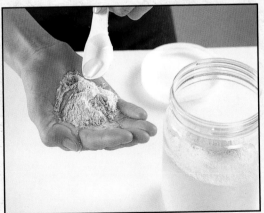

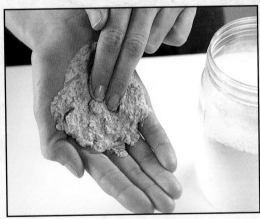

3. and 4. Get ready to scrub. To use, pour about two tablespoons of the mixture into your hand, add water to make a thin paste, and scrub your face and upper body gently. Rinse and follow with a toner.

(continued)

A Daily Regimen for Smoother, Fresher-Looking Skin—Continued

PROTECT WITH AN HERBAL TONER

After cleansing, scrubbing, or applying a mask to your face, it's time for a toner. This simple toner relies on skin-calming herbs and apple-cider vinegar, ingredients that have been used in cosmetics for centuries.

"Whenever I meet an older woman with beautiful skin, I ask her what she uses," says Shatoiya de la Tour, herbalist and founder of Dry Creek Herb Farm and Learning Center in Auburn, California, who presents workshops on herbal body care at the annual Women's Herb Conference in Peterbor-ough, New Hampshire. "Often, the answer is simply apple-cider vinegar. It helps whether your skin is dry, normal, or oily. And don't be afraid that you'll smell like a salad. The vinegar is diluted, and the smell goes away in minutes."

Customize this basic toner, devised by de la Tour, with your choice of soothing herbs. She suggests comfrey leaves, plantain, calendula, red roses, chamomile, nettle, lemon balm, lavender, scented geranium leaves, mullein, yarrow, rosemary, or thyme.

What You'll Need

Here's everything you'll need to make your herbal toner.

✓ Dried or fresh herbs of your choice
✓ A pint jar with a tight-fitting lid
✓ A fine-mesh strainer
✓ A bowl
✓ Plastic containers with tight-fitting lids
✓ Distilled water
✓ A measuring cup
✓ A funnel
✓ 2 cups apple-cider vinegar
✓ Witch hazel or witch hazel tincture

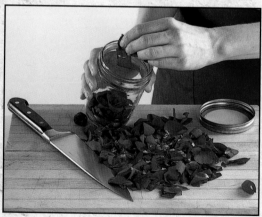

1. Fill a jar. Pack the herbs into a pint jar. If you're using fresh herbs, chop or bruise them slightly, then loosely layer them to the top of the jar. If you're using dried herbs, fill the jar halfway.

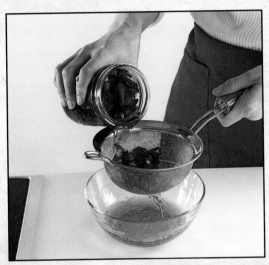

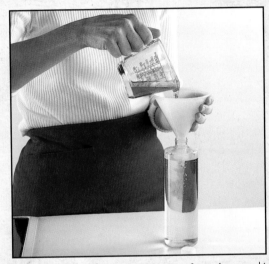

2. Get ready to steep. Pour vinegar into the jar and close it tightly. Let it steep for 3 to 6 weeks, then pour it through a strainer into a bowl. Add 2 tablespoons of witch hazel or tincture of witch hazel for every ⅔ quart of vinegar.

3. Bottle and store. Using a funnel, pour ¼ cup of the vinegar and witch hazel mixture and 2 cups of distilled water into plastic bottles. Shake well before using. This mixture will keep for a year or more. (A slimy coating called a mother vinegar may grow on the surface, but it can be removed and doesn't affect the quality of the toner.) Apply the toner with a cotton ball or pad or store it in a misting bottle and spritz your face when you need a pick-me-up.

Wrinkles

To Subtract Years, Add Herbs

Wrinkles are a small price to pay for hearing a good joke. Or snuggling up to a big, fluffy pillow as you sleep. Or smiling into the sun as you watch boats, birds, or balloons drift by.

In fact, if you've lived at all, you've probably got wrinkles—or will in the years to come, says Kathlyn Quatrochi, N.D., a naturopathic physician and herbalist in Oak Glen, California, and author of *The Skin Care Book: Simple Herbal Recipes.*

Some wrinkles are part of living, some aren't. Some wrinkles, called intrinsic wrinkles, show up as the collagen and elastin (protein fibers that give skin support and elasticity) break down over time. Others, called extrinsic wrinkles, are directly linked to "optional" activities like smoking or sunbathing.

Everything you do—or don't do—is reflected in your skin, it seems. "Your skin reflects the interior state of your body as you age," says Amanda McQuade Crawford, a practicing herbalist in Ojai, California, professional member of the American Herbalists Guild, member of Britain's National Institute of Medical Herbalists, president of the American College of Integrative Medicine in Albuquerque, and author of *Herbal Remedies for Women.* "Smoking ages your skin prematurely—it constricts blood vessels and impairs circulation to the skin. That's why lifestyle improvements are so worthwhile," she says.

Herbal Support for Mature Skin

"It's difficult to avoid or erase wrinkles completely," says Dr. Quatrochi. "But there are plenty of herbal options for minimizing them and making dehydrated or sun-damaged skin look its best." Like other herbalists (and many physicians), Dr. Quatrochi suggests skin-friendly lifestyle changes first, to help smooth and soften wrinkles. Among them: Drink plenty of water (at least eight eight-ounce glasses a day), don't smoke, wear sunscreen, avoid tanning salons, get regular physical activity, and include some healthy fats in your diet, such as olive or canola oil and fatty fish like mackerel and salmon. "Take these steps, and your skin will have more of a glow and feel more supple," she says. Then try these herbal wrinkle fighters.

Get your rose hips. High in vitamin C, rose hips help prompt your body to build collagen, the supportive substance that helps keep skin looking smooth and youthful, says Dr. Quatrochi. "Take capsules or tablets of rose hips (available at health food stores and some drugstores) and follow the package directions," she says.

Use a gentle herbal peel. Botanical face peels remove the upper layers of dead skin and over time can minimize wrinkles by encouraging the growth of new skin, says Dr. Quatrochi. "Herbal peels vary in intensity. Some are as strong as the chemical peels doc-

Rehydrate Wrinkles with Essential Oils

More than good scents, pure essential oils can help smooth and plump wrinkled skin, says Amanda McQuade Crawford, a practicing herbalist in Ojai, California, professional member of the American Herbalists Guild, member of Britain's National Institute of Medical Herbalists, president of the American College of Integrative Medicine in Albuquerque, and author of *Herbal Remedies for Women*.

Start with an ounce of honey or a cup of cooled herbal tea. (Chamomile tea soothes the skin, while nettle tea nourishes it, McQuade Crawford says. And don't worry— once dried or cooked, nettle quickly loses its sting.) Then add a drop or two of sandalwood, lavender, clary sage, or chamomile essential oil, she suggests. For oily skin, try a citrus variety such as lemon or tangerine. For dry skin, make it rose, she says. "This helps moisturize and brings blood flow to the surface of the skin. And remember, less is more. You only need a few drops of essential oil."

Smoothed on the skin several times a week, this formula can begin to improve the look of wrinkled skin in six to eight weeks, says McQuade Crawford. Remember to keep essential oils and formulas that contain them away from your eyes and mouth.

tors perform," she says. "Others are much milder."

Before you attempt a face peel, check with your dermatologist. If you have lupus or broken capillaries, a face peel may aggravate your skin.

To prepare your face for an herbal peel, clean your skin with a nonoily cleanser. Then pat the peeling mixture on your face with your fingers. Don't get any in your eyes or on your lips. "Make sure your hands are clean, too," notes Dr. Quatrochi. Here are several herbal peels to try.

Herbal mix. Mix 1 teaspoon each of dried parsley, chamomile, and rose hips in ¼ cup of hot water. Steep for 15 minutes, or until cool.

Mashed fruit. Puree apples and strawberries.

Lemon and water. Mix equal parts of lemon juice and distilled water. This is a strong peel and is useful for pronounced wrinkles. After two weeks, you can use 2 parts lemon juice to 1 part water.

"Your face should feel a little puckery and may even sting very slightly," says Dr. Quatrochi. Leave the peel in place for up to five minutes, but remove it sooner if it stings too much, she says. Rinse it off and apply a non-petroleum moisturizer.

"Use a peel three times a week until you like what you see," Dr. Quatrochi says. "Within three months, you may see a major difference in your skin, without the use of synthetic chemicals. Small wrinkles may diminish completely. You're peeling the outer layers of skin where the fine wrinkles have formed."

Tighten with egg. An egg facial will tighten wrinkles temporarily, acting as a

An Herbal Steam Facial

STEAM YOUR FACE, RAISE YOUR SPIRITS

Rose and calendula petals slowly unfurl in the hot water. Fragrant steam rises, opening pores and delighting the nose. Soft music plays in the background.

"A weekly or monthly facial steam is not only a good way to clean your pores, it's a lovely time to relax and pamper yourself," says Donna Bryant, an herbalist in Pembroke, New Hampshire, who teaches at Sage Mountain herbal education center in East Barre, Vermont. "You'll quickly discover that herbs are good for your spirit as well as for your skin." The herbs can be customized for your skin type.

For normal to dry skin: Bryant suggests combining 2 parts calendula flowers, 2 parts borage, 1 part lavender, 1 part chamomile, 1 part roses, and ½ part fennel seeds. "These herbs help to soften dry, rough skin," she says.

For oily skin: Try 2 parts comfrey, 2 parts calendula, 2 parts witch hazel, 1 part yarrow, and 1 part rosemary. "These are soothing and astringent herbs that will help ease oil production," notes Bryant. Add 1 part peppermint for a refreshing zing.

What You'll Need

Assemble the following materials for your steam facial.
- ✓ A teakettle
- ✓ A heatproof bowl
- ✓ Fresh or dried herbs chosen for your skin type
- ✓ A large towel

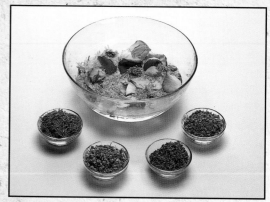

1. Heat it up. Place 3 cups of water in a teakettle and bring it to a boil, then carefully pour the steaming water into a heatproof bowl, as shown. Add about a cup of herb blend.

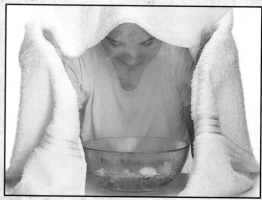

2. Steam away. Drape a large towel over your head and lean over the bowl, close enough to feel the steam (about 12 inches away), but not so close that it burns. "You simply want to build up a rolling sweat on your skin," says Bryant. Steam for 5 to 20 minutes, then pat your face dry. Follow with a mask for more cleansing or with a toner and moisturizer.

short-term face-lift to make skin smooth for four to five hours, Dr. Quatrochi says. For oily skin, use only the egg white, and for normal or dry skin, use one whole egg. "Whip it up with 1 teaspoon of dried or fresh lavender flowers, which are a good antibacterial that soothes the skin," she says. "Apply to clean skin and leave until the egg is hardened."

To remove, wet a washcloth with tepid water and lay it on your face, allowing the water to soften the egg. Then glide the egg off with a very wet washcloth. "This is great before going out to a special event, when you want to look really nice," Dr. Quatrochi notes. Always follow with a toner and a non-petroleum moisturizer.

Plump wrinkles with steam. You can temporarily rehydrate wrinkled skin with a fennel facial steam, according to Stephanie Tourles, a licensed aesthetician in Hyannis, Massachusetts, and author of *The Herbal Body Book*. Crush 1 tablespoon of fennel seeds and boil 3 cups of water. Carefully pour the water into a heat-resistant bowl and place it on a sturdy table. Add the crushed seeds and 2 drops of essential oil (rose, lavender, sandalwood, or rose geranium are all nice). Put a towel over your head and hold your face at least 12 inches away from the steam for 10 minutes. Follow with a moisturizer.

"This steam has a slippery, moisturizing quality," Tourles says. "It's also good for rough, chapped skin." If you have acne, acne roseacea, or spider veins, however, you should not steam your face, as it could further aggravate the condition. Tourles suggests using warm compresses of fennel tea instead.

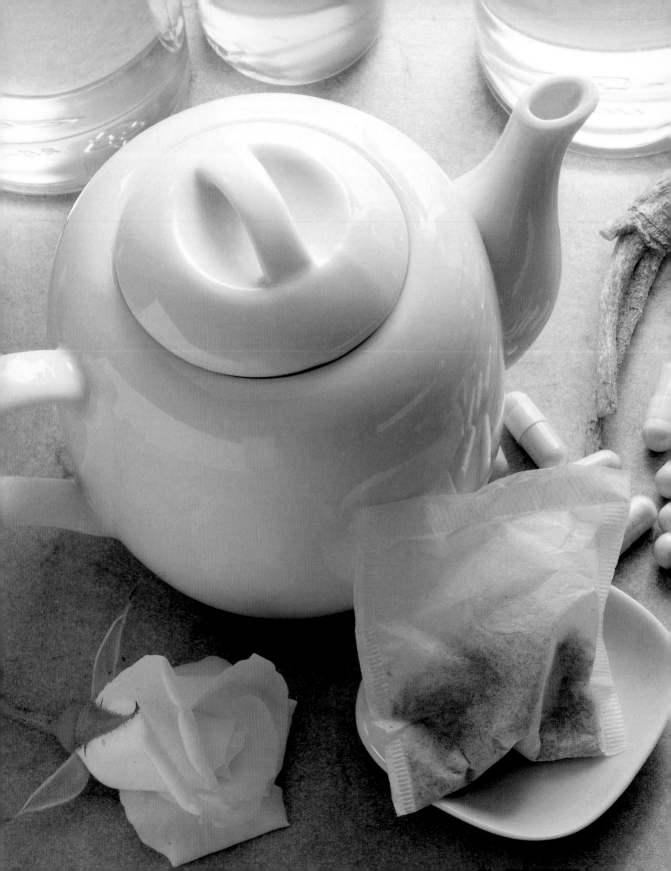

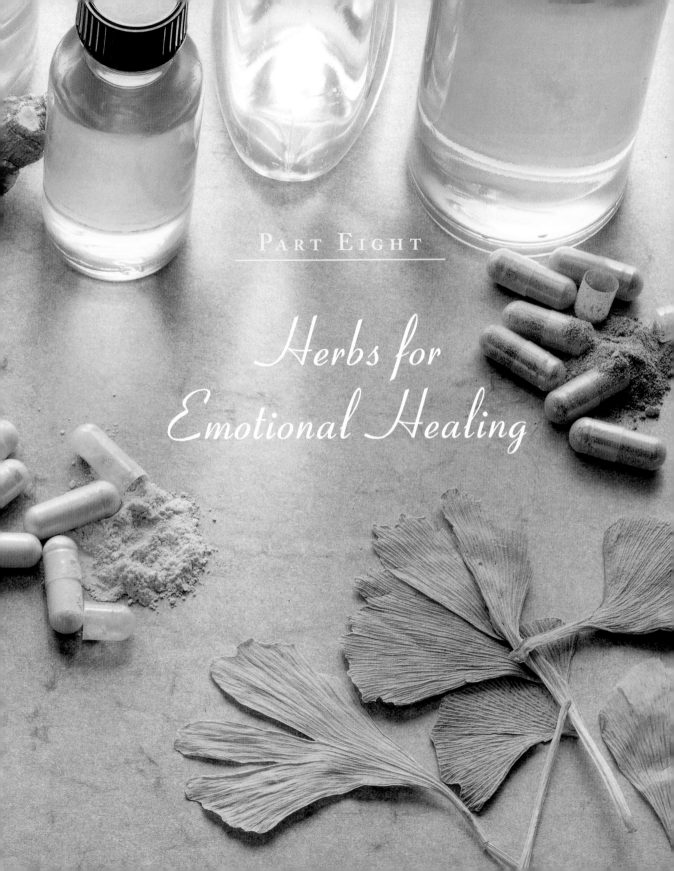

PART EIGHT

Herbs for Emotional Healing

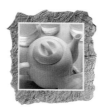

A Holistic Look at Herbal Therapy

Botanical medicine has so much to offer by way of remedies for physical ills—ginger for motion sickness, echinacea for colds and flu, black cohosh for hot flashes. So reaching for an herbal remedy when you feel emotionally unwell also seems natural enough. And indeed, herbalists have much to offer in the way of botanical support for emotional ills. St.-John's-wort for mild to moderate depression. Kava-kava for anxiety. Damiana for stress.

Just as with physical complaints, however, herbal medicine works best if you address the underlying cause of your distress, not just the symptoms.

"Herbal healing doesn't suppress the symptoms of turmoil," says Candis Cantin-Packard, a professional member of the American Herbalists Guild (AHG) and director of the Evergreen Herb Garden and Learning Center in Placerville, California. "I believe symptoms like depression, anxiety, and other problems are gateways to growth, as painful as that growth may occasionally be."

According to Cantin-Packard, herbs not only help support you when you're going through an emotional crisis, they also help strengthen you so that you'll be healthier when the crisis is over. Instead of trying to medicate emotional problems away, naturally or pharmaceutically, herbalists say that we should pay attention to what those problems are trying to tell us.

"Stress, depression, anxiety—these conditions should make us ask ourselves, 'Are these problems to get rid of . . . or messages to listen to?'" says David Hoffman, a founding and professional member of the AHG, a fellow of Britain's National Institute of Medical Herbalists, assistant professor of integral health studies at the California Institute of Integral Studies in Santa Rosa, and author of *The New Holistic Herbal.*

Even then, herbs aren't automatically better than prescription medications for emotional problems. "For serious situations, prescription medicines may or may not be more appropriate," says Toni Bark, M.D., who practices holistic medicine in Glencoe, Illinois. Severe depression, manic-depression, schizophrenia, phobias, panic, and disabling anxiety all call for medical attention, Dr. Bark adds.

For mild to moderate anxiety, herbal therapy can be effective, and for some women, it may be a better choice than prescription medication, says Harold H. Bloomfield, M.D., a psychiatrist in private practice in Del Mar, California, and author of *How to Heal Depression*.

Another downside of taking prescription medications for emotional problems is the issue of dependency and side effects, Dr. Bloomfield notes. "There's far less dependency with herbs than with tranquilizers like Valium and Xanax, for example," he says.

Stepping-Stones, Not Crutches

Hoffman is quick to point out that, contrary to popular opinion, herbs are not without side effects. True, the side effects of herbs are likely to be gentler and less unwelcome than those sometimes experienced with prescription drugs, especially drugs like diazepam (Valium) and fluoxetine (Prozac). "Sure, doctors can prescribe herbs the way they prescribe prescription drugs," says Dr. Bark. "For example, St.-John's-wort works a lot like Prozac, with fewer side effects. So if you're going to use one or the other, I'd rather use St.-John's-wort. But I'd also rather find out what's really going on."

"Say you have a high-stress job," says Hoffman. "Perhaps you should consider other options, like not going to work on a particular day or considering a line of work that's not so stressful."

"For women, using herbs appropriately can help begin the process of self-healing," Hoffman continues. "When used as a stepping-stone toward taking charge of your life, herbs have a tremendous amount to offer," he says. "But if you use herbs as remedies in the same way you use prescription drugs, you'll experience no real health advantage."

Garden Your Way to Serenity

Growing your own herbs adds yet another dimension to their healing potential. "That's a rather devious way of getting people back in touch with nature," Hoffman notes wryly.

"You can't grow your own Valium," he says. But getting your hands in the dirt helps counteract alienation from nature and the environment and therefore reduces much of the cultural malaise that can lead to emotional problems, he believes.

Balancing life with nature is just one path to emotional well-being. A healthy diet and lifestyle are vital. So is living in a creative, supportive, and fulfilling environment, Hoffman notes.

"To rely on herbal medicine without supporting yourself with a good diet is a grave mistake," says Glenn Gurman, a licensed acupuncturist, professional member of the AHG, founder of the Holistic Health Care Clinic in Norwich, Vermont, and author of *The Eight Treasures of Health*. "That means centering your diet around nourishing foods that build and strengthen blood production, including foods rich in iron and the B vitamins."

"The body and the mind aren't separate," says Brigitte Mars, a professional member of the AHG who teaches at the Rocky Mountain School of Botanical Medicine in Boulder, Colorado. "I practice an East/West approach to medicine, which teaches us that our physical and emotional parts are intertwined. For example, it is believed that when the liver is out of balance, you can feel angry or frustrated," she explains.

Herbal Counseling

Visit an herbalist for your feelings of depression, your high anxiety, your mood swings, or your concentration problems, and you're likely to experience first-hand the difference between traditional medical care and the way herbalists help you work with emotional problems.

Say you consult Kathleen Gould, a professional member of the AHG in Indialantic, Florida, for example. She'd invite you to take a seat in her cozy shop, the Herb Corner.

You'd tell her your troubles, and she'd probably brew you a cup of oatstraw, lemon balm, and chamomile tea. You would participate in the process.

"I'll show a woman the herbs, tell her why I'm selecting herbs specifically for her, and teach her what to do with them," says Gould. "I'll walk her through how to use them, then I'll back away so that she can take responsibility for her own healing. I tell her to find a pretty teapot to make her tea in, make lavender and oatmeal baths, write in a journal, and generally make some time for herself. And the more a woman complains that she doesn't have time for all that, the more I know she needs to make the time," Gould says.

Anxiety

TAKE THE EDGE OFF EDGINESS

Most women have plenty to worry about. An occasional prickle-in-the-back-of-the-mind worry that strikes in the middle of the night. Omnipresent worry about children, careers, or aging parents. And once-in-a-while worries about missing a connecting flight or forgetting to turn off the iron. They're all perfectly normal, in normal amounts.

But when worry goes awry, it becomes anxiety. Anxiety is a response beyond your control, a physical response to danger. When you feel particularly anxious, your body releases chemicals called catecholamines,

which stimulate the central nervous system. As a result, your sympathetic nervous system, designed to help you cope when you're under attack, kicks in: Alertness increases, your heart rate quickens, and your muscles tense.

Sedatives from Nature

In our have-to-get-it-done-right-this-minute culture, our sympathetic nervous systems can get stuck permanently in the "on" mode, making anxiety an all-too-constant companion, says Hyla Cass, M.D., assistant clinical professor of psychiatry at the Univer-

Kava-Kava: Herbal Anxiety Insurance

If you're gripped by anxiety, insomnia, or pain, kava-kava, with its sharply odd, resin-like flavor, may become a taste you'll decide to acquire.

"I think kava is the herb for our present-day stressful lifestyle. It allows relaxation while maintaining alertness," says Hyla Cass, M.D., assistant clinical professor of psychiatry at the University of California, Los Angeles, UCLA School of Medicine.

Native to tropical forests, kava-kava is a staple at Polynesian religious rites, in which it's drunk as a fermented liquor. Natives believe that it relaxes the mind and produces restful sleep without mind-numbing mental impairment or hangover.

Scientists have identified a number of active ingredients in kava-kava, including two pain-relieving chemicals thought to be as effective as aspirin. Kava is available in tinctures (sometimes called extracts) and capsules wherever herbal products are sold.

Do not take kava-kava if you are pregnant or nursing, and do not exceed the dosage on the product labels. Taking it with alcohol or barbiturates may increase their effect.

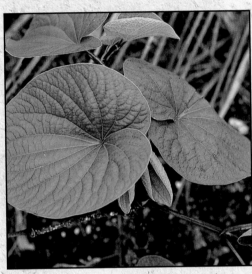

Kava-kava is yet another nondrug option to help relieve sleep problems and nervous tension.

sity of California, Los Angeles, UCLA School of Medicine. When the sympathetic nervous system starts cranking, you feel tired but you can't sleep, your whole body is tense, and you live in a perpetual state of edginess.

A class of herbs called nervines, including kava-kava, California poppy, and chamomile, is believed to ease anxiety by nudging the parasympathetic nervous system into action. That's the part of our nervous systems that winds us down and helps us to relax, says Dr. Cass.

Simply sipping a cup of chamomile tea at day's end can help, she says, as one of its actions is that of a nervine. Herbal sedatives are safer than prescription sedatives like alprazolam (Xanax) and diazepam (Valium), which make you sleepy and can lead to dependency, says Dr. Cass.

Here's what herbalists recommend for anxiety.

Tea for one. "I've had high-powered executives say, 'My doctor wants to put me on Xanax,'" says Patricia Howell, a professional member of the American Herbalists Guild (AHG) and director of the Living with

Herbs Institute in Atlanta. "Instead, I put them on chamomile tea, and they've told me that they felt their lives were theirs again."

But the chamomile tea that Howell recommends is much stronger than the average brew. To make this chamomile infusion, put 2 to 3 ounces of dried chamomile flowers in a jar and cover it with freshly boiled water. Let it steep overnight. Then strain out the herb and drink about ¼ cup of this fairly strong infusion as needed for anxiety and accompanying digestive upset. "It is a very strong preparation and can be taken as often as needed," she says. "It can be diluted with hot water to make a weaker tea."

Reach for some kava. "Kava is a fantastic anti-anxiety herb," says Howell. As a nervine herb, it relaxes the body while the mind stays alert, so that you can see clearly."

To use kava, start out with ½ teaspoon of kava tincture (also called an extract) if you weigh between 130 and 175 pounds, advises Howell. Use a bit more or less if you fall over or under that range. Put the tincture in a little water and sip. "If you like the way the kava makes you feel, you can take another dose as soon as you feel the anxiety return," says Howell.

Make mine skullcap, please. "I use skullcap, another nervine herb, for the 'hamster in a cage' feeling that we get when our minds start whirling around and around with worry, like a hamster on a wheel," says Howell. "I think of it as a mother's cool hand on the forehead, and I call it the 'there, there' herb. Use the same dosage recommendations as for kava tincture: ½ teaspoon if your weight is within the 130-to-175-pound range. Take it three or four times a day," suggests Howell.

Banish panic with passionflower. "Some people are beset by anxiety attacks that come on during the night," says Ellen Hopman, a member of the AHG who practices in Amherst, Massachusetts. "These are the night terrors that literally make your heart palpitate. You may awake from a bad dream feeling like you've been chased. The Chinese call this feeling 'the three fires in the home'—in your dream, you've been fleeing, fighting, or nearly consumed by fire. To the Chinese, dreams like this could be symptoms of high blood pressure, allergies, or nervous exhaustion."

The best remedy? Passionflower, yet another nervine herb. According to Hopman, you can brew passionflower into a tea. Steep 2 teaspoons of the dried herb for 30 minutes in a cup of freshly boiled water. Strain the tea before drinking. You can brew a larger amount and store it in the refrigerator in a tightly closed glass jar for up to a week, Hopman adds. Drink ¼ cup four times a day between meals so it absorbs more directly.

You can also take passionflower tincture: 20 drops in water four times a day between meals. Continue taking passionflower until your anxiety subsides, and then take it for a day or two longer. But passionflower should not be taken for more than two weeks in a row, Hopman notes.

Two anti-anxiety formulas are better than one. "Easing anxiety takes more than a quick fix," says Kathleen Gould, a professional member of the AHG and director of the Herb Corner, an herbal education center in Indialantic, Florida. So she often offers two herbal formulas, one that works quickly to help you relax and a second that strengthens the adrenal system over time to make coping with anxiety easier.

To ease anxiety in the short term, Gould recommends a blend of either tinctures or dried herbs consisting of equal parts of passionflower, skullcap, lemon balm, and oat-straw, all of which are nervines. For mental clarity, she might add equal parts of gotu kola or ginkgo to the blend in order to promote blood flow to the brain, she says.

If you use tinctures, take ¾ teaspoon of the formula in a little water two to four times a day, Gould advises. If you use dried herbs, fill "00" gelatin capsules with the mixture and take two capsules three or four times a day, she says.

The second formula that Gould recommends includes adaptogenic (long-term) herbs like Siberian ginseng and astragalus combined with nervine (short-term) herbs like damiana and gotu kola. "I have women take a formula like this three or four times a day for a few months to balance the nervous system," she says. She balances the blend individually, depending on a particular woman's needs. Gould may blend equal parts of Siberian ginseng, skullcap, passionflower, lemon balm, and gotu kola, for example, to tame anxiety.

Try a quick calm-down formula. If you experience an occasional bout of uncomfortable anxiety due to a particularly stressful situation, this tonic should give you some peace, says Candis Cantin-Packard, a professional member of the AHG and director of the Evergreen Herb Garden and Learning Center in Placerville, California.

"A combination of 1 ounce each of dried Siberian ginseng, licorice root, and skullcap and ½ ounce each of marshmallow and valerian may be helpful in strengthening the adrenal glands as well as soothing and nourishing nerves," Cantin-Packard says. "You can make a tea with herbs that have been cut in small pieces and sifted herbs. Put all the herbs in a wide-mouth jar and then scoop out 1 teaspoon of the combination.

Let steep in hot water for 10 minutes, strain, and drink one to three cups per day as needed." Avoid valerian if you are taking other sleep-enhancing or mood-regulating medications such as Valium or amitriptyline (Elavil).

For those who prefer herbal tinctures, you can purchase an ounce of each of the above herbs, Cantin-Packard adds. Add 5 to 10 drops of each tincture to a little water and take one to three times a day, she says.

Sniff ylang-ylang and other soothing scents. Research indicates that the very expensive essential oil of neroli, made from the flowers of the bittersweet orange tree, is very useful for anxiety, says Jane Buckle, R.N., an aromatherapist in Hunter, New York, and author of *Clinical Aromatherapy in Nursing*. Also good—and less costly—is essential oil of petitgrain, made from the leaves of the same tree, notes Buckle. "And I find ylang-ylang very relaxing," she says. "I always travel with it and put a mixture of ylang-ylang and lavender on a tissue inside my pillowcase to help me sleep when I am in a different time zone. You can use the tissue the same way for anxiety—just sniff it when you're feeling tense."

Other Anti-Anxiety Aids

Herbs work best if you also take into account other contributing factors in anxiety. Here's what else herbalists recommend.

Do the caffeine wean. Caffeine is a major cause of anxiety and nervous tension, stresses Dr. Cass. "I urge everyone who has an anxiety problem to wean themselves off all beverages containing caffeine."

Pair herbs with B vitamins. That B vitamins are essential for a healthy nervous system is a matter of medical fact. A niacin deficiency, for example, can cause nervousness, irritability, apprehension, and even paranoia. Too little riboflavin, and you risk mood swings from depression to hysteria to lethargy. And vitamin B_{12} is a catalyst that enables the entire nervous system to function at peak efficiency.

"Most adults in our culture are probably a little deficient in the B vitamins, so I usually advise people to take one good B-complex vitamin a day, always with food, so the vitamins are properly absorbed," says David Hoffman, a founding and professional member of the AHG, a fellow of Britain's National Institute of Medical Herbalists, assistant professor of integral health studies at the California Institute of Integral Studies in Santa Rosa, and author of *The New Holistic Herbal*.

Depression

PLANTS TO EASE YOUR ACHING PSYCHE

No blood test, CAT scan, or other high-tech tool exists to diagnose depression, the silent emotional illness that strikes women far more fiercely than men. Consider the numbers: One in four women is likely to experience depression during her lifetime. And depression can strike twice: Once hit with depression, the chances are 50-50 that a woman will have a second bout.

Depression resembles the feelings of grief and mourning that usually follow bereavement. Typical symptoms include feelings of low self-esteem, guilt, and self-reproach; withdrawal from others; overeating or loss of appetite; and sleep problems. Feelings associated with depression range from simple sadness or discouragement (the "common cold" of emotional health) to a suicidal sense of despair.

The loss of a loved one, a serious chronic disease, or other severe emotional or physical strain can spark a bout. Sometimes, depression seems to have no source at all and is known as endogenous depression, or depression that arises from within.

The trickiest thing about fighting depression is that many women don't realize that it's treatable, for three key reasons.

    Depression creates low self-esteem, so a woman feels defective rather than in need of treatment.

    Depressed women are often pessimistic and believe that nothing can make them feel better.

    Depression can be so exhausting that it prevents a woman from seeking the help she needs.

The Chemistry of Depression

When the brain's ten billion cells function smoothly, they transmit billions of messages every second. Biochemical messengers such as dopamine, serotonin, and norepinephrine, which are collectively called neurotransmitters, are responsible for the actual sending and receiving of this "correspondence" (you could call it B-mail). When all circuits are working as they should and neurotransmitters are adequate, we feel just fine—confident, hopeful, and secure.

A deficiency of these neurotransmitters, research indicates, may be linked to depression, just as too many could ignite the manic phase of manic-depression. So the medical approach to depression involves strategies to restore the chemical imbalance that causes the neurotransmitter deficiency, usually with drugs (antidepressants).

In Search of a Drug-Free Antidepressant

A veritable rainbow of pills exists to fight depression. Fluoxetine (Prozac), paroxetine (Paxil), venlafaxine (Effexor), and sertraline (Zoloft) are some of the best-known of the 80-plus medications dispensed by pharmacists. Known as selective serotonin reuptake inhibitors (SSRIs), they work by raising brain levels of serotonin. Others like phenelzine (Nardil) and tranylcypromine (Parnate), known as monoamine oxidase (MAO) inhibitors, also increase serotonin levels, but in a slightly different way. The tab for Prozac and other high-tech antidepressants can run upward of $200 a month.

Add to that the physical cost: Antidepressants come with troubling side effects. Discomforts and annoyances like anxiety, insomnia, drowsiness, decreased sexual desire, and impaired sexual function drive users to explore nondrug alternatives, including herbs.

"Women are leading the way in finding alternatives to Prozac," says Harold H. Bloomfield, M.D., a psychiatrist in private practice in Del Mar, California, and author of *How to Heal Depression*. "Studies show that 50 percent of women who take serotonin-enhancing antidepressants like Prozac report feeling a decrease in sexual interest. Other common side effects of this drug include nausea, diarrhea, insomnia, agitation, vivid dreams or nightmares, feelings of fogginess, drowsiness, and persistent yawning."

St.-John's-Wort to the Rescue

The common, yellow-flowered plant called St.-John's-wort (also known as hypericum) is emerging as nature's weapon in the battle against depression. Hardly a new medicine, St.-John's-wort has been healing people for more than two millennia, since the era of Hippocrates, the father of medicine.

Researchers in Munich, Germany, conducted a methodical review of 23 randomized trials of the use of St. John's-wort for depression, examining its effect on 1,757 people with mild to moderately severe depressive symptoms. They concluded that St.-John's-wort works as well as standard antidepressants for the treatment of mild to moderately severe depression. (Both worked better than a placebo.)

"For women using St.-John's-wort for mild to moderate depression, it works as well as prescription antidepressants," says Donald J. Brown, N.D., a naturopathic doctor in Seattle and author of *Herbal Prescriptions for Better Health*.

"Both the research and my experience indicate that St.-John's-wort is as effective for

Herbs or Medication?

Research indicates that St.-John's-wort is "effective for the treatment of mild to moderate depression," says Harold H. Bloomfield, M.D., a psychiatrist in private practice in Del Mar, California, and author of *Hypericum and Depression*. But if you're depressed, how do you know whether the problem is mild, moderate, or severe? To clear up any confusion, Dr. Bloomfield offers these guidelines.

Mild depression. If you just don't feel very good mentally and physically, and you feel that way all the time, you may have low-grade depression, says Dr. Bloomfield. "You may not feel as if you're suffering, but you don't experience any joy, either."

Moderate depression. "If you struggle along in your relationships and accomplish daily tasks with some degree of difficulty, you may be moderately depressed," says Dr. Bloomfield. You're experiencing some degree of mental suffering. Whether you're feeling mildly or moderately depressed, don't wait more than a few weeks to get help if you don't begin to feel better, he says.

Severe depression. "If you can't get out of bed, your social relationships break down, and you isolate yourself from friends and loved ones, your depression is disabling," says Dr. Bloomfield. "And if you have suicidal thoughts, the condition is life-threatening."

If you suspect your depression is severe or have suicidal thoughts that you think you might act upon, don't rely on herbs. Get help immediately. "Call your physician, your therapist, your religious counselor, a suicide hotline, or 911 immediately," Dr. Bloomfield urges. "A number of drugs treat severe depression very successfully," he notes.

treating mild to moderate depression as prescription drugs," says Dr. Bloomfield, who also wrote *Hypericum and Depression*. What's more, he says, "St.-John's-wort has none of the side effects that prescription antidepressants do. And it costs significantly less to use than Prozac does—about 30 or 40 cents a day compared to about $4 a day for Prozac." So herbal healers say they have good reason to recommend St.-John's-wort to people they treat for depression.

"When it comes to effectively treating mild to moderate depression with alternative therapies, St.-John's-wort is in a class by itself," says Dr. Brown.

"St.-John's-wort is remarkable," says Hyla Cass, M.D., assistant clinical professor of psychiatry at the University of California, Los Angeles, UCLA School of Medicine and author of *St.-John's-Wort: Nature's Blues Buster*. "In my experience, I have found St.-John's-wort to help many women for whom drugs were ineffective or had intolerable side effects," she says.

St.-John's-wort isn't an immediate cure for depression, and it isn't for every woman. "You have to give it time," says Dr. Bloomfield. "Relief from the symptoms of depression may take as long as four to six weeks. And 20 to 25 percent of depressed women will remain depressed, because St.-John's-wort just doesn't work for everyone. No one medicine ever does.

"Don't despair if St.-John's-wort doesn't help you," he says. "And don't feel any stigma whatsoever if you are advised to take prescription medications for your depression. After all, the side effects of depression are far worse than the side effects of depression medication."

How Does "Herbal Prozac" Lift Mood?

As for how and why St.-John's-wort works, researchers look to the chemistry of plants and people. When you're under stress, your adrenal glands secrete cortisol, a substance that helps the body deal with stress. If you're under chronic stress, your cortisol levels stay high and can not only dampen the immune response but also lead to depression and other problems, says Dr. Cass.

A compound in St.-John's-wort appears to normalize levels of cortisol secretions. According to Dr. Bloomfield, evidence suggests that St.-John's-wort also stimulates secretions of dopamine, which is known as the pleasure hormone.

"At first, doctors and scientists mistakenly thought that St.-John's-wort was an MAO inhibitor," says Dr. Bloomfield. "Learning otherwise is important, because we used to tell people that some drugs, and even certain foods and beverages, like aged cheese and wine, shouldn't be taken with MAO inhibitors. Now we believe that there are no drug-to-St.-John's-wort interactions to worry about." But there's more to St.-John's-wort than intricate medical science.

"St.-John's-wort comes from an age-old folk medicine tradition," says Dr. Bloomfield.

"It grew ubiquitously near humans and has been used medicinally since time immemorial. That means that the genes of the plant evolved alongside the genes of human beings. So it's no accident that we tolerate St.-John's-wort so well."

Pill, Extract, or Tincture?

Herbalists and medical doctors who prescribe St.-John's-wort disagree over what form works best—capsules, extracts, or tinctures.

An M.D.'s Rx. Dr. Bloomfield prefers capsules standardized to 0.3 percent hypericin. That way, you know exactly how much of the active ingredient you're getting. He recommends slowly building the dosage to one 300-milligram capsule three times a day. (A few notes on taking St.-John's-wort: Do not use it with other antidepressants without medical approval. And be careful about exposure to direct sunlight if you are fair-skinned—this herb may cause sun sensitivity.)

Although some women have reported feeling better within a week's time, Dr. Bloomfield suggests that you should expect to use St.-John's-wort for four to six weeks before you see results. You can also use a tincture, as long as you take 300 milligrams standardized to 0.3 hypericin three times a day, notes Dr. Bloomfield. You can take the tincture in a little water if you like. If you don't begin to feel better after six weeks, you should seek professional help, Dr. Bloomfield adds.

The case for extracts. Arguing that hypericin is just one of the active ingredients in St.-John's-wort and that a healing plant's power emanates from all of its constituents rather than from a single chemical, some herbalists advise against standardizing St.-John's-wort to 0.3 percent hypericin.

"The 0.3 percent standardized product works fine for some people, but not for everyone, because it misses some of the plant's healing components," says Christopher Hobbs, a fourth-generation herbalist who practices in Santa Cruz, California, professional member of the American Herbalists Guild (AHG) and author of *Stress and Natural Healing* and *St.-John's-wort: The Mood-Enhancing Herb*. "I get better results in my clinic with the whole plant extract."

If you grow your own St.-John's-wort, it's easy to make your own highly potent dried extract, says Hobbs. Here's how: Harvest the top five inches of the plants in flower. Take as much of the fresh plant as you have and juice it in a juicer. To the juice, add enough Siberian ginseng powder to make a thin, creamy mixture (to 8 ounces of juice, for example, you'd add 4 ounces of ginseng powder). Then pour the juice into the "fruit leather" tray of a food dehydrator and process according to the manufacturer's instructions until dry. Powder the dried extract and fill empty "00" gelatin capsules with it. Take one or two capsules twice a day, Hobbs recommends.

The Tincture Route

You may also want to try St.-John's-wort in tincture form. Here's what herbal experts recommend.

Make it or buy it. You can make St.-John's-wort tincture from the top five inches of your home-grown plants, says Hobbs. You can also tincture dried St.-John's-wort that you've purchased from a health food store or by mail (see "Where to Buy Herbs and Herbal Products" on page 462), he says. Whether you use fresh plant material or dried, follow the instructions for making a plant tincture in "Tinctures" on page 92.

You can also buy St.-John's-wort tincture (sometimes labeled as an extract) at health food stores and from mail-order sources.

Go for rich red. "No matter whether you make or buy St.-John's-wort tincture, make sure it's richly red or purple red in color," says Hobbs, noting that good tincture will have a slightly astringent taste.

Take the right amount. No matter which kind of tincture you use, the dosage is the same, says Hobbs: Take four dropperfuls in a little water in the morning and three in the evening. If you still feel depressed after two or three weeks, increase the dosage to a teaspoon morning and evening, says Hobbs. If, after raising the dose, you still don't feel better after two months, then St.-John's-wort probably won't work for you, Hobbs says.

Add some California poppy. "I often combine equal parts of St.-John's-wort tincture and California poppy tincture to treat depression," says Hobbs. "California poppy is the best anti-anxiety herb I've found, and it works quickly, often within three hours." It is non-narcotic and non-habit-forming, and it's safe enough even for children, adds Hobbs. Don't take California poppy while pregnant or while taking other MAO inhibitor drugs without your doctor's permission.

Beyond St.-John's-Wort

Although St.-John's-wort works fine for many women, it is by no means the only botanical ally for those who are beset by the blues. Here are some strategies offered by America's most respected clinical herbalists to help women deal with depression.

Sip dandelion tea. Sometimes, depression arises when women suppress anger, suggests Patricia Howell, a professional member of the AHG and director of the Living with Herbs Institute in Atlanta. "For many women, suppressing anger leads to a subtle depression that's hard to pinpoint," she says. "When women report this sad, uneasy feeling to their doctors, they're frequently told, 'It's all in your head.' And that makes them feel even worse," she says.

"These women keep their emotions in check for such a long time that they become numb, and as a result, they feel down and depressed."

Howell uses a very simple herbal remedy to ease depression caused by suppressed anger: dandelion. "I have depressed women sip tea made from dandelion root two or three times a day, and it seems to be very helpful," she says. One woman drank dandelion root tea for a day or so and called Howell to joyfully report that she'd actually been able to get really angry at someone and vent. "She was delighted and felt much better," recalls Howell (for directions on brewing herbal tea, see "Teas and Infusions" on page 89).

Brew the "happy" herbs. "A simple, easy formula containing oatstraw, lemon balm, and damiana has helped many women beat the blues," says Kathleen Gould, a professional member of the AHG and director of the Herb Corner, an herbal education center in Indialantic, Florida.

Oatstraw contains calcium and helps strengthen the nervous system. Lemon balm, the "gladdening herb," lifts the heart and spirit. Damiana is known throughout the Southwest as "the happy herb." It is a gentle, hormone-balancing herb, says Gould.

To make happy tea, combine equal parts of dried oatstraw, lemon balm, and damiana and brew a tea. Drink one to three cups a day. According to Gould, most women will feel better within a week or two.

Give yourself an herbal foot massage. Massage, especially of the feet, is one calming element in Ayurvedic medicine, a healing system with origins in India. "A foot massage can be as soothing as a full-body massage," says Candis Cantin-Packard, a professional member of the AHG, Ayurvedic lifestyle counselor, author of *The Pocket Guide to Ayurvedic Healing*, and director of the Evergreen Herb Garden and Learning Center in Placerville, California.

To 1 ounce of sesame oil, which is considered the most calming oil (although almond oil is a good substitute), add 10 drops each of essential oil of lavender and rose geranium. These oils are specific for depression. Take plenty of time. Working slowly, gently massage each foot with the oil before bedtime, suggests Cantin-Packard.

Spritz your home with lavender. "Lavender is very uplifting," says Gould. "You can use the essential oil of lavender all over your home when you're feeling down. Put it on lamp rings, add three to four drops to your bathwater, or dab a drop on your wrists and temples."

Don't miss meals. "When you're depressed, you might not feel like eating, but skipping meals creates a feeling of emptiness, which may make depression and anxiety feel worse," says Cantin-Packard. "Aim to eat cooked, easily digested foods like soups, steamed vegetables, well-cooked grains, and small amounts of organic meats," she advises.

Energy Drain

BOTANICAL BOOSTS FOR FATIGUE

When it comes to treating exhaustion, herbalists and medical practitioners have lots in common. Both agree that if you're too tired to get through the day or enjoy life, you need to find out why before you turn to any kind of pick-me-up, herbal or otherwise. Like physicians, responsible herbalists believe in curing the causes of fatigue rather than stimulating you out of your exhaustion.

"Plenty of young mothers and working women come in asking me for some kind of safe herbal stimulant to help them get through the day," says Kathleen Gould, a professional member of the American Herbalists Guild (AHG) and director of the Herb Corner, an herbal education center in Indialantic, Florida. "Unfortunately, no safe instant remedy exists. When I get requests like these, I generally tend to work backward, determining what the woman needs. I usually help her develop long-range plans that include nourishing herbal tonics," says Gould.

In Search of a Safe Stimulant

As is sometimes the case, just because an herbal stimulant is natural doesn't automatically mean that it's safe or desirable. A case in point: The most universally consumed herbal stimulant is caffeine, which occurs naturally in coffee beans and other plants. It can give you a temporary lift, but it won't cure an out-and-out energy drain. And it could upset your stomach or keep you awake when you need to sleep.

Then there are more powerful herbs like ephedra, or ma huang, sort of a natural amphetamine that's frequently touted as a not-very-secret ingredient in weight-loss formulas and even recreational drugs (like Herbal Ecstasy). Taking ephedra is a risky way to try to shore up flagging energy levels: It can cause insomnia and anxiety, and it may even aggravate high blood pressure. Several people who have taken large overdoses of ephedra-containing commercial products have died. And if you're tired because you're stressed out—as is often the case—the last thing you need is a powerful stimulant that jeopardizes your health.

No Quick Fixes

"Fatigue and energy drain are symptoms," says Patricia Howell, a professional member of the AHG and director of the Living with Herbs Institute in Atlanta. "We live in a culture that's very pill-oriented, but it's my job as an herbalist to offer a whole different system of healing. To treat people effectively, you have to alter things at a constitutional level, in terms of both lifestyle and body function."

So before you reach for a quick fix, herbal or otherwise, ask yourself a couple of questions, says Donald J. Brown, N.D., a naturopathic doctor in Seattle and author of *Herbal Prescriptions for Better Health*. How long have

Restorative Chinese Herbal Soup

An elaborate but effective elixir brewed with soup stock is a powerful tool to support yourself during periods of nasty stress, says Glenn Gurman, a licensed acupuncturist, professional member of the American Herbalists Guild, founder of the Holistic Health Care Clinic in Norwich, Vermont, and author of The Eight Treasures of Health.

"This slightly bittersweet mixture of Chinese and American herbs helps the body restore its energy reserves," says Gurman. "To add more nourishment and flavor to the soup, brew the herbs in chicken, beef, or vegetable broth instead of water. Use real broth rather than instant cubes. Begin taking the tonic the day after your period ends and take it for three weeks, then give your body a week off."

You need to take a break because, Gurman says, "this tonic helps build and support the blood, spleen, and kidneys, which helps strengthen the body. Just prior to and during a woman's menstrual period—her moon phase—herbal wisdom dictates that you let the body normalize itself. You begin taking tonic again when your period ends."

Gurman says that you can take the tonic for three cycles, and if you still feel fatigued, you should consult a qualified herbalist.

Do not eat dairy products, cold vegetables, or sprouts with this formula, Gurman says. Also, do not use this soup if you are pregnant or have high blood pressure, he adds.

"Very rarely, drinking these herbs can cause stomach upset, nausea, diarrhea, or, even more rarely, a skin rash," says Gurman. "If that occurs, discontinue using these herbs and consult a qualified health-care practitioner. "Be sure to eat well, reduce or eliminate caffeine, and drink green tea rather than coffee if you use caffeine," Gurman says. "Attend to gentle exercise, plenty of water, good sleep, and fresh air, and go out of your way to laugh."

If you generally feel warm more often than cool, add a little bit of peppermint or any other mint. If you generally feel cool more often than warm, add a little ginger and a little cinnamon.

The unusual herbs used in this recipe—he shou wu and dang shen (also known as codonopsis)—along with astragalus and chen pi (dried, aged orange peel) are available by mail order (see "Where to Buy Herbs and Herbal Products" on page 462).

Here's his recipe.

3	quarts water or chicken, beef, or vegetable broth
2	parts gotu kola
2	parts dried nettle
I	part American ginseng
3	parts he shou wu
2	parts dang shen
2	parts chen pi
I	part astragalus
¼	part dang gui

Combine the ingredients in a large glass or ceramic pot, then cover and simmer gently for a minimum of 25 minutes to an hour.

Drink a small teacup of the soup twice a day before breakfast and lunch, adding five drops of reishi mushroom tincture to each dose. Refrigerate the formula in the pot and bring to a simmer again each time you use it.

you been tired? Have you been under a lot of stress for a long time? Then get a checkup right away.

"I'm adamant about getting to the root of a person's fatigue by taking a thorough medical history and recommending a few standard medical tests to rule out thyroid problems, anemia, or other conditions common in women," says Dr. Brown.

The reasons for your fatigue will dictate which herbs may help. "If fatigue is stress-related, I may recommend tonic herbs, such as licorice, that help support adrenal function," Dr. Brown says. He may also select Korean ginseng or Siberian ginseng, two other herbs used for long-term adrenal support.

Gentle Pick-Me-Ups from Nature

If you're basically healthy and just want to restore your energy levels, herbalists offer the following suggestions.

Snare some ginseng. One of the oldest, most widely used remedies for boosting energy reserves is ginseng, says Dr. Brown. "My first choice in energy-boosting tonics for women of menstrual age is Siberian ginseng. Women nearing or past menopause can also use Korean ginseng. I recommend taking two to three grams of Siberian ginseng in capsule form or 100 to 200 milligrams of Korean ginseng in standardized extract capsules a day." To prevent irritability, avoid consuming caffeine and other stimulants while using ginseng.

Make a nourishing energy tea. "I treat fatigue with nourishing herbs," says Howell. "For busy women who don't have a lot of time to brew special teas every few hours, I often make a tincture (also called an extract)

that they can carry with them and use as needed. The exact formula depends on the women and their needs."

If you can spare the time, Howell recommends a nourishing tea made with equal parts of dried nettle, red clover, oatstraw, and red raspberry. Combine the dried herbs in a tea canister. Use 1 teaspoon per cup of water (follow the directions in "Teas and Infusions" on page 89). You can also combine equal parts of tinctures of these herbs rather than making the tea, Howell says.

According to Howell, this formula balances endocrine function and calms the adrenals. "Drinking a cup a day will make a significant difference in your energy level— and your health," she says.

Blast off with basil. "One of the best remedies I know for relieving mental fatigue is basil," says Howell. "I use the essential oil of basil in a diffuser all the time when I'm teaching, and I still have energy left at the end of the day. It relieves that feeling of exhaustion when your brain stops clicking, even though you're still awake and alert." (Diffusers are small devices that release essential oils into the air of a room. They are available in some health food stores and through mail order; see "Where to Buy Herbs and Herbal Products" on page 462.)

Make a minty mister. Add about 20 drops of essential oil of peppermint to a four-ounce spray mister filled with water. "When they need a mental energy boost, we have the students here at school close their eyes, then we pass around the mint mister and everyone gives themselves a gentle blast," says Brigitte Mars, a professional member of the AHG who teaches at the Rocky Mountain School of Botanical Medicine in Boulder, Colorado. Avoid spraying the mist into your eyes.

Low Sexual Desire

HERBAL LOVE POTIONS

*I*magine wanting your mate so badly your teeth ache. Your breasts tingle. You just can't wait. Imagine feeling that way—tonight.

"Take the phone off the hook, lock the door, put on some romantic music, and share an herbal aphrodisiac," says Margi Flint, a professional member of the American Herbalists Guild (AHG) from Marblehead, Massachusetts, who teaches herbal approaches to health at Tufts University School of Medicine in Boston. "Think about how you and your partner have a beautiful relationship. Then have some fun," adds Flint, who is also a practicing herbalist at Atlanti-Care Hospital in Lynn, Massachusetts.

Scents-uality Unleashed

Herbalists say that you can recapture that "swept away" feeling with the help of herbal potions, oils, and teas. But first, a brief reality check.

"Sometimes problems that have nothing to do with sex can get in the way of a great sex life," notes Flint. "If you're approaching menopause, you may have vaginal dryness, for example. Or you could have recurring vaginal infections. That can really put a damper on sexual relations. So can depression and anxiety." (For herbal remedies for these conditions, see "Menopause" on page 281, "Vaginal Problems" on page 367, "Anxiety" on page 428, and "Depression" on page 432.)

Sometimes, inhibited sexual desire, or lack of libido, is rooted in unresolved psychological issues that need attention. But if you've worked through all of the medical and psychological factors and still yearn for more sexual intimacy, herbalists say that botanicals can help. One caution, however: Libido-enhancing herbs are not recommended for pregnant women.

Breathe a sensual aroma. Set the stage for passion by scenting the bedroom (or any room) with a few potent droplets of sandalwood, rose, or amber essential oil (available in health food stores or through mail order; see "Where to Buy Herbs and Herbal Products" on page 462), suggests Aviva Romm, a certified professional midwife, herbalist, and professional member of the AHG who practices in Bloomfield Hills, Michigan, and is the author of *The Natural Pregnancy Book* and *Natural Healing for Babies and Children.*

"Sandalwood is a traditional aphrodisiac. It makes you feel very centered in your body, very aware of physical sensation," Romm says. "Rose and amber both have long associations with love and sensuality."

Here are three simple ways to subtly "perfume" the air with sensuality: add a few droplets of your chosen essential oil to a diffuser ring, an inexpensive aromatherapy device (available in health food stores or by mail) that sits over a light bulb and relies on the bulb's heat to release fragrance. Simpler still, just add a few drops of essential oil to a cup of warm water (the heat will re-lease the aroma) or place five drops of es-sential oil and ½ cup of water in an atomizer, then shake and spray into the air. Romm suggests.

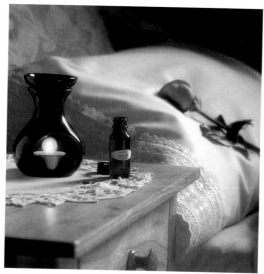

Scenting your bedroom with rose, sandalwood, or other sensual aromas creates a passionate atmosphere.

Take massage to new heights. The same essential oils, when added to massage oil, bring new sensual dimensions to a full-body massage before lovemaking, Romm says. "You need only a few drops of essential oil to scent a massage oil," she says. "For ex-ample, to an ounce of jojoba oil (available at health food stores), add a total of 8 or 9 drops of sandalwood, rose, or amber or a combina-tion of them." Massage each other from head to toe; concentrate first on relaxation by working on tense spots such as the upper back, then let your touch become slower, more caressing, even arousing. Include erogenous zones like the backs of the knees and the inner thighs.

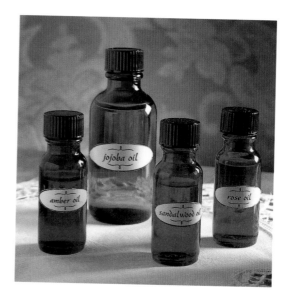

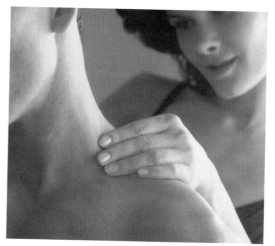

Added to massage oils and stroked on erogenous zones, ylang-ylang and other essential oils help enhance arousal during lovemaking.

Sip damiana tea. Damiana has a long reputation in folk medicine as an aphrodisiac. "It seems to lower anxiety and open the door to sensual expression," notes Flint.

To make a quick damiana tea, steep 1 tea-spoon of dried leaves in a cup of boiling water for 10 minutes. Or use damiana tincture (also called an extract). "If you want to take damiana (available at health food stores) regularly as a tonic, use 15 to 20 drops of tincture three times a day," Romm notes. "To boost passion for a sexual encounter, try 20 to 30 drops in ¼ cup of warm water, taken about an hour in advance."

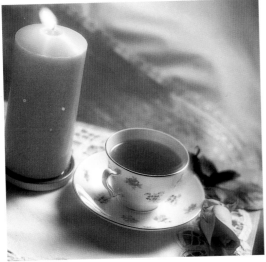

Damiana has a long-standing reputation in folk medicine as an aphrodisiac.

Sip a stimulating tea. Simple herbal stimulants that get blood circulation flowing enhance sexual feelings in women, Romm notes. "With more blood flow to the pelvis, you'll feel more aroused," she notes.

Her recipe? Simmer the following herbs in 2 cups of water for 20 minutes: 1 tablespoon of grated gingerroot, 7 to 10 cloves, 2 or 3 cinnamon sticks, 4 or 5 black peppercorns, and 7 to 10 cardamom pods. Strain and add small amounts of milk and honey to taste. "For a really nice touch, add ¼ teaspoon of vanilla. Vanilla comes from the orchid family, and orchids are incredibly sensual flowers."

Sip the tea after a meal and see what happens, Romm suggests. "It's especially good after a nice, spicy meal, which also gets the blood flowing," she notes. "What could be better than getting into a warm bath with beautiful candles, sipping this tea together, and seeing where it leads? But don't drink this tea before sleep. It really is stimulating."

To enhance passion, try tonic herbs. Herbalists who incorporate Traditional Chinese Medicine into their practices may suggest that women begin building passion with tonic herbs that strengthen and warm the kidneys and adrenal glands, Romm says. "Among Chinese practitioners, these organs are seen as the seat of sexuality."

Romm recommends taking daily doses of angelica, dang gui, ginseng, chasteberry, or saw palmetto as tinctures. "Use ½ teaspoon to 1 full teaspoon in ¼ cup of warm water twice a day," she says. "You can take them for three months or longer, since tonic herbs can be used safely for longer periods. But give your body a break. For one day a week, don't take the herb, then every three weeks, take a week off."

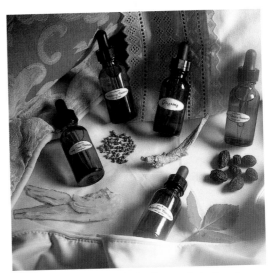

Taken regularly, tonic herbs can help boost passionate feelings.

12 Top Herbs for the Man You Love

If you're like many women, you find that you're the caretaker not only of your own health but of your partner's as well. And if you use herbs, you're probably eager to press them into service to help your partner stay healthy, too. Here's a short list of common herbs and suggestions for ways that they may help the man in your life prevent or relieve some common male health concerns, including some that can affect your relationship and even your sex life.

Herb	Botanical Name	Healing Potential
Garlic	*Allium sativum*	May help lower cholesterol (see "Heart Health" on page 245)
Ginseng	*Panax ginseng*	Can help relieve fatigue and boost energy (see "Energy Drain" on page 438)
Hawthorn	*Crataegus oxycantha*	Dilates coronary arteries to help strengthen the heart (see "Heart Health")
Lemon balm	*Melissa officinalis*	Helps regulate blood pressure (see "Heart Health")
Milk thistle	*Silybum marianum*	May protect the liver and regenerate damaged liver cells (see "Milk Thistle" on page 66)
Peppermint	*Mentha piperita*	Relieves indigestion (see "Digestive Problems" on page 203)
St.-John's-wort	*Hypericum perforatum*	Relieves mild to moderate depression (see "Depression" on page 432)
Saw palmetto	*Serenoa repens*	May increase sperm count and improve sperm motility; helps maintain health of the prostate gland and nourishes male sexual organs
Skullcap	*Scutellaria laterifolia*	Helps relieve anxiety and stress (see "Anxiety" on page 428 and "Stress" on page 451)
Tea tree oil	*Melaleuca* species	Relieves athlete's foot when applied to the skin (see "Athlete's Foot" on page 170)
White willow	*Salix alba*	Can help relieve muscle strain (see "Muscle Strains and Sprains" on page 313)
Yarrow	*Achillea millefolium*	Helps maintain health of male sexual organs and urinary tract (see "Yarrow" on page 80)

Add nourishing herbs. "Herbs that strengthen a woman's system in general will help with sexuality and passion," Romm notes. "Herbs such as nettle and red clover can be used for very long periods of time." Over time, Romm says a woman who uses these herbs may gain a feeling of well-being and emotional stability. She may also notice more vaginal lubrication. "You should start feeling results after about a month," she says.

Among her favorites for building and sustaining passion is ashwaganda (available through mail order), a kidney-nourishing botanical. "Add about $\frac{1}{2}$ teaspoon of ashwaganda powder to a cup of milk, bring it just to a boil, then sweeten with honey," she says. "You can drink this every day." Don't use this herb during pregnancy, however.

Or try shatavari. The Hindu name of his Indian herb (available through mail order) means "she who possesses 100 husbands," Romm says. "You could combine it with the ashwaganda in milk, using $\frac{1}{2}$ teaspoon to 1 full teaspoon of shatavari. Or mix that amount of shatavari with a little honey and eat it as a sweet paste."

Memory Problems and Poor Concentration

HERBS FOR SHARPER RECALL AND FOCUS

Don't be too quick to blame the aging process for forgetfulness and fuzzy thinking. More than likely, you can trace problems with recall and focus to stress, fatigue, or outright exhaustion, says Glenn Gurman, a licensed acupuncturist, professional member of the American Herbalists Guild (AHG), founder of the Holistic Health Care Clinic in Norwich, Vermont, and author of *The Eight Treasures of Health*.

"Stress acts like poison to the brain," says Dharma Singh Khalsa, M.D., director of the Alzheimer's Prevention Foundation in Tucson and author of *The Great Brain Longevity*. When stimulated by stress, the adrenal glands release cortisol, a powerful hormone that helps get you through sudden emergencies, such as swerving to avoid a child on a bike when you're driving your car (that's good). Over time, though, frequent or unrelenting stress can gradually kill or injure billions of brain cells (that's not good). If stress continues unchecked, it can eventually interfere with your ability to think, says Dr. Khalsa.

Besides stress, diet and lifestyle can influence how well you can concentrate and remember.

"When a woman comes to me complaining that she can't concentrate or that she's forgetful, the first thing I ask her to do is keep a food journal for a week," says Brigitte Mars, a professional member of the AHG who teaches at the Rocky Mountain School of Botanical Medicine in Boulder, Colorado. She also asks clients to bring any medications, nutritional supplements, or herbs that they may be taking. "Before I suggest that she put anything more into her body, I need to find out what's going on in her life. Is she a hairstylist, breathing in chemical fumes every day? Has she recently had her home repainted or recarpeted? Environmental toxins and pollutants may interfere with concentration and memory," says Mars.

Some women report that their thinking slows down when they hit menopause, says Donald J. Brown, N.D., a naturopathic doctor in Seattle and author of *Herbal Prescriptions for Better Health*.

Ginkgo and Other "Brain Herbs"

Once you've ruled out (and corrected) external factors that can blunt your thinking, herbalists say that you can try these herbal helpers.

Go for the ginkgo. "Ginkgo tops the list of herbs that help keep you mentally sharp," says Dr. Brown. "For one thing, it stimulates blood flow. Also, evidence suggests that ginkgo has the ability to boost brain function." Ginkgo contains a unique blend of terpene lactones that enable extracts of this herb to increase circulation to the brain and other

parts of the body. These substances also help protect nerve cells, says Dr. Brown. Take the recommended dose, which is usually 120 to 240 milligrams a day, divided into two daily doses, he says.

Choose the right ginkgo. Look for ginkgo tablets that are standardized to contain 24 percent ginkgo flavone glycosides and 6 percent terpene lactones, Dr. Brown suggests.

Rely on rosemary. "When my daughter was studying for her college chemistry final, I told her to dab some essential oil of rosemary in her hair," recalls Mars. "She also dabbed on the oil just before taking the test. Smelling the scent during the test reminded her of the material she'd studied, so she was able to remember what she'd learned. It helped tremendously." You could also place one to three drops of essential oil of rosemary on a cotton ball or tissue, tuck it in your sleeve, and inhale as needed for the same effect.

"Rosemary is one of the best essential oils to help memory," says Jane Buckle, R.N., an aromatherapist in Hunter, New York, and author of *Clinical Aromatherapy in Nursing*. "It can even be useful after stroke when speech has been impaired," she says. So those with only slightly impaired memory should also benefit.

Buckle recommends Aromavera, a particularly gentle essential oil of rosemary; it's less stimulating than other forms of rosemary oil. Just apply one to three drops on a tissue and inhale as needed. Never take it by mouth, however, as many essential oils are quite toxic, and never apply it undiluted to the skin, because the oils are so concentrated that they will cause irritation, Buckle warns. In addition, you should avoid using it after 6:00 P.M. because it can keep you awake, she says.

Bring on the basil. "The essential oil of basil (available at health food stores) makes a pretty good memory stimulant," says Buckle. "Be sure to choose an essential oil made from European rather than Asian basil," she says. If the label says "exotic," it's the wrong kind. Your supplier should know if the oil is European or Asian, so be sure to ask, she suggests. Asian basil essential oil can have nerve-damaging effects if used for prolonged periods of time, but inhaling one to three drops of European basil essential oil when needed is perfectly safe, Buckle notes. (For specific advice about how to use essential oils, see "Aromatherapy" on page 134.)

Blend a memory tincture. "I make up this formula and keep it in the classroom when my students are taking exams," says Kathleen Gould, a professional member of the AHG and director of the Herb Corner, an herbal education center in Indialantic, Florida. Use dried or fresh herbs, if available. Blend equal parts of gotu kola, ginkgo, peppermint, and rosemary. Tincture them in vodka for a couple of weeks (longer is better, Gould notes). Then take ½ teaspoon of the tincture, diluted in a small amount (⅛ cup) of water, twice a day, she suggests. (For complete instructions on preparing a tincture, see "Tinctures" on page 92.)

Try a peach- or apricot-flavored tincture. "I sometimes like to tincture herbs in either peach or apricot brandy," says Gould. "It makes a better-tasting formula, which is helpful when herbs are bitter or people don't care for their flavor," she adds.

Midafternoon Slump

GET READY FOR HERBAL PICK-ME-UPS

Call it the Black Hole of your day. Between 1:00 and 5:00 P.M., energy fades like a battery on a cell phone that's checked voice mail a few too many times. Or you hit a wall of unproductiveness smack-dab in the middle of a busy day. Your brain and body are functioning on minimum power.

You won't find midafternoon slump in any medical text. But millions of women (and men) vouch for its existence. Mental focus fades. Blood sugar levels plummet. Nerves fray at the edges. And your adrenal glands struggle to keep up with unflagging demands on your brain and body.

Reaching for coffee or a candy bar isn't the answer, says Gayle Eversole, R.N., Ph.D., a nurse practitioner, medical herbalist, and professional member of the American Herbalists Guild (AHG) in Everett, Washington. "Coffee or junk food may restore your zip, but in a way that can be harmful. Blood sugar levels and energy levels rise, then drop. And neither coffee nor candy helps the underlying causes of low energy."

Sagging blood sugar levels are just one

possible cause of midafternoon slump. Stress pileups can leach energy from every cell. So can sitting transfixed at a computer screen for hours or trying to function in the heat.

When energy sags between lunch and dinner, herbs may help restore your mental focus, balance plummeting blood sugar levels, nourish frazzled nerves, and even support the overworked glands that pump out stress hormones and regulate energy levels, herbalists say.

An Herbal Rescue Plan

Assuming that your doctor has ruled out an underlying medical cause and you're getting enough rest, herbalists suggest these herbal pick-me-ups for midday slump.

Take a tea break. Dragging your tail? Say no to coffee and yes to an afternoon cup of mint tea, suggests Margi Flint, a professional member of the AHG from Marblehead, Massachusetts, who teaches herbal approaches to health at Tufts University School of Medicine in Boston and is a practicing herbalist at AtlantiCare Hospital in Lynn, Massachusetts.

"Peppermint, spearmint, or lemon balm, which is also in the mint family, will help revive your energy," says Flint. Lemon balm also has the power to calm and soothe, which makes it perfect for times when you feel tired yet stressed, she adds. Use 1 teaspoon of your chosen herb per cup of boiling water. Steep for 5 to 15 minutes, covered. Or you can combine herbs and use 1 teaspoon of the mix per cup. (Peppermint and lemon balm are especially tasty together.)

Customize your blend. Go beyond the mint family and personalize your tea-time blend by adding other herbs to your basic brew that soothe frazzled nerves, nourish your body, and calm cranky feelings, Flint suggests. For an added lift, serve your special tea in a pretty mug. Flint recommends the following herbs.

Nettle, which adds a deep flavor and delivers extra calcium and trace minerals to your body.

Rose hips, for a pleasantly tart taste and added vitamin C.

Oatstraw, for a mild, sweet flavor and soothing action. "Oatstraw calms the little fibers on nerve endings that get frazzled when you're on edge," Flint says.

Chamomile or linden, both time-honored nerve soothers. Chamomile imparts a pleasant flowery, lemony flavor.

Gotu kola, to ease the emotional irritation that can come with menopause.

Prepare your special blend by mixing equal parts of your chosen dried herbs in a jar. When you're ready for a nice cup of tea, scoop the blend into a tea ball or tea strainer, place it in your cup, and add boiling water. Use 1 teaspoon of tea mix per cup of boiling water and steep for about 15 minutes. If you find you prefer a stronger flavor, increase the amount of tea per cup.

Fill up your Thermos. If you're tired every afternoon, make a Thermos of your tea blend in advance (at home or first thing in the morning when you get to work) and sip it slowly throughout the day, suggests Flint. "This tea may help treat the underlying problem and protect your nervous system all day long," she says.

Sweeten with stevia. If you have reason to believe that roller-coaster blood sugar levels are responsible for afternoon lethargy (if having a candy bar gives you an energy boost, for example, but leaves you tired again quickly), add a tiny pinch of stevia to the tea blend, Flint suggests. "Stevia is sweet without

Gotu Kola: An Herbal Energizer

In ancient China, gotu kola was a principal ingredient in an infamous elixir called *Fo Ti Tieng*, a brew that had a dubious "Fountain of Youth" reputation.

What isn't dubious is this: Gotu kola, which has been called an apothecary shop in one herb, offers impressive benefits. For one thing, it is believed to accelerate the healing process. In tests in which gotu kola extract was applied to 20 people with slow-healing wounds, 64 percent of the wounds healed completely and another 16 percent improved considerably.

In India, where it grows widely, gotu kola is a traditional remedy for skin problems. People there also take it to create inner peace before practicing yoga or meditating. In the West, herbalists sometimes use gotu kola in modern elixirs to boost memory, ease anxiety, increase energy, and protect against stress. And in fact, in the laboratory, the herb appears to have the ability to relieve stress and fatigue, increase general mental ability, and improve memory. It is available at health food stores in the form of teas, tinctures, and capsules.

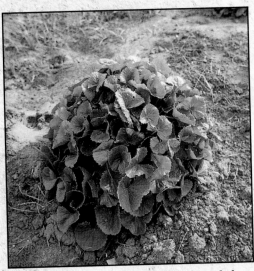

Used widely in India and China, gotu kola acts like a vitamin for the brain.

containing sugar," she says. "And it can help balance blood sugar levels so that you feel more consistent energy." You can buy boxes of stevia, which is known as "the sweet herb of Paraguay," at health food stores.

Dip into dandelion. Dandelion-root tea also balances blood sugar and helps support liver function, says Dr. Eversole. "Sluggishness can be caused by too many snack foods and too much coffee. When you eat and drink that way, blood sugar plummets, and your liver might need help clearing those residues from the body. Dandelion root is a big help." Boil 1 heaping teaspoon of dried dandelion root in 1½ cups of water for 15 to 20 minutes. "Dried roots need to be boiled to extract the full medicinal properties of the herb," she says.

Pair herbs with protein. Herbs aren't the only way to deal with blood sugar–related energy dips. Diet counts, too. Dr. Eversole and other herbalists suggest eating or drinking a protein-rich snack at mid-morning or midafternoon. Protein can give you an energy boost, balance blood sugar levels, and support the thyroid gland, which regulates energy levels in the body, Dr. Eversole notes.

Try whole-wheat crackers with a dab of peanut butter or a cup of plain yogurt mixed with fresh fruit, or sip Dr. Eversole's quick favorite. "I like organic or sodium-free tomato or vegetable juice with a tablespoon or two of protein-rich nutritional yeast mixed into it," she says. You can start with 1 teaspoon a day and gradually build up to more yeast from there, she adds. Two tablespoons of nutritional yeast (available at health food stores) supplies six grams of protein—more than a slice of turkey breast lunch meat.

Brew up some ginseng. Herbs like ginseng are adrenal tonics—that is, they buffer the negative effects of stress on your adrenal glands. Located just above the kidneys, your adrenal glands produce hormones that regulate vital body functions. Continuous stress can exhaust and deplete these important glands and even cause them to shrink. Without properly functioning adrenal glands, your body cannot react to stress in a healthy way.

"If your energy levels are strong in the morning but flag in the afternoon, then supporting your adrenal glands with the right herbs can help in the long run," says Christopher Hobbs, a fourth-generation herbalist who practices in Santa Cruz, California, professional member of the AHG, and author of *Stress and Natural Healing*.

According to Hobbs, Siberian and Korean ginseng are good adrenal tonics. So are reishi—a red mushroom that's gained a place of honor in herbal medicine for its calming and strengthening qualities—and rehmannia, a root used in Traditional Chinese Medicine that also supports the adrenal glands. "These herbs are available as powdered extracts or in capsule form, which may be a simpler way to take them on a long-term basis. Take the powdered extract, following package directions, two or three times a day, or take three capsules three times a day," Hobbs says. "Over three months, you should feel much steadier, calmer energy."

Nix computer tension. Hours of typing and staring at a computer screen can build tension in your neck, leading to an afternoon drop in energy, Flint says. Revive your taut, tired muscles with a mist concocted from isopropyl rubbing alcohol or vodka and some dried sage, she suggests.

Combine 1 pint of rubbing alcohol or vodka with a handful of sage in a quart glass jar with a tight-fitting lid. "Let it steep for two weeks and shake it every day," she says. "Strain and discard the herb, then transfer the herb-alcohol mixture to a clean spray bottle and mist your neck and arms when you need it. (Avoid contact with your eyes.) It just melts away muscle tension. You can take this into the restroom, take off your blouse, and mist your upper arms and upper back as well."

Spritz yourself with an essential oil mist. When you feel wilted by high heat and beating sun in summer, perk up with a cooling mist, says Flint.

Add 30 drops each of essential oils of birch, frankincense, and sandalwood to a bottle of isopropyl rubbing alcohol or vodka Shake well, then transfer the mixture to a spray bottle. "When you're feeling hot, sticky, and exhausted by the heat, spray this on your arms, your legs, or your neck," she suggests. "The essential oils will make you feel revived and calm. The alcohol takes away the grimy feeling if you've been sweating." (Avoid contact with your eyes.)

You could substitute essential oils of lavender, rose, or rosemary, Flint adds. "They're also uplifting and stimulating."

Stress

Stress is a word that gets passed around these days as freely as a fruitcake in late December. And it's just about as unwelcome (not to mention as unavoidable) as any citron-studded holiday loaf.

But what exactly is this ubiquitous force that seems to shadow so many women's lives? Simply put, stress is any pressure that disturbs our status quo, whether it's internal (a cold or joint pain), external (loud noise or crowds), or emotional (guilt or worry). How your body reacts to stress can also be stressful: If you overreact or react inappropriately, your health is jeopardized.

Herbalists say that it's unrealistic to assume that herbs, on their own, can erase the stress-caused angst that comes from wearing way too many hats for your own good. But herbal medicine does help—in a significant way, say herbalists—when you make it part of a holistic approach for managing stress. In other words, making a cup of herbal tea won't magically wipe out stress. You also need to pay attention to what you eat, how you spend your time, how much time you take for leisure, and how you cultivate your spiritual well-being.

Herbs for Damage Control

Nature has blessed us with two different types of herbs—adaptogens and nervines—to help the body deal with stress, says David Hoffman, a founding and professional member of the American Herbalists Guild (AHG), a fellow of Britain's National Institute of Medical Herbalists, assistant professor of integral health studies at the California Institute of Integral Studies in Santa Rosa, and author of *Herbs to Relieve Stress*.

Simply put, an adaptogen helps the body adapt to the external pressures that can lead to illness. "Adaptogenic herbs help the body deal with stress by supporting the adrenal glands, and that seems to increase the body's ability to resist stress-related damage," says Hoffman.

The concept of adaptogenic herbs is a legacy of Eastern medical traditions, especially Traditional Chinese Medicine, which emphasizes prevention of disease, says Hoffman. As such, adaptogenic herbs aren't antidotes to stress, to be swilled after a confrontation with a teenager over curfews. Rather, they are used as tonics, over time, to help the body normalize itself, he says. "Because adaptogenic herbs work on the adrenal glands and don't alter brain chemistry, there's little chance of dependency."

Among the herbs that Hoffman feels are most helpful when it comes to dealing with stress are familiar herbs like ginseng and Siberian ginseng as well as more exotic herbs such as ashwaganda, shiitake, and schisandra.

Press ginseng into service. Of the adaptogens mentioned, Hoffman recommends Siberian ginseng most highly. He says that the usual dose is $\frac{1}{2}$ to $\frac{3}{4}$ teaspoon of tincture (also called an extract) three times a day. He

Too Stressed for Sex?
Damiana Might Help

Judging by one of its Latin names, *Turnera aphrodisiaca*, you can pretty much guess what kind of problem the herb damiana is used for. Grown in Mexico and the Southwest, the herb has a reputation for upping a woman's sexual interest (and as a bonus, perhaps inducing erotic dreams) when sipped at bedtime.

Damiana's reputation as a love potion has yet to be laboratory-tested. It contains a bitter substance called damianin, but no one knows what it does, if anything. So it may not be a true aphrodisiac. Maybe it simply piques erotic urges.

More often, damiana is used for depression and anxiety, which together can dampen sexual desire, says David Hoffman, a founding and professional member of the American Herbalists Guild, a fellow of Britain's National Institute of Medical Herbalists, assistant professor of integral health studies at the California Institute of Integral Studies in Santa Rosa, and author of *Herbs to Relieve Stress*. Damiana is considered safe, although it may have a laxative effect. It's usually taken three times a day as an infusion or a tincture.

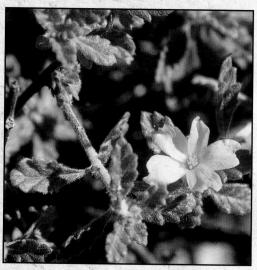

Damiana may enhance sexual desire and trigger erotic dreams.

recommends taking the herb daily for six weeks, followed by a two-week break. You can repeat the regimen for as long as necessary, he says.

Relax with Nerve Tonics

The second category of herbs that help us cope with stress are appropriately called nervines. They affect the nervous system in one of three ways, says Hoffman. Nervines can either relax you, stimulate you, or nourish damaged nerves. The nervines that Hoffman considers most useful for dealing with stress range from mildly relaxing herbs (notably lemon balm, chamomile, and lavender) to somewhat stronger herbs (such as damiana, skullcap, and St.-John's-wort) to highly relaxing herbs (such as valerian, passionflower, hops, and California poppy).

Stress can and does affect various systems of the body—the heart, lungs, digestive system, reproductive system, muscles, and skin—as well as the nerves. And it can wreak havoc with your sex life. So the herb of choice partly depends on what symptoms stress triggers for you. Nevertheless, the following formulas, designed to cover all the bases, may go a long way toward helping to buffer the effects of stress.

Try this gentle anti-stress combo. For dealing with basic stress, Hoffman suggests this gentle herbal combination, made from herbal tinctures. The formula contains 2 parts skullcap, 2 parts valerian, and 1 part oats. Take one teaspoon of the tincture in a little water anytime you feel as if stress is getting the best of you, he recommends.

Blend a batch of super-stress tincture. If you find yourself dealing with a seriously stressful situation that causes indigestion and palpitations, try a tincture blend of 2 parts each of skullcap and valerian plus 1 part each of motherwort, chamomile, and mugwort, suggests Hoffman.

The motherwort helps you relax and calms palpitations, and the chamomile aids digestion, notes Hoffman. Take a teaspoon of tincture as needed, he recommends.

Soothing Stress with Aromatherapy

Imagine slipping into a warm bath spiked with essential oil of lavender. Or being slowly and gently massaged with an aromatic blend of the essential oils of chamomile and lemongrass. Just thinking about the scents can help take the edge off a trying day.

"Stress causes many different physical and mental symptoms, and in my experience, these symptoms can usually be relieved with the right essential oil," says Jane Buckle,

R.N., an aromatherapist in Hunter, New York, and author of *Clinical Aromatherapy in Nursing*.

The best anti-stress essential oils are those high in chemical components called esters and aldehydes, says Buckle. Think of essential oils as very complicated chemical storehouses, each containing between 100 and 400 chemicals. "Those who study or use herbs have noted that when an essential oil contains a large proportion of esters or aldehydes, it will have calming, soothing properties," says Buckle. "Oils high in alcohols, on the other hand, tend to be more stimulating."

Clary sage, lavender, marjoram, and Roman chamomile are high in esters. Aldehydes are found in lemongrass, lemon balm, and eucalyptus. (For more details on how to reap the anti-stress benefits of essential oils, see "Aromatherapy" on page 134.)

Stress-Relief Tips from the East

"In dealing with prolonged stress, the key issue is resiliency," says Glenn Gurman, a licensed acupuncturist, professional member of the AHG, founder of the Holistic Health Care Clinic in Norwich, Vermont, and author of *The Eight Treasures of Health*. "We have to treat the whole woman over the long haul rather than take a short-term, cookbook approach that 'this herb recipe cures stress.'"

Traditional Chinese Medicine teaches that, in order to strengthen your long-term resiliency against stress, you need to consider the relationship of three organs: the kidneys, the spleen, and the liver.

"In Chinese medicine, the kidneys are thought to be a storehouse of energy, not unlike the battery in your car," says Gurman. "Excesses like smoking, drinking, staying up too late, overusing sexual energy, and other emotional challenges overtax the kidneys' reserves of energy. Traditional Chinese healers call the kidneys the gate of life and the root of health,. So to nurture the root of health, healers use herbs that support the kidneys," says Gurman.

The first steps in any program to help your body deal with stress are to pay attention to your diet and to add activities like tai chi or yoga that help reduce stress, says Gurman. "Using herbs without supporting your body—and your mind—is a shallow path," he says.

Eat meat, gingerly. "The Taoists believe that small quantities of red meat, combined with fresh ginger, help counteract blood deficiencies," says Gurman. (Taoism is a Chinese religion that focuses on harmony.) "So many delicious oriental meals are enhanced by ginger," Gurman adds.

To add ginger to food, simply grate, slice, or chop 3 to 7 tablespoons of fresh ginger. Then add other ingredients, such as vegetables and small amounts of meat, and steam or stir-fry them.

Make yourself a tonic. To help the body resist the ravages of stress, Gurman recommends a bittersweet, earthy-tasting, nurturing tonic. It's meant to be taken for the week before and the two weeks right after your period every month, for about three or four months. Stop taking the tonic if you feel a cold or flu coming on, says Gurman. "Otherwise, it will drive the cold or flu deeper into your system," he adds.

In this formula, dang shen, or codonopsis, and bai zhu, or atractylodes, are Chinese herbs; chen pi is dried, aged orange peel (for purchasing sources, see "Where to Buy Herbs and Herbal Products" on page 462).

2	quarts water
1	ounce dried nettle
1	tablespoon dried yellow dock root
4 or 5	pieces (5 inches long) dang shen
4	slices bai zhu
½	teaspoon chen pi
1	small, thin sliver dang gui root

If you generally feel warm more often than cool, add a little bit of peppermint or any other mint. If you generally feel cool more often than warm, add a little ginger and a little cinnamon.

Place the herbs and water in a glass or ceramic pot and simmer, covered, without boiling them, for a minimum of 25 minutes. Take one cup with breakfast and another with lunch. Refrigerate the formula in the pot and bring it to a simmer again each time you use it; there should be enough for about a week. Do not eat dairy products, cold vegetables, or sprouts with this formula, Gurman says, and do not use this tonic while pregnant.

Sip an anti-stress tincture. "When you're facing an acute period of stress, when everything's hit the wall but you still have to deal with it, try this nervine tincture," Gurman says. "You should feel its calming effects within two days. If you feel no positive effect after a couple of weeks, consult an herbalist or a qualified health-care practitioner." (The Chinese herbs used in the following formula are available by mail order.)

½	ounce black haw bark
1	ounce chamomile
⅛	ounce dried or fresh gingerroot
1	ounce gotu kola
½	ounce lemon balm

1 ounce hops
½ ounce skullcap
¼ ounce gou qi zi
8–10 da zao (Chinese jujube dates)
⅛ ounce suan zao ren
⅛ ounce zhi zi
Vodka

Combine the herbs in a ½-gallon canning jar and fill it with enough vodka to cover the herbs by 2 inches. Place it in a warm, dark place for at least two weeks. The longer you let the mixture steep, the stronger it gets. It will last for a few years, Gurman says. Strain enough to fill a tincture bottle and use as needed for short episodes of intense stress, up to four dropperfuls four times a day in a little hot water, says Gurman. Alternately, you could use a few drops on the tongue as needed. Don't use this tincture while pregnant or before operating heavy machinery, he says.

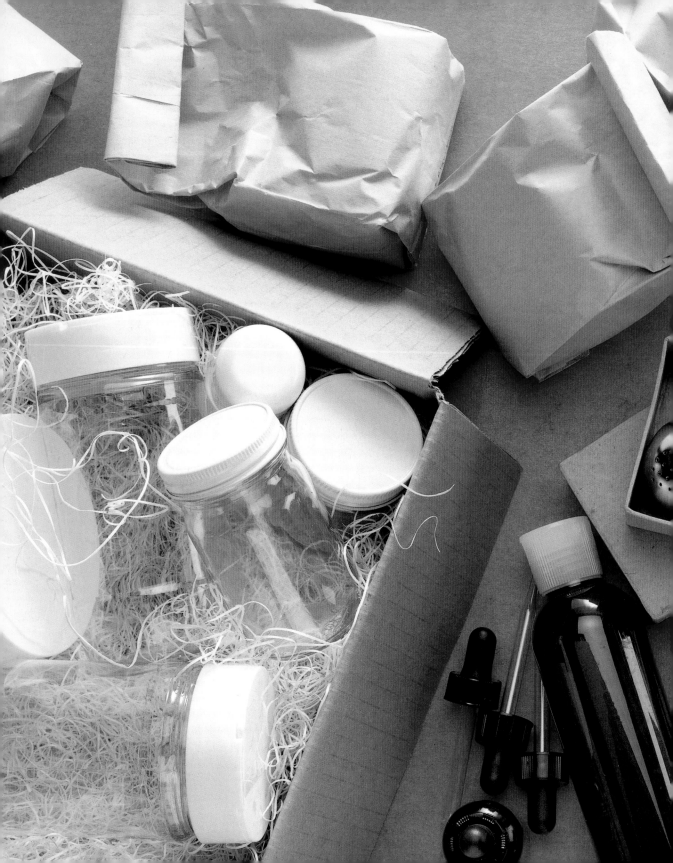

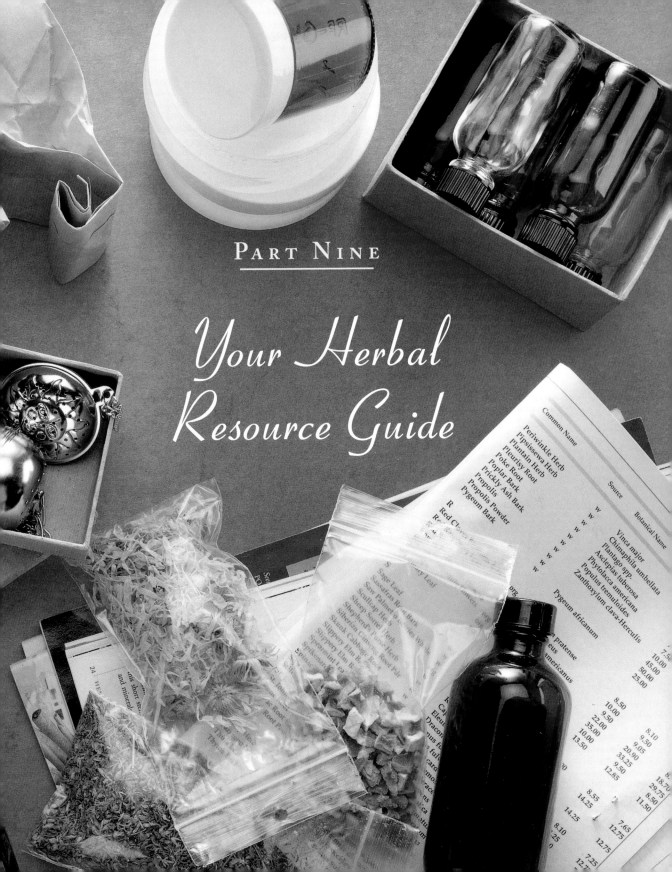

PART NINE

Your Herbal Resource Guide

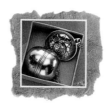

Botanical Names
of the Healing Herbs

A

Agrimony: *Agrimonia eupatoria*
Alfalfa: *Medicago sativa*
Allspice: *Pimenta dioica*
Aloe: *Aloe barbadensis*
American ginseng: *Panax quinquefolium*
Angelica: *Angelica archangelica*
Aniseed: *Pimpinella anisum*
Arbor vitae: *Thuja occidentalis*
Arnica: *Arnica montana*
Artichoke: *Cynara scolymus*
Ashwaganda: *Withania somnifera*
Astragalus: *Astragalus membranaceous*

B

Balsam: *Abies balsamea*
Barberry: *Berberis vulgaris*
Basil: *Ocimum basilicum*
Bay: *Laurus nobilis*
Bee balm: *Monarda didyma*
Beet leaf: *Beta vulgaris*
Benzoin: *Styrax benzoin*

Bergamot: *Citrus bergamotia*
Beth root: *Trillium erectum*
Betony: *Stachys officinalis*
Bilberry: *Vaccinium myrtillus*
Birch: *Betula* spp.
Blackberry root: *Rubus occidentalis*
Black cohosh: *Cimicifuga racemosa*
Black haw: *Viburnum prunifolium*
Black horehound: *Ballota nigra*
Black pepper: *Piper nigrum*
Bladderwrack: *Fucus vesiculosus*
Blessed thistle: *Cnicus benedictus*
Bloodroot: *Sanguinaria canadensis*
Blue cohosh: *Caulophyllum thalictroides*
Boneset: *Eupatorium perfoliatum*
Borage: *Borago officinalis*
Buchu: *Barosma crenulata*
Buckwheat: *Fagopyrum occulentum*
Bupleurum: *Bupleurum* spp.
Burdock: *Arctium lappa*
Butcher's broom: *Ruscus aculeatus*
Butternut: *Juglans cinerea*

C

Calendula: *Calendula officinalis*
California poppy: *Eschscholzia californica*
Camphor: *Cinnamonum camphora*
Caraway: *Carum carvi*
Cardamom: *Elettaria cardamomum*
Carrot: *Daucas carota*
Cascara sagrada: *Rhamnus purshianus*
Castor oil: *Ricinus communis*
Catnip: *Nepeta cataria*
Cayenne: *Capsicum annuum; C. frutescens*
Cedarwood: *Cedrus atlantica*
Centaury: *Erythraea centaurium*
Cerato: *Ceratostigma willmottianna*
Chamomile: *Matricaria recutita*
Chasteberry: *Vitex agnus-castus*
Chickweed: *Stellaria media*
Chicory: *Cichorium intybus*
Chinese skullcap: *Scutellaria baicalensis*
Cinnamon: *Cinnamomum zeylanicum*
Citronella: *Cymbopogon nardu*
Clary sage: *Salvia sclarea*
Cleavers: *Galium aparine*
Clematis: *Clematis vitalba*
Clove: *Syzygium aromaticum*
Coffee: *Coffea arabica*
Coltsfoot: *Tussilago farfara*
Comfrey: *Symphytum officinale*
Coriander: *Coriandrum sativum*
Cornsilk: *Zea mays*
Couch grass: *Agropyron repens*
Cramp bark: *Viburnum opulus*
Cranberry: *Vaccinium macrocarpon*
Cucumber: *Cucumis sativus*
Cumin: *Cuminum cyminum*
Cypress: *Cupressus sempervirens*

D

Damiana: *Turnera diffusa; T. aphrodisiaca*
Dandelion: *Taraxacum officinale*
Dang gui: *Angelica sinensis*
Dang shen: *Codonopsis pilosula; C. tangshen*

Dill: *Anethum graveolens*
Dwarf pine: *Pinus mugo*

E

Echinacea: *Echinacea angustifolia; E. purpurea*
Elderberry: *Sambucus canadensis; S. nigra*
Elecampane: *Inula helenium*
Ephedra: *Ephedra sinica*
Eucalyptus: *Eucalyptus globulus*
Evening primrose: *Oenothera biennis*
Eyebright: *Euphrasia officinalis*

F

False unicorn root: *Chamaelirium luteum*
Fennel: *Foeniculum vulgare*
Fenugreek: *Trigonella foenum-graecum*
Feverfew: *Chrysanthemum parthenium;
    Tanacetum parthenium*
Figwort: *Scrophularia marilandica*
Flax: *Linum usitatissimum*
Foxglove: *Digitalis purpurea*
Frankincense: *Boswellia carteri*

G

Garlic: *Allium sativum*
Gentian: *Gentiana lutea*
Geranium: *Geranium maculatum*
Germander: *Teucrium chamaedrys*
Ginger: *Zingiber officinale*
Ginkgo: *Ginkgo biloba*
Ginseng: *See* American ginseng; Korean
    ginseng; Siberian ginseng
Goat's rue: *Galega officinalis*
Goldenrod: *Solidago virgaurea*
Goldenseal: *Hydrastis canadensis*
Gotu kola: *Centella asiatica*
Gou qi zi: *Lycium chinensis*
Grindelia: *Grindelia robusta*
Guggul: *Commiphora mukul*

H

Hawthorn: *Crataegus oxycantha; C. laevigata;
    C. monogyna*

Helichrysum: *Helichrysum bracteatum*
Heliotrope: *Heliotropium arborescens*
Helonias: *Chamaelirium luteum*
He shou wu: *Polygonum multiflorum*
Hibiscus: *Hibiscus sabdariffa*
Hops: *Humulus lupulus*
Horehound: *Marrubium vulgare*
Horse chestnut: *Aesculus hippocastanum*
Horseradish: *Armoracia rusticana*
Horsetail: *Equisetum* spp.
Hyssop: *Hyssopus officinalis*

I

Impatiens: *Impatiens glandulifera*

J

Jamaican dogwood: *Piscidia erythrina*
Jasmine: *Jasminum officinale*
Jewelweed: *Impatiens capensis*
Juniper: *Juniper* spp.

K

Kava-kava: *Piper methysticum*
Korean ginseng: *Panax ginseng*

L

Lady's-mantle: *Alchemilla vulgaris*
Lavender: *Lavandula officinalis*; *L. angusti-folia*; *L. vera*
Lemon: *Citrus limon*
Lemon balm: *Melissa officinalis*
Lemongrass: *Cymbopogon citratus*
Lemon verbena: *Aloysia triphylla*
Licorice: *Glycyrrhiza glabra*
Lime: *Citrus aurantiifolia*
Linden flower: *Tilia* × *europaea*
Lovage: *Levisticum officinale*

M

Maitake: *Grifola frondosa*
Marjoram: *Origanum majorana*
Marshmallow: *Althaea officinalis*

Meadowsweet: *Filpendula* spp.
Menthol: *Mentha* × *piperita*
Milk thistle: *Silybum marianum*
Mimulus: *Mimulus guttatus*
Morning glory: *Ipomoea nil*; *I. pupurea*;
    I. tricolor
Motherwort: *Leonurus cardiaca*
Mugwort: *Artemisia vulgaris*
Mullein: *Verbascum thapsus*
Myrrh: *Commiphora myrrha*
Myrtle: *Cyrilla racemiflora*

N

Neroli: *Citrus aurantium*
Nettle: *Urtica dioica*
Nutmeg: *Myristica fragrans*

O

Oak: *Quercus* spp.
Oatstraw: *Avena sativa*
Onion: *Allium cepa*
Oregano: *Origanum heracleoticum*
Oregon grape root: *Mahonia aquifolium*
Osha: *Ligusticum potreri*

P

Parsley: *Petroselinum crispum*
Partridgeberry: *Mitchella repens*
Passionflower: *Passiflora incarnata*
Patchouli: *Pogostemon cablin*
Pau d'arco: *Tabebuia impetiginosa*
Pennyroyal: *Mentha pulegium*; *Hedeoma pulegioides*
Peppermint: *Mentha piperita*
Plantain: *Plantago lanceolata*; *P. major*;
    P. media
Pleurisy root: *Asclepias tuberosa*
Poke: *Phytolacca americana*
Poplar: *Populus tremuloides*
Potentilla: *Potentilla canadensis*
Prickly ash: *Zanthoxylum americanum*
Psyllium: *Plantago ovata*

Q
Queen Anne's lace: *Daucus carota*

R
Red clover: *Trifolium pratense*
Red mandarin: *Citrus reticulata*
Red raspberry: *Rubus idaeus*
Rehmannia: *Rehmannia glutinosa*
Reishi: *Ganoderma lucidum*
Rhubarb: *Rheum officinale*
Rockrose: *Helianthemum nummularium;
    H. canadense*
Roman chamomile: *Anthemis nobilis*
Rose: *Rosa* spp.
Rose geranium: *Pelargonium graveolens*
Rose hips: *Rosa canina*
Rosemary: *Rosmarinus officinalis*
Rosewood: *Tipuana tipu*

S
Sage: *Salvia officinalis*
St.-John's-wort: *Hypericum perforatum*
Sandalwood: *Santalum album*
San qi ginseng: *Panax notoginseng*
Sarsaparilla: *Smilax orata*
Sassafras: *Sassafras albidum*
Savory: *Satureja* spp.
Saw palmetto: *Serenoa repens*
Schisandra: *Schisandra chinensis*
Scleranthus: *Scleranthus annuus*
Senna: *Cassia senna*
Sesame: *Sesamum indicum*
Shatavari: *Asparagus racemosus*
Shepherd's purse: *Capsella bursa-pastoris*
Shiitake: *Lentines edodes*
Siberian ginseng: *Eleutherococcus
    senticosus*
Skullcap: *Scutellaria laterifolia*
Slippery elm: *Ulmus fulva*
Spearmint: *Mentha spicata*
Spikenard: *Arialia racemosa*
Staphisagria: *Delphinium staphisagria*

Stevia: *Stevia rebaudiana*
Strawberry: *Fragaria vesca*
Suan zao ren: *Ziziphus spinosa*

T
Tea: *Camellia sinensis*
Tea tree: *Melaleuca quinquenervia*
Thyme: *Thymus vulgaris*
True unicorn root: *Aletris farinosa*
Turmeric: *Curcuma domestica*

U
Usnea: *Usnea barbata*
Uva-ursi: *Arctostaphylos uva-ursi*

V
Valerian: *Valeriana officinalis*
Vanilla: *Vanilla planifolia*
Vervain: *Verbena officinalis*
Violet: *Viola adunca*

W
Water lily: *Nymphaea odorata*
Water violet: *Hottonia palustris*
White grapefruit: *Citrus × paradisi*
White peony: *Paeonia lactiflora*
White pine: *Pinus stroba*
White willow bark: *Salix alba*
Wild indigo: *Baptisia tinctoria*
Wild yam: *Discorea villosa*
Wintergreen: *Gaultheria procumbens*
Witch hazel: *Hamamelis virginiana*

Y
Yarrow: *Achillea millefolium*
Yellow dock: *Rumex crispus*
Yerba santa: *Eriodictyon californicum*
Ylang-ylang: *Cananga odorata*

Z
Zhi zi: *Gardenia jasminoides*

Where to Buy Herbs and Herbal Products

You may find all the herbs and herbal products you need in your local health food store, garden center, or aromatherapy shop. These days, herbs are even crowding the shelves of supermarkets, drugstores, and large discount chain stores. Still, there may be times when you cannot find exactly what you need. A product is out of stock. An unusual herb isn't available. A raw ingredient for an infused oil or special shampoo cannot be found.

Luckily, there is a wealth of mail-order suppliers that carry everything from bulk herbs (including Chinese and Ayurvedic herbs) to live roots for planting and exotic essential oils, from jars for holding your home-made herbal products to premade herbal formulas. This resource guide represents just a sampling of the many companies that carry herbal products and supplies for growing herbs and making your own botanical remedies.

The fact that a company is listed does not imply that we endorse it. Also, this list is not meant to be all-inclusive: If a company has been omitted, that doesn't mean it's not reputable. Rather, this directory is provided as a convenience to point you in the right direction and give you an idea of the types of products each can offer.

To request catalogs, write to the addresses below or call directory assistance for phone numbers. (Some companies may charge a small fee for their catalogs.) Many companies also have Web sites on the Internet. One note: The descriptions included here are just an overview; many of these companies carry additional items.

Abundant Life Seed Foundation
P. O. Box 772
Port Townsend, WA 98368
Seeds for medicinal and culinary herbs.

Aroma Vera
5901 Rodeo Road
Los Angeles, CA 90016-4312
Essential oils; aromatherapy diffusers, candles, and mists; jewelry; hair- and skin-care products; and spa products.

Avena Botanicals
219 Mill Street
Rockport, ME 04856
Tinctures (extracts), infused oils, bulk herbs, and books.

Ayurveda Holistic Center
82-A Bayville Avenue
Bayville, NY 11709
Ayurvedic dried herbs and herbal blends, including several women's herbal-blend caplets.

Barney's Ginseng Patch
Rt. 2, Box 43HGM
Montgomery City, MO 63361
Ginseng and goldenseal seeds and roots for planting.

Black Kat Herbals
P. O. Box 271
Smithville, TN 37166
Tinctures (extracts), capsules, salves, teas, herbal soaps, and massage oils.

Blessed Herbs
109 Barre Plains Road
Oakham, MA 01068
Bulk herbs and skin-care products.

Botanic Health
P. O. Box 5
Hammond, IN 46325-0005
Herbal formulas as capsules and tablets; also skin- and hair-care products.

Catskill Mountain Herbals
P. O. Box 1426
Olive Bridge, NY 12461
Tinctures (extracts), herbal vinegars, infused oils, salves, and some dried herbs.

Cedarbrook Herb Farm
1345 South Sequim Avenue
Sequim, WA 98382
Seeds, live plants, and books.

Chef's Catalog
P. O. Box 620048
Dallas TX 75262-0048
Coffee grinders, electric tea infusers, and food dehydrators.

Cheryl's Herbs
836 Hanley Industrial Court
St. Louis, MO 63144
Essential oils, aromatherapy products, and dried herbs.

The Chopra Center for Well-Being
7630 Fay Avenue
La Jolla, CA 92037
Books, audio and video tapes, Ayurvedic herbal formulas as tablets and jam; also massage oils, teas, skin-care products, and shatavari.

Christopher's Original Formulas
P. O. Box 777
Springville, UT 84663
Herbal formulas created by John R. Christopher, N.D., as capsules, powders, syrups, herb blends, tinctures (extracts), and ointments; also dried herbs and essential oils.

Companion Plants
7247 North Coolville Ridge Road
Athens, OH 45701
Herb seeds and plants.

The Cook's Garden
P. O. Box 5010
Hodges, SC 29653-5010
Herb seeds and gardening supplies.

Dancing Willow Herbs
960 Main Avenue
Durango, CO 81301
Extracts (tinctures), tea blends, essential oils, herb-infused oils, salves, and liniments.

Day's Organic Herb Farm
129 Bakes Road
Vevay, IN 47043-9691
Herb plants, dried herbs, and body-care products.

Devonshire Apothecary
2105 Ashby Avenue
Austin, TX 78703
Tinctures (extracts), teas, salves, bath herbs, aromatherapy supplies, and books.

Dragon River Herbals
P. O. Box 28
El Rito, NM 87530
Tinctures (extracts).

Dry Creek Herb Farm and Learning Center
13935 Dry Creek Road
Auburn, CA 95602
Bulk herbs, tea blends, books, tapes, tinctures (extracts), essential oils, skin-care products, and supplies for making cosmetics and salves.

Earth Essentials
6349 Filbert Avenue
Orangevale, CA 95662
Essential oils.

East Earth Herb, Inc.
P. O. Box 2802
Eugene, OR 97402
Tablets and alcohol extracts.

East Earth Trade Winds
P. O. Box 493151
Redding, CA 96049-3151
Chinese herbal products and patent medicines, dried herbs, essential oils, special-order Chinese remedies, and books.

Eclectic Institute, Inc.
14385 Southeast Lusted Road
Sandy, OR 97055-9549
Tinctures (extracts), including flavored tinctures; freeze-dried herbs in capsules; and chewable herb tablets.

Elixir Farm Botanicals, LLC
Brixey, MT 65618
Chinese and indigenous medical plant seeds and bare-root plants.

Fragrant Earth
c/o Samarkand Trading Company
936 Peace Portal Drive #98
Blaine, WA 98231-8014
Essential oils and aromatherapy diffusers.

The Gaia Garden Herbal Dispensary
2672 West Broadway
Vancouver, BC V6K 2G3
Canada
Tinctures (extracts), dried herbs, essential oils, salves, skin- and hair-care products, and books.

Gaia Herbs
108 Island Ford Road
Brevard, NC 28712
Tinctures (extracts), including Ayurvedic, Chinese, and rain forest liquid herbal extracts; solid extracts; salves; and herb-infused oils.

Ginseng Select Products, Inc.
611 Druid Road East, Suite 711
Clearwater, FL 33756
Ginseng in many forms.

Green Terrestrial
328 Lake Avenue
Greenwich, CT 06830
Herb-infused oils, salves, herbal tea blends, and dried herbs.

Grovel's
P. O. Box 281
Port Perry, ON L9L 1A3
Canada
Essential oils, dried herbs, and body-care products.

Harris Seeds
P. O. Box 22960
Rochester, NY 14692
Herb seeds and gardening accessories.

Healing Spirits Organically Grown and Wildcrafted Medicinal Herbs
9198 State Route 415
Avoca, NY 14809
Dried herbs and fresh herbs by special order.

Herbalist and Alchemist
P. O. Box 553
Broadway, NJ 08808

Tinctures (extracts), including Chinese, Ayurvedic, and mushroom extracts; dried Chinese herbs and tea blends; infused oils and ointments; and books.

Herbally Yours, Inc.
P. O. Box 26
Changewater, NJ 07831

Bathtub blends, skin- and hair-care products, essential oils, cosmetics ingredients, dried herbs, tea blends, tinctures (extracts), and books.

The Herb Cupboard
12 South Broadway
Scottdale, PA 15683

Tinctures (extracts), capsules, salves, teas, body-care products, and books.

The Herb Farm
323 Parleeville Road, RR 4
Norton, NB E0G 2N0
Canada

Dried herbs and tea blends.

The Herb Garden
P. O. Box 773-RD
Pilot Mountain, NC 27041

Herb plants.

Herb Hill
71 Ferris Lane
Poughkeepsie, NY 12601

Herbal salves.

Herb Pharm
P. O. Box 116
Williams, OR 97544

Tinctures (extracts), herb-infused oils, and books.

The Herb Shoppe
4372 Chris Greene Lake Road
Charlottesville, VA 22911

Dried herbs, including Chinese herbs and custom-order combinations; special-order Ayurvedic herbs and formulas; herbal oils; liniments; and Ayurvedic beauty products.

HomeHealth
3890 Park Central Boulevard, North
Pompano Beach, FL 33064

Herb supplements, skin- and hair-care products, castor oil, and white wool flannel (for making castor-oil packs).

Horizon Herbs
P. O. Box 69
Williams, OR 97544

Seeds for medicinal herbs; also live roots.

Indian River Herb Farm
RD 4, Box 268A
Riverdale Park
Millsboro, DE 19966

Ceremonial herbs, teas, tinctures (extracts), dried herbs, and aromatherapy products.

Indiana Botanic Gardens, Inc.
3401 West 37th Avenue
Hobart, IN 46342

Dried herbs, teas, essential oils, and books.

Inner Balance
360 Interlocken Boulevard, Suite 300
Broomfield, CO 80021

Castor oil, unbleached wool flannel (for making castor-oil packs), and natural bath/body products.

Interweave Press
201 East Fourth Street
Loveland, CO 80537-5655

Publishes Herbs for Health *and* The Herb Companion *magazines as well as the books* Herbs for Your Health, The Herb Companion Wish Book and Resource Guide, *and others.*

Johnny's Selected Seeds
Foss Hill Road
Albion, ME 04910
Seeds.

Land Reformers Nursery and Landscapes
35703 Loop Road
Rutland, OH 45775
Prairie herbs and flowers as seeds and small plants.

Lavender Lane
7337 #1 Roseville Road
Sacramento, CA 95842
Bottles, jars, and tins for homemade herbal products; essential oils; vegetable oils; beeswax; and aromatherapy diffusers.

Liberty Seed Company
P. O. Box 806
New Philadelphia, OH 44663
Seeds.

Lin Sister Herb Shop, Inc.
4 Bowery
New York, NY 10013
Chinese herbal remedies.

Longevity Herb Company
1549 Jewett
White Salmon, WA 98672
Herb tincture presses.

Materia Medica, LLC
112 Hermosa, Southeast
Albuquerque, NM 87108
Tinctures (extracts), creams, capsules, tablets, essential oils, and vegetable oils.

Mountain Herbals
7 Langdon Street
Montpelier, VT 05602-2908
Dried herbs, tinctures (extracts), and made-to-order customized formulas.

Mountain Rose Herbs
20818 High Street
North San Juan, CA 95960
Infused herbal oils; tinctures (extracts); essential oils; cream and salve supplies, vegetable oils; flower waters; glass bottles and jars for homemade herbal preparations; coffee grinders; tea-brewing supplies; dried herbs; dream pillows; and herb seeds.

Mountain Spirit
P. O. Box 368
Port Townsend, WA 98368
Tinctures (extracts), teas, bath herbs, massage and baby oils, and herbal birthing supplies.

National College of Naturopathic Medicine
Natural Health Centers
11231 Southeast Market Street
Portland, OR 97216
Tinctures (extracts), capsules, dried herbs, essential oils, and flower essences.

Natural Products Co-op
P. O. Box 299
Norway, IA 52318
Dried herbs, tinctures (extracts), herb capsules, salves, essential oils, Chinese herb teas, and skin- and hair-care products.

Nature's Meadow
P. O. Box 510
Gainesville, MO 65655
Tinctures (extracts).

Nichols Garden Nursery
North Pacific Highway, Northeast
Albany, OR 97321-4580
Herb seeds, plants, gardening tools, and books.

Original Swiss Aromatics
P. O. Box 6842
San Rafael, CA 94903
Essential oils, massage oils, and aromatherapy diffusers.

Otto Richter and Sons
357 Highway #47
Goodwood, ON L0C 1E0
Canada
Herb seeds, plants, dried herbs, teas, essential oils, and books.

Pacific Botanicals
4350 Fish Hatchery Road
Grants Pass, OR 97527
Organic dried herbs and sea vegetables.

Raven's Nest Herbals
P. O. Box 370
Duluth, GA 30136
Custom-blended dried herbs and oils.

Redwood City Seed Company
P. O. Box 361
Redwood City, CA 94064
Seeds.

Sage Mountain Herbs
P. O. Box 420
East Barre, VT 05649
Tinctures (extracts), formulas, and beauty products.

Sage Woman Herbs
2211 West Colorado Avenue
Colorado Springs, CO 80904
Herbal formulas in capsules, tea blends, tea-brewing supplies, dried herbs, tinctures (extracts), supplies for making castor-oil packs, essential oils, vegetable oils, herbal soaps, supplies for preparing and storing homemade herbal products, salves, skin- and hair-care products, and flower essences.

St. John's Herb Garden, Inc.
P. O. Box 70
Bowie, MD 20720
Herb plants, dried herbs, teas, essential oils, Chinese herbs, and extracts.

San Francisco Herb Company
250 14th Street
San Francisco, CA 94103
Dried herbs.

Second Opinion Products
P. O. Box 69046
Portland, OR 97201
Dried herbs and tea blends.

Seeds of Change
P. O. Box 15700
Santa Fe, NM 87506-5700
Herb seeds, gardening supplies, and books.

Shepherd's Garden Seeds
30 Irene Street
Torrington, CT 06790
Herb seeds and plants and gardening supplies.

SKS Bottle and Packaging
3 Knaber Road
Mechanicville, NY 12118
Glass and plastic bottles and jars.

Ten Ren Tea and Ginseng Company
75 Mott Street
New York, NY 10013

135-18 Roosevelt Avenue
Flushing, NY 11354

825-G Rockville Pike
Rockview, MD 20852
Ginseng and Chinese teas.

Tieraona's Herbals
112 Hermosa Southeast
Albuquerque, NM 87108
Tinctures (extracts), tea blends, creams, salves, capsules, essential oils, and vegetable oils.

Turtle Island Herbs
2825 Wilderness Place, Suite 350
Boulder, CO 80301
Tinctures (extracts), syrups, and salves.

The Ultimate Herb and Spice Shoppe
Box 395
Duenweg, MO 64841
Dried herbs, soaps, and massage oils.

Unitea Herbs
1705 14th Street, Suite 318
Boulder, CO 80302
Tea blends.

Walnut Acres Organic Farms
Penns Creek, PA 17862-0800
Organic foods, supplements, and some natural household products.

Well-Sweep Herb Farm, Inc.
205 Mt. Bethel Road
Port Murray, NJ 07865
Herb plants and seeds, dried herbs, essential oils, skin-care products, and books.

Western Botanicals
7122 Almond Avenue
Orangevale, CA 95662
Herbal formulas as capsules, powders, teas, tinctures (extracts), and massage oils; also some dried herbs.

Wild Weeds
1302 Camp Weott Road
Ferndale, CA 95536
Tea blends, tea-brewing supplies, herbal salves and oils, skin- and hair-care products, tinctures (extracts), dried herbs, supplies for preparing and storing homemade herbal products, essential oils, and books

Wise Woman Herbals
P. O. Box 279
Creswell, OR 97426
Tinctures (extracts), salves, solid extracts, capsules, suppositories, herbal oils, essential oils, and bottles.

Credits

Photographs

A-Z Botanical Collection Ltd.: Page 449

Pallava Bagla/A-Z Botanical Collection Ltd.: Page 251

Candace M. Billman/Rodale Images: Page 147 (impatiens)

Geoff Bryant/Photo Researchers: Page 146 (cerato)

G. Büttner/Naturbild/OKAPIA/Photo Researchers: Page 202

David Cavagnaro: Page 200

John D. Cunningham/Visuals Unlimited: Page 147 (scleranthus)

Alan and Linda Detrick/Photo Researchers: Page 147 (rockrose)

Steven Foster: Pages 179, 196 (aloe), 304, and 324

Gilbert S. Grant/Photo Researchers: Page 429

Farrell Grehan/Photo Researchers: Page 147 (gentian)

Dan Guravich/Photo Researchers: Page 147 (mimulus)

Mimi Kamp: Pages 136, 310, and 452

Erich Lessing/Art Resource, NY: Page 20

Francois Merlet/A-Z Botanical Collection Ltd.: Pages 147 (vervain) and 324

Mitch Mandel: Pages xvi–1, 23, 27, 28–29, 32–81, 82–83, 88–89, 91, 93–94, 97–98, 100, 102–3, 105–7, 109, 111–12, 132–33, 136, 138, 141, 150–51, 160–61, 196 (arnica), 197, 273, 309, 330, 340, 359, 371, 376, 378–79, 390–91, 399, 407–8, 417–19, 422, 424–25, 442 (left and top right), 443, 456–57

Diane Rawson/Photo Researchers: Page 269 (citronella)

Rodale Images: Pages 146 (clematis), 224, and 442 (bottom right)

Dan Sams/A-Z Botanical Collection Ltd.: Page 175

Kjell B. Sandved/Visuals Unlimited: Page 237

Peter Skinner/Photo Researchers: Page 371

Jan Staples/A-Z Botanical Collection Ltd.: Page 147 (water violet)

Joseph G. Strauch Jr.: Pages 146 (chicory), 193 (yarrow), 263, 288, 324, 339, and 345

Aleksandra Szywala: Page 146 (agrimony)

Mary M. Thacher/Photo Researchers: Page 244

Norm Thomas/Photo Researchers: Page 193 (chickweed)

Mark Turner: Pages 182 and 193 (plantain)

John Watney/Photo Researchers: Pages 146 (centaury) and 207

Chris Wheeler/A-Z Botanical Collection Ltd.: Page 373

George Whiteley/Photo Researchers: Page 269 (pennyroyal)

Roger Wilmshurst/Photo Researchers: Page 349

Illustrations

Virge Kask: Pages 11 and 15

Wendy Smith: Pages 32–81

Index

Blue gum. *See* Eucalyptus
Boneset, *345*
 for fever, 231–32
 safety guidelines for, **126**
 uses for, 345
Botanical names, of herbs, 31, 119, 458–61
Bottles, for storing herbal remedies, 85
Bramble. *See* Red raspberry
Breastfeeding
 herbs to avoid during, 125
 problems
  cracked, sore nipples, 175–76
  engorged breasts, 176
  insufficient milk, 174–75
Breasts
 engorged, from breastfeeding, 176
 herbs for, 26
 painful, 175–76, 177–81
  caffeine and, 177, 186
Bronchitis, 344–46
Bruises, 181–83
Bruisewort. *See* Comfrey
Buchu, for urinary tract infections, 366
Buckwheat, for varicose veins, 374
Bugbane. *See* Black cohosh
Bupleurum, for irregular menstrual cycles, 308
Burdock, 38, *38*
 for treating
  acne, 382
  arthritis, 168–69
  breast pain, 180
  dandruff, 394
  eczema, 225
  heavy menstrual bleeding, 311
  herpes, 257
  hot flashes, 287
  menstrual cramps, 306
  oily hair, 410
  psoriasis, 341
Burns, 184–85
Butcher's broom, *373*
 for varicose veins, *373*, 374
Butternut, for hemorrhoids, 255–56
B vitamins, for preventing anxiety, 431–32

C

Cabbage, for acne, 385
Caffeine
 anxiety from, 431
 as endometriosis risk factor, 230
 as energy booster, 438
 reducing premenopausal intake of, 286
Caffeine addiction, 186–88
Calcium
 for PMS, 303
 for reducing menstrual cramps, 305
Calendula, 39, *39, 359*
 for herbal first-aid kit, 22
 for treating
  acne, 382–83, 385
  athlete's foot, 171–72
  bad breath, 173
  bruises, 183
  burns, 184, 185
  canker sores, 189
  cesarean incision, 338
  cracked nipples, 176
  cuts and scrapes, 194, *197*, 198
  dry skin, 397, 400, 401
  perineum, after childbirth, 335
  psoriasis, 340
  scars, 359
  sunburn, 362
  urinary tract infections, 364
  vaginal infections, 370
  wounds, 359–60, 359
 uses for, 10
 for washing wounds, *197*
California poppy
 as flower essence, 148
 safety guidelines for, **127**
 for treating
  depression, 436
  endometriosis, 227
Camphor, for insect bites and stings, 269–70
Canker sores, 188–89
Capillaries, broken, on face, 400
Capsaicin
 for improving digestion, 320
 for pain relief, 4
 for psoriasis, 341
 for increasing metabolism, 320
Capsules
 purchasing, 124
 storing, 124
 vs. teas and tinctures, 119
Cardamom
 for bad breath, 173
 for preventing indigestion, 212
Cardiac glycosides, effects of, 246
Carrier oils, for diluting essential oils, 136–37,
  142–43

Carrot seed oil
  for age spots, 387–88
  in aromatherapy, 138, *138*
Carrot seed, wild, for birth control, 265
Castor oil, for treating
  breast pain, 178
  chapped lips, 391
  dry cuticles, 402
  endometriosis, 228
Catnip, for treating
  insomnia, 274
  nicotine withdrawal, 317
Cayenne, 40, *40*
  for preventing
    digestive problems, 208
    gas, 210
  safety guidelines for, **127**
  seaweed supplements taken with, 321
  for treating
    cold hands and feet, 294
    gum problems, 236–37
    toothaches, 202–3
  for weight loss, 320
Centaury, as flower essence, 146, *146*
Cerato, as flower essence, 146, *146*
Cervical changes, 189–92
Cervical dysplasia
  conventional treatment of, 190–91
  from human papillomavirus, 190
  naturopathic treatment of, 191–92
Cesarean section, healing after, 336–38
Chamomile, 41, *41*
  for herbal first-aid kit, 22
  for minimizing wrinkles, 421
  miscarriage from, 333
  for preventing indigestion, 212–13
  research validating uses for, 13
  safety guidelines for, **127**
  for treating
    acne, 385
    anxiety, 429–30
    breastfeeding problems, 174
    broken capillaries, 400
    canker sores, 189
    diarrhea, 214
    digestive problems, 206, 212–13, 331
    dull, brittle nails, 402
    eczema, 223
    engorged breasts, 176
    fever, 233
    gas, 210
    gum problems, 236
    heartburn, 209

indigestion during pregnancy, 331
    insomnia, 272, 274, 333
    irritable bowel syndrome, 218
    midafternoon slump, 448
    motion sickness, 312–13
    nausea, 220
    nicotine withdrawal, 317
    PMS, 301, 303
    puffy eyes, 413–14, 415
    stomach ailments, 162
    stress, 453, 454–55
    tension headaches, 243
  uses for, 135, 136, 139
Chamomile oil, in aromatherapy, 139
Chapped lips, 388–91
Chasteberry 42, *42*
  safety guidelines for, **127**
  for treating
    acne, 382–83
    endometriosis, 229
    hot flashes, 287
    infertility, 261–62, 264
    low sexual desire, 443
    menopausal problems, 295, 296
    menstrual problems, 214–15, 289, 296, 306, 307
    PMS, 298, 299–300
Cheese, gas from, 210
Chen pi, for treating
  energy drain, 439
  stress, 454
Chicken soup, for colds and flu, 347, 350
Chickweed, for treating
  cuts and scrapes, 193, *193*
  dry skin, 401
  insect bites and stings, 267
  mood swings, 291
  urinary tract infections, 364
Chicory
  for caffeine addiction, 187, 188
  as flower essence, 146, *146*
  for liver health, 187
Chili pepper. *See* Cayenne
China, herbs used in, 2, 9
Chinese medicine. *See* Traditional Chinese
  Medicine
Cholesterol
  estrogen and, 283
  high, preventing, 247–52
Cinnamon, 43, *43*
  for treating
    cold hands and feet, 294
    colds and flu, 351
    diarrhea, 214, 219

Essential oils *(continued)*
    production of, 137
    safety guidelines for, 143–44
    selecting, 137, 139
    for treating
        dry hair, 395–96
        dry skin, 400–401
        jet lag, 275
        labor pain, 335
        low sexual desire, 441–42
        memory problems, 446
        midafternoon slump, 450
        stress, 453
    understanding labels on, 141
Estrogen
    heart disease and, 246, 283
    insomnia and, 271
    menopause and, 282, 283
    migraines and, 240
Eucalyptus, 50, *50*
    safety guidelines for, **128**
Eucalyptus oil
    for herbal first-aid kit, 22
    for treating
        colds and flu, 350
        coughs, 355
        jet lag, 275
Eugenol, in clove oil, 202, *202*
Europe, herbalism in, 2, 9, 13, 16, 17
Evening primrose oil, 51, *51*
    after cesarean section, 337
    for treating
        breast pain, 178
        dry hair, 395
        eczema, 225
        PMS, 303
        vaginal dryness, 290
Exercise
    for preventing atherosclerosis, 247
    for treating
        insomnia, 271
        menopausal problems, 292–93
        stress, 248
Exhaustion, 438–40
Extracts. *See* Tinctures
Eye balm. *See* Goldenseal
Eyebright, *244*
    for treating
        hay fever, 356
        puffy eyes, 414, 415
        sinus headaches, 244–45
    uses for, 244
Eyes, puffy, 413–15

F

Facial peels, for minimizing
    crow's-feet, 392–93
    wrinkles, 420–21
False unicorn root, *263*
    safety guidelines for, **128**
    for treating
        infertility, 262, 263
        menopausal problems, 294, 295
Fatigue, 438–40
    from midafternoon slump, 447–50
FDA, on classification of herbal products, 114
Featherfew. *See* Feverfew
Feet, cold, 291, 294
Fennel, 52, *52*
    after cesarean section, 337
    for minimizing wrinkles, 423
    multiple actions of, 7
    during pregnancy, 327
    for preventing indigestion, 212, 213
    safety guidelines for, **128**
    for treating
        breastfeeding problems, 174–75
        gas, 210–11
        heartburn during pregnancy, 331
        heavy menstrual bleeding, 311
        irritable bowel syndrome, 217
        puffy eyes, 414
Fen-phen, herbal, cautions with, 319
Fenugreek, for improving digestion, 206
Ferrous sulfate, for anemia, 165–66
Fertility, herbs for increasing, 259–60
FES, 148
Fever, 231–35
Feverfew, 53, *53*
    for migraines, 234, 240–41
    research validating uses for, 13
    safety guidelines for, **128**
Fever tree. *See* Eucalyptus
Fiber
    for hemorrhoid relief, 255
    for preventing digestive problems, 208
    supplements, 320
    for weight loss, 319–20
Fibrocystic breast disease, 177, 186
Field mint. *See* Peppermint
Figwort
    for hemorrhoids, 256
    safety guidelines for, **128**
First-aid kit, herbal, 22, *23*, *196–97*
Flatulence. *See* Gas

Flavonoids
    for asthma, 343
    benefits of, _14_
Flaxseed, for treating
    constipation, 216, 332
    eczema, _224_, *224*
    endometriosis, 228
    menopausal problems, 286
    splinters, _194_
Flirtwort. *See* Feverfew
Flower essences, 145–49
    effectiveness of, 148–49
    for emotional healing, 145, 148, 149
    modern uses of, 148
    origin of, 145, 148
    reasons for using, 149
Flower Essence Society (FES), 148
Flu, 21, 347–51
Fluoxetine (Rx), side effects of, 433
Foal-foot. *See* Coltsfoot
Folic acid, for cervical dysplasia, 192
Folklore, herbal, modern herbalists and, 9
Food and Drug Administration (FDA), on
        classification of herbal products, 114
Food sensitivity, irritable bowel syndrome
        confused with, 217
Forgetfulness, 445–47
Foxglove, heart affected by, 246
Fox's clote. *See* Burdock
France, herbal medicine in, 17
Frankincense, for treating
    jet lag, 275
    midafternoon slump, 450
Fruits, dried, for anemia, 167

G

Garden lavender. *See* Lavender
Gargle, for treating
    bad breath, 173
    sore throat, _354_
Garlic, 54, *54*
    in capsules, 250
    multiple actions of, 7
    in pesto, _249_
    for preventing digestive problems, 208
    research validating uses for, 13
    as tonic herb, 152, 153
    for treating
        athlete's foot, 171
        bronchitis, 346

colds and flu, 21, _350_, 351
    cuts and scrapes, 195
    ear infections, 221
    gas, 211
    high cholesterol, 248–50, **444**
    infections, 21
    insect bites and stings, 267–69
    low immunity, _280_
    uses for, _10_
Gas, 210–11
    with PMS, 301
Genital warts, 189–92
Gentian
    as flower essence, _147_, *147*
    for improving digestion, 206, _207_, *207*, 211,
        _212_
    safety guidelines for, **128**
Geranium, for treating
    heavy menstrual bleeding, 310–11
    wounds, 358
Geranium oil, in aromatherapy, 139–40
German chamomile. *See* Chamomile
German chamomile oil, conditions helped by,
        _135_
Germany, herbal medicine in, 17
Ginger, 55, *55*
    for herbal first-aid kit, _22_
    for preventing
        gas, 210
        indigestion, 213
        migraines, 241
    research validating uses for, 17
    safety guidelines for, **128**
    for treating
        altitude sickness, 164–65
        colds and flu, 351
        congestion, 351–52, 352
        diarrhea, 215
        digestive problems, 206
        fever, 233
        gas, 211
        high blood pressure, 250
        high cholesterol, 250–51
        irritable bowel syndrome, 217
        menstrual cramps, 306
        morning sickness, 329–31
        motion sickness, 18, 311–12
        nausea, 218, 219
        PMS, 301–2
        stress, 454–55
        varicose veins, 374
        vomiting, 218–19
Gingivitis, 235

menopausal problems, 285
varicose veins, 374
Hay fever, 355–56
Headaches, 238–45
with altitude sickness, 165
causes of, 238–39
dream pillows for, 273
herbs for, 26
migraine, 234, 239–42
as side effect of herbs, 159
sinus, 243–45
tension, 242–43
Healing-herb. *See* Comfrey
Heart, herbs for, 26
during pregnancy, 331, 332
Heart disease
herbs for preventing, 246–54
hawthorn, 158
incidence of, in women, 245–46
menopause and, 246, 283
Heart heal. *See* Motherwort
Heart medications, hawthorn interacting with,
163
Helichrysum oil
in aromatherapy, 138, *138*
for treating
age spots, 387
broken capillaries, 400
dry skin, 397, 400
Helmet flower. *See* Skullcap
Hemorrhoids, 255–56
Henna, coloring hair with, 404
Herbal folklore, modern herbalists and, 9
Herbalism
origins of, 2–3
reasons for popularity of, 4–5
Herbal medicine, origins of, 7, 9
Herbal practitioners, choosing, 116–17
Herbal products, mail-order sources of, 462–68
Herbal remedies
allergic reactions to, 120, 159
from ancient civilizations, 2, 9, 13
benefits of
effectiveness, 17–18
fewer side effects, 18, 21
preventive medicine, 21, 24
renewed connection to nature, 25
for women, 24–25
dangerous, 121
discussing with doctors, 118
as family tradition, 3
figuring correct doses of, 121–23

herbal combinations for, 119
homemade
benefits of, 84–85
equipment for, 85
interacting with prescription medicines, 120–21,
122–23
labeling on, 114
from local plants, 10
purchasing tips for, 124
research validating use of, 13, 17
safety of
guidelines for, **126–31**
for minor vs. serious problems, 115
tips for ensuring, 119–21, 158–59, 163
selecting, 112–14, 118–19
standardized, 120
storing, 124
when not to use, 115–18
Herbal tonics. *See* Tonic herbs
Herbal wisdom, 13, 24, 173, 187, 195, 219, 241,
257, 285, 297, 306, 312, 317, 321, 326, 357,
362, 369
Herb-drug interactions, 120–21, **122–23**, 163, 242,
243, 246
Herb of the angel. *See* Angelica
Herbs. *See also specific herbs*
active ingredients in, 14–15
botanical names of, 31, 119, 458–61
common names of, 31, 119, 458–61
drying, 86–88, 88, *88*
harvesting, 86, 87
healing compounds in, 5
multiple actions of, 5, 7
mail-order sources of, 462–68
parts of, healing potential of, 119
quality of, 157
storing, 88
wild, gathering, 87
Herpes, 256–58
cold sores from, 188, 256
He-shou-wu
safety guidelines for, **129**
for treating
energy drain, 439
infertility, 263, 264
High blood pressure, 252–54
High cranberry. *See* Cramp bark
Hive vine. *See* Partridgeberry
Holy Trinity flower. *See* Passionflower
Hops, 60, *60*
for improving digestion, 207, 213
safety guidelines for, **129**

Menopause, 281–96
 aromatherapy for, 136
 black cohosh for, 169
 heart disease after, 246
 herbal protection during, 284–86, 294–96
 hormonal changes during, 282–83
 hormone replacement therapy during, 283, _293_
 insomnia during, 271
 naturopathic approach to, _292–93_
 phytoestrogens for, 284
 problems during
  cold hands and feet, 291, 294
  hot flashes, 286–87
  irregular periods and flooding, 289–90
  mood swings, 290–91
  night sweats, 287–88
  vaginal dryness, 290
 as transition, 281–82
Menstrual cycle
 breast changes during, 177
 herb use and, _157_
 insomnia and, 271
 jet lag disrupting, 275
 migraines during, 240
 sense of smell affected by, 136
Menstrual problems, 296–311
 cramps, 304–6
 dang gui for, 158
 heavy bleeding, 289–90, 309–11
 irregular cycles, 289–90, 306–8
 from liver congestion, _205_
 premenstrual syndrome, 297–303
 stool irregularities, 214–15
Menstruum, for making tinctures, 92, 95
Menthol, for insect bites and stings, 269–70
Midafternoon slump, 447–50
Migraines, 239–42
 feverfew for, _234_
Milk, gas from, 210
Milk production, insufficient, in breastfeeding, 174–75
Milk thistle 66, _66_
 for improving digestion, _207_
 for treating
  breastfeeding problems, 174–75
  breast pain, 180
  caffeine addiction, 188
  endometriosis, _229_
  heavy menstrual bleeding, 311
  high blood pressure, 253
  liver damage, 18, **444**
  psoriasis, 341
Milky oats, for tension headaches, 243

Millefoil. _See_ Yarrow
Mimulus, as flower essence, _147, 147_
Mint. _See also specific types_
 for insomnia, 274
 uses for, _10_
Miscarriage, herbs causing, 327, 333
Missouri snakeroot. _See_ Echinacea
Moisturizers
 for acne, 385
 for oily skin, 412–13
Monkey flower, as flower essence, _147, 147_
Monk's pepper. _See_ Chasteberry
Mood swings
 during menopause, 290–91
 from riboflavin deficiency, 432
Moon root. _See_ Valerian
Morning glory, for alertness, 145
Morning sickness, 329–31
Mother herb. _See_ Motherwort
Mother's cordial, for increasing fertility, 262
Motherwort, 67, _67_
 for treating
  hot flashes, 287
  menopausal problems, 294, 295, 296
  strains and sprains, 316
  stress, 453
Motion sickness, 18, 311–13
Mountain box. _See_ Uva-ursi
Mountain tea. _See_ Partridgeberry
Mouth, herbs for, _26_
Mouthwash
 plant-based antiseptic in, 4
 for treating
  canker sores, 189
  gum problems, 236
Mucilage, benefits of, _15_
Mugwort, _324_
 for preventing poison-plant rashes, 323, _324_
 for stress, 453
Mullein, for treating
 bronchitis, 345–46, 346
 coughs, 353
 ear infections, 221
Muscle(s)
 herbs for, _26_
 sore, during pregnancy, 334
 strains and sprains, 313–16
 tension, 450
Mushrooms
 maitake, for strengthening immunity, 279–80
 reishi
  as adrenal tonic, 450
  for preventing colds and flu, 348, 351

nicotine withdrawal, 317
stress, 158
Obesity, 318–21
Oils. *See* Carrier oils; Essential oils; Infused oils;
specific herbal oils
Ointments, 110–11
making, <u>111–12</u>, *111–12*
Olive oil
for dry hair, 396
for making infused oils, 101
Onions
for cholesterol reduction, 248, 250
for congestion, 352
honey and, for coughs, 355
Orange-blossom water, for treating
dry skin, 397
oily skin, 411
Orange oil, for broken capillaries, <u>400</u>
Orange rind, for menopausal problems,
296
Orange root. *See* Goldenseal
Oregon grape root, *339*
for treating
breast pain, 180
burns, 184
cuts and scrapes, 194
poison ivy, oak, and sumac, 323
psoriasis, <u>339</u>, 341
sinus infections, 245
Organic products, for endometriosis, 230
Osha, for insect bites and stings, 270
Osteocomplex, for bone health, <u>293</u>
Osteoporosis
after menopause, 283
supplements for preventing, <u>293</u>
Overweight, 318–21

P

Papaya facial peel, for crow's-feet, 392
Papoose root. *See* Blue cohosh
Pap smear, cervical dysplasia detected by, 190
Parsley
for minimizing wrinkles, 421
safety guidelines for, **130**
for treating
age spots, 387
bad breath, 173
bruises, <u>183</u>
urinary tract infections, 364–65
water retention, 377

Partridgeberry, 70, *70*
after cesarean section, 337
for treating
endometriosis, <u>229</u>
infertility, <u>261</u>, 262, 264
Passionflower, 71, *71*
for treating
anxiety, 430, 431
endometriosis, 227
herpes, 258
insomnia, 274, 334
irritability from poison-plant rashes, 325
labor pain, 335
PMS, 301
strains and sprains, 316
tension headaches, 243
Passion-vine. *See* Passionflower
Patchouli, added to shampoo, 405
Patch test, for sensitivity to essential oils, 143
Pau d'arco, *304*
as hormone balancer, <u>304</u>
Peels, facial, for minimizing
crow's-feet, 392–93
wrinkles, 420–21
Pennyroyal, *269*
as insect repellent, <u>268–69</u>
for menstrual cramps, 305
Peppermint, 72, *72*
for preventing indigestion, 211–12
for treating
bad breath, 173
caffeine addiction, 188
congestion, 352
digestive problems, 206, **444**
fever, <u>232</u>, 233
gas, 210
memory problems, 447
midafternoon slump, 448
motion sickness, 312
nausea, 219–20
oily skin, 411
Peppermint oil, for treating
acne, 385
energy drain, 440
insect bites and stings, 267
irritable bowel syndrome, 217
jet lag, 275
labor pain, 335
morning sickness, 329
Perineum
postpartum rinse for, 335–36
softening, for childbirth, 335
Periodontitis, 235

Red raspberry, 74, *74*
    after cesarean section, 337
    for labor and childbirth preparation,
        335
    for postpartum recovery, 336
    during pregnancy, 327, 328
    for treating
        diarrhea, 214
        endometriosis, 227
        energy drain, 440
        infertility, 260, 261
        menopausal problems, 285
    uses for, 10
Reflux, heartburn and, 208–10
Rehmannia, as adrenal tonic, 450
Reishi mushrooms
    as adrenal tonic, 450
    for preventing colds and flu, 348, 351
    safety guidelines for, **130**
    for treating
        endometriosis, 228
        low immunity, 279
Remifemin, for menopausal problems, 293
Reproductive health, herbs for, 26, 259–60
Rescue Remedy
    effectiveness of, 149
    for herbal first-aid kit, 22, 199
    for treating
        emotional upset, 199
        pimples, 384
Resins, plant, benefits of, 14–15
Respiratory problems, 341–57
    asthma, 342–44
    benefits of herbal treatment for, 342
    bronchitis, 344–46
    colds, 347–51
    congestion, 351–52
    coughs, 352–53, 355
    flu, 347–51
    hay fever, 355–56
    herbs for, 26
    sinus problems, 356–57
Riboflavin deficiency, mood swings from,
    432
RICE, for sprains and strains, 314
Rice water, for diarrhea, 215
Rinses, hair, 405, 410
    making, 408–9, **408**, *409*
Rockrose, as flower essence, 147, *147*
Romans, herbs used by, 9
Root of life. *See* Ginseng
Root of the Holy Ghost. *See* Angelica
Rose elder. *See* Cramp bark

Rose geranium oil
    conditions helped by, 135
    in hair rinse, 405, 410
    as insect repellent, 269
    for treating
        endometriosis, 228
        menstrual cycle disruption, from jet lag, 275
Rose hips
    for minimizing wrinkles, 420, 421
    in pregnancy tea, 328
    for treating
        crow's-feet, 392–93
        infertility, 260
        midafternoon slump, 448
Rosemary
    darkening hair with, 403
    for preventing migraines, 241
    for treating
        breast pain, 180
        congestion, 352
        dandruff, 394
        fever, 233
        memory problems, 447
        perineum, after childbirth, 335, 336
Rosemary oil, for treating
    jet lag, 275
    memory problems, 446
Rose oil
    in aromatherapy, 142
    for treating
        broken capillaries, 400
        low sexual desire, 441, 442
Rose water, for oily skin, 411
Rubdown, for arthritis, 168

S

Safety, of herbs
    during breastfeeding, 125
    guidelines for, 119–21, **126–31**, 158–59, 162–63
    for minor vs. serious conditions, 115
    during pregnancy, 125, 326–28
Sage
    darkening hair with, 403
    safety guidelines for, **130**
    for treating
        bad breath, 173
        fever, 233
        menopausal problems, 295–96
        muscle tension, 450
        night sweats, 288, 288

Tiredness, 438–40
  with midafternoon slump, 447–50
Toners, for treating
  acne, 385
  dry skin, 397, 400–401
  oily hair, 410
  oily skin, 411
  tired skin, 415, _418_, *418–19*
Tonic herbs, 152–59
  avoiding side effects from, 158–59
  criteria for, 153
  customized, _154–57_
  for health protection, 21
  helper, **156**
  primary, **155**
  purpose of, 152–53
  qi, 153, 158
  for strengthening endocrine system, 295–96,
    450
  system-specific, 153, 158
  teas from, _156_
  tinctures from, _156–57_
  tips for using, _157_
  for treating
    low sexual desire, 443
    menopausal problems, 284–85
    stress, 454
Toothaches, 201–3
Traditional Chinese Medicine
  conditions treated in
    headaches, 238–39
    low sexual desire, 443
    reproductive problems, 308
    stress, 453–54
  principles of, _8_
Tree primrose. *See* Evening primrose oil
True lavender. *See* Lavender
True unicorn root, for menopausal problems, 294
Turmeric
  for heartburn, 209
  safety guidelines for, **130**
12 Healers, The, _146–47_, *146–47*

U

Urinary tract
  herbs for, _26_
  infections, 363–66
Usnea, for treating
  dull, brittle nails, 402
  lip blisters, 391
  vaginal infections, 372
Utensils, for preparing herbal remedies, 85

Uva-ursi, 78, *78*
  research validating uses for, 17
  safety guidelines for, **130**
  for treating
    mood swings, _291_
    urinary tract infections, 364, _365_
    water retention, 377

V

Vaginal problems, 367–72
  causes of, 367–68
  dryness, 290
Valerian, 79, *79*
  active ingredients in, 7
  drugs interacting with, 243
  multiple actions of, 7
  safety guidelines for, **130**
  for treating
    anxiety, 431
    endometriosis, 227, _229_
    insomnia, 18, 271–72, 301
    irritability from poison-plant rashes, 325
    menstrual cramps, 305
    PMS, 301
    strains and sprains, 315, 316
    stress, 453
    tension headaches, 243
Valium (Rx), valerian interacting with, 243
Vanilla scent, for reducing anxiety, 136
Varicose veins, 18, _26_, 372–74
Vervain
  as flower essence, _147_, *147*
  for herpes, 257
  for postpartum recovery, 336
Vetter-voo. *See* Feverfew
Vinegar
  for making tinctures, 95
  for treating
    anemia, 167
    dandruff, 394
    dry skin, 397, 400
    sunburn, 362
    vaginal infections, 371–72
Violets, for puffy eyes, 414
Vitamin A suppository, for cervical dysplasia,
  191
Vitamin B_{12}, for nervous system function, 432
Vitamin C
  after cesarean section, 337
  for preventing broken capillaries, _400_

Vitamin C *(continued)*
   for treating
      canker sores, 189
      cervical dysplasia, 191
      colds and flu, 350
Vitamin E
   after cesarean section, 337
   for treating
      dry skin, 396, 397
      hot flashes, 293
Vitamin E oil, for treating
   cesarean incision, 338
   dry skin, 397, 400
   vaginal dryness, 290
Vitex. *See* Chasteberry
Vodka, in astringent for oily skin, 411–12
Volatile oils, benefits of, 14
Vomiting, 218–20
   from morning sickness, 329–31
von Bingen, Hildegard, 20

W

Warfarin (Rx), willow bark interacting with,
   242
Warts, genital, 189–92
Water
   for aiding digestion, 208
   increasing intake, for water retention,
      290–91
Water elder. *See* Cramp bark
Water retention, 375–77
   during menopause, 290–91
   premenstrual, 301, 375
Water violet, as flower essence, 147, *147*
Weight control, herbs for, 26
Weight loss, 318–21
   harmful products for, 319
White peony root, *309*
   for irregular menstrual cycles, 309
Whitethorn. *See* Hawthorn
White willow bark. *See* Willow
Wild chicory. *See* Dandelion
Wildcrafting, 87
Wild oats. *See* Oatstraw
Wild spinach. *See* Nettle
Wild yam, for treating
   endometriosis, 229
   hot flashes, 287
   infertility, 263, 264
   irritable bowel syndrome, 218

   menopausal problems, 294, 295–96
   menstrual cramps, 306
   PMS, 302–3
Willow
   drugs interacting with, 242
   safety guidelines for, **131**
   for treating
      arthritis, 168
      endometriosis, 227, 228
      fever, 233–34
      migraines, 242
      strains and sprains, 314, **444**
Winter clover. *See* Partridgeberry
Wise Woman tradition of healing, 6
Witch hazel
   for herbal first-aid kit, 22
   for treating
      cuts and scrapes, 194
      dry skin, 400–401
      hemorrhoids, 255
      skin irritation, *197*
      sprains, 314, 315
      strains, 315
      vaginal dryness, 290
      varicose veins, 374
      wounds, 358
Women's Phase II, for menopausal problems, 287, 293
Wood betony, for insomnia, 274
Wounds, slow-healing, 358–60
Wrinkles, 420–23

X

Xanax (Rx), willow bark interacting with, 242

Y

Yarrow, 80, *80*
   safety guidelines for, **131**
   for treating
      acne, 385
      cesarean incision, 338
      congestion, 352
      cuts and scrapes, 193, *193*
      endometriosis, 229
      fever, 232–33, *232*
      flu, 219
      heavy menstrual bleeding, 310–11
      male health problems, **444**

Z